Acute presentations

Reference ranges

Haematological values

Haemoglobin	13–18 g/dL
	11.5–16 g/dL
Mean cell volume (MCV)	76–96 fL
Platelets	150–400 × 10⁹/L
White cell count (WCC)	4–11 × 10⁹/L
Neutrophils	2.0–7.5 × 10⁹/L
Eosinophils	0.04–0.44 × 10⁹/L
Lymphocytes	1.3–3.5 × 10⁹/L

Biochemistry values

Sodium	135–145 mmol/L
Potassium	3.5–5.0 mmol/L
Creatinine	70–150 μmol/L
Urea	2.5–6.7 mmol/L
Calcium (total)	2.12–2.65 mmol/L
Albumin	35–50 g/L
Protein	60–80 g/L
Alanine aminotransferase (ALT)	5–35 iu/L
Alkaline phosphatase	30–150 u/L
Bilirubin	3–17 μg/L
Gamma-glutamyl-transpeptidase (γGT)	11–51 iu/L
	7–33 iu/L
Thyroid stimulating hormone (TSH)	0.5–5.7 mu/L
Thyroxine (T4)	70–140 nmol/L
Thyroxine (free)	9–22 pmol/L
Tri-iodothyronine (T3)	1.2–3.0 nmol/L
Vitamin B12	0.13–0.68 nmol/L
Folate	2.1 μg/L
Glucose (fasting)	3.5–5.0 mmol/L
Prolactin	<450 u/L
	<600 u/L
Creatinine kinase (CK)	25–195 iu/L
	25–170 iu/L
Osmolality	278–305 mosmol/kg

Urine

Osmolality	350–1000 mosmol/kg
Sodium	100–250 mmol/24h
Protein	<150 mg/24h
Hydroxymethylmandelic acid (HMMA, VMA)	16–48 mmol/24h

Reference ranges for selected drugs

Lithium	0.8–1.2 mmol/L	(p. 328)
	0.6–0.8 mmol/L (as an augmentative agent)	
Valproate	50–125 mg/L	(p. 332)
Carbamazepine	4–12 mg/L	(p. 334)
	(>7 mg/L may be more efficacious in bipolar disorder)	
Clozapine	350–500 μg/L (0.35–0.5 mg/L)	(p. 218)
Nortriptyline	50–150 μg/L	

OXFORD MEDICAL PUBLICATIONS

Oxford Handbook of
Psychiatry

ALIND SRIVASTAVA

BGH & EH

Oxford Handbooks

Oxford Handbook of
Psychiatry

David Semple

Consultant Psychiatrist,
Hairmyres Hospital, East Kilbride
and Honorary Fellow,
Division of Psychiatry, University of Edinburgh, UK

Roger Smyth

Consultant Psychiatrist,
St John's Hospital at Howden, West Lothian, UK

Jonathan Burns

Community Psychiatrist,
Nelson Mandela School of Medicine,
University of KwaZulu-Natal, South Africa

Rajan Darjee

Lecturer in Forensic Psychiatry,
Division of Psychiatry, University of Edinburgh, UK

Andrew McIntosh

Lecturer in Psychiatry,
Division of Psychiatry, University of Edinburgh, UK

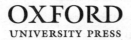

OXFORD

UNIVERSITY PRESS

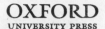

OXFORD
UNIVERSITY PRESS

YMCA Library Building, Jai Singh Road, New Delhi 110001

Oxford University Press is a department of the University of Oxford.
It furthers the University's objective of excellence in research, scholarship
and education by publishing worldwide in
Oxford   New York
Auckland   Cape Town   Dares Salaam   Hong Kong   Karachi   Kuala Lumpur   Madrid
Melbourne   Mexico City   Nairobi   New Delhi   Taipei   Toronto   Shanghai
With Offices in
Argentina   Austria   Brazil   Chile   Czech Republic   France   Greece   Guatemala
Hungary   Italy   Japan   South Korea   Poland   Portugal   Singapore   Switzerland
Thailand   Turkey   Ukraine   Vietnam

Oxford is a registered trade mark of Oxford University Press
in the UK and in certain other countries.

Published in the United States
by Oxford university Press, inc., New York

First published 2005
First Indian edition 2005

A catalogue record for this title is available from the British Library
Library of Congress Cataloging in Publication Data
Oxford handbook of psychiatry/David Semple
Includes bibliographical refrences and index.

ISBN-13: 978- 0-19-567265-7
ISBN-10: 0-19-567265-8

Reprinted by arrangement with Oxford University Press
Oxford for sale in India, Bangladesh, Nepal, Bhutan, Sri Lanka and
Myanmar only and not for export therefrom. Not for sale in Pakistan.

Typeset by Newgen Imaging Systems (P) Ltd., Chennai, India

Printed in India Anand Binders, New Delhi - 110031
and published by Manzar Khan, Oxford University Press
YMCA Library Building, Jai Singh Road, New Delhi 110001

Preface

Every medical student and doctor is familiar with that strange mixture of panic and perplexity which occurs when, despite having spent what seems like endless hours studying, one is completely at a loss as to what to do when confronted with a real patient with real problems. For doctors of our generation that sense of panic was eased somewhat by the reassuring presence in the white coat pocket of the original *Oxford Handbook of Clinical Medicine*. A quick glance at one of its pages before approaching the patient served to refresh factual knowledge, guide initial assessment, and highlight 'not to be missed' areas, allowing one to enter the room with a sense of at least initial confidence which would otherwise have been lacking.

The initial months of psychiatric practice are a time of particular anxiety, when familiar medical knowledge seems of no use and the patients and their symptoms appear baffling and strange. Every new psychiatrist is familiar with the strange sense of relief when a 'medical' problem arises in one of their patients'—'finally something I know about'. At this time, for us, the absence of a similar volume to the *Oxford Handbook of Clinical Medicine* for psychiatrists was keenly felt. This volume attempts to fulfil the same function for medical students and doctors beginning psychiatric training or practice. The white coat pocket will have gone, but we hope that it can provide that same portable reassurance.

2004

D. M. S.
R. S. S.
J. K. B.
R. D.
A. M. M.

Acknowledgements

In preparing this *Handbook*, we have benefited from the help and advice of a number of our more senior colleagues, and we would specifically like to thank Prof. E.C. Johnstone, Prof. K.P. Ebmeier, Prof. D.C.O. Cunningham-Owens, Prof. M. Sharpe, Dr S. Gaur, Dr S. Lawrie, Dr J. Crichton, Dr L. Thomson, Dr H. Kennedy, Dr F. Browne, Dr C. Faulkner, and Dr A. Pelosi for giving us the benefit of their experience and knowledge. Also our SpR colleagues: Dr G. Ijomah, Dr D. Steele, Dr J. Steele, Dr J. Smith, and Dr C. McIntosh, who helped keep us on the right track.

We 'piloted' early versions of various sections with the SHOs attending the Royal Edinburgh Hospital for teaching of the MPhil course in Psychiatry (now reborn as the MRCPsych course). In a sense they are all contributors, through the discussions generated, but particular thanks go to Dr J. Patrick, Dr A. Stanfield, Dr A. Morris, Dr R. Scally, Dr J. Hall, Dr L. Brown, and Dr J. Stoddart.

Other key reviewers have been the Edinburgh medical students who were enthusiastic in reading various drafts for us: Peh Sun Loo, Claire Tordoff, Nadia Amin, Stephen Boag, Candice Chan, Nancy Colchester, Victoria Sutherland, Ben Waterson, Simon Barton, Anna Hayes, Sam Murray, Yaw Nyadu, Joanna Willis, Ahsan-Ul-Haq Akram, Elizabeth Elliot, and Kave Shams.

Finally, we would also like to thank the staff of OUP for their patience, help, and support.

Contents

Symbols and abbreviations

Other abbreviations are given on pages where they occur.

Abbreviations can be a useful form of shorthand in both verbal and written communication. They should be used with care however, as there is the potential for misinterpretation when people have different understandings of what is meant by the abbreviation (e.g. PD may mean personality disorder or Parkinson's disease; SAD may mean seasonal affective disorder or schizoaffective disorder).

⚠	Warning
▶	Important
▶▶	Don't dawdle
♂	Male
♀	Female
∴	Therefore
~	Approximately
≈	Approximately equal to
±	Plus/minus
↑	Increased
↓	Decreased
→	Leads to
1°	Primary
2°	Secondary
α	Alpha
β	Beta
γ	Gamma
δ	Delta
σ	Sigma
💣	Bomb (controversial topic)
AA	Alcoholics Anonymous
ABC	Airway / breathing / circulation (initial resuscitation checks)
ABG	Arterial blood gas
ACh	Acetylcholine
AChE(Is)	Acetylcholinesterase (inhibitors)
ACTH	Adrenocorticotrophic hormone
ADH	Antidiuretic hormone
ADHD	Attention deficit hyperactivity disorder

ADLs	Activities of daily living
AED	Anti-epileptic drug
AF	Atrial fibrillation
AFP	Alpha-fetoprotein
AIDS	Acquired immunodeficiency syndrome
AJP	American Journal of Psychiatry
aka	Also known as
ANF	Antinuclear factor
APA	American Psychiatric Association
APD	Antisocial personality disorder
ApoE	Apolipoprotein E
ARDS	Acute respiratory distress syndrome
BAC	Blood alcohol concentration
bd	Bis die (twice daily)
BDZ	Benzodiazepine
BJP	British Journal of Psychiatry
BMI	Body mass index
BMJ	British Medical Journal
BNF	British National Formulary
BP	Blood pressure
BPD	Borderline personality disorder
C&A	Child and adolescent
Ca^{2+}	Calcium
cAMP	Cyclic adenosine monophosphate
CBF	Cerebral blood flow
CBT	Cognitive behavioural therapy
CC	Creatinine clearance
CCF	Congestive cardiac failure
CCK	Cholecystokinin
CD	Conduct disorder
CFS	Chronic fatigue syndrome
CJD	Creutzfeldt-Jakob Disease
C(P)K	Creatine (phospho)kinase
Cl^-	Chloride
CMV	Cytomegalovirus
CNS	Central nervous system
CO	Carbon monoxide
COAD	Chronic obstructive airways disease
CPA	Criminal Procedures Act; Care Programme Approach
CPN	Community psychiatric nurse

CRF	Corticotropin-releasing factor; chronic renal failure
CRH	Corticotropin-releasing hormone
CRP	C-reactive protein
CSA	Childhood sexual abuse
CSF	Cerebrospinal fluid
CT	Computed tomography
CVA	Cerebrovascular accident
CVS	Cardiovascular system
CXR	Chest X-ray
d	Day(s)
DA	Dopamine
DAT	Dementia of the Alzheimer type
DBT	Dialectical behavioural therapy
DLB	Dementia with Lewy bodies
DMST	Dexamethasone suppression test
DNA	Deoxyribonucleic acid
DSH	Deliberate self-harm
DSM-IV	Diagnostic and Statistical Manual, 4th edition
DTs	Delirium tremens
DZ	Dizygotic
E/P	Extrapyramidal
EBM	Evidence-based medicine
EBMH	Evidence-based mental health
EBV	Epstein-Barr virus
ECAS	European Catchment Area Survey
ECG	Electrocardiogram
Echo	Echocardiogram
ECT	Electro-convulsive therapy
EEG	Electroencephalogram
ELISA	Enzyme-linked immunosorbant assay
EMG	Electromyograph
EMW	Early morning wakening
ESR	Erythrocyte sedimentation rate
EPSEs	Extrapyramidal side-effects
FBC	Full blood count
fMRI	Functional magnetic resonance imaging
FSH	Follicle-stimulating hormone
g	Gram
GABA	Gamma-aminobutyric acid
GAD	Generalised anxiety disorder

GCS	Glasgow Coma Scale
GFR	Glomerular filtration rate
GGT	Gamma glutamyl transferase
GH	Growth hormone
GI(T)	Gastrointestinal Tract
GMC	General Medical Council
GnRH	Gonadotropin-releasing hormone
GP	General practitioner
GU	Genitourinary
h	Hour
HAV	Hepatitis A virus
Hb	Haemoglobin
HBV	Hepatitis B virus
Hct	Haematocrit
HCV	Hepatitis C virus
HD	Huntington's disease (chorea)
HDV	Hepatitis D virus
HIV	Human immunodeficiency virus
HPA	Hypothalamic-pituitary-adrenal (axis)
HR	Heart rate
HRT	Hormone replacement therapy
HSV	Herpes simplex virus
HVS	Hyperventilation syndrome
Hz	Hertz (cycles per second)
5-HT	5-hydroxytryptamine (serotonin)
5-HTP	5-hydroxytryptophan
IBS	Irritable bowel syndrome
ICD-10	International Classification of Diseases, 10th revision
ICP	Intracranial pressure
ICU	Intensive care unit
IDDM	Insulin-dependent diabetes mellitus
IHD	Ischaemic heart disease
IM	Intramuscular
INR	International normalised ratio (prothrombin ratio)
IPCU	Intensive psychiatric care unit
IPT	Interpersonal therapy
IQ	Intelligence quotient
iu	International unit
IVDU	Intravenous drug user
IV(I)	Intravenous (infusion)

JAMA	Journal of the American Medical Association
K⁺	Potassium
kg	Kilogram
L	Litre; left
LD	Learning disability
LFTs	Liver function tests
LH (RH)	Luteinising hormone (releasing hormone)
LOC	Loss of consciousness
LP	Lumbar puncture
LRTI	Lower respiratory tract infection
LSD	Lysergic acid diethylamide
LTM	Long-term memory
LTP	Long-term potentiation
μg	Microgram
mane	In the morning
MAOI	Monoamine oxidase inhibitor
MCV	Mean cell volume
MDD	Major depressive disorder
MDMA	Methylenedioxymethamphetamine (ecstasy)
ME	Myalgic encephalomyelitis
MEG	Magnetoencephalogram
mg	Milligram
Mg²⁺	Magnesium
mGluR	Regional metabolism of glucose
MHA	Mental Health Act
MI	Myocardial infarction
min(s)	Minute(s)
ml	Millilitre
mmHg	Millilitres of mercury
MMSE	Mini mental state examination
MND	Motor neurone disease
MRI	Magnetic resonance imaging
MRS	Magnetic resonance spectroscopy
MS	Mutiple sclerosis
MSE	Mental state examination
MSLT	Multiple sleep latency test
MZ	Monozygotic
NA	Noradrenaline
Na²⁺	Sodium
NAD	No abnormality detected

NARI	Noradrenaline reuptake inhibitor
NaSSA	Noradrenaline and specific serotonin antagonist
NCS	(US) National Comorbidity Study
NEJM	New England Journal of Medicine
n	Sample size, number of subjects
ng	Nanogram
NG(T)	Nasogastric (tube)
NICE	National Institute for Clinical Excellence (*www.nice.org.uk*)
NIDDM	Non-insulin dependent diabetes mellitus
NIMH	National Institute of Mental Health (US)
NMDA	*N*-methyl-*D*-aspartate
NMR	Nuclear magnetic resonance
NMRS	Nuclear magnetic resonance spectroscopy
NMS	Neuroleptic malignant syndrome
NNT	Number needed to treat
NO	Nitric oxide
NPH	Normal pressure hydrocephalus
NSAIDs	Non-steroidal anti-inflammatory drugs
nvCJD	New variant Creutzfeldt-Jakob disease
N&V	Nausea and vomiting
OCD	Obsessive-compulsive disorder
od	Omni dei (once daily)
OD	Overdose
ODD	Oppositional defiant disorder
OPD	Outpatient department
OR	Odds ratio
OT	Occupational therapy
P_aCO_2	Partial pressure of carbon dioxide in arterial blood
P_aO_2	Partial pressure of oxygen in arterial blood
PANSS	Positive and Negative Symptom Scale
PCP	*Pneumocystis carinii* pneumonia; phencyclidine
PD	Personality disorder; panic disorder; Parkinson's disease
PDD	Pervasive developmental disorder; premenstrual dysphoric disorder
PE	Pulmonary embolism
PET	Positron emission tomography
pHVA	Plasma homovanillic acid
PKU	Phenylketonuria
PL	Prolactin
PMDD	Premenstrual dysphoric disorder

PMH	Past medical history
PMS	Premenstrual syndrome
PND	Paroxysmal nocturnal dyspnoea; post-natal depression
PO	*Per os* (by mouth, orally)
PO$_4$	Phosphate
PR	*Per rectum* (by the rectum); pulse rate
PRL	Prolactin (or PrL)
PRN	*Pro re nata* (as required)
PrP	Prion protein
PSA	Prostate specific antigen
PSE	Present state examination
PSNP	Progressive supranuclear palsy
PTA	Post-traumatic amnesia
PTH	Parathyroid hormone
PTSD	Post-traumatic stress disorder
PTT	Prothrombin time
PV	*Per vagina* (by the vagina)
qds	*Quarter die sumendus* (four times daily)
qid	*Quarter in die* (four times daily)
R	Right
RA	Rheumatoid arthritis; retrograde amnesia
RAS	Reticular activating system
RBC	Red blood cell
rCBF	Regional cerebral blood flow
RCT	Randomised controlled trial
REM	Rapid eye movement (sleep)
RET	Rational emotive therapy
RIMA	Reversible inhibitor of monoamine oxidase
RSBD	REM sleep behaviour disorder
RTA	Road traffic accident
RTI	Respiratory tract infection
R$_x$	Recipe (treat with)
s	Second (or sec)
S	Section (of MHA)
SAD	Seasonal affective disorder
SARI	Serotonin antagonist and reuptake inhibitor
SC	Subcutaneous
SD	Standard deviation
SDH	Subdural hematoma
SIADH	Syndrome of inappropriate antidiuretic hormone secretion

SL	Sublingual
SLE	Systemic lupus erythematosis
SNRI	Serotonin and noradrenaline reuptake inhibitor
SPECT	Single photon emission computed tomography
SPET	Single photon emission tomography
SR	Slow release (or modified release, or XL)
SSPE	Subacute sclerosing panencephalitis
SSRI	Selective serotonin reuptake inhibitor
stat	*Statim* (immediately)
STD	Sexually transmitted disease
STI	Sexually transmitted infection
STM	Short-term memory
SWS	Slow wave sleep
SXR	Skull X-ray
T°	Temperature
$t_{1/2}$	Biological half-life
T_3	Triiodothyronine
T_4	Thyroxine
TB	Tuberculosis
TCA	Tricyclic antidepressant
TD	Tardive dyskinesia
tds	*Ter die sumendus* (three times daily)
TFTs	Thyroid function tests
TGA	Transient global amnesia
THC	Tetrahydrocannabinol
TIA	Transient ischaemic attack
tid	*Ter in die* (three times daily)
TLE	Temporal lobe epilepsy
TPR	Temperature, pulse, respirations (general observations)
TRH	Thyroid-releasing hormone
TS	(Gilles de la) Tourette's syndrome
TSH	Thyroid-stimulating hormone
U	Units
U&E	Urea and electrolytes
URT	Upper respiratory tract
URTI	Upper respiratory tract infection
US(S)	Ultrasound (scan)
UTI	Urinary tract infection
vCJD	Variant Creutzfeldt-Jakob Disease
VDRL	Venereal Disease Research Laboratory (test for syphilis)

VEP	Visual evoked potential
VMA	Vanillyl mandelic acid
WBC	White blood cell
WCC	White cell count
WFMH	World Federation for Mental Health
WHO	World Health Organisation
wk(s)	Week(s)
WPA	World Psychiatric Association
yr(s)	Year(s)

Chapter 1

Thinking about psychiatry

First thoughts

In the stanzas opposite, satirist Alexander Pope captured the essence of the then ongoing European enlightenment, inspiring his readers to use their sense of reason to replace irrationality in their exploration of the world. This period also saw the re-emergence of attempts to use the same method of thinking to study mental illness, whose sufferers had then spent more than a thousand years as objects of fear and superstition. Pope's words resonate even today, 250 years later, when—confronted with patients thinking 'too little or too much' or in 'chaos of thought and passion all confused'—we are still struggling to use science to guide the exploration of this 'riddle of the world'.

Psychiatry has often been derided as the 'Cinderella' specialty: poorly funded, exiled to outside hospitals, a victim of rushed political experiments, castigated by anti-psychiatrists, its intellectual basis ridiculed, and the self confidence of its practitioners lowered. As a trainee psychiatrist you will have to cope with questions like 'are you a real doctor?' In addition, the general public (and sometimes other medical professionals) frequently misunderstand the types and severity of illnesses that you deal with. Either they picture you spending all of your time tending to 'Woody Allen'-like self-obsessed, befuddled neurotics, or guarding 'Hannibal Lecter'-like murdering psychopaths. The reality is that psychiatrists deal with the most common human disorders which cause the greatest morbidity worldwide.

Psychiatry considers all aspects of human experience over the whole of the life span: elation, grief, anxieties, flights of fancy, confusion, despair, perception and misperception, and memory and its loss. We see the mother with a healthy baby, perplexed and frightened by her tearfulness and inability to cope, and terrified by her thoughts of harming her child. We see the family of a young man who have watched him become a stranger, muttering wild accusations about conspiracies. And we aim to be the doctors who know what best to do in these circumstances. The specialty of psychiatry is (or should be) the most 'human' specialty—devoted to the understanding of the whole person in health and illness. Indeed, it is the only medical specialty without a veterinary counterpart.

It is certainly true that the level of knowledge about causation and treatment of mental disorders is less advanced than for other branches of medicine. In some ways, however, this is an attraction. In other specialities much of what was formerly mysterious is now understood, and interventions and diagnostic methods once fantastic are now quotidian. Psychiatry offers a 'final frontier' of diagnostic uncertainty and an 'undiscovered country' of aetiology to explore. Perhaps the lack of progress made in psychiatry, compared with the other specialties, is not because of lack of will or intelligence of the practitioners but due to the inherent toughness of the problems. To put this another way, all scientists 'stand on the shoulders of giants', and in psychiatry we have no fewer and no shorter giants, just a higher wall to peer over.

The proper study of mankind

Know then thyself, presume not God to scan
The proper study of mankind is man
Placed on this isthmus of a middle state
A being darkly wise, and rudely great
With too much knowledge for the sceptic side
With too much weakness for the stoic's pride
He hangs between, in doubt to act, or rest
In doubt to deem himself a God, or Beast
In doubt his mind or body to prefer
Born but to die, and reasoning but to err
Alike in ignorance, his reason such
Whether he thinks too little, or too much
Chaos of thought and passion, all confused
Still by himself abuse, or disabuse
Created half to rise, and half to fall
Great lord of all things, yet a prey to all
Sole judge of truth, in endless error hurled
The glory, jest, and riddle of the world

Go, wondrous creature!
Mount where Science guides
Go, measure earth, weigh air and state the tides
Instruct the planets in what orbs to run
Correct old time, and regulate the sun
Go, soar with Plato to the empyreal sphere
To the first good, first perfect, and first fair
Or tread the mazy round his followers trod
And quitting sense call imitating God
As Eastern priests in giddy circles run
And turn their heads to imitate the Sun
Go, teach Eternal Wisdom how to rule
Then drop into thyself, and be a fool

Superior being, when of late they saw
A mortal man unfold all Nature's law
Admired such wisdom in an earthly shape
And showed a Newton as we show an Ape
Could he, whose rules the rapid comet bind
Describe or fix one movement of his mind
Who saw its fires here rise, and there descend,
Explain his own beginning, or his end?
Alas what wonder! Man's superior part
Unchecked may rise, and climb from art to art
But when his own great work is but begun
What reason weaves, by passion is undone

Trace science then, with modesty thy guide
First strip off all her equipage of pride
Deduct what is but vanity, or dress
Or learning's luxury, or idleness
Or tricks to show the stretch of human brain
Mere curious pleasure, ingenious pain
Expunge the whole, or lop the excrescent parts
Of all, our vices have created arts
Then see how little the remaining sum
Which served the past, and must the times to come!

From Alexander Pope (1688–1744). *An Essay on Man.*
As reproduced in *Poetical Works*, ed. Cary HF (London: Routledge, 1870), 225–6.

What is disease?

Most mental diagnoses have had their validity questioned at several points in their history. Diagnosed by doctors on the basis of symptoms alone, some people find their 'presence' difficult to accept in a field which has been almost universally successful in finding demonstrable physical pathology or infection.

Disease in medicine as a whole was not always based on pathology. The microscope was developed long after doctors began to make disease attributions. Thomas Sydenham developed the medico-pathological model based on symptoms, but it has grown to incorporate information obtained from post-mortem and tissue examination. This model of disease has become synonymous in many peoples' mind with a model based solely on demonstrably abnormal structure. Thomas Szasz (p. 19) has criticised psychiatry in general by suggesting that its diseases fail when this model is applied.

This argument that psychiatric diagnoses are invalid still strikes a chord with many doctors and non-medical academics. The *BMJ* conducted a recent survey of non-disease[1] (see opposite). Many people thought depression to be a non-disease, although schizophrenia and alcoholism fared somewhat better. It is clear from the graph that many conditions rated as real diseases have a characteristic pathology, although some do not (alcoholism, epilepsy). Similarly, many people regard head injury and duodenal ulcer as non-disease, although their pathology is well described.

There are several models of disease in existence (see table below). No single model is adequate by itself and diseases may move from one group to another. Models based on aetiology or pathology have been found to be the most useful, but the reality may be that 'disease' is a concept which will tend to change over time and has no real existence in itself.

Models of disease

Model	Summary of assumptions
Medical-pathological definition (Sydenham 1696; Szasz 1960)	Assumes diseases are associated with a necessary cause (e.g. bacterial infection) or have a replicable morbid anatomy.
Biological disadvantage (Scadding 1972)	Assumes that sufferers from a disease have a common characteristic to place them at a biological disadvantage.
Plan of action (Linder 1965)	Assumes disease labels are justifications for treatments and further investigations.
Syndrome with characteristic symptoms/outcome (Kendell 1975)	Assumes diseases represent circumscribed concepts distinguished from others by a bimodal distribution of scores on a discriminant function.
Disease as imperfection (Cohen 1943, 1953)	Assumes diseases are quantitative or qualitative deviations from a desirable norm.
Disease as 'concept' (Aristotle)	Assumes diseases are man-made abstractions with no independent existence.

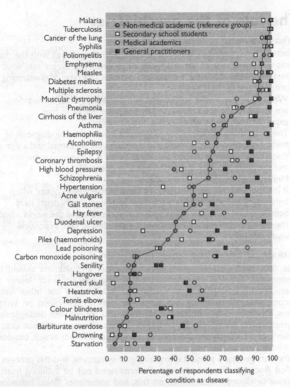

Malaria
Tuberculosis
Cancer of the lung
Syphilis
Poliomyelitis
Emphysema
Measles
Diabetes mellitus
Multiple sclerosis
Muscular dystrophy
Pneumonia
Cirrhosis of the liver
Asthma
Haemophilia
Alcoholism
Epilepsy
Coronary thrombosis
High blood pressure
Schizophrenia
Hypertension
Acne vulgaris
Gall stones
Hay fever
Duodenal ulcer
Depression
Piles (haemorrhoids)
Lead poisoning
Carbon monoxide poisoning
Senility
Hangover
Fractured skull
Heatstroke
Tennis elbow
Colour blindness
Malnutrition
Barbiturate overdose
Drowning
Starvation

○ Non-medical academic (reference group)
□ Secondary school students
○ Medical academics
■ General practitioners

0 10 20 30 40 50 60 70 80 90 100
Percentage of respondents classifying
condition as disease

Percentage of respondents classifying a condition as a disease Figure appears
in *BMJ* (1; 2); reproduced with permission of BMJ Publishing Group.

1 Smith R (2002) In search of 'non-disease'. *BMJ* **324**, 883–5.

2 Campbell EJ, Scadding JG, Roberts RS (1979) The concept of disease. *BMJ* **29**,
757–62.

The role of the psychiatrist

What is illness?

Doctors, being generally practical people, busy themselves with the diagnosis and treatment of various types of illness. They rarely ask 'what is illness?' or 'what is health?' For several reasons this type of questioning is more germane for psychiatrists:

- While all illnesses have subjective components, psychiatric disorders are usually completely diagnosed by the patient's subjective experiences rather than objective abnormalities.
- There is a non-absolute, value judgement involved in the diagnosis of mental disorder—e.g. wheeze and dyspnoea are abnormal and a sign of disease, but some degree of anxiety at times is a common experience and the point at which it is pathological is debatable.
- Mental illnesses have legal consequences.
- It is important that psychiatrists are clear in themselves about which behaviours and abnormalities are their province. Psychiatrists have been involved in human rights abuses in states around the world when the definitions of mental illness were expanded to take in political insubordination.

Disease, sickness, and illness behaviour

The distinction between disease (or disorder) and sickness should be understood. Disease encompasses either the specific tissue lesion or characteristic constellation of symptoms. Sickness, on the other hand, encompasses the suffering and functional deficit consequent on symptoms. One may exist without the other—e.g. a patient with undiagnosed, asymptomatic breast cancer undoubtedly has disease but is not sick; a patient with CFS may see themselves (and be considered) as sick, but does not have an identifiable lesion.

Patients generally present complaining of symptoms, and this process is called illness or illness behaviour. Patients need not be suffering from a disease or disorder in order to do this, and sometimes illness behaviour may be abnormal (even when the patient does have a disease). Subject to certain social conventions (e.g. attending a doctor), they are then afforded the 'sick role' which allows them to relinquish some of their normal obligations. This is a man-made concept, encompassing the special rights and expected behaviour of both someone who is sick and the doctor who is treating them (see box). Difficulties arise when a person adopts the sick role to gain the rights afforded to them, whilst neglecting their duties. Another concern relates to the process of diagnosis—causing someone who is not currently ill to adopt the 'sick role'. Doctors should understand their special responsibility to act in the patient's best interests and not to stray outside their area of expertise.

The rights and duties of patients and doctors	
Patient	**Doctor**
Rights	
• Exemption from blame	• To be considered an expert
• Exemption from normal duties whilst in the sick role	• To have privileged access to patient information and person
• To expect the doctor to act in their best interests	• To direct (and sometimes insist on) a course of action
	• To validate the sick role
Duties	
• To seek help	• To act in the patient's best interests
• To be open and honest	• To maintain confidentiality
• To comply with treatment	• To keep up to date
• To give up the sick role once well	• To act, where possible, in society's interests

Clarity of roles

It is all too easy for psychiatrists to slip into other roles than that which is properly theirs—an expert in mental disorder. These may include: substitute parent, 'friend', guardian of public morals, predictor of future criminality, arbiter of normal behaviour. Psychiatrists have special training and experience in mental disorder, and should avoid being drawn outside this remit in their professional role.

Mental health and mental illness

Psychiatrists are properly occupied in the business of diagnosing and treating significant psychiatric disorders. As gatekeepers to mental health resources there are often pressures to validate distress or medicalise normal experience. Saying that someone does not satisfy criteria for a specific mental disorder does not mean that they do not have significant problems; rather, the problems do not fall within the scope of psychiatry and would probably be best deal with by help or advice elsewhere. In general, psychiatrists should not spend their time advising people on 'good mental health' or how to live their lives—this is the self-appointed remit of 'popular psychology'.

Good mental health is more than simply the absence of mental disorder, it requires:

• A sense of self sufficiency, self esteem, and self worth.
• The ability to put one's trust in others.
• The ability to give and receive friendship, affection, and love.
• The ability to form enduring emotional attachments.
• The ability to experience deep emotions.
• The ability to forgive others and oneself.
• The ability to examine oneself and consider change.
• The ability to learn from experience.
• The ability to tolerate uncertainty and take risks.
• The ability to engage in reverie and fantasy.

Diagnosis in psychiatry

Labels People have a natural enthusiasm to be seen as individuals rather than members of a class: 'I'm a person, not a label'. This desire for the recognition of individuality and uniqueness is a part of the public reaction against race, class, and gender related value judgements. Doctors, on the other hand, appear to love labels and classification, and in their enthusiasm can sometimes appear like the stereotypical Victorian butterfly collector who cannot deal with life unless it is named, categorised, and safely inert behind glass. Labels in medicine are based on characteristic combinations of symptoms and signs, but these are viewed differently by patient and doctor. Symptoms are important to patients because of their *individual* nature; that this strange and atypical thing is happening to *them*. Symptoms are important to doctors because they indicate *diagnosis* and are features which make this patient similar to others we have seen or read about.

Diagnosis The naming of a thing is the first step towards understanding it. We seek to identify disorders (diagnosis) in order that we should be able to suggest treatments (management) and predict their course (prognosis). Ultimately, the aim is to identify the physical abnormality (pathology) and the cause of the disease (aetiology) and so develop means of prevention and cure. The ideal diagnostic system labels diseases according to aetiology. The aetiology of most mental disorders is unknown and so we tend towards a diagnostic system based upon common clinical features, shared natural history, common treatment response, or a combination of all three. Diagnosis leads to the consideration of individual diseases as members of groups contained within a hierarchy: a form of classification system.

Why make a diagnosis? Why allocate the patient, with his individual and unique history, experience, and range of signs to a single label, with the inevitable compromises and loss of information this entails? Diagnosis must be justified on a general and an individual basis. Generally, the process of establishing a diagnosis is essential to allow succinct communication with colleagues, to help predict prognosis, and to carry out valid research on pathological mechanisms and on treatments. Remember, however, that allocation of a patient to a diagnostic category can only be justified if it will bring him benefit, not harm.

Classification in psychiatry Over the past century within psychiatry there has been a debate about the value of, and method of, psychiatric classification. On one hand the academic and biological psychiatrists worried that psychiatric diagnosis was insufficiently reliable and valid, with a wide variety of terms being used in imprecise or idiosyncratic ways; on the other hand psychodynamic practitioners emphasised the importance of unique patient factors and the degree of detail lost by the reductionism of the diagnostic method. The first concern was tackled by the development of *operational criteria*—clearly defined clinical descriptions of the disorders, together with explicit inclusion and exclusion criteria and details of the number and duration of symptoms required for diagnosis. The second concern was met by the development of *multi-axial diagnosis*, where, in addition to the primary mental disorder coded on axis-I, additional axes code information about the patient's psychosocial problems, personality factors, medical health, and degree of disability.

International classification

In psychiatric classification, there are two systems in use world wide the International Classification of Diseases (ICD-10), produced by the World Health Organisation; and the Diagnostic and Statistic Manual of Mental Disorders (DSM-IV), produced by the American Psychiatric Association.

The International Classification of Diseases (ICD-10)

The ICD-10 is a general medical classification system intended for worldwide, multi-specialty use. It includes 21 chapters, each identified by a roman numeral and an arabic letter. Psychiatric classification is Chapter V, and psychiatric disorders are identified by the letter F. An index of the disorders described in this book, together with their ICD-10 coding, is given on pp. 923–42.

Coding The disorders are identified using an open alpha-numeric system in the form Fxx.xx. The letter 'F' identifies the disorder as a mental or behavioural disorder; the first digit refers to the broad diagnostic grouping (e.g. psychotic, organic, substance-induced); and the second digit refers to the individual diagnosis. The digits which follow the decimal point code for additional information specific to the disorder such as sub-type, course, or type of symptoms. When used as second or third digits, '8' codes for 'other' disorders while '9' codes for 'unspecified'.

Versions Four versions of the ICD-10 classification of mental disorders exist, suitable for different purposes. *ICD-10: clinical descriptions and diagnostic guidelines* ('the blue book') is used by psychiatric practitioners and gives clinical descriptions of each disorder together with the diagnostic criteria. *ICD-10: diagnostic criteria for research* ('the green book') contains more restrictive and clearly defined clinical features with explicit inclusion, exclusion, and time-course criteria, and is suitable for identification of homogenous patient groups for research purposes. The *primary care version* focuses on those disorders prevalent in primary care settings and contains broad clinical descriptions, diagnostic flow-charts, and treatment recommendations. A *short glossary* containing the coding together with brief descriptions can be used as a quick reference by practitioners, as well as by administrative and secretarial staff.

Axial-diagnosis The multi-axial version of ICD-10 uses three axes to broaden the assessment of the patient's condition. Axis 1 describes the mental disorder (including personality disorder and mental handicap); axis 2 describes the degree of disability; and axis 3 describes current psychosocial problems.

The Diagnostic and Statistical Manual of Mental Disorders (DSM-IV)

While ICD-10 is a wider general medical classification, DSM-IV describes only mental disorders. The two classifications are broadly similar, having undergone a degree of convergence and 'cross-fertilisation' with subsequent revisions. Relevant DSM-IV codes corresponding to ICD-10 disorders are given on pp. 923–42. DSM-IV uses a closed, numeric coding system of the form xxx.xx (mostly in the range 290.xx–333.xx). A single version of DSM-IV is used for both clinical and research purposes. DSM-IV is a multi-axial diagnostic system using five axes. Axis 1 describes the clinical disorder or the current clinical problem; axis 2 describes any personality disorder and any mental handicap; axis 3, general medical conditions; axis 4, current psychosocial problems; and axis 5, a global assessment of functioning.

Why don't psychiatrists look at the brain?

Psychiatrists, with the exception of those doing academic research projects, are the only medical specialists who rarely directly examine the organ they treat. The chances that a patient with a serious psychiatric disorder (e.g. schizophrenia, bipolar disorder, severe depression) has ever had a brain scan are fairly slim. Psychiatrists prescribe antipsychotics, antidepressants, mood stabilisers, ECT—all of which have a major impact on brain function—but do not know beforehand which areas of the brain are working well, and which are not functioning properly. Why is this?

As a medical student, a medical practitioner, or even as a trainee psychiatrist, this situation does seem somewhat at odds with the medical training we receive. Imagine the outcry if an orthopaedic surgeon were to set fractures without first taking an X-ray, or a cardiologist diagnosed coronary artery disease without ECG, angiography, or CT. Imagine if, based on your description of the problem, a car mechanic replaced the radiator in your car (at great expense to you) without even bothering to look under the bonnet first. How can it be that the state of the art in psychiatry is not to look at the brain?

Looking at this issue another way it is perhaps not surprising. If I were a patient, who presented to a psychiatrist with a catalogue of recent losses (including both my parents, and a recent redundancy), low mood, sleep problems, loss of appetite, and a feeling of general hopelessness about the future, I would probably be somewhat perturbed if my psychiatrist declared that they could not help me until they had taken half an armful of blood, performed a painful LP, and arranged an MRI/SPET of my brain (which might take a few months). I might be impressed at their thoroughness, but over the following weeks as I fretted even more about the results of my brain scan, I might contemplate the wisdom of approaching someone who just seems to have added to my worries. When the final results came in and the psychiatrist declared that I was suffering from depression, I might seriously question their abilities, when I could have told them that three months ago!

In the main, psychiatrists base diagnosis and treatment on symptom clusters, not brain imaging or other investigations. This is not to say that it is not good clinical practice to perform a physical examination and some routine blood tests (or even an EEG or CT/MRI when indicated by the history or clinical signs). Rather, these are generally investigations of *exclusion* (sometimes a *negative* result can be useful—a point that is often lost on other clinicians when psychiatrists do request investigations which are reported as 'normal'). Psychiatric disorders (with the exception of the organic brain disorders, e.g. dementia) are predominantly disorders of brain *function*; there are rarely observable changes in brain *structure* which would aid diagnosis. At present there are no 'gold standard' diagnostic tests for psychiatric disorders. This is not to say that in the future functional imaging of the brain might not play a role in psychiatric diagnosis, but at present (and despite the fact that high-resolution SPECT and PET scans of the brain have been available for more than 15 years) it's not yet time to use these imaging tools in *routine* psychiatric practice. More research is needed to determine the specificity and sensitivity of these imaging tools, even though there are hundreds of articles on functional brain imaging in a variety of psychiatric disorders (as a Medline search will quickly reveal).

Does this relegate psychiatry to the lower divisions of medical specialties? No. Rather, the doctor practicing in psychiatry needs a firm grounding in general medicine (to recognise *when* a condition may have an organic basis), sharply honed interviewing skills (to elicit important psychiatric symptoms), a firm grasp of psychopharmacology (to differentiate between symptoms of disease and drug-related problems), and an appreciation of the psychosocial problems that may affect an individual in the society in which they live.

Psychiatry is not about *medicalising* normal experience; it is the ability to recognise *symptoms of disease,* as they are manifest in abnormalities of emotion, cognition, and behaviour. *Psychopathology* reveals as much to a trained psychiatrist as *pathology* does to his medical or surgical colleagues. Psychiatrists may not (yet) examine the brain directly, but they are certainly concerned with the functioning of the brain in health and disease.

Treating patients against their will

Psychiatric patients may have treatment, hospitalisation, and other measures imposed on them against their wishes. The power to impose such measures does not sit comfortably with the usual doctor-patient relationship, and psychiatrists may find 'sectioning' patients unpleasant. The existence of these powers means that under some circumstances psychiatrists will be damned if they do (criticised for being agents of social control, disregarding a person's autonomy, and being 'heavy handed') and damned if they don't (neglecting their duties, not giving patients the necessary care, and putting the public at risk). Although it may not seem so, 'sectioning' a patient may, in fact, be a very *caring* thing to do: akin to lifting and holding a two-year-old having a tantrum and at risk of hurting themselves and then soothing them. Such a (literally) paternalistic view may appall some people, but historically, paternalism has had a major influence in this area.

When we consider why it is that we have such powers, we might argue that because psychiatric illness may affect insight and judgement (i.e. a person's *capacity*) sometimes patients might not be capable of making appropriate decisions about their care and treatment. Although to modern ears this may sound ethically sensible, we have had mental health legislation for over 200 years, and it is only recently that explicit consideration of such matters has influenced mental health legislation.

Mental health legislation has its origins in 18th-century laws allowing for the confinement of 'lunatics' and the regulation of private madhouses. The main concerns at that time were the proper care of lunatics, fear of lunatics wandering free, and paternalistic sentiments that lunatics as a group did not know what was best for them and so others should determine this. Large county asylums were built in the 19th century and became the old mental hospitals of the 20th. Until 1930, all patients were detained; there was no such thing as a voluntary or informal patient. If you were insane your relatives (if you were rich) or the poor law receiving officer (if you were poor) would apply to a justice of the peace with the necessary medical certification and you would be confined to an asylum—because this was deemed to be the best place for you. Our current legislation has its ancestral roots in such procedures—reform has never led to redrafting from scratch; vestiges of old laws are passed on through the centuries.

Another question often raised is why should we deal with psychiatric illnesses any differently from physical illnesses? After all, physicians cannot detain their patients in order to manage their medical problems, can they? Interestingly, in certain circumstances, they can. Although it is unusual, under Sections 37 and 38 of the Public Health Act, the compulsory detention of patients with infectious tuberculosis of the respiratory tract is allowed—however, the patient cannot be treated against their wishes. Patients with physical illness can only be treated against their wishes if they lack capacity (which may be due to psychiatric disorder).

Is it right that psychiatric patients can be treated against their wishes even when they have capacity to make such decisions? In the 21st century paternalism is dead and autonomy rules. A patient with motor neuron disease is allowed to have their life support machine turned off, despite the wishes of their doctors—why not the same right for psychiatric patients? This does seem to raise interesting ethical questions about whether interventions can ever be justified by principles of paternalism or public protection, when a mentally disordered person has capacity. A pertinent example is that of a currently well patient with a diagnosis of bipolar disorder, who wishes to stop their mood stabiliser, despite past episodes of dangerous driving when unwell.

Let's return to the 'public health' argument of public protection. Infectious patients with tuberculosis may pose a risk to others, and some psychiatric patients may also pose a risk to others. However, most people with mental disorder (even severe cases) are never violent; violence is difficult to predict, and many other people who pose a public risk (those who drink heavily or drive fast) are not subject to such special measures. Potentially dangerous behaviour is not *in itself* a justification for the existence of mental health legislation, but instead provides one criterion for the use of such measures when a person meets other criteria (namely having a mental disorder) and needs care and treatment.

We need to be very wary of how our special powers to detain and treat patients against their wishes might be extended and misused. It is not the role of psychiatric services (including forensic psychiatric services) to detain dangerous violent offenders and sex offenders just to prevent them from re-offending. That is not to argue that psychiatrists should not have a role in the assessment and management of such individuals; just that we should not have primary responsibility for their 'care'. This is a current area of controversy, particularly with the imminent introduction of the new Mental Health Act in England and Wales and the recent development of Dangerous and Severe Personality Disorder (DSPD) Units.

In the 21st century we should be clear of our role: to care for individuals with psychiatric illnesses, without necessarily being paternalistic. We should treat our patients in such a way as to prevent harm to them and to others, but this should not be our raison d'être. The primary justification for the existence of mental health legislation should be to ensure the provision of care and treatment for people who, because of mental disorder, have impaired ability to make appropriate decisions for themselves. We should not be able to forcibly intervene unless this is the case and, when we do, our interventions should be for *their* benefit.

Perceptions of psychiatry

Since the beginning of recorded history, the public imagination has been fascinated and provoked by the mentally afflicted. Of equal interest have been the social and political responses to mental illness and the mechanisms that have emerged to manage and control the 'mad' among us. In general, public perceptions have tended towards polar extremes: on the one hand fear, ignorance, ridicule, and revulsion; on the other, idealisation, romanticism, and a voyeuristic curiosity. The social constructions of madness throughout history have coloured both lay and professional notions of mental illness and its treatment in the present age. These varying perceptions are represented in the arts, the media, and the political discourse of our societies.

In the ancient world, mental illness came from the Gods. Nebuchadnezzar's delusions, the senseless violence of Homer's Ajax, and the suicidal depression of Saul were the result of angry or meddling deities and 'furies'. In Deuteronomy (vi:5) it is written 'The Lord will smite thee with madness'. The first to situate mental suffering within the brain were the sages of the classic world: Hippocrates, Aristotle, and Galen. However, the dark age of medieval Europe saw a return to magical and spiritual interpretations of mental disturbance—madness was the work of demonic forces and witchcraft. Thus, Joan of Arc and countless others were burnt at the stake or drowned for their sins. With the dawn of the Enlightenment, Cartesian notions of rationality and a mind that resided separate from the body displaced the supernatural and laid a foundation for modern concepts of mental illness. Insanity represented 'the flight of reason' and religious moralism gave way to scientific moralism—instead of being one possessed the unfortunate sufferer was now a 'degenerate'. The Romantic era provided a foil to the empiricist veneration of reason. Byron, Blake, Rousseau, Shelley—these were the figures that epitomised in the public mind the archetypal union of madness and genius. 'Great wits are sure to madness near allied; And thin partitions do their bounds divide' wrote Dryden, while in a 17th-century etching, Melancolicus proclaims 'the price of wisdom is melancholy'. The age of asylums and shackles (portrayed by Hogarth in his series depicting 'Rake's Progress' through Bedlam and condemned by Foucault as 'the great confinement') came to an end when, in the spirit of the French Revolution, Pinel struck off the chains from his charges.

The beginning of the 20th century witnessed Freud's description of the unconscious and the birth of medical psychiatry. It was to be a century of controversy and intense soul-searching as psychiatry became equated in the public imagination with 'shock therapy', lobotomies, and the political abuses of Nazi and Soviet regimes. This provided fodder for Laing and Cooper and the anti-psychiatry movement, while skirmishes continue to this day between psychoanalytic and biological paradigms. Finally, in the age of mass media, the actions of a handful of mentally ill stalkers and assassins such as Hinckley (who shot Reagan), Mark David Chapman (who shot John Lennon), and Tsafendas (who killed Verwoerd, the architect of apartheid) have kindled in the public mind the smouldering image of the crazed killer into a blaze of prejudice and stigma.

At the dawn of the 3rd millennium we are the inheritors of these historical constructs of mental illness. Our individual notions of madness and perceptions of psychiatry are derived in part from this varied bequest. Supernatural, romantic, biological, and psychological notions of madness abound, while the historic tensions between the belief that psychiatry is fundamentally benevolent and the conviction that it is inherently repressive continue into the present. The public mind is exposed to portrayals of madness and psychiatry in art, literature, film, and the media and these are powerful influences in shaping individual and collective perceptions. There are many examples of our contrasting notions within popular art. For example, The Crucible illustrates the mentally afflicted as cursed and invokes witchcraft as the agent of causation. By comparison, Quills and The Madness of George III portray the sick as mentally impaired, disordered, degenerate (with differing degrees of historical accuracy). Similarly, in literature, Don Quixote and King Lear depict the anti-hero as simple or incomplete. The neurologist Oliver Sacks has done much to counter this stereotype with his sympathetic portrayal of neuropsychiatric conundrums, for example in Awakenings. The mad genius archetype appears in A Beautiful Mind, The Hours, and Shine, while Joyce's 'Nighttown' chapter of Ulysses and Nietzche's Thus Spake Zarathustra celebrate the gift of unfettered thought. Nietzche defines madness as the 'eruption of arbitrariness in feeling, seeing and hearing, the enjoyment of the mind's lack of discipline, the joy in human unreason.'[1] In Hannibal Lecter (Silence of the Lambs), Raskolnikov (Crime and Punishment), and the villainous Hyde of Dr Jekyll and Mr Hyde, we see the stereotype of the crazed and dangerous killer. Finally, artistic critiques of psychiatry abound, but the champions surely include One Flew over the Cuckoo's Nest, The Snake Pit, and Sylvia Plath's The Bell Jar.

The challenge for us in this post-modern era is to consider our own constructs of what mental suffering means and to reflect upon how we should portray our psychiatric profession in society. In doing so, it is worth remembering the ideas we have inherited from our ancestors and how these ideas pervade current discourse. In sifting the grain from the chaff we would do well to proceed cautiously—since most ideas contain at least some grains of wisdom.

1 Nietzche F (1974) The Gay Science (trans. W Kaufmann). New York: Vintage.

Stigma

Stigma is a Greek word meaning 'mark' and originally referred to a sign branded onto criminals or traitors in order to publicly identify them. The plural, stigmata, when used in medical settings, means the collection of symptoms and signs by which a particular disorder may be identified. In its wider, modern sense, stigma refers to the sense of collective disapproval and group of negative perceptions attached to a particular people, trait, condition, or lifestyle. Stigmatisation describes the process by which the characteristics of the group in question are identified and discriminated against.

Stigmatisation can be thought of as a three-stage process: firstly, the individual is marked out as different by his actions or appearance; secondly, society develops a series of beliefs about the affected individual; finally, society changes its behaviour towards these individuals in a way consistent with those beliefs, often to the detriment of the stigmatised individuals. Stigma can become self-reinforcing as it can be associated with avoidance of the stigmatised individuals, leaving no opportunity for society to confront and change its beliefs.

Fear of the unknown, fear of contamination, and fear of death or the sight of death have led to diseases of all kinds being stigmatising throughout history. This is a particularly true of infectious diseases, diseases causing disfigurement, and mental disorders. As the infectious and disfiguring diseases have become both more treatable and better understood, sufferers from mental disorders have remained uniquely vulnerable to stigmatisation.

One marker of this has been the ease with which originally neutral, descriptive terms for mental disorders have taken on a pejorative and disparaging meaning: cretin, maniac, spastic, imbecile. All have been abandoned in an attempt to free affected individuals from the approbation the name had acquired. Unfortunately, stigmatisation involves fundamental and widely held beliefs and is not usually amenable to simple cures such as changes of name of conditions or organisations.

For the person affected by mental illness, the name of the condition and their abnormalities of experience and behaviour will mark them out as different, and are the root cause of their distress. However, the wider societal beliefs, expressed as stigmatisation, will add to the burden of morbidity, and may in themselves prolong the condition. For example, the belief that depression is 'all in the mind' and could be resolved if the affected individual would only 'pull themselves together', may cause people to behave less sympathetically towards the sufferer, but it may also hinder the sufferer from seeking appropriate help.

There is no simple answer to the problem of stigma. We can certainly learn from the increasingly successful approach to the problem of the stigmatisation which initially attached to those individuals suffering from HIV infection. Increased public awareness of the cause of the disease, its method of transmission, the plight of its sufferers, and its means of treatment appear to be associated with less, not more stigmatisation. The Royal College of Psychiatrists, with its recent 'Defeat Depression' campaign, has been active in this regard.

On an individual basis we can:
- **Challenge our own prejudices** These may exist, particularly in connection with patients with personality disorder and patients with substance misuse problems.
- **Avoid stigmatising language** There is no place for forced political correctness in medicine, but we should consider whether calling an individual 'a schizophrenic' describes them as a single, unfavourable characteristic, rather than as a person with an illness.
- **Challenge lack of knowledge within the profession** A surprising lack of knowledge of mental disorders is often seen in our colleagues in other specialties. This may be expressed in, for example, a lower aspiration for treatment in individuals with mental handicap or chronic psychotic illness.
- **Be advocates for political change** Professional conservatism should not halt us from being at the forefront of moves to improve the autonomy of patients, their involvement in society, and their legal protection.

Anti-psychiatry

One view of medicine is that it is an applied science whose object of scientific curiosity is the understanding of the causes and processes of human illness and the study of methods of preventing or ameliorating them. In the scientific method there are no absolute truths, only theories which fit the observed facts as they are currently known. All scientists must be open to the challenging of firmly established theories as new observations are made and new experiments reported.

All psychiatrists should retain this healthy scientific scepticism and be prepared to question their beliefs about the causes and cures of mental illness. Developments (and hence improvements in patient care) come from improvement in observation methods and trials of new treatment modalities. A result of this may be the enforced abandonment of cherished beliefs and favoured treatments. Always remember that insulin coma therapy* was at one time believed to be an effective treatment for psychotic illnesses.

While rigorous examination of the basic and clinical sciences of psychiatry is essential if the specialty is to progress, psychiatry as a medical specialty has, over the last fifty years, been subject to a more fundamental criticism—that the empirical approach and the medical model are unsuited to the understanding of mental disorder and that they cause harm to the individuals they purport to treat. This basic belief, known as 'anti-psychiatry', has been expressed by a variety of individuals over the years, reaching a peak in the late sixties. Although the central arguments of the 'anti-psychiatry movement' have largely been discredited in the mainstream scientific literature, they have retained currency in some areas of the popular press, within some patient organisations, and in certain religious cults. They are presented here for historic interest and so that the sources for modern-day advocates of these ideas can be identified.

Central anti-psychiatry beliefs
- The mind is not a bodily organ and so cannot be diseased.
- The scientific method cannot explain the subjective abnormalities of mental disorder as no direct observation can take place.
- Mental disorder can best be explained by social, ethical, or political factors.
- The labelling of individuals as 'ill' is an artificial device used by society to maintain its stability in the face of challenges.
- Medication and hospitalisation are harmful to the individual so treated.

The anti-psychiatry movement did raise some valid criticisms of then contemporary psychiatric practice; in particular, pointing out the negative effects of institutional living, criticising stigma and labelling, and alerting psychiatrists to the potential use of political change in improving patient care. It was, however, fatally flawed by a rejection of empiricism, an overreliance on single case reports, domination by a small number of personalities with incompatible and deeply held beliefs, and an association with half-baked political theory of the Marxist–Leninist strain.

Prominent anti-psychiatrists

- **Szasz** Rejected compulsory treatment. Author of *Pain and pleasure* and *The myth of mental illness*. Viewed disease as a bodily abnormality with an observable pathology which, by its nature, the brain was immune to. Saw mental illness as conflict between individuals and society. Rejected the insanity defence and committal to hospital. Accepted patients for voluntary treatment for drug-free analysis on payment of fee and acceptance of treatment contract.
- **Scheff** Worked in labelling theory. Wrote *Being mentally ill*. Hypothesised that mental illness was a form of social rule breaking. Labelling such individuals as mentally ill would stabilise society by sanctioning such temporary deviance.
- **Goffman** Wrote *Asylums*. Described the 'total institution' observed as a result of an undercover study. Commented on the negative effects of institutions segregated from the rest of society and subject to different rules.
- **Laing** Author of *The divided self*, *Sanity, madness and the family*, and *The politics of experience*. Developed probably the most complete anti-psychiatry theory. He saw the major mental illnesses as arising from early family experiences, in particular from hostile communication and the desire for 'ontological security'. He saw newborns as housing potential which was diminished by the forced conformity of the family and the wider society. Viewed normality as forced conformity and illness as 'the reality which we have lost touch with'.
- **Cooper** Revived anti-psychiatry ideas. A committed Marxist, he saw schizophrenia as a form of social repression.
- **Busaglia** Wrote *The deviant majority*. Held that diagnosis didn't aid understanding of the patient's experience. Believed that social and economic factors were crucial. Successful in pressing for significant reform of the Italian mental health system.
- **Schull** Wrote *Museums of madness*. Saw mental health systems as part of 'the machinery of the capitalist system'.
- **Breggin** Modern advocate of anti-psychiatry views. Author of *Toxic psychiatry* which views psychopharmacology as 'disabling normal brain function'. Rejects results of systematic reviews.

---

* In 1933 Manfred Sakel introduced insulin coma therapy for the treatment of schizophrenia. This involved the induction of a hypoglycaemic coma using insulin, the rationale being that a period of decreased neuronal activity would allow for nerve cell regeneration. In the absence of alternative treatments, this was enthusiastically adopted by practitioners worldwide. However, with the advent of antipsychotics in the 1950s and the emergence of RCTs, it became clear that the treatment had no effect above placebo and it was subsequently abandoned.

A brief history of psychiatry

Ancient times ~4000 B.C. Sumerian records describe the euphoriant effect of the poppy plant. **~1700 B.C.** First written record concerning the nervous system. **460–379 B.C.** Hippocrates discusses epilepsy as a brain disturbance. **387 B.C.** Plato teaches that the brain is the seat of mental processes. **280 B.C.** Erasistratus notes divisions of the brain. **177** Galen lectures On the Brain.

Pre-modern 1649 Descartes describes the pineal as a control centre of body and mind. **1656** Bicêtre and Salpêtrière asylums established by Louis XIV in France. **1755** Perry publishes A Mechanical Account and Explication of the Hysteric Passion. **1758** Battie publishes his Treatise on Madness. **1773** Cheyne publishes his book English Malady, launching the idea of 'nervous illness'. **1774** Mesmer introduces 'animal magnetism' (later called hypnosis). **1793** Pinel is appointed to the Bicêtre and directs the removal of chains from the 'madmen'. **1794** Chiarugi publishes On Insanity specifying how a therapeutic asylum should be run.

1800–1850s 1808 Reil coins the term 'psychiatry'. **1812** Rush publishes Medical Inquiries and Observations upon the Diseases of the Mind. **1817** Parkinson publishes An Essay on the Shaking Palsy. ● Esquirol lectures on psychiatry to medical students. **1813** Heinroth links life circumstances to mental disorders in Textbook of Mental Hygiene. **1825** Bouillaud presents cases of aphonia after frontal lesions. ● Todd discusses localisation of brain functions. **1827** Heinroth appointed as the first professor of 'psychological therapy' in Leipzig. **1832** Chloral hydrate discovered. **1843** Braid coins the term 'hypnosis'. **1848** Phineas Gage has his brain pierced by an iron rod with subsequent personality change.

1850–1900s 1856 Morel describes 'démence précoce'—deteriorating adolescent psychosis. **1863** Kahlbaum introduces the term 'catatonia'. ● Friedreich describes progressive hereditary ataxia. **1864** Hughlings Jackson writes on aphonia after brain injury. **1866** Down describes 'congenital idiots'. **1868** Griesinger describes 'primary insanity' and 'unitary psychosis'. **1869** Galton claims that intelligence is inherited in Hereditary Genius. **1871** Hecker describes 'hebephrenia'. **1872** Huntington describes symptoms of a hereditary chorea. **1874** Wernicke publishes Der Aphasische Symptomenkomplex on aphasias. **1876** Ferrier publishes The Functions of the Brain. ● Galton uses the term 'nature and nurture' to describe heredity and environment. **1877** Charcot publishes Lectures on the Diseases of the Nervous System. **1883** Kraepelin coins the terms 'neuroses' and 'psychoses'. **1884** Gilles de la Tourette describes several movement disorders. **1885** Lange proposes use of lithium for excited states. **1887** Korsakoff describes characteristic symptoms in alcoholics. **1892** American Psychological Association formed. **1895** Freud and Breuer publish Studies on Hysteria. **1896** Kraepelin describes 'dementia praecox'. **1899** Freud publishes The Interpretation of Dreams.

1900s 1900 Wernicke publishes Basic Psychiatry in Leipzig. **1903** Barbiturates introduced. ● First volume of Archives of Neurology and Psychiatry published in USA. ● Pavlov coins the term 'conditioned reflex'.

1905 Binet and Simon develop their first IQ test. **1906** Alzheimer describes 'presenile degeneration'. **1907** Adler's *Study of Organ Inferiority and its Physical Compensation* published. ● Origins of group therapy in Pratt's work supporting TB patients in Boston. **1909** Brodmann describes 52 cortical areas. ● Cushing electrically stimulates human sensory cortex. ● Freud publishes the case of Little Hans in Vienna.

1910s 1911 Bleuler publishes his textbook *Dementia Praecox or the Group of Schizophrenias*. **1913** Jaspers describes 'non-understandability' in schizophrenia thinking. ● Syphilitic spirochaete established as cause of 'generalized paresis of the insane'. ● Jung splits with Freud forming the school of 'analytic psychology'. ● Mental Deficiency Act passed in UK. ● Goldmann finds blood–brain barrier impermeable to large molecules. **1914** Dale isolates acetylcholine. ● The term 'shell shock' is coined by British soldiers. **1916** Henneberg coins the term 'cataplexy'. **1917** Epifanio uses barbiturates to put patients with major illnesses into prolonged sleep. ● Wager-Jauregg discovers malarial treatment for neurosyphilis.

1920s 1920 Moreno develops 'psychodrama' to explore individual problems through re-enactment. ● Watson and Raynor demonstrate the experimental induction of phobia in 'Little Albert'. ● Crichton-Miller found the Tavistock Clinic in London. ● Klein conceptualises development theory and the use of play therapy. ● Freud's *Beyond the Pleasure Principle* published. **1921** Rorschach develops the inkblot test. **1922** Klaesi publishes results of deep-sleep treatment, which is widely adopted. **1923** Freud describes his 'structural model of the mind'. **1924** Jones uses the first example of systematic desensitisation to extinguish a phobia. **1927** Jacobi and Winkler first apply pneumoencephalography to the study of schizophrenia. ● Wagner-Jauregg awarded the Nobel Prize for malarial treatment of neurosyphilis. ● Cannon-Bard describes his 'theory of emotions'. **1929** Berger demonstrates first human electroencephalogram.

1930s 1930 First child psychiatry clinic established in Baltimore, headed by Kanner. **1931** Hughlings-Jackson describes positive and negative symptoms of schizophrenia. ● Reserpine introduced. **1932** Klein publishes *The Psychoanalysis of Children*. **1933** Sakel introduces 'insulin coma treatment' for schizophrenia. **1934** Meduna uses chemical convulsive therapy. **1935** Moniz and Lima first carry out 'prefrontal leucotomy'. ● Amphetamines synthesised. **1936** Mapother appointed as England's first Professor of Psychiatry. ● Dale and Loewi share Nobel Prize for work on chemical nerve transmission. **1937** Kluver and Bucy publish work on bilateral temporal lobectomies. ● Papez publishes work on limbic circuits and develops 'visceral theory' of emotion. **1938** Cerletti and Bini first use 'electroconvulsive therapy'. ● Skinner publishes *The Behaviour of Organisms* describing operant conditioning. ● Hoffmann synthesises LSD.

1940s 1942 Freeman and Watts publish *Psychosurgery*. **1943** Antihistamines used in schizophrenia and manic depression. **1946** Freeman introduces 'transorbital leucotomy'. ● Main publishes *Therapeutic Communities*. **1948** Foulkes' *Introduction to Group Analytical Psychotherapy* published. ● *International Classification of Diseases* (ICD) first published by WHO. ● Jacobsen and Hald discover the use of disulfiram.

1949 Cade introduces lithium for treatment of mania. ● Penrose publishes *The Biology of Mental Defect.* ● Moniz awarded Nobel Prize for treatment of psychosis with leucotomy. ● Hess receives Nobel Prize for work on the 'interbrain'. ● Magoun defines the reticular activating system. ● National Institute of Mental Health is established. ● Hebb publishes *The Organization of Behaviour: A Neuropsychological Theory.*

1950s 1950 First World Congress of Psychiatry held at Paris. ● Chlorpromazine (compound 4560 RP) synthesised by Charpentier. ● Roberts and Awapara independently identify GABA in the brain. **1951** Papaire and Sigwald report efficacy of chlorpromazine in psychosis. **1952** *Diagnostic and Statistical Manual* (DSM-I) introduced by the APA. ● Eysenck publishes *The Effects of Psychotherapy.* ● Delay and Deniker treat patients with psychological disturbance using chlorpromazine. ● Delay, Laine, and Buisson report isoniazid use in the treatment of depression. **1953** Lurie and Salzer report use of isoniazid as an 'antidepressant'. **1954** Kline reports that reserpine exerts a therapeutic benefit on both anxiety and obsessive-compulsive symptoms. ● Delay and Deniker, Noce and Steck report favourable effects of reserpine on mania. ● First community psychiatric nurse post established in UK. **1955** Chlordiazepoxide, the first benzodiazepine, synthesised by Sternbach for Roche. ● Kelly introduces his 'personal construct therapy'. ● Shepherd and Davies conduct the first prospective placebo-controlled, parallel-group randomised controlled trial in psychiatry, using reserpine in anxious-depressive out-patients (with definite benefit.) **1957** Imipramine as an antidepressant. ● Iproniazid launched as an antidepressant. ● Delay and Deniker describe the characteristics of neuroleptics. **1958** Carlsson *et al* discover dopamine in brain tissues and identify it as a neurotransmitter. ● Janssen develops haloperidol, the first butyrophenone neuroleptic. ● Lehman reports first (successful) trial of imipramine in USA. **1959** Russell Barton's *Institutional Neurosis in England* draws attention to the adverse effects of institutional regimes. ● Diazepam first synthesised by Roche. ● Schneider defines his 'first rank symptoms' of schizophrenia. ● English Mental Health Act of 1959 allows voluntary admission to psychiatric hospitals.

1960s 1960 Merck, Roche, and Lundbeck all launch versions of amitriptyline. **1961** Knight, a London neurosurgeon, pioneers stereotactic subcaudate tractotomy. ● Founding of the World Psychiatric Association. ● Thomas Szasz publishes *The Myth of Mental Illness.* **1962** Ellis introduces 'rational emotive therapy'. ● US Supreme Court declares addiction to be a disease and not a crime. **1963** Beck introduces his 'cognitive behavioural therapy.' ● Carlsson shows that neuroleptics have effects on cathecholamine systems. **1966** Gross and Langner demonstrate effectiveness of clozapine in schizophrenia. **1968** Strömgren describes 'brief reactive psychosis' ● Ayllon and Azrin describe the use of 'token economy' to improve social functioning. ● Publication of DSM-II and ICD-8.

1970s 1970 Laing and Esterson publish *Sanity, madness and the family.* ● Rutter publishes the landmark Isle of Wight study on the mental health of children. ● Janov publishes *Primal Scream.* ● Maslow describes his 'hierarchy of needs'. ● Axelrod, Katz, and Svante von Euler share Nobel Prize for work on neurotransmitters. **1971** British Misuse of Drugs Act passed.

• Carlsson, Corrodi et al develop zimeldine, the first of the SSRIs. **1972** Feighner et al describe St Louis criteria for diagnosis of schizophrenia. **1973** International pilot study of Schizophrenia uses narrow criteria and finds similar incidence of schizophrenia across all countries studied. **1974** Hughes and Kosterlitz discover enkephalin. **1975** Research diagnostic criteria (RDC) formulated by Spitzer et al in the USA. • Clozapine withdrawn following episodes of fatal agranulocytosis. **1976** Johnstone uses CT to study schizophrenic brains **1977** Guillemin and Schally share Nobel Prize for work on peptides in the brain. **1979** Russell describes bulimia nervosa.

1980s 1980 DSM-III published by the APA. • Crow publishes his two syndrome (type I and type II) hypothesis of schizophrenia. **1984** Klerman and Weissman introduce 'interpersonal psychotherapy.' • Smith et al first use MRI to study cerebral structure in schizophrenia. • Andreasen develops scales for the assessment of positive and negative symptoms in schizophrenia (SAPS and SANS). **1987** Liddle describes a three-syndrome model for schizophrenia. • Fluvoxamine introduced. • Mednick publishes first prospective cohort study of schizophrenia using CT. **1988** The 'harm minimisation' approach to drug misuse introduced in Britain. • Kane et al demonstrate efficacy of clozapine in treatment-resistant schizophrenia.

1990s 1990 Sertraline introduced. • Ryle introduces 'cognitive analytical therapy.' **1991** Paroxetine introduced. **1992** Moclobemide introduced as first RIMA. • The False Memory Syndrome Society Foundation formed in the USA. • Publication of ICD-10. **1993** Huntington's disease gene identified. • Launch of risperidone as an 'atypical' antipsychotic. • Linehan first describes her 'dialectical behaviour therapy'. **1994** Publication of DSM-IV. • Launch of olanzapine. • Gilman and Rodbell share the Nobel Prize for their discovery of G-protein coupled receptors and their role in signal transduction. **1995** Citalopram (SSRI), nefazodone (dual action SSRI), venlafaxine (first SNRI) all introduced. **1999** Hodges publishes first results from prospective Edinburgh High Risk (Schizophrenia) Study using MRI.

2000s 2000 Carlsson, Greengard, and Kandel share Nobel Prize for their work on neurotransmitters.

Psychiatric assessment

The clinical interview

In most branches of clinical medicine, diagnoses are made largely on the basis of the patient's history, with physical examination and investigation playing important but subordinate roles. In psychiatry, physical examination and investigations are rarely of diagnostic value and diagnosis is based on the clinical interview and, to a lesser extent, the later course of the patient's illness. Clinical interviewing is thus the central skill of the psychiatrist and development of clinical interviewing skills is the main aim of basic psychiatric training.

The clinical interview includes both history taking and mental state examination. The mental state examination is a systematic record of the patient's current psychopathology. In addition to its role in diagnosis, the clinical interview begins the development of a therapeutic relationship and is, in many cases, the beginning of treatment.

Clinical interview skills cannot be learned from a textbook. This chapter is intended as a guide to the doctor developing skills in interviewing psychiatric patients. As a trainee psychiatrist you should also take the opportunity to observe experienced clinicians as they interview patients; to review your own videotaped consultations with a tutor; and most importantly, carry out many clinical interviews and present the results to your seniors. Skills in this area, as with all others, come with experience and practice.

This chapter describes a model for the assessment of general adult and old-age psychiatry patients on the wards or in the outpatient clinic. For special patient populations, modifications or extensions to the standard interview are described in the appropriate chapter: drug and alcohol problems (pp. 510–11, pp. 548–9); forensic (pp. 666–7); child and adolescent (pp. 568–71); learning disability (p. 690); and psychotherapy (p. 766).

The student or doctor coming to psychiatric interviewing for the first time is likely to be apprehensive. The symptoms which the patient describes may seem bizarre or incomprehensible, and the examiner may struggle for understanding and knowledge of which further questions to ask. Remember that the interviewer is not like a lawyer or policeman trying to 'get at the truth' but rather an aid to the patient telling the story in their own words. Start by listening, prompting only when necessary, and aim to feel at the end of the interview that you really understand the patient's problems and their perception of them.

The following pages describe the standard structure for a routine history, mental state examination, and case summary; there are then pages devoted to the different symptom areas in adult psychiatry with suggested probe questions. These are intended as guides to the sort of questions to ask the patient (or to ask yourself about the patient) and may be rephrased in your own words.

Always consider your personal safety when interviewing

There is a risk of aggression or violence in only a small minority of psychiatric patients. In the vast majority of patients the only risk of violence is towards themselves. However, the fact that violence is rare can lead to doctors putting themselves at risk due to thoughtlessness. To combat this it is important to think about the risk of violence before every consultation with a new patient or with a familiar patient with new symptoms.

Before interviewing a patient, particularly for the first time, consider: **who** you are interviewing, **where** you are interviewing, and **with whom**. Ensure that the nursing staff have this information.

- If possible, review the patient's records noting previous symptomatology and episodes of previous violence (the best predictor of future violence).
- A number of factors will increase the risk of violence including: previous history of violence, psychotic illness, intoxication with alcohol or drugs, frustration, feeling of threat (which may be delusional or relate to 'real world' concerns).
- The ideal interview room has two doors, one for you and one for the patient. If this is not available sit so that the patient is not between you and the door. Remove all potential weapons from the interview room.
- Familiarise yourself with the ward's panic alarm system *before you first need to use it.*
- If your hospital organises 'break-away' or aggression management training courses, attend these regularly to keep your skills up-to-date.

Setting the scene

Introductions Observe the normal social forms when meeting someone for the first time. Introduce yourself and any accompanying staff members by name and status. Ensure that you know the names and relationships of any people accompanying the patient (and ask the patient if they wish these persons to be present during the interview). It is best to introduce yourself by title and surname and refer to the patient by title and surname. Do not use the patient's Christian name except at their request.

Seating The traditional 'consultation room', with the patient facing the doctor across a desk is inappropriate in psychiatry. Use two or more comfortable chairs, of the same height, orientated to each other at an angle. This is less confrontational but allows direct eye contact as necessary. A clipboard will allow you to write notes as you go along.

Explanation Inform the patient of your status and specialty and explain the purpose of the interview. Explain the reasons for referral as you understand them and inform the patient of the information you have been told by the referrer. Patients often imagine you know more about them than you do. It is helpful to indicate to the patient how long the interview will last; this will allow both of you to plan your time so as not to omit vital topics. Advise them that you may wish to obtain further information after the interview from other sources, and obtain their consent to talk to any informants accompanying them if this would add to your assessment.

Documentation For all clinical interviewing a written account is crucial, both as a way of recording and communicating information and as a medico-legal record. It is best to write up the account as you go along. This saves time afterwards and allows for a more accurate account of the patient's own words. The record should be legible, signed, and dated, and ordered in a standard fashion. Initially you may find it helpful to write out the standard headings on sheets of paper beforehand.

Interviewing non-English speaking patients Where the doctor and the patient do not speak a common language, an interpreter is essential. Even in situations where the patient appears to speak some English, sufficient for day-to-day conversation, an interpreter is still highly desirable because idiomatic language and culturally specific interpretations of psychological phenomena may confuse understanding. Where possible the interpreter should share not only a language but also a cultural background with the patient, as many descriptions of psychiatric symptoms are culture specific. Do not use members of a patient's family as interpreters except where unavoidable (e.g. in emergency situations). It is unethical to use children as interpreters.

Interviewing psychiatric patients

Interview structure

The exact internal structure of the interview will be decided by the nature of the presenting complaint. However, the interview will generally go through a number of more or less discrete phases:

Initiation Introduce yourself and explain the nature and purpose of the interview. Describe how long the interview will last and what you know about the patient already.

Patient led history Invite the patient to tell you about their presenting complaint. Use general opening questions and prompt for further elaboration. Let the patient do most of the talking: your role is to help them to tell the story in their own words. During this phase you should note down the major observations in the MSE. Having completed the history of the present complaint and the MSE you will be able to be more focused when taking the other aspects of the history.

Doctor-led history Clarify the details in the history thus far with appropriate questions. Clarify the nature of diagnostic symptoms (e.g. are these true hallucinations? Is there diurnal mood variation?) Explore significant areas not mentioned spontaneously by the patient.

Background history Complete the history by direct enquiry. This is similar to standard medical history taking, with the addition of a closer enquiry into the patient's personal history.

Summing-up Recount the history as you have understood it back to the patient. Ensure there are no omissions or important areas uncovered. Indicate if you would like to obtain other third-party information, emphasising that this would add to your understanding of the patient's problems and help you in your diagnosis.

Questioning techniques

Open vs. closed questions An open question does not suggest the possible answers; a closed question expects a limited range of replies (cf. 'can you tell me how you are feeling?' and 'is your mood up or down at the moment?'). In general, begin the interview with open questions, turning to more closed questions to clarify details or factual points.

Non-directive vs. leading questions A leading question directs a patient towards a suggested answer (e.g. 'is your mood usually worse in the mornings?' rather than 'is your mood better or worse at any time of day?') Just as lawyers are reprimanded for 'leading a witness' we should in general avoid leading our patients to certain replies, as the desire to please the doctor can be a very powerful one.

Giving advice

Aim to leave at least the last quarter of the available interview time for discussion of the diagnosis, your explanation to the patient of your understanding of the nature and cause of their symptoms, and your detailing of your plans for treatment or further investigation or referral as indicated. The patient's confidence in your diagnosis will be improved by their belief that you really understand 'what is going on' and spending time detailing exactly what you want them to do will pay dividends in increased compliance.

As a junior trainee you may have to break at the end of the history-taking segment in order to present the case to your senior and get advice on management.

After the interview

The process of assessment does not of course end with the initial clinical interview. In psychiatry, all diagnoses are to some extent provisional. You should follow your initial interview by gathering information from relatives, GP, previous case records, and clarifying symptoms observed by nursing staff. In the emergency situation a modification of this technique, focusing mainly on the acute problem, is more appropriate, with re-interviewing later to 'fill in the blanks' if required.

Discussing management

In psychiatry, more than any other specialty, it is essential for successful management that the patient has a good understanding of their disorder and its treatment. There is no equivalent in psychiatry of the 'simple fracture' where all that is required of the patient is to 'lie back and take the medicine'. The treatment of any psychiatric disorder begins at the initial interview, where in addition to the assessment, the doctor should aim to establish the therapeutic alliance, effectively communicate the management plan, instil a sense of hope in the patient, and encourage self-help strategies.

Establish a therapeutic relationship

- Aim to listen more than you speak (especially initially).
- Show respect for the patient as an individual (e.g. establish their preferred mode of address, ask permission for anyone else to be present at the interview).
- Explicitly make your actions for the benefit of the patient.
- Do not argue; 'agree to disagree' if consensus cannot be reached.
- Accept that in some patients trust may take time to develop.

Communicate effectively

- **Be specific** Explain what you think the diagnosis is and what the management should be.
- **Avoid jargon** Use layman's language or explain specialist terms which you use.
- **Avoid ambiguity** Clarify precisely what you mean and what your plans are. Be explicit in your statements to patients (e.g. say 'I will ask one of our nurses to visit you at home on Monday morning', rather than 'I'll arrange some community support for you').
- **Connect the advice to the patient** Explain why you think what you do and what it is about the patient's symptoms that suggests the diagnosis to you.
- **Use repetition and recapitulation** Use the 'primacy/recency' effect to your advantage. Restate the important information first and repeat it at the end.
- **Break up/write down** Most of what is said to patients in medical interviews is rapidly forgotten or distorted. Make the information easier to remember by breaking it up into a numbered list. Consider providing personalised written information, in addition to any advice leaflets etc. that you give the patient. This is imperative if the advice is complex and specific (e.g. dosage regimes for medication).

Instil hope

- Patients with mental health problems often feel extremely isolated and 'cut off' from others, and may feel that they are the only people ever to experience their symptoms. Reassure them that you recognise their symptoms as part of a pattern representing a treatable illness.
- Convey to the patient your belief that this illness is understandable and that there are prospects for recovery.

- Counteract unrealistic beliefs (e.g. fear of 'losing my mind' or 'being locked away forever').
- Where 'cure' is not possible, emphasise that there is still much that can be done to manage the illness and ameliorate symptoms.

Encourage self-help
- Be clear to the patient what they can do to help themselves. For example, maintain treatment adherence (pp. 850–1), avoid exacerbating factors (e.g. drug or alcohol misuse), consider lifestyle changes (e.g. house move, relationship counselling).
- Provide written self-help materials appropriate to the current disorder (p. 921).
- Where appropriate, encourage contact/attendance at voluntary treatment organisations, self-help groups, or patient organisations (pp. 916–18). Develop knowledge of, and links with, local resources and aim to have their contact numbers and location information available at the consultation.

History

The history should, as far as possible, be gathered in the standard order presented here. This provides structure and logical coherence to the questioning, both for the doctor and the patient, and it is less likely that items will be omitted.

Basic information Name, age, and marital status. Current occupation. Route of referral. Current legal status (detained under Mental Health Act?).

Presenting complaints Number and brief description of presenting complaints. Which is the most troublesome symptom?

History of presenting complaints For each individual complaint record its nature (in the patient's own words as far as possible); chronology; severity; associated symptoms and associated life events occurring at or about the same time. Note precipitating, aggravating, and relieving factors. Have these or similar symptoms occurred before? To what does the patient attribute their symptoms?

Past psychiatric and medical history Previous psychiatric diagnoses. Chronological list of episodes of psychiatric inpatient, day hospital, and outpatient care. Current medical conditions. Chronological list of episodes of medical or surgical illness. Episodes of symptoms for which no treatment was sought. Any illnesses treated by GP.

Drug history List names and doses of current medication (have they been taking it?) Previous psychiatric drug treatments. History of adverse reactions or drug allergy. Any non-prescribed or alternative medications taken.

Family history Family tree (see opposite) detailing names, ages, relationship, and illnesses of 1st and 2nd degree relatives. Are there any familial illnesses?

Personal history

Childhood Were there problems during their pregnancy or delivery? Did they reach development milestones normally? Was their childhood happy? In what sort of family were they raised?

Education Which primary and secondary schools did they attend? If more than one of each, why was this? Did they attend mainstream or specialist schools? Did they enjoy school—if not, why? At what age did they leave school and with what qualifications? Type of further education and qualifications attained. If they left higher education before completing the course—why was this?

Employment Chronological list of jobs. Which job did they hold for the longest period? Which job did they enjoy most? If the patient has had a series of jobs—why did they leave each? Account for periods of unemployment in the patient's history. Is the type of job undertaken consistent with the patient's level of educational attainment?

Relationships Sexual orientation. Chronological account of major relationships. Reasons for relationship breakdown. Are they currently in a relationship? Do they have any children from the current or previous relationships? Who do the children live with? What relationship does the patient have with them?

Forensic (pp. 666–7) Have they been charged or convicted of any offences? What sentence did they receive? Do they have outstanding charges or convictions at the moment?

Social background information Current occupation. Are they working at the moment? If not, how long have they been off work and why? Current family/relationship situation. Alcohol and illicit drug use (pp. 510–11, pp. 548–9). Main recreational activities.

Premorbid personality How would they describe themselves before they became ill? How would others have described them?

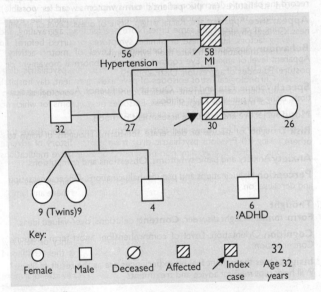

Family tree diagram

Mental state examination

The mental state examination (MSE) is an ordered summary of the examining doctor's observations as to the patient's mental experiences and behaviour at the time of interview. Its purpose is to suggest evidence for and against a diagnosis of mental disorder, and if mental disorder is present, to record the current type and severity of symptoms. The information contained should, together with the psychiatric history, enable a judgement to be made regarding the presence of and severity of any mental disorder and the risk of harm to self or others.

The required information can be obtained during the course of history taking or in a systematic fashion afterwards. The MSE should be recorded and presented in a standardised format, although the information contained may derive from material gained in different ways. It is helpful to record the patient's description of significant symptoms word for word.

Appearance Apparent age. Racial origin. Style of dress. Level of cleanliness. General physical condition.

Behaviour Appropriateness of behaviour. Level of motor activity. Apparent level of anxiety. Eye contact. Rapport. Abnormal movement or posture. Episodes of aggression. Distractibility.

Speech Volume, rate, and tone. Quantity and fluency. Abnormal associations, clang and punning. Flight of ideas.

Mood Subjective and objective assessment of mood.

Risk Thoughts of suicide or deliberate self-harm. Thoughts of harm to others.

Anxiety Anxiety and panic symptoms. Obsessions and compulsions.

Perception Hallucinations and pseudo-hallucinations. Depersonalisation and derealisation.

Thought
Form: formal thought disorder. **Content**: delusions, over-valued ideas.

Cognition Orientation. Level of comprehension. Short-term memory. Concentration.

Insight Does the patient feel his experiences are as the result of illness? Will he accept medical advice and treatment?

Case summary

The written and oral presentation of the results of clinical interview should follow a standard format—history, MSE, results of physical examination, and case summary. The case summary can take a variety of forms but the structure suggested here is suitable for most situations. You should include a brief synopsis of the case, a differential diagnosis with your favoured working diagnosis, and a comment on aetiological factors in this patient.

Synopsis This should be a short paragraph summarising the salient points of the preceding information. Mention the basic personal information, previous psychiatric diagnosis, description of presentation, description of current symptoms, positive features on MSE, suicide risk, and attitude to illness.

Differential diagnosis This will usually be a short list of two or three possibilities. In an exam situation, mention other less likely possibilities you would consider in order to exclude. Your presentation should have directed you towards choosing one as your working diagnosis.

Formulation For general psychiatric patients the formulation should include comment on why the person has become ill and why now. You should identify the 'three P's'—predisposing, precipitating, and perpetuating factors for the current illness. This information will be important in guiding a suitable management plan. So, for example, in a patient with depressed mood following the birth of a baby: predisposing factors could be family history of depressive illness, female sex; precipitating factors could be the post-natal period, job loss, change of role, and feelings of inadequacy; and prolonging factors could be disturbed sleep, unsupportive partner.

Management plan Following the presentation of history, MSE, physical examination, and formulation you would normally go on to present or to document your initial management plan, including necessary investigations, initial drug treatment, instructions to nursing staff, and comment on potential risks and whether or not, in your opinion, the patient is currently detainable under the Mental Health Act.

Observations of appearance and behaviour

The greater part of the MSE consists of empathic questioning about the patient's internal experiences. Nonetheless, important information regarding mental state can be obtained from careful observation of the patient's appearance, behaviour, and manner, both during the interview and in some cases, later on the ward. This is particularly important in some situations, for example with a patient who may be concealing the presence of psychotic symptoms, or where there is reason to doubt the patient's account.

Take time to observe the patient during the interview and ask yourself the following questions. If possible, ask nursing staff about behaviour on the ward (e.g. does he have any abnormal movements or mannerisms; how does he interact with other patients; does he appear to be responding to unseen voices or commands?)

What is the patient's appearance? Describe the patient's physical appearance and racial origin. Compare what age they appear with their actual age (i.e. biological vs. chronological age). What is their manner of dress? Patients with manic illnesses may dress in an excessively formal, flamboyant, or sexually inappropriate manner. Patients with cognitive impairment may have mismatched or wrongly buttoned clothing.

What is the patient's behaviour during the interview? Are there episodes of tearfulness? Do they attend to the interview or do they appear distracted? Do they maintain an appropriate level of eye contact? Do you feel that you have established rapport?

What is the patient's level of activity during the interview? Does the patient appear restless or fidgety? Do they settle to a chair or pace during interview? Is there a normal level of gesticulation during conversation?

Is there any evidence of self-neglect? Does the patient have lower than normal standards of self-care and personal hygiene? Are they malodorous, unshaven, or dishevelled? Are their clothes clean? Are there cigarette burns or food stains on their clothes?

Is the patient's behaviour socially inappropriate? Is there embarrassing, overly familiar, or sexually forward behaviour? All are seen in manic illness or where there is cognitive impairment.

Is the patient's behaviour threatening, aggressive, or violent? In manner or in speech does the patient appear hostile or threatening? Do you feel at risk? Is there aggressive or violent behaviour on display during the interview? What prompts it?

Are there any abnormal movements? Does the patient have repetitive or rocking movements or bizarre posturing (stereotypies)? Do they perform voluntary, goal-directed activities in a bizarre way (mannerisms)? What is their explanation for this? For patients on neuroleptic medication, is there evidence of side-effects (e.g. stiffness, rigidity, tremor, akathisia)?

Is the patient distractible or appear to be responding to hallucinations? Does the patient appear to be attending to a voice other than yours? Are they looking around the room as if for the source of a voice? Are they murmuring or mouthing soundlessly to themselves? Are there episodes of giggling, verbal outbursts, or other unexplained actions?

Speech

The content of the patient's speech (i.e. what they say) will be our major source of information for their history and mental state. The form of their speech (i.e. how they say it) is abnormal in a number of mental disorders and should be observed and commented upon.

Is there any speech at all? A small number of patients are mute during interview. Here the doctor should aim to comment on apparent level of comprehension (does the patient appear to understand what is said e.g. shakes or nods head appropriately), level of alternate communication (can they write answers down, do they point or use gestures?), and level of structural impairment of the organs of speech (a patient who can cough on demand is demonstrably able to oppose both vocal cords normally).

What is the quantity of speech? Are answers unduly brief or monosyllabic? Conversely, are they inappropriately prolonged? Does the speech appear pressured? (i.e. there is copious, rapid speech, which is hard to interrupt).

What is the rate of speech? There is a wide variation in normal rates of speech across even the regions of the UK. Is the patient's speech unusually slow or unusually rapid, given the expected rate? This may reflect acceleration or deceleration in the speed of thought in affective illnesses.

What is the volume and quality of speech? Does the patient whisper? Or speak inappropriately loudly? Is there stuttering or slurring or speech?

What is the tone and rhythm of speech? Even in a non-tonal language like English, normal speech has a musical quality with the intonation of the voice and rhythm of the sentences conveying meaning (i.e. the rise in tone at the end of a question). Loss of this range of intonation and rhythmic pattern is seen in chronic psychotic illnesses.

How appropriate is the speech? Is the content of the speech appropriate to the situation? Does the patient answer questions appropriately? Are there inappropriate or pointless digressions? Can the meaning of the speech always be followed?

Is there abnormal use of language? Are there word-finding difficulties, which may suggest an expressive dysphasia? Are there neologisms (i.e. made up words, or normal words used in an idiosyncratic manner)?

Abnormal mood

In describing disorders of mood we draw a distinction between affect (the emotional state prevailing at a given moment) and mood (the emotional state over a longer period). To use a meteorological analogy, affect represents the weather, where mood is the climate. Variations in affect, from happiness to sadness, irritability to enthusiasm are within everyone's normal experience. Assessment of pathological abnormality of affect involves assessing the severity, longevity, and ubiquity of the mood disturbance and its association with other pathological features suggestive of mood disorder.

Depressed mood is the most common symptom of the mood disorders and in its milder forms has been experienced by most people at some point. Its experience is personal and is described in a variety of ways by different people: sometimes as a profound lowering of spirits, subjectively different from normal unhappiness; sometimes as an unpleasant absence of emotions or emotional range; and sometimes as a more physical symptom of 'weight' or 'blackness' weighing down on the head or chest. Increasingly, severe forms of depressed mood are indicated by the patient's rating of greater severity as compared with previous experience, increased pervasiveness of the low mood to all situations, and decreased reactivity of mood (i.e. decreased ability of the mood to be lightened by pleasurable or encouraging events).

The two central clinical features of depressive illness are (1) pervasively depressed and unreactive mood and (2) anhedonia—the loss of pleasure in previously pleasurable activities. The clinical picture also includes the 'biological features of depression', thoughts of self-harm, and, in more severe cases, mood-congruent psychotic features. The biological features include disturbance of sleep (particularly early morning waking and difficulty getting off to sleep), reduced appetite, loss of libido, reduced energy levels, and subjective impression of poorer concentration and memory. Many depressed patients will have thoughts of deliberate self-harm or ending their lives as a way of ending their suffering. With increasingly severe depressed mood there are increasingly frequent and formed plans of suicide. The development of a sense of hopelessness towards the future is a worrying sign.

Mania and depression are often thought of as two extremes of illness with 'normality' or euthymia 'in the middle'. Morbid change in mood (either elevation or depression) can more accurately be considered as being on one side of a coin with normality on the other. Some patients display both manic and depressive features in the one episode—a 'mixed affective state'. Manic and depressive illnesses have, in common, increased lability (i.e. susceptibility to change) of mood, increased irritability, decreased sleep, and an increase in subjective anxiety.

The core clinical features of manic illnesses are sustained and inappropriate elevation in mood (often described as feeling 'on top of the world') and a distorted or inflated estimate of one's importance and abilities. The clinical picture also includes increased lability of mood, increased irritability, increased activity levels, disturbed sleep pattern with a sense of diminished need for sleep, and subjectively improved memory and concentration despite objective deterioration in these skills. With increasingly severe episodes of manic illness there is loss of judgement, an increase in inappropriate and risky behaviour, and the development of mood-congruent delusions.

Asking about depressed mood

'How has your mood been lately?' Patients vary in their ability to introspect and assess their mood. Beginning with general questioning allows a more unbiased account of mood problems. Report any description of depression in the patient's own words. Ask the patient to assess the depth of depression (e.g. 'on a scale of one to ten, where ten is normal and one is as depressed as you have ever felt, how would you rate your mood now?'). How long has the mood been as low as this? Enquire about any notable discrepancy between the patient's report of mood and objective signs of mood disturbance.

'Does you mood vary over the course of a day?' Clarify if the mood varies as the day goes on. If mood improves in the evening, does it return completely to normal? Does anything else change as the day goes on to account for the mood change (e.g. more company available in the evenings)?

'Can you still enjoy the things you used to enjoy?' By this point of the interview you should have some idea about the activities the patient formerly enjoyed. Depressed patients describe lack of interest in their previous pursuits, decreased participation in activities, and a sense of any participation being more of an effort.

'How are you sleeping?' Many patients will simply describe their sleep as 'terrible'. They should be asked further about time to bed, time falling asleep, wakefulness throughout the night, time of waking in the morning, quality of sleep (is it refreshing or not?), and any daytime napping.

'What is your appetite like at the moment?' Patients reporting a change in their appetite should be asked about reasons for this (loss of interest in food, loss of motivation to prepare food, or swallowing difficulties?) Has there been recent weight loss? Do their clothes still fit?

'How is your concentration?' Clarify any reported decline by asking about ability to perform standard tasks. Can they read a newspaper? Watch a TV show? Ask about work performance.

'What is your memory like at the moment?' Again, clarify any reported decline.

'How is the sexual side of your relationship?' Potentially embarrassing topics are best approached in a professional and matter-of-fact way. It is important to enquire about this directly as the symptom of loss of libido can cause considerable suffering for patient and partner and is less likely than other symptoms to be mentioned spontaneously. During treatment this symptom should again be asked about as many psychotropic drugs negatively affect sexual performance.

'Do you have any worries on your mind at the moment?' Characteristic of depressive illness is a tendency to preferentially dwell on negative issues.

'Do you feel guilty about anything at the moment' Patients with depressive illnesses often report feelings of guilt or remorse about current or historical events. In severe illnesses these feelings can become delusional. Aim to assess the presence and nature of guilty thoughts.

Asking about thoughts of self-harm

Completed suicide is an unfortunately common outcome in many psychiatric conditions. Thoughts of deliberate self-harm occur commonly and should always be enquired about. The majority of patients with illness of any severity will have had thoughts of deliberate self-harm at some stage. It should be emphasized that asking about deliberate self-harm *does not* 'put the idea in their head', and indeed many patients will welcome the opportunity to discuss such worrying thoughts.

The assessment is not only of the presence of suicidal thoughts, but their severity and frequency and the likelihood of them being followed by suicidal action. One suggested method involves asking about behaviours and thoughts associated with increasing suicide risk. This tactful enquiry can be made in addition to an estimate of risk. The aim is not to trap the patient into an unwanted disclosure but to assess the severity of suicidal intent and hence the attendant risk of completed suicide.

'How do you feel about the future?' Many patients will remain optimistic of improvement despite current severe symptoms. A description of hopelessness towards the future and a feeling that things will never get better is worrying.

'Have you ever thought that life was not worth living?' A consequence of hopelessness is the feeling that anything, even nothingness, would be better.

'Have you ever wished you could go to bed and not wake up in the morning?' Passive thoughts of death are common in mental illness and can also be found in normal elderly people towards the end of life, particularly after the deaths of spouses and peers.

'Have you had thoughts of ending your life?' If yes, enquire about the frequency of these thoughts—are they fleeting and rapidly dismissed; or more prolonged? Are they becoming more common?

'Have you thought about how you would do it?' Enquire about methods of suicide the patient has considered. Particularly worrying are violent methods that are likely to be successful (e.g. shooting, hanging, or jumping from a height).

'Have you made any preparations?' Aim to establish how far the patient's plans have progressed from ideas to action—have they considered a place, bought pills, carried out a final act (e.g. suicide note, or begun putting their affairs in order).

'Have you tried to take your own life?' Has there been a recent concealed attempt (e.g. OD)? If so, consider whether current medical assessment is required.

Self-injurious behaviours Some patients report causing harm to themselves, sometimes repeatedly, without reporting a desire to die (e.g. lacerate their arms, legs, or abdomen; burn themselves with cigarettes). In these cases, enquire about the reasons for this behaviour, which may be obscure even to the person concerned. In what circumstances do they harm themselves? What do they feel and think before harming themselves? How do they feel afterwards?

Asking about elevated mood

'How has your mood been lately?' As for enquiries about depressed mood, begin with a very general question. Report the patient's description of their mood in their own words. Clarify what the patient means by general statements such as 'on top of the world'.

'Do you find your mood is changeable at the moment?' Besides general elevation in mood, patients with mania often report lability of mood, with tearfulness and irritability as well as elation. The pattern and type of mood variation should be noted if present.

'What is your thinking like at the moment?' Patients with mania often report a subjective increase in the speed and ease of thinking, with many ideas occurring to them, each with a wider variety of associated thoughts than normal. This experience, together with the nature of their ideas should be explored and described.

'Do you have any special gifts or talents?' A characteristic feature of frank mania is the belief that they have exceptional abilities of some kind, (e.g. as great writers or painters) or that they have some particular insight to offer the world (e.g. the route to achieving world peace). These beliefs may become frankly delusional, with the patient believing they have special or magical powers. The nature of these beliefs and their implications and meaning for the patient should be described.

'How are you sleeping?' Manic patients describe finding sleep unnecessary or a distraction from their current plans. Enquire about the length and quality of sleep.

'What is your appetite like at the moment?' Appetite is variable in manic illnesses. Some patients describe having no time or patience for the preparation of food; others eat excessively and spend excessively on food and drink. Ask about recent weight gain or loss and about a recent typical day's food intake.

'How is your concentration?' Typically, manic patients have impaired concentration and may report this; in this case the complaint should be clarified by examples of impairment. Some manic patients overestimate their concentration, along with other subjective estimates of ability. Report on objective measures of concentration (e.g. attention to interview questioning or ability to retain interest in newspapers or TV while on the ward).

'How is the sexual side of your relationship?' Again, this topic should be broached directly and straightforwardly. Manic patients sometimes report increased interest in sexual activity. Clarify the patient's estimate of his or her own sexual attractiveness and recent increase in sexual activity or promiscuity.

Anxiety symptoms

Anxiety symptoms are the most common type of symptoms seen in patients with psychiatric disorders. They are the core clinical features of the ICD-10 neurotic disorders (which are indeed called 'Anxiety Disorders' in DSM-IV), and are also prominent clinical features in psychotic illnesses, affective illness, organic disorders, and in drug and alcohol use and withdrawal.

Anxiety has two components: **psychic anxiety**—an unpleasant affect in which there is subjective tension, increased arousal, and fearful apprehension; and **somatic anxiety**—bodily sensations of palpitations, sweating, dyspnoea, pallor, and abdominal discomfort. The sensations of anxiety are related to autonomic arousal and cognitive appraisal of threat which were adaptive primitive survival reactions.

Anxiety symptoms are part of normal healthy experience, particularly before novel, stressful, or potentially dangerous situations. Moderate amounts of anxiety can optimise performance (the so-called 'Yerkes-Dobson' curve—plotting performance level against anxiety shows an 'inverse-U' shape). They become pathological when they are abnormally severe, abnormally prolonged, or if they are present at a level out of keeping with the real threat of the situation.

Anxiety symptoms may be present at a more or less constant level—**generalised anxiety;** or may occur only episodically—**panic attacks**. Anxiety symptoms may or may not have an identifiable stimulus. Where a stimulus can be identified it may be very specific, as in a simple phobia (e.g. fear of cats or spider); or may be more generalised, as in social phobia and agoraphobia. In phobias of all kinds there is avoidance of the feared situation. Because this avoidance is followed by a reduction in unpleasant symptoms it is reinforced and is liable to be repeated. Breaking of this cycle is the basis of desensitisation methods of treating phobias (p. 784).

The repetition of behaviours in order to achieve reduction in the experience of anxiety is also seen in the symptoms of **obsessions** and **compulsions**. Here, the patient regards the thoughts (obsessions) and/or actions (compulsions) as purposeless, but is unable to resist thinking about them or carrying them out. Resistance to their performance produces rising anxiety levels, which are diminished by repeating the resisted behaviour.

Asking about anxiety symptoms

In enquiring about anxiety symptoms, aside from the nature, severity, and precipitants of the symptoms, it is important to establish in all cases the impact they are having on the person's life. Record what particular activities or situations are avoided because of their symptoms and, in the case of obsessional symptoms, note how much time the patient spends on them.

'Would you say you were an anxious person?' There is a wide variation in the normal level of arousal and anxiety. Some people are inveterate 'worriers', while others appear relaxed at all times.

'Recently, have you been feeling particularly anxious or on edge?' Ask the patient to describe when the symptoms began. Was there any particular precipitating event or trauma?

'Do any particular situations make you more anxious than others?' Establish whether the symptoms are constant or fluctuating. If the latter, enquire about those situations that cause worsening or improvement.

'Have you ever had a panic attack?' Ask the patient to describe to you what they mean by this. A classical panic attack is described as sudden in onset with gradual resolution over 30–60 minutes. There are physical symptoms of dyspnoea, tachycardia, sweating, chest tightness/ chest pain, and paraesthesia (related to over-breathing); coupled with psychological symptoms of subjective tension and apprehension that 'something terrible is going to happen'.

'Do any thoughts or worries keep coming back to your mind even though you try to push them away?'

'Do you ever find yourself spending a lot of time doing the same thing over and over—like checking things, or cleaning—even though you've already done it well enough?' Besides identifying the type of repetitive thought or action involved it is important to establish that the thoughts or impulses are recognised as the person's own (in contrast with thought insertion in psychotic illness) and that they are associated with resistance (although active resistance may diminish in chronic OCD). Patients with obsessional thoughts often worry that they are 'losing their mind' or that they will act on a particular thought (e.g. a mother with an obsessional image of smothering her baby). Where the symptom is definitively that of an obsession the patient can be reassured that they will not carry it out.

Abnormal perceptions

Abnormal perceptual experiences form part of the clinical picture of many mental disorders. Equally, the range of normal perceptual experience is very wide. Patients vary in their ability to explain their subjective perceptual experiences.

The brain constantly receives large amounts of perceptual information via the five special senses of vision, hearing, touch, taste, and smell; the muscle, joint, and internal organ proprioceptors; and the vestibular apparatus. The majority of this information is processed unconsciously and only a minority reaches conscious awareness at any one time. An *external object* is represented internally by a *sensory percept* that combines with memory and experience to produce a *meaningful internal percept* in the conscious mind. In health, we can clearly distinguish between percepts which represent real objects and those which are the result of internal imagery or fantasy, which may be vividly experienced in the mind but are recognised as not real.

Abnormal perceptual experiences may be divided into two types:
- Altered perceptions—including sensory distortions and illusions—in which there is a distorted internal perception of a real external object.
- False perceptions—including hallucinations and pseudo-hallucinations—in which there is an internal perception without an external object.

Sensory distortions are changes in the perceived intensity or quality of a real external stimulus. They are associated with organic conditions and with drug ingestion or withdrawal. **Hyperacusis** (experiencing sounds as abnormally loud) and **micropsia** (perceiving objects as smaller and further away, as if looking through the wrong end of a telescope) are examples of sensory distortions.

Illusions are altered perceptions in which a real external object is combined with imagery to produce a false internal percept. Both lowered attention and heightened affect will predispose to experiencing illusions.

Affect illusions occur at times of heightened emotion (e.g. while walking through a dangerous area late at night a person may see a tree blowing in the wind as an attacker lunging at them).

Completion illusions rely on our brain's tendency to 'fill-in' presumed missing parts of an object to produce a meaningful percept and are the basis for many types of optical illusion. Both these types of illusions resolve on closer attention.

Pareidolic illusions are meaningful percepts produced when experiencing a poorly defined stimulus (e.g. seeing faces in a fire or in clouds).

Hallucinations A hallucination is defined as 'a percept without an object' (Esquirol, 1838). As symptoms of major mental disorder, hallucinations are the most significant type of abnormal perception. It is important to appreciate that the subjective experience of hallucination is that of experiencing a normal percept in that modality of sensation. A *true hallucination* will be perceived as being in external space, distinct from imagined images, outside conscious control, and as possessing relative permanence. A *pseudo-hallucination* will lack one or all of these characteristics and be subjectively experienced as internal or 'in my head'. The only characteristic of true perceptions which true hallucinations lack is publicness; hallucinating patients may accept that their experiences are not shared by others around them in the same way as a normal sensory experience.

Auditory hallucinations are most frequently seen in functional psychoses. Three experiences of auditory hallucinations are first-rank symptoms in schizophrenia. These are:

- Hearing a voice speak one's thoughts aloud.
- Hearing a voice narrating one's actions.
- Hearing two or more voices arguing.

Visual hallucinations are associated with organic disorders of the brain and with drug and alcohol intoxication and withdrawal. They are very rarely seen in psychotic illness alone but are reported in association with dementias, cortical tumours, stimulant and hallucinogen ingestion, and, most commonly, in delirium tremens. The visual hallucinations seen in delirium tremens are characteristically 'Lilliputian hallucinations' of miniature animals or people.

Olfactory and gustatory hallucinations may be difficult to distinguish and occur in a wide range of mental disorders. Olfactory hallucinations are seen in epileptic auras, in depressive illnesses, (where the smell is described as unpleasant or repulsive to others), and in schizophrenia. They may also occur in association with a persistent delusion of malodourousness.

Hypnagogic/hypnopompic hallucinations are transient false perceptions which occur on falling asleep (hypnagogic) or on waking (hypnopompic). They may have the characteristics of true or pseudo-hallucinations and are most commonly visual or auditory. While they are sometimes seen in narcolepsy and affective illnesses they are not indicative of ill health and are frequently reported by healthy people.

Elemental hallucinations are the hallucinatory experience of simple sensory elements, such as flashes of light or unstructured noises. They are associated with organic states.

Extracampine hallucinations are those false perceptions where the hallucination is of an external object beyond the normal range of perception of the sensory organs.

Functional hallucinations are hallucinations of any modality that are experienced simultaneously with a normal stimulus in that modality (e.g. a patient who only experiences auditory hallucinations when he hears the sound of the ward's air conditioning).

Reflex hallucinations are hallucinations in one modality of sensation experienced after experiencing a normal stimulus in another modality of sensation.

Asking about abnormal perceptions

Asking patients about their experience of abnormal perceptions and abnormal beliefs (e.g. hallucinations and delusions) presents a number of problems for the examiner. Unlike symptoms such as anxiety, these symptoms are not part of normal experience, and so the examiner will not have the same degree of empathic understanding. Patients will often fear the reaction of others to the revelation of psychotic symptoms (fear of being thought 'mad') and so conceal them. When such symptoms are not present, patients may resent such questioning or regard it as strange or insulting.

As with most potentially embarrassing topics, the best approach is frankness, lack of embarrassment, and straightforwardness. If the interview thus far has not led to report of psychotic symptoms, the examiner should begin by saying something like:

'Now I want to ask you about some experiences which some- times people have, but find difficult to talk about. These are questions I ask everyone.' This makes clear that these questions are not as a result of suspicion in the examiner's mind or an indicator of how seriously he regards the patient's problems.

'Have you ever had the sensation that you were unreal—or that the world had become unreal?' The symptoms of depersonal- isation and derealisation are non-specific symptoms in a variety of affective and psychotic conditions. Many patients find them difficult or impossible to explain clearly, commonly describing the experience as 'like being in a play'. Patients often worry about these experiences fearing they presage 'going mad'. They may therefore be reluctant to mention them sponta- neously.

'Have you ever had the experience of hearing noises or voices when there was no-one about to explain it?' If the patient agrees, then this experience should be further clarified: When did this occur? Was the patient fully awake? How often? Where did the sound appear to come from? If a voice was heard, what did it say? Did the patient recognise the voice? Was there more than one? How did the voice refer to the patient (e.g. as 'you' or 'him')? Can the patient give examples of the sort of things the voice said?

'Have you seen any visions?' Again, clarify when and how often the experience occurred. What were the circumstances? Was the vision seen with the 'mind's eye' or perceived as being in external space? Was it distinct from the surroundings or seen as part of the wallpaper or curtain pattern?

'Do you ever notice smells or tastes that other people aren't bothered by?' Again, clarify the details surrounding any positive response. Aim to distinguish olfactory hallucinations (where there is the experience of an abnormal odour) from a patient who has a delusion that he is malodorous.

Asking about abnormal perceptions

Abnormal beliefs

Examination of the patient's ideas and beliefs will form an important part of the MSE. Abnormal or false beliefs include primary and secondary delusions and over-valued ideas. More so than other symptoms of mental ill health, a patient with delusions fits the common preconceptions of 'madness'. Delusions are important symptoms in the diagnosis of the major psychoses.

Delusions

A delusion is a pathological belief which has the following characteristics:
- It is held with absolute subjective certainty and cannot be rationalised away.
- It requires no external proof and may be held in the face of contradictory evidence.
- It has personal significance and importance to the individual concerned.
- It is not a belief which can be understood as part of the subject's cultural or religious background.

N.B. Although the content of the delusion is usually demonstrably false and bizarre in nature, this is not invariably so.

A **secondary delusion** is one whose development can be understood in the light of another abnormality in mental state (e.g. the development of delusions of poverty in a severely depressed patient). A **primary delusion** cannot be understood in this way and must be presumed as arising directly from the pathological process. Delusions can be categorised by their content or by the manner in which they are perceived as having arisen (p. 86).

Over-valued ideas

An over-valued idea is a non-delusional, non-obsessional abnormal belief. Here, the patient has a belief which is in itself acceptable and comprehensible but which is preoccupying and comes to dominate their thinking and behaviour. The idea is not perceived as 'external' or 'senseless' but will generally have great significance to the patient. Over-valued ideas may have a variety of contents in different disorders (e.g. concern over physical appearance in dysmorphophobia; concern over weight and body shape in anorexia nervosa; concern over personal rights in paranoid personality disorder).

Asking about abnormal beliefs

Both at the initial interview and during subsequent treatment, professional staff dealing with a deluded patient should avoid colluding in the delusional belief system. The doctor should not be drawn into arguments about the truth of the delusion—by their nature delusions cannot be argued or rationalised away and arguments of this type will damage rapport. Nonetheless, the doctor should always make clear to the patient that he regards the delusional symptom as a symptom of mental ill health, albeit one which is very real and important to the patient concerned.

Delusional ideas vary in their degree of detail and in their intensity over the course of an illness episode. In evolving psychotic illness there will often be a perplexing sense of 'something not being right' and ill-formed symptoms such as a vague sense that they are being spied upon or persecuted in some way. As the delusion becomes more fully formed it comes to dominate the person's thinking and becomes more **elaborated**—more detailed and with more 'evidence' produced to support the belief. With treatment the delusion will hopefully fade in importance and the person may come to appreciate the belief as false or, despite holding to its initial truth, will regard it as no longer important.

'Do you have any particular worries preying on your mind at the moment?' Beginning with a very general question like this offers the patient an opportunity to broach a topic which may have been concerning them but which they have been putting off mentioning.

'Do you ever feel that people are watching you or paying attention to what you are doing?' Ask the patient to describe this sensation and an episode of its occurrence. Distinguish normal self-consciousness or a patient's awareness of genuinely notable abnormality from referential delusions. A delusion will generally have further elaboration of the belief—there will be some 'reason' why the reported events are happening. Elaboration may take the form of other beliefs about cameras, bugs, etc.

'When you watch the television or read the newspapers do you ever feel that the stories refer to you directly, or to things that you have been doing?' Invite the patient to elaborate further on a positive response. Again, probe for further elaboration of the belief and seek examples of when it has occurred.

'Do you ever feel that people are trying to harm you in any way?' Persecutory delusions are among the most common features of psychotic illness. There is potential for diagnostic confusion with paranoid personality traits, with suspicion and resentfulness towards medical and nursing staff and with genuine fears, understandable in the context of the patient's lifestyle (e.g. of retribution from drug dealers or money lenders). Explore the nature and basis of the beliefs and the supporting evidence that the patient advances for them.

'Do you feel that you are to blame for anything, that you are responsible for anything going wrong?' Delusions of guilt are seen in psychotic depression, in addition to the psychotic disorders. The affected individual may believe that they are responsible for a crime, occasionally one which has been prominently reported. On occasions these individuals may 'turn themselves in' to the police rather than seeking medical help.

'Do you worry that there is anything wrong with your body or that you have a serious illness?' Hypochondriacal delusions show diagnostic overlap with normal health concerns, hypochondriacal over-valued ideas, and somatisation disorder. Clarify this symptom by examining the patient's evidence for this belief and the firmness with which it is held.

Asking about the first-rank symptoms of schizophrenia

The first-rank symptoms are a group of symptoms which have special significance in the diagnosis of schizophrenia. There is no symptom that is pathognomic of schizophrenia. The first-rank symptoms are useful because they occur reasonably often in schizophrenia and more rarely in other disorders and it is not too difficult to tell whether they are present or not. They can all be reported in other conditions (e.g. organic psychoses, manic illnesses). They do not give a guide to severity or prognosis of illness (i.e. a patient with many first-rank symptoms is not 'worse' than one with few) and they may not occur at all in a patient who undoubtedly has schizophrenia. There are 11 first-rank symptoms, organised into four categories according to type (see also pp. 91–2 and p. 179 for Schneider's original list).

Auditory hallucinations
- 'Voices heard arguing'
- Thought echo
- 'Running commentary'

Delusions of thought interference
- Thought insertion
- Thought withdrawal
- Thought broadcasting

Delusions of control
- Passivity of affect
- Passivity of impulse
- Passivity of volitions
- Somatic passivity

Delusional perception
- A primary delusion of any content that is reported by the patient as having arisen following the experience of a normal perception.

'Do you ever hear voices commenting on what you are doing? Or discussing you between themselves? Or repeating your own thoughts back to you?' For this symptom to be considered first-rank, the experience must be that of a true auditory hallucination where the hallucinatory voice refers to the patient in the 3rd person (i.e. as 'him' or 'her' rather than 'you'). Distinguish these experiences from internal monologues.

'Do you ever get the feeling that someone is interfering with your thoughts—that they are putting thoughts into your head or taking them away? Or that your thoughts can be transmitted to others in some way?' It is the experience itself that renders this symptom first-rank. The patient may describe additional delusional elaboration (e.g. involving implanted transmitters or radio waves). The important point to clarify with the patient is that the experience is really that of thoughts being affected by an external agency and that it is not simple distraction or absent mindedness. For thought broadcasting, ensure that the patient is not simply referring to the fact that they are 'easily read' or that they give away their emotions or thoughts by their actions.

'Do you ever get the feeling that you are being controlled? That your thoughts or moods or actions are being forced on you by someone else?' Again, there may be delusional elaboration of this symptom but it is the experience itself, of an external controller affecting things which are normally experienced as totally under one's own control which makes this symptom first rank. Clarify that the actions are truly perceived as controlled by an outside agency, rather than, for example, being directed by auditory hallucinations.

Disorders of the form of thought

In describing psychopathology we draw a distinction between the content and the form of thought. Content describes the meaning and experience of belief, perception, and memory, while form describes the subjective experience of the thinking process itself. In addition to abnormalities of perception and belief, mental disorders can produce abnormality in the normal form of thought processes. This abnormality may be suggested by abnormalities in the form of speech, the only objective representation of the thoughts, or may be revealed by empathic questioning designed to elicit the patient's subjective experiences.

Among the psychiatric symptoms which are outside normal experience, thought disorder is the most difficult to understand and the most difficult for the doctor to have empathy with. It may be helpful to consider a model of normal thought processes and use this to simplify discussions of abnormalities. In this model we visualise each thought, giving rise to a constellation of associations (i.e. a series of related thoughts). One of these is pursued, which in turn gives rise to a further constellation and so on. This sequence may proceed towards a specific goal driven by a *determining tendency* (colloquially the 'train of thought') or may be undirected as in daydreaming ('letting one's mind wander'). Disturbances in the form of thought may affect the rate or the internal associations of thought as follows.

Accelerated tempo of thought is called *flight of ideas*. It may be reflected in the speech as pressure of speech or may be described by the patient. The sensation is of the thoughts proceeding more rapidly than can be articulated and of each thought giving rise to more associations than can be followed up. Flight of ideas is a feature of manic illnesses. In mild forms the determining tendency in the thoughts can be followed (increased follow-up of side associations is referred to as *circumstantiality*), but in more severe cases there is *loosening of associations*, where the normal semantic connection between ideas is weakened, lost, or replaced by associations based on punning, alliteration, or the sound of words (*clang associations*).

Decelerated tempo of thought, or *psychic retardation*, occurs in depressive illnesses. Here the subjective speed of thought and the range of associations are decreased. There may be decreased rate of speech and absence of spontaneous speech. In addition, the remaining thoughts tend towards gloomy themes. In both accelerated and decelerated thought there may be an increased tendency for the determining tendency of thought to be lost, (referred to as *increased distractibility*).

Disturbances of the associations between the thoughts are closely associated with schizophrenia and may be referred to as *schizophrenic thought disorder*. Four disturbances are classically described: snapping-off (entgleiten), fusion (verschmelzung), muddling (faseln), and derailment (entgleisen).

- Snapping-off or *thought blocking* describes the subjective experience of the sudden and unintentional stop in a chain of thought. This may be unexplained by the patient or there may be delusional elaboration (e.g. explained as *thought withdrawal*).

- Derailment or *knight's move thinking* describes a total break in the chain of association between the meanings of thoughts.
- Fusion is when two or more related ideas from a group of associations come together to form one idea.
- Muddling is a mixture of elements of fusion and derailment. *Drivelling* refers to the resulting speech.

Assessing symptoms of thought disorder

Patients will rarely directly complain of the symptoms of thought disorder. In assessing the first-rank symptoms of schizophrenia the doctor will have enquired about delusions of the control of thought and about the passivity delusions. Both these symptom areas require the patient to introspect their thought processes; however, they will more rarely be aware of disorders which affect the form as opposed to the content of their thoughts. They can be asked directly about the symptoms of acceleration and deceleration of thought and these symptoms may be directly observable in acceleration or deceleration of speech. Observation and recording of examples of abnormal speech is the method by which formal thought disorder is assessed. Record examples of the patient's speech as verbatim quotes, particularly sentences where the meaning or the connection between ideas is not clear to you during the interview. Following recovery, patients can sometimes explain the underlying meaning behind examples of schizophrenic speech.

Abnormal cognitive function

All mental disorders affect cognition as expressed in affect, beliefs, and perceptions. The organic mental illnesses directly affect the higher cognitive functions of conscious level, clarity of thought, memory, and intelligence.

Level of consciousness This can range from full alertness through to clouding of consciousness, sopor, and coma (**pathological unconsciousness**); or from full alertness through to drowsiness, shallow sleep, and deep sleep, (**physiological unconsciousness**).

Confusion Milder forms of brain insult are characterised by a combination of disorientation, misinterpretation of sensory input, impairment in memory, and loss of the normal clarity of thought—together referred to as confusion. It is the main clinical feature of delirium (p. 86) and is also present during intoxication with psychotropic substances and occasionally as part of the clinical picture of acute psychotic illnesses.
- **Disorientation** An unimpaired individual is aware of who he is and has a constantly updated record of where he is and when it is. With increasing impairment there is disorientation for time, then place, and lastly, with more severe confusion, disorientation for person.
- **Misinterpretation** With confusion there is impairment of the normal ability to perceive and attach meaning to sensory stimuli. In frank delirium there may be hallucinations, particularly visual, and secondary delusions, particularly of a persecutory nature.
- **Memory impairment** With confusion there is impairment in both the registration of new memories and recall of established memories. Events occurring during the period of confusion may be unable to be recalled, or may be recalled in a distorted fashion, indicating a failure of registration.
- **Impaired clarity of thought** The layman's 'confusion'. A variable degree of impairment in the normal process of thought with disturbed linkages between meaning, subjective and objective slowing of thought, impaired comprehension, and bizarre content.

Memory Beyond the ephemeral contents of our minds, containing our current thoughts and current sensorium, our memory contains all records of our experience and personality.
- **Working memory** A very short-term, limited group of registers for information at the 'front of the mind'. Used for such purposes as holding a telephone number while dialing it. Most people have between 5 and 9 'spaces' available, with an average of 7 (the 'magic number'). New information will enter at the expense of the old.
- **Short-term memory** Used to hold recent memories and experiences. Some short-term memory material may be transferred to long-term memory—a process taking time.
- **Long-term memory** Store for permanent memories with apparently unlimited capacity. There appear to be separate storage areas for information (**episodic memory**), learned skill (**procedural memory**), and emotional associations with people, places, or events (**emotional memory**), which can be differentially affected by disease process.

Intelligence A person's intelligence refers to their ability to reason, solve problems, apply previous knowledge to new situations, learn new skills, think in an abstract way, and formulate solutions to problems by internal planning. It is stable through adult life unless affected by a disease process. Intelligence is measured by the intelligence quotient (IQ), a unitary measure with a population mean of 100 and a normal distribution. There is a 'hump' on the left-hand side of the population curve for IQ representing those individuals with congenital or acquired lowered IQ. No pathological process produces heightened IQ.

Acute vs. chronic brain failure Despite its great complexity the brain tends to respond to insults, whatever their source, in a variety of stereotyped ways (e.g. delirium, seizure, coma, dementia). These present as clinically similar or identical whatever their underlying cause. Acute brain failure (delirium) and chronic brain failure (dementia) are two characteristic and stereotyped responses of the brain to injury. In common with other organ failure syndromes there is an 'acute on chronic' effect, where patients with established chronic impairment are susceptible to developing acute impairment following an insult which would not cause impairment in a normal brain (e.g. the development of florid delirium in a woman with mild dementia who develops a UTI).

Assessing cognitive function

Assessing level of consciousness The **Glasgow coma scale (GCS)** is a rapid, clinical measure of the conscious level (see opposite). In delirium both the conscious level and the level of confusion may vary rapidly on an hour-by-hour basis and may present as apparently 'normal' on occasions. Patients with symptoms suggestive of delirium should therefore be re-examined regularly.

Assessing confusion Assess orientation by direct questioning. Some degree of uncertainty as to date and time can be expected in the hospitalised individual who is away from his normal routine. Directly enquire about episodes of perceptual disturbance and their nature. Document examples of confused speech and comment on the accompanying affect.

Assessing memory Working memory can be assessed by giving the patient a fictitious address containing six components, asking them to repeat it back to ensure registration, and asking for it after approximately five minutes. In assessing short-term memory by testing the patient's recall of recent events ensure you can verify that the patient's answers are in fact correct.

Mini mental state examination (MMSE) The MMSE (p. 66) allows a standardised assessment of orientation, memory, concentration, and performance.

Level of intelligence In most cases formal IQ testing will not be used and the IQ is assessed clinically. Clinical assessment of IQ is by consideration of the highest level of educational achievement reached and by assessment of the patient's comprehension, vocabulary, and level of understanding in the course of clinical interview. To some extent this technique relies upon experience giving the doctor a suitable cohort of previous patients for comparison, and allowance should be made for apparent impairment that may be secondary to other abnormalities of the mental state. In any case, if there is significant doubt about the presence of mental impairment more formal neuropsychological testing should be undertaken.

Glasgow coma score (GCS)[1]

The GCS is scored between 3 and 15, 3 being the worst (you cannot score 0), and 15 the best. It is composed of three parameters:

[E] Best eye response (maximum score = 4)
1. No eye opening
2. Eye opening to pain
3. Eye opening to verbal command
4. Eyes open spontaneously

[V] Best verbal response (maximum score = 5)
1. No verbal response
2. Incomprehensible sounds
3. Inappropriate words
4. Confused but converses
5. Orientated and converses

[M] Best motor response (maximum score = 6)
1. No motor response
2. Extension to pain
3. Flexion to pain
4. Withdrawal from pain
5. Localising pain
6. Obeys commands

Notes:
- The phrase 'GCS of 11' is essentially meaningless; the figure should be broken down into its components (e.g. E3 V3 M5 = GCS 11).
- A GCS of 13 or more correlates with a mild brain injury; 9–12 is a moderate injury; and 8 or less, a severe brain injury.

1 Teasdale G and Jennett B (1974) *Lancet* **2**: 81–4.

Mini mental state examination (MMSE)[1]

Orientation
'Which day of the week is it? What is the date? The month? The season? The year?' (One point for each correct response)
'What is the name of this building? What floor are we on? What town are we in? What county are we in? What country are we in?' (One point for each correct response)

Maximum 10 points

Registration/concentration/recall
'I am going to give you a list of 3 objects to remember. I want you to repeat them back to me and I will ask you to repeat them again later. [Say 'apple', 'penny', 'table'.] Repeat the list until the patient has learned all 3 words, up to a maximum of 3 tries. (Score 1 point for each word learned after first repetition)
'Spell the word 'WORLD' backwards.' (D L R O W) (Score 1 point for each letter in the correct place)
'What were the 3 objects I asked you to remember a few moments ago?' (Score 1 point for each object recalled)

Maximum 11 points

Language/drawing
'I am going to show you an instruction. I want you to read it and do what it says'. [Show card with CLOSE YOUR EYES written on it.] (Score 1 point if the instruction is carried out. If the patient reads the sentence aloud, prompt: 'now do what it says.')
'Write a complete sentence on this piece of paper.' [Offer pen and piece of paper.] (Score 1 point if the patient writes a meaningful sentence with a verb. Incorrect spelling and grammar do not matter.)
'Please make a copy of this drawing.' [Show figure/drawing from pg. 67.] (Score 1 point if the patient draws two five-sided figures intersecting at a four-sided figure)
'I am going to give you a sentence and I want you to repeat it back to me: No ifs ands or buts'. (Score 1 point if repeated correctly)
'What are the names of these objects?' [Show a pen and a wristwatch]. (Score 1 point for each object correctly named)
'I am going to give you a piece of paper. When I do, take the paper in your right hand; fold the paper in half with both hands; and put the paper on your lap.' [Offer piece of paper.] (Score 1 point for each of the 3 actions)

Maximum 9 points
Note: *The test is scored out of a maximum of 30 points. A score of >27 is normal. A score of <25 is suggestive of a diagnosis of dementia. Scoring may also be lowered by depressive illness or acute confusional state.*

1 Folstein MF et al (1975) *J Psychiatr Res* **12**, 196–8.

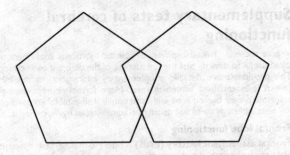

CLOSE YOUR
EYES

Supplementary tests of cerebral functioning

Where there is clinical suspicion of specific functional impairment, it is often useful to directly test the functioning of the different cerebral lobes. This provides more detailed supplementary information to the MMSE (which is essentially a screening test). More formal neuropsychological assessment may be required with additional, well-established psychological tests, although these will usually be administered by psychologists.

Frontal lobe functioning

Frontal assessment battery (FAB) A brief (10-minute) test of executive function (opposite), which essentially regroups tests often used when testing executive function at the bedside. These tests are associated with specific areas of the frontal lobes (i.e. conceptualisation with dorsolateral areas; word generation with medial areas). and inhibitory control with orbital or medial areas. The maximum score is 18 and a cut-off score of 12 in patients with dementia has been shown to have a sensitivity of 79% for frontotemporal dementia vs. Alzheimer's disease. However, any performance below 17 may indicate frontal lobe impairment.

The Wisconsin card sorting task The patient has to determine the rule for card allocation and allocate cards accordingly. When the rule changes, a patient with frontal lode dysfunction is likely to make more errors (tests response inhibition and set shifting).

Digit span Short-term verbal memory is tested with progressively longer number sequences, first forwards (normal maximum digit span 6 ± 1) and, subsequently, in reverse order (normal maximum 5 ± 1).

Trail making test A 'join the dots' test of visuomotor tracing testing conceptualisation and set shifting. Test A is a simple number sequence; Test B is of alternating numbers and letters (more sensitive for frontal lobe dysfunction).

Cognitive estimate testing The patient is asked a question that requires abstract reasoning and cannot be answered by general knowledge alone (e.g. 'how many camels are there in the UK?').

Parietal lobe functioning

Tests for dominant lesions

Finger agnosia Patient cannot state which finger is being touched with their eyes closed.

Astereoagnosia Patient unable to recognise the feel of common objects (e.g. coin, pen) with their eyes closed.

Dysgraphaethesia Inability to recognise letters or numbers written on the hand.

(N.B. Although of disputed clinical value, Gerstmann syndrome is classically described as: right-left disorientation, finger agnosia, dysgraphia, and dyscalculia; due to a lesion of the dominant (usually left) parietal lobe.)

Tests for non-dominant lesions

Asomatognosia Patient does not recognise parts of their body (e.g. hand, fingers).

Constructional dyspraxia Inability to draw shapes or construct geometrical patterns.

Other problem areas
- Visual fields (as optic tracts run through the parietal lobe to reach the occipital lobe).
- Speech—alexia, receptive dysphasia (Wernicke area); conduction aphasia (cannot repeat a phrase, but does understand the meaning).
- Reading/writing (angular gyrus lesions).

Frontal assessment battery (FAB)

Domain	Instructions	Score
Similarities (*Concepts*)	'In what way are they alike?' A banana and an apple; A table and a chair; A tulip, a rose, and a daisy	Three correct: 3 Two correct: 2 One correct: 1 None correct: 0
Lexical fluency (*Mental flexibility*)	'Say as many words as you can beginning with the letter 'S', except surnames or proper nouns' (If no response for 5 sec, say 'for instance, snake'; do not count repetitions, variations)—time 60 sec	>9 words: 3 6–9 words: 2 3–5 words: 1 <3 words: 0
Motor series (*Programming*)	'Look carefully at what I'm doing'. The examiner performs 3 times the fist-palm-edge series. 'Now, with your right hand, do the same series, first with me, then alone'.	6 correct consecutive series alone: 3 3 correct consecutive series alone: 2 3 correct consecutive series with the examiner: 1 <3 correct consecutive series with the examiner: 0
Conflicting instructions (*Sensitivity to interference*)	'Tap twice when I tap once'. (Make 3 trials of 1-1-1 and 2-2-2 to make sure that patient has understood) Test series: 1-1-2-1-2-2-2-1-1-2	No error: 3 1-2 errors: 2 >2 errors: 1 4 consecutive errors: 0
Go/no go (*Inhibitory control*)	'Tap once when I tap once, do not tap when I tap twice'. (a series of 3 trials is run with 1-1-1 and 2-2-2) Test series: 1-1-2-1-2-2-2-1-1-2	No error: 3 1-2 errors: 2 >2 errors: 1 4 consecutive errors: 0
Prehension behaviour (*Environmental autonomy*)	'Do not take my hands' The examiner brings his hands close to the patient's hands (that are resting palms face upwards on his knees) and touches the palms of patitent's hands. Repeat instructions and try again if patient takes the hands.	Does not take the examiner's hands: 3 Hesitates and asks what he has to do: 2 Takes the hands: 1 Takes the hands even after being told not to: 0

Frontal assessment battery (FAB), Dubois B *et al.* (2000) *Neurology* **55**, 1621–6.

Insight

The question of whether the patient has insight into the nature of their symptoms tends only to arise in psychiatric illnesses. In general, a patient with physical illness knows that their symptoms represent abnormality and seeks their diagnosis and appropriate treatment. In contrast, a variety of psychiatric illnesses are associated with impairment of insight and the development of alternative explanations by the patient as to the cause of their symptoms, for example:

- An elderly man with early dementia who is unable to recall where he leaves objects and attributes this to someone stealing them. He angrily accuses his son of the 'crime'.
- An adolescent, with developing schizophrenia, who believes his auditory hallucinations and sense of being watched are caused by a neighbour who has planted cameras and loudspeakers into his flat. He repeatedly calls the police and asks them to intervene.
- A middle-aged woman with worsening depression who develops the delusion that she is bankrupt and is shortly about to be evicted from her home in disgrace.

Impairment of insight is not specific to any one psychiatric condition and is not a generally a diagnostically important symptom. It tends to occur in psychotic and organic illnesses and in the more severe forms of depressive illness. Neurotic illnesses and personality disorders are generally not associated with impairment of insight. Impairment of insight can give a crude measure of severity of psychotic symptoms and regaining of insight into the pathological nature of psychotic beliefs can give a similarly crude measure of improvement with treatment.

Insight can be defined succinctly as 'the correct attitude to morbid change in oneself'. It is a deceptively simple concept that includes a number of beliefs about the nature of the symptoms, their causation, and the most appropriate way of dealing with them. Insight is sometimes reported as an 'all or nothing' measure—as something an individual patient either does or does not have. In fact, insight is most usefully inquired about and reported as a series of health beliefs:

- Does the patient believe that their abnormal experiences are symptoms?
- Does the patient believe their symptoms are attributable to illness?
- Do they believe that the illness is psychiatric?
- Do they believe that psychiatric treatment might benefit them?
- Would they be willing to accept advice from a doctor regarding their treatment?

Beyond the simple question of whether the patient has impairment of insight or not it is vital to understand how the patient views their symptoms as this will tend to influence their compliance and future help-seeking behaviour. It is important to emphasise that disagreement with the doctor as to the correct course of action does *not* necessarily indicate lack of insight. A patient may very well not agree to be admitted to hospital or to take a particular medication despite having full insight into the nature of their symptoms. In these cases the doctor should be sure to clarify that the patient has all the necessary information to make a suitable decision before considering the possible need for compulsory treatment.

Physical examination

Examination of the patient's physical condition is an integral part of a comprehensive psychiatric assessment. There are five main reasons why this is so:

- Physical symptoms may be a direct result of psychiatric illness (e.g. alcohol dependency—see pp. 532–3; eating disorders—see pp. 378–9; physical neglect in severe depression, schizophrenia, etc.)
- Psychiatric drugs may have physical side-effects (e.g. EPSEs and antipsychotics, hypothyroidism and lithium, withdrawal syndromes—see pp. 872–3).
- Physical illnesses can cause or exacerbate mental symptoms.
- Occult physical illness may be present.
- In the case of later development of illness (or more rarely, medico-legal issues) it is helpful to have baseline physical findings documented.

Physical examination is all too often deferred and then not done, or not done as thoroughly as is indicated. It may well be acceptable to defer full examination on occasions (e.g. a distressed and paranoid man seen in A&E), but a minimal investigation can be done and completed as the situation allows.

A routine physical examination has the aim of documenting the patient's baseline physical state, noting the presence or absence of abnormal signs which could be associated with mental or physical illness, and highlighting areas requiring further examination or investigation.

General condition Note height and weight. Does the patient look well or unwell? Are they underweight or are there signs of recent weight loss? Note bruising or other injuries and estimate their age.

Cardiovascular Radial pulse—rate, rhythm, and character. Blood pressure. Carotid bruits? Heart sounds. Pedal oedema.

Respiratory Respiratory rate. Expansion. Percussion note. Breath sounds to auscultation.

Abdominal Swelling or ascites. Masses. Bowel sounds. Hernias.

Neurological Pupilliary response and other cranial nerves. Wasting. Tone. Power. Sensation. Reflexes. Gait. Involuntary movements.

Some physical signs in psychiatric illness, and possible causes

General examination

'Parkinsonian facies'	Antipsychotic drug treatment
	Psychomotor retardation (depression)
Abnormal pupil size	Opiate use
Argyll-Robertson pupil	Neurosyphilis
Enlarged parotids	Bulimia nervosa
('hamster face')	(secondary to vomiting)
Hypersalivation	Clozapine treatment
Goitre	Thyroid disease
Multiple forearm scars	Borderline personality disorder
Multiple tattoos	Dissocial personality disorder
Needle tracks/phlebitis	IV drug use
Gynaecomastia	Antipsychotic drug treatment
	Alcoholic liver disease
Russell's sign (knuckle callus)	Bulimia nervosa
	(secondary to inducing vomiting)
Lanugo hair	Anorexia nervosa
Piloerection ('goose flesh')	Opiate withdrawal
Excessive thinness	Anorexia nervosa

Cardiovascular

Rapid/irregular pulse	Anxiety disorder
	Drug/alcohol withdrawal
	Hyperthyroidism
Slow pulse	Hypothyroidism

Abdominal

Enlarged liver	Alcoholic liver disease
	Hepatitis
Multiple surgical scars	Somatisation disorder
('checker-board' abdomen)	
Multiple self-inflicted scars	Borderline personality disorder

Neurological

Resting tremor	Increased sympathetic drive
	(anxiety, drug/alcohol misuse)
	Antipsychotic drug treatment
	Lithium treatment
Involuntary movements	Antipsychotic drug treatment
	Tic disorder
	Huntingtons's/Sydenhams's chorea
Abnormal posturing	Antipsychotic-induced dystonia
	Catatonia
Festinant (shuffling) gait	Antipsychotic drug treatment
Broad-based gait	Cerebellar disease (alcohol, lithium toxicity)

Clinical investigation

Clinical investigations, including blood testing, imaging techniques, and karyotyping, play a smaller role in psychiatry than in other medical specialties. They are mainly carried out to exclude medical conditions which may be part of the differential diagnosis (such as hypothyroidism as a cause of lethargy and low mood) or which may be comorbid. They should generally be carried out as a result of positive findings in the history or physical examination or in order to exclude serious and reversible occult disorders (such as syphilis as a cause of dementia).

'Routine' investigations may be carried out to assess general physical health, and to provide a 'baseline' measure prior to commencing medication known to have possible adverse effects (e.g. FBC and LFTs and antipsychotic medication; U&Es, creatinine clearance, TFTs prior to lithium therapy). Specific screening and monitoring tests are detailed in specific sections. It is good practice to screen new patients with some standard tests, and the usual test battery will include: FBC (and differential), U&Es, LFTs, TFTs, glucose. Where there is suspicion of drug or alcohol misuse/dependency, MCV, B_{12}/folate, and toxicology screening may be added.

Other physical investigations are rarely requested (with perhaps the exception of ECG for patients on specific or high-dose antipsychotics) unless clinical examination indicates the possibility of an underlying (undiagnosed) physical disorder. Performance of a lumbar puncture, for example, is reserved for situations where there is clear evidence to suggest a neurological disorder presenting with psychiatric symptoms (e.g. suspected meningitis or encephalitis; multiple sclerosis) and, more often than not, in these circumstances a referral will be made for a medical review.

Use of other tools, such as EEG, CT, or MRI (and SPECT or PET where available) require justification on the grounds of diagnostic need. EEG is frequently overused by psychiatrists, and may be difficult to interpret as psychotropic medications may 'muddy the waters'. EEG may be useful where epilepsy is suspected (on clinical grounds), to monitor some acute (toxic) confusional states, to assess atypical patterns of cognitive impairment, to aid diagnosis in certain dementias (e.g. HIV, vCJD), to evaluate particular sleep disorders, or as the 'gold standard' for seizure monitoring during ECT. EEG should not be used as a general screening tool.

Similarly, brain imaging adds little to the diagnosis of primary psychiatric disorders, and should only be used where there is good evidence for possible neurological problems (e.g. history of significant head injury, epilepsy, multiple sclerosis, previous neurosurgery) or where history and clinical examination indicate the possibility of a space-occupying lesion (e.g. localising neurological signs, unexplained fluctuating level of consciousness, severe headache, marked and unexplained acute behavioural change.) With the exception of organic disorders (e.g. the dementias —where diagnostic imaging techniques may add useful information to inform diagnosis, management, and prognosis), the sensitivity and specificity of imaging findings for most psychiatric conditions have yet to be established.

As a general rule comorbid or causative disorders will be suspected due to other symptoms and signs or by the atypical nature of the psychiatric picture, and the likelihood of revealing a totally unexpected diagnosis is small.

Common assessment instruments

The diagnosis of psychiatric disorders is largely clinical, with assessment tools only useful in a minority of cases (e.g. IQ tests in the diagnosis of learning disability). Nonetheless, a huge variety of assessment tools is available for the diagnosis of psychiatric disorders in general, for the diagnosis and assessment of severity of individual disorders, and for the monitoring of progress and treatment response in established cases. Their primary use is in research, in order to ensure heterogeneous patient groupings and reliably standardised diagnosis. Hundreds of tools are available, some only being used in a single study. Examples of the more commonly found general and specific tests are given here.

General Health Questionnaire (GHQ) Self-rated questionnaire used as screening instrument for presence of psychiatric illness. Patient is asked to report the presence of a list of symptoms in the preceding weeks. Four versions are available using 12, 28, 30, and 60 items. Takes 5-15 minutes to complete depending on version.

Present State Examination (PSE) Clinician-administered semi-structured clinical interview yielding clinical diagnoses.

Schedule for Assessment in Neuropsychiatry (SCAN) Development of PSE. Semi-structured interview for use by experienced clinicians. Consists of interview schedule, glossary with symptom definitions, and past history questionnaire. Interview takes 60-90 minutes to complete.

Structured Clinical-Interview for DSM-IV (SCID) Clinician-administered semi-structured clinical interview for use with patients in whom a psychiatric diagnosis is suspected. Interviewer should have sufficient experience to make clinical diagnoses without the use of a structured interview. Interview consists of probe questions and follow-up questions for nine diagnostic groupings with interviewer-rated diagnostic criteria for 51 DSM-IV axis-I diagnoses. Kappa values for test-retest reliability for the DSM-III version of the SCID were ~0.7.

Diagnostic Interview Schedule (DIS) Non-clinician-administered fully-structured interview. Takes 45–60 minutes.

Global Assessment of Functioning Scale (GAF) 100-item, self-report rating scale measuring overall psychosocial functioning.

Health of the Nation Outcome Scales (HoNoS) Health-practitioner rating scale consisting of 12 items scored 0-5. Provides measure of health and clinical need, not diagnosis or prognosis. Used in general population screening or for monitoring clinical recovery.

Quality of Life Interview (QOLI) Non-clinician-administered fully-structured interview available in full and brief versions with 158 and 78 items respectively. Suitable for assessment of quality of life in those with enduring and severe mental illnesses.

Hamilton Rating Scale for Depression (HAM-D) Interviewer-rated, 17-item rating scale for depressive illness. Not a diagnostic instrument; used to measure changes (e.g. as a result of drug treatment). 17 items scored according to severity, producing total score.

Montgomery-Asberg Depression Rating Scale (MADRaS) 10-item observer-rated scale. Each item rated 0-6 with total score obtained.

Beck Depression Inventory (BDI) Self-rated questionnaire containing 21 statements with four possible responses for each. Total score is quoted with >17 indicating moderate and >30 indicating severe depression.

Positive and Negative Symptom Scale (PANSS) Clinician-administered rating scale for assessment of severity and monitoring of change of symptoms in patients with a diagnosis of schizophrenia. 30 items covering positive symptoms, negative symptoms, and general psychopathology.

Hamilton Anxiety Rating scale (HARA) Clinician-administered rating scale for generalised anxiety disorder. 14 items each rated on a 5-point scale.

Yale-Brown Obsessive-Compulsive Scale (Y-BOCS) Clinician-administered semi-structured interview allowing rating of severity in patients with a pre-existing diagnosis of OCD.

Cage Questionnaire Brief screening test for alcohol problems consisting of 4 yes/no questions, a score of 2 or more indicating the need for further assessment.

Minnesota Multiphasic Personality Inventory (MMPI) Self-report questionnaire consisting of 567 questions covering 8 areas of psychopathology, 2 additional areas of personality type, and 3 scales assessing truthfulness. Results are compared with normative data from non-clinical populations. Results generate information useful for a broad range of clinical applications.

International Personality Disorder Examination (IPDE) Semi-structured clinical interview for use by clinicians producing ICD-10-personality disorder diagnosis. 67 standardised probe questions. 57-item true/false questionnaire also included for screening purposes.

Symptoms of psychiatric illness

Symptoms of psychiatric illness

In general medicine, **symptom** refers to an abnormality reported by the patient, while **sign** refers to an abnormality detected by the doctor by observation or clinical examination. In psychiatry, the terms symptom and sign tend to be used synonymously because abnormalities of mental state can only be elicited by exploring, with the patient, their internal experiences.

Psychopathology is the study of abnormalities in mental state and is one of the core sciences in clinical psychiatry. **Descriptive psychopathology** is one method for describing the subjective experience and behaviour of patients and is the basis for our current clinical descriptions of mental disorder. It is atheoretical, and does not rest on any particular explanation for the cause of the abnormal mental state. In this it contrasts with **dynamic (Freudian) psychopathology** which attempts to describe and then to explain these states.

Descriptive psychopathology includes close observation of the patient's behaviour and empathic exploration of their subjective experience. The latter is called **phenomenology**. The following general terms are used as qualifiers for symptoms described in the following pages:

- **Subjective vs. objective** Objective signs are those noted by an external observer; subjective signs are those reported by the patient.
- **Form vs. content** A distinction is drawn between the *form* and *content* of abnormal internal experiences. For example, a patient may believe that he is continually under surveillance by agents of MI5 who are plotting to frame him for another's crimes. Here, the *content* of the symptom is the belief about the name and methods of the persecutor; the *form* is that of a persecutory delusion. *Content* is culture and experience related, whereas *form* is attributable to the type of underlying mental illness.
- **Primary vs. secondary** Primary symptoms are considered as arising directly from the pathology of the mental illness; secondary symptoms arise as an understandable response to some aspect of the disordered mental state (e.g. a patient with severe depression developing a *secondary delusion* of being wicked and deserving punishment). Secondary symptoms can be understood in the light of knowledge of the patient's symptoms; primary symptoms can be empathised with but not fully understood.
- **Endogenous vs. reactive** These terms have been largely made redundant by developments in understanding of mental disorders, but are still seen occasionally. It was formerly thought that some conditions arose in response to external events (e.g. depression arising after job loss) (*reactive*), while others arose spontaneously from within (*endogenous*).
- **Psychotic vs. neurotic** In present classifications these terms are used purely descriptively to describe two common types of symptoms that may occur in a variety of mental disorders. Previously, they were used to distinguish those disorders characterised by impairment of insight, abnormal beliefs, and abnormal perceptual experiences from those where there was preserved insight but abnormal affect.

- **Congruent vs. incongruent** This is an observation made regarding the apparent 'appropriateness' of a patient's affect towards their symptoms or their symptoms to their mood. A patient with apparent cheerfulness despite persecutory beliefs is described as having '*incongruent* affect'; a patient with profoundly depressed mood developing a delusion that they were mortally ill is described as possessing a '*mood-congruent* delusion'.
- **Structural vs. functional** A distinction formerly made between those brain disorders with observable structural abnormalities on post-mortem (e.g. Alzheimer's disease) and those without (e.g. schizophrenia). This usage has diminished since the discovery of definite observable brain changes in those disorders formerly called '*functional psychoses*'. Nowadays, the term is more often used in neurology/ neuropsychiatry to distinguish syndromes which generally have abnormal investigation findings (e.g. multiple sclerosis) from those without (e.g. conversion paralysis).

Dictionary of psychiatric symptoms

Abnormal beliefs A category of disturbance which includes **delusions** and **overvalued ideas.**

Abnormal perceptions A category of disturbance which includes **sensory distortions** and **false perceptions.**

Acute confusional state See **delirium**.

Affect The emotional state prevailing in a patient at a particular moment and in response to a particular event or situation. Contrasted with **mood** which is the prevailing emotional state over a longer period of time.

Affect illusion See **illusion**.

Agitated depression A combination of depressed **mood** and **psychomotor agitation**, contrasting with the more usual association of depressed mood with **psychomotor retardation.** A common presentation of depressive illness in the elderly.

Agitation See **psychomotor agitation.**

Agoraphobia A generalized **phobia** in which there is fear of open spaces, social situations, crowds, etc. Associated with **avoidance** of these stimuli.

Akathisia A subjective sense of uncomfortable desire to move, relieved by repeated movement of the affected part (usually the legs). A side-effect of treatment with neuroleptic drugs.

Alexithymia The inability to describe one's subjective emotional experiences verbally. May be a personality characteristic but is also associated with **somatisation.**

Alogia Poverty of thoughts as observed by absence of spontaneous speech. A **negative symptom** of schizophrenia and a symptom of depressive illness.

Ambitendency A **motor symptom of schizophrenia** in which there is an alternating mixture of **automatic obedience** and **negativism.**

Amnesia Loss of the ability to recall memories for a period of time. May be **global** (complete memory loss for the time period), or **partial** (patchy memory loss with 'islands' of preserved memory).

Anergia The subjective feeling of lack of energy and sense of increased effort required to carry out tasks. Associated with depressive illness.

Anhedonia The feeling of absent or significantly diminished enjoyment of previously pleasurable activities. A core symptom of depressive illness, also a **negative symptom** of schizophrenia.

Anorexia Loss of appetite for food. Seen in depressive illness and many general medical conditions. Interestingly, patients with anorexia nervosa often do not have anorexia as so defined. They commonly describe themselves as very hungry—controlling their desire for food by supreme effort in order to control their weight.

Anterograde amnesia The period of **amnesia** between an event (e.g. head injury) and the resumption of continuous memory. The length of anterograde amnesia is correlated with the extent of brain injury.

Anxiety A normal and adaptive response to stress and danger which is pathological if prolonged, severe or out of keeping with the real threat of the external situation. Anxiety has two components: psychic anxiety, which is an affect, characterised by increased arousal, apprehension, sense of vulnerability, and **dysphoria**; and somatic anxiety, in which there are bodily sensations of palpitations, sweating, dyspnoea, pallor, and abdominal discomfort.

Aphonia Loss of the ability to vocalise. May occur with structural disease affecting the vocal cords directly, the 9th cranial nerve, or higher centres. May also occur in functional illness where the underlying vocal cord function is normal. This can be demonstrated by asking the patient to cough—a normal cough demonstrates the ability of the vocal cords to oppose normally.

Asyndesis Synonym for **loosening of associations.**

Ataxia Loss of coordination of voluntary movement. Seen in drug and alcohol intoxication and organic disorders, particularly cerebellar.

Athetosis Sinuous, writhing involuntary movements.

Aura Episode of disturbed sensation occurring before an epileptic event. Wide range of manifestations although usually stereotyped for each individual.

Autochthonous delusion A primary **delusion** which appears to arise fully formed in the patient's mind without explanation (e.g. a patient suddenly becomes aware that he has inherited a large estate in the Scottish Highlands and will thus have the funds to settle score with all those who have ever wronged him).

Automatic obedience A **motor symptom of schizophrenia** in which the patient obeys the examiner's instructions unquestioningly. This cooperation may be 'excessive', with the patient going beyond what is asked (e.g. raising both arms and both legs when asked to raise an arm).

Automatism Behaviour which is apparently conscious in nature which occurs in the absence of full consciousness (e.g. during a temporal lobe seizure).

Autoscopy The experience of seeing a visual **hallucination** or **pseudohallucination** of oneself. Also known as 'phantom mirror image'. Uncommon symptom reported in schizophrenia and in temporal lobe epilepsy.

Avoidance The action of not exposing oneself to situations which generate anxiety (e.g. a patient with **agoraphobia** remaining at home or a patient with PTSD following an RTA refusing to drive). Can be understood in terms of an operant conditioning model where actions with reward—in this case reduction of anxiety—are repeated.

Belle indifference A surprising lack of concern for, or denial of, apparently severe functional disability. It is part of classical descriptions of hysteria and continues to be associated with operational descriptions of conversion disorder. It is also seen in medical illnesses (e.g. CVA) and is a rare and non-specific symptom of no diagnostic value.

Biological features of depression Symptoms of moderate to severe depressive illness which reflect disturbance of core vegetative function. They are **depressive sleep disturbance, anorexia, loss of libido, anergia,** and subjective impression of deteri~ ation in memory and concentration.

Blunting of affect Loss of the normal degree of emotional sensitivity and sense of the appropriate emotional response to events. A **negative symptom** of schizophrenia.

Broca's dysphasia A type of **expressive dysphasia** due to damage to the posterior part of the inferior frontal gyrus of the dominant hemisphere (Broca's language area).

Bulimia Increased appetite and desire for food and/or excessive, impulsive eating of large quantities of usually high-calorie food. Core symptom of bulimia nervosa and may also be seen in mania and in some types of learning disability.

Capgras syndrome A type of **delusional misidentification** in which the patient believes that a person known to them has been replaced by a 'double' who is to all external appearances identical, but is not the 'real person'.

Catalepsy A rare **motor symptom of schizophrenia**. Describes a situation in which the patient's limbs can be passively moved to any posture which will then be held for a prolonged period of time. Also known as **waxy flexibility** or **flexibilitas cerea.** See also **psychological pillow.**

Cataplexy Symptom of narcolepsy in which there is sudden loss of muscle tone leading to collapse. Usually occurs following emotional stress.

Catastrophic reaction Response occasionally seen in patients with **dementia** who are asked to perform tasks beyond their, now impaired, performance level. There is sudden agitation, anger, and occasionally violence.

Catatonia Increased resting muscle tone which is not present on active or passive movement (in contrast to the rigidity associated with Parkinson's disease and **extra-pyramidal side-effects**). A **motor symptom of schizophrenia.**

Chorea Sudden and involuntary movement of several muscle groups with the resultant action appearing like part of a voluntary movement.

Circumstantial thinking A disorder of the form of thought where irrelevant details and digressions overwhelm the direction of the thought process. This abnormality may be reflected in the resultant speech. It is seen in mania and in anankastic personality disorder.

Clang association An abnormality of speech where the connection between words is their sound rather than their meaning. May occur during manic **flight of ideas.**

Clouding of consciousness Conscious level between full consciousness and coma. Covers a range of increasingly severe loss of function with drowsiness and impairment of concentration and perception.

Command hallucination An auditory hallucination of a commanding voice, instructing the patient towards a particular action. Also known as **teleological hallucination**.

Completion illusion See **illusion.**

Compulsion A behaviour or action which is recognised by the patient as unnecessary and purposeless but which he cannot resist performing repeatedly (e.g. hand washing). The drive to perform the action is recognised by the patient as his own (i.e. there is no sense of 'possession' or passivity) but it is associated with a subjective sense of need to perform the act, often in order to avoid the occurrence of an adverse event. The patient may resist carrying out the action for a time at the expense of mounting **anxiety.**

Concrete thinking The loss of the ability to understand abstract concepts and metaphorical ideas leading to a strictly literal form of speech and inability to comprehend allusive language. Seen in schizophrenia and in dementing illnesses.

Confabulation The process of describing plausibly false memories for a period for which the patient has **amnesia**. Occurs in Korsakoff psychosis, dementia, and following alcoholic **palimpsest.**

Confusion The core symptom of delirium or acute confusional state. There is **disorientation, clouding of consciousness** and deterioration in the ability to think rationally, lay down new memories, and to understand sensory input.

Conversion The development of features suggestive of physical illness but which are attributed to psychiatric illness or emotional disturbance rather than organic pathology. Originally described in terms of psychoanalytic theory where the presumed mechanism was the 'conversion' of unconscious distress to physical symptoms rather than allowing its expression in conscious thought.

Coprolalia A 'forced' vocalisation of obscene words or phrases. The symptom is largely involuntary but can be resisted for a time, at the expense of mounting **anxiety.** Seen in Gilles de la Tourette Syndrome.

Cotard syndrome A presentation of psychotic depressive illness seen particularly in elderly people. There is a combination of severely depressed mood with **nihilistic delusions** and/or **hypochondriacal delusions**. The patient may state that he is already dead and should be buried, that his insides have stopped working and are rotting away, or that he has stopped existing altogether.

Couvade syndrome A **conversion** symptom seen in partners of expectant mothers during their pregnancy. The symptoms vary but mimic pregnancy symptoms and so include nausea, vomiting, abdominal pain, and food cravings. It is not delusional in nature; the affected individual does not believe they are pregnant (c.f. **pseudocyesis**). This behaviour is a cultural norm in some societies.

Craving A subjective sense of need to consume a particular substance (e.g. drugs or alcohol) for which there may be **dependence**.

Cyclothymia A personality characteristic in which there is cyclical mood variation to a lesser degree than in bipolar disorder.

De Clérambault syndrome A form of **delusion of love.** The patient, usually female, believes that another, higher-status individual is in love with them. There may be an additional **persecutory delusional** component where the affected individual comes to believe that individuals are conspiring to keep them apart. The object may be an employer or doctor, or in some cases a prominent public figure or celebrity.

Déjà vu A sense that events being experienced for the first time have been experienced before. An everyday experience but also a non-specific symptom of a number of disorders including temporal lobe epilepsy, schizophrenia, and anxiety disorders.

Delirium A clinical syndrome of **confusion**, variable degree of **clouding of consciousness**, visual **illusions**, and/or visual **hallucinations**, **lability of affect**, and **disorientation**. The clinical features can vary markedly in severity hour by hour. Delirium is a stereotyped response by the brain to a variety of insults and is similar in presentation whatever the primary cause.

Delirium tremens The clinical picture of acute confusional state secondary to alcohol withdrawal. Comprises **confusion, withdrawals, visual hallucinations**, and, occasionally, **persecutory delusions** and **Lilliputian hallucinations.**

Delusion An abnormal belief which is held with absolute subjective certainty, which requires no external proof, which may be held in the face of contradictory evidence, and which has personal significance and importance to the individual concerned. Excluded are those beliefs which can be understood as part of the subject's cultural or religious background. While the content is usually demonstrably false and bizarre in nature, this is not invariably so.

Primary delusions are the direct result of psychopathology, while **secondary delusions** can be understood as having arisen in response to other primary psychiatric conditions (e.g. a patient with severely depressed mood developing delusions of poverty or a patient with progressive memory impairment developing a delusion that people are entering his house and stealing or moving items). Primary delusions can be subdivided by the method by which they are perceived as having arisen or into broad classes based on their content.

If the patient is asked to recall the point when they became aware of the delusion and its significance to them, they may report that the belief arose: 'out of the blue' (*autochthonous delusion*); on seeing a normal percept (*delusional perception*); on recalling a memory (*delusional memory*); or on a background of anticipation, odd experiences, and increased awareness (*delusional mood*).

Based on their content, 12 types of primary delusion are commonly recognised: persecutory delusions, grandiose delusions, delusions of control, delusions of thought interference, delusions of reference, delusions of guilt, delusional misidentification, hypochondriacal delusions, delusional jealousy, delusions of love, nihilistic delusions, and delusions of infestation.

Delusional atmosphere Synonym for **delusional mood.**

Delusional elaboration Secondary delusions which arise in a manner which is understandable as the patient attempting to find explanations for primary psychopathological processes (e.g. a patient with persistent auditory hallucinations developing a belief that a transmitter has been placed in his ear).

Delusional jealousy A delusional belief that one's partner is being unfaithful. This can occur as part of a wider psychotic illness, secondary to organic brain damage (e.g. following the 'punch drunk syndrome' in boxers), associated with alcohol dependence, or as a monosymptomatic delusional disorder (**'Othello syndrome'**). Whatever the primary cause, there is a strong association with violence, usually towards the supposedly unfaithful partner. For this type of delusion the content is not bizarre or inconceivable and the central belief may even be true.

Delusional memory A primary **delusion** which is recalled as arising as a result of a memory (e.g. a patient who remembers his parents taking him to hospital for an operation as a child becoming convinced that he had been implanted with control and monitoring devices which have become active in his adult life).

Delusional misidentification A delusional belief that certain individuals are not who they externally appear to be. The delusion may be that familiar people have been replaced with outwardly identical strangers (**Capgras syndrome**) or that strangers are 'really' familiar people (**Frégoli syndrome**). A rare symptom of schizophrenia or of other psychotic illnesses.

Delusional mood A primary **delusion** which is recalled as arising following a period when there is an abnormal mood state characterised by anticipatory anxiety, a sense of 'something about to happen', and an increased sense of the significance of minor events. The development of the formed delusion may come as a relief to the patient in this situation.

Delusional perception A primary **delusion** which is recalled as having arisen as a result of a perception (e.g. a patient who, on seeing two white cars pull up in front of his house became convinced that he was therefore about to be wrongly accused of being a paedophile). The percept is a real external object, not a hallucinatory experience.

Delusions of control A group of delusions which are also known as **passivity phenomena** or delusions of bodily passivity. They are considered **first-rank symptoms** of schizophrenia. The core feature is the delusional belief that one is no longer in sole control of one's own body. The individual delusions are that one is being forced by some external agent to feel emotions, to desire to do things, to perform actions, or to experience bodily sensations. Respectively these delusions are called: **passivity of affect, passivity of impulse, passivity of volition, and somatic passivity.**

Delusions of guilt A delusional belief that one has committed a crime or other reprehensible act. A feature of psychotic depressive illness (e.g. an elderly woman with severe depressive illness who becomes convinced that her child, who died by cot death many years before, was in fact murdered by her).

Delusions of infestation A delusional belief that one's skin is infested with multiple, tiny mite-like animals. As a monosymptomatic delusional disorder this is called **Ekbom syndrome**. It is also seen in acute confusional states (particularly secondary to drug or alcohol withdrawal), in schizophrenia, in dementing illnesses, and as **delusional elaboration** of tactile hallucinatory experiences.

Delusions of love A delusion where the patient believes another individual is in love with them and that they are destined to be together. A rare symptom of schizophrenia and other psychotic illnesses, one particular sub-type of this delusion is **de Clérambault syndrome**.

Delusions of reference A delusional belief that external events or situations have been arranged in such a way as to have particular significance for, or to convey a message to the affected individual. The patient may believe that television news items are referring to him or that parts of the bible are about him directly.

Delusions of thought interference A group of delusions which are considered **first-rank symptoms** of schizophrenia. They are **thought insertion**, **thought withdrawal**, and **thought broadcasting**.

Dementia Chronic brain failure—in contrast with delirium (which is acute brain failure). In dementia, there is progressive and global loss of brain function. It is usually irreversible. Different dementing illnesses will show different patterns and rate of functional loss but, in general, there is impairment of memory, loss of higher cognitive function, perceptual abnormalities, **dyspraxia**, and disintegration of the personality.

Dependence The inability to control intake of a substance to which one is addicted. The dependence syndrome (p. 502) is characterised by primacy of drug-seeking behaviour, inability to control intake of the substance once consumption has started, use of the substance to avoid **withdrawals**, increased tolerance to the intoxicating effects of the substance, and re-instigation of the pattern of use after a period of abstinence. Dependence has two components: **psychological dependence**, which is the subjective feeling of loss of control, cravings, and preoccupation with obtaining the substance; and **physiological dependence**, which is the physical consequences of withdrawal and is specific to each drug. For some drugs (e.g. alcohol) both psychological and physiological dependence occur; for others (e.g. LSD) there are no marked features of physiological dependence.

Depersonalisation An unpleasant subjective experience where the patient feels as if they have become 'unreal'. A non-specific symptom occurring in many psychiatric disorders as well as in normal people.

Depressed mood The core feature of depressive illness. Milder forms of depressed mood are part of the human experience, but in its pathological form it is a subjective experience. Patients describe variously: an unremitting and pervasive unhappiness; a loss of the ability to experience the normal range of positive emotions ('feeling of a lack of feeling'); a sense of hopelessness and negative thoughts about themselves, their situation, and the future; somatic sensations of 'a weight' pressing down on head and body; and a sort of 'psychic pain' or wound.

Depressive sleep disturbance Characteristic pattern of sleep disturbance seen in depressive illness. It includes **initial insomnia** and **early morning waking**. In addition, sleep is described as more shallow, broken, and less refreshing. There is increased REM latency, where the patient enters REM sleep more rapidly than normal and REM sleep is concentrated in the beginning rather than the end of the sleep period.

Derailment A symptom of **schizophrenic thought disorder** in which there is a total break in the chain of association between the meaning of thoughts. The connection between the two sequential ideas is apparent neither to the patient nor to the examiner.

Derealisation An unpleasant subjective experience where the patient feels as if the world has become unreal. Like **depersonalisation** it is a non-specific symptom of a number of disorders.

Diogenes syndrome Hoarding of objects, usually of no practical use, and the neglect of one's home or environment. May be a behavioural manifestation of an organic disorder, schizophrenia, depressive disorder, or obsessive-compulsive disorder; or reflect a reaction late in life to stress in a certain type of personality.

Disinhibition Loss of the normal sense of which behaviours are appropriate in the current social setting. Symptom of manic illnesses and occurs in the later stages of dementing illnesses and during intoxication with drugs or alcohol.

Disorientation Loss of the ability to recall and accurately update information as to current time, place, and personal identity. Occurs in delirium and dementia. With increasing severity of illness, orientation for time is lost first, then orientation for place, with orientation for person usually preserved until dysfunction becomes very severe.

Dissociation The separation of unpleasant emotions and memories from consciousness awareness with subsequent disruption to the normal integrated function of consciousness and memory. **Conversion** and **dissociation** are related concepts. In **conversion** the emotional abnormality produces physical symptoms; while in **dissociation** there is impairment of mental functioning (e.g. in **dissociative fugue** and **dissociative amnesia**).

Distractibility Inability to maintain attention or the loss of vigilance on minimal distracting stimulation.

Diurnal variation A variation in the severity of a symptom depending on the time of day (e.g. depressed mood experienced as most severe in the morning and improving later in the day).

Double depression A combination of **dysthymia** and depressive illness.

Dysarthria Impairment in the ability to properly articulate speech. Caused by lesions in brain stem, cranial nerves, or pharynx. Distinguished from **dysphasia** in that there is no impairment of comprehension, writing, or higher language function.

Dyskinesia The impairment of voluntary motor activity by superimposed involuntary motor activity.

Dyslexia Inability to read at the level normal for one's age or intelligence level.

Dysmorphophobia A type of **over-valued idea** where the patient believes one aspect of his body is abnormal or conspicuously deformed.

Dysphasia Impairment in producing or understanding speech (**expressive dysphasia** and **receptive dysphasia** respectively) related to cortical abnormality, in contrast with **dysarthria** where the abnormality is in the organs of speech production.

Dysphoria An emotional state experienced as unpleasant. Secondary to a number of symptoms (e.g. **depressed mood, withdrawals**).

Dyspraxia Inability to carry out complex motor tasks (e.g. dressing, eating) although the component motor movements are preserved.

Dysthymia Chronic, mildly depressed mood and diminished enjoyment, not severe enough to be considered depressive illness.

Early morning waking (EMW) Feature of **depressive sleep disturbance**. The patient wakes in the very early morning and is unable to return to sleep.

Echo de la pensée Synonym for **thought echo.**

Echolalia The repetition of phrases or sentences spoken by the examiner. Occurs in schizophrenia and mental retardation.

Echopraxia Motor symptom of schizophrenia in which the patient mirrors the doctor's body movements. This continues after being told to stop.

Eidetic imagery Particular type of exceptionally vivid visual memory. Not a **hallucination**. More common in children than adults, c.f. **flashbacks**.

Ekbom syndrome A monosymptomatic delusional disorder where the core delusion is a **delusion of infestation.**

Elation Severe and prolonged **elevation of mood.** A feature of manic illnesses.

Elemental hallucination A type of hallucination where the false perceptions are of very simple form (e.g. flashes of light or clicks and bangs). Associated with organic illness.

Elevation of mood The core feature of manic illnesses. The mood is preternaturally cheerful, the patient may describe feeling 'high', and there is subjectively increased speed and ease of thinking.

Entgleisen Synonym for **derailment.**

Entgleiten Synonym for **thought blocking** or **snapping off.**

Erotomania Synonym for **delusions of love.**

Euphoria Sustained and unwarranted cheerfulness. Associated with manic states and organic impairment.

Euthymia A 'normal' mood state, neither depressed nor manic.

Expressive dysphasia Dysphasia affecting the production of speech. There is impairment of word-finding, sentence construction, and articulation. Speech is slow and 'telegraphic', with substitutions, 'null' words, and **perseveration.** The patient characteristically exhibits considerable frustration at his deficits. Writing is similarly affected. Basic comprehension is largely intact and emotional utterances and rote learned material may also be surprisingly preserved.

Extracampine hallucination A hallucination where the percept appears to come from beyond the area usually covered by the senses (e.g. a patient in Edinburgh 'hearing' voices seeming to come from a house in Glasgow).

Extra-pyramidal side-effects (EPSE) Side-effects of rigidity, tremor, and dyskinesia caused by the anti-dopaminergic effects of psychotropic drugs, particularly neuroleptics. Unlike in idiopathic Parkinson's disease, bradykinesia is not prominent.

Ey syndrome Synonym for **Othello syndrome.**

False perceptions Internal perceptions which do not have a corresponding object in the external or 'real' world. Includes **hallucinations** and **pseudo-hallucinations.**

Faseln Synonym for **muddling.**

First-rank symptoms (of schizophrenia) A group of symptoms originally described by Schneider which are useful in the diagnosis of schizophrenia. They are neither pathognomic for, nor specific, to schizophrenia and are also seen in organic and affective psychoses. There are 11 symptoms in 4 categories:

Auditory hallucinations
- 'Voices heard arguing'
- Thought echo
- 'Running commentary'

Delusions of thought interference
- Thought insertion
- Thought withdrawal
- Thought broadcasting

Delusions of control
- Passivity of affect
- Passivity of impulse
- Passivity of volitions
- Somatic passivity

Delusional perception

- A primary delusion of any content that is reported by the patient as having arisen following the experience of a normal perception.

Flashbacks Exceptionally vivid and affect-laden re-experiencing of remembered experiences. Flashbacks of the initial traumatic event occur in PTSD and flashbacks to abnormal perceptual experiences initially experienced during LSD intoxication can occur many years after the event.

Flattening of affect Diminution of the normal range of emotional experience. A **negative symptom** of schizophrenia.

Flexibilitas cerea Synonym for **catalepsy**.

Flight of ideas Subjective experience of one's thoughts being more rapid than normal with each thought having a greater range of consequent thoughts than normal. Meaningful connections between thoughts are maintained.

Folie à deux Describes a situation where two people with a close relationship share a delusional belief. This arises as a result of a psychotic illness in one individual with development of a delusional belief, which comes to be shared by the second. The delusion resolves in the second person on separation, the first should be assessed and treated in the usual way.

Formal thought disorder A term which is confusingly used for three different groups of psychiatric symptoms:
- To refer to all pathological disturbances in the form of thought.
- As a synonym for **schizophrenic thought disorder.**
- To mean the group of **first-rank symptoms** which are delusions regarding thought interference, (i.e. **thought insertion**, **thought withdrawal**, and **thought broadcasting).**

The first of these uses is to be preferred.

Formication A form of tactile **hallucination** in which there is the sensation of numerous insects crawling over the surface of the body. Occurs in alcohol or drug withdrawal, particularly from cocaine.

Free-floating anxiety Anxiety occurring without any identifiable external stimulus or threat (cf. **phobia**).

Frégoli syndrome A type of **delusional misidentification** in which the patient believes that strangers have been replaced with familiar people.

Functional hallucination A hallucination experienced only when experiencing a normal percept in that modality (e.g. hearing voices when the noise of an air conditioner is heard).

Fugue A **dissociative** reaction to unbearable stress. Following a severe external stressor (e.g. marital break-up) the affected individual develops global **amnesia** and may wander to a distant location. Consciousness is unimpaired. Following resolution there is amnesia for the events which occurred during the fugue.

Fusion A symptom of **schizophrenic thought disorder** in which two or more unrelated concepts are brought together to form one compound idea.

Ganser symptom The production of 'approximate answers'. Here the patient gives repeated wrong answers to questions which are nonetheless 'in the right ballpark' (e.g. 'what is the capital of Scotland?'—'Paris'). Occasionally associated with organic brain illness it is much more commonly seen as a form of **malingering** in those attempting to feign mental illness (e.g. in prisoners awaiting trial).

Gedankenlautwerden Synonym for **thought echo**.

Globus hystericus The sensation of a 'lump in the throat' occurring without oesophageal structural abnormality or motility problems. A symptom of anxiety and somatisation disorders.

Glossolalia 'Speaking in tongues'. Production of non-speech sounds as a substitute for speech. Seen in dissociative and neurotic disorders and accepted as a sub-cultural phenomenon in some religious groups.

Grandiose delusion A delusional belief that one has special powers, is unusually rich or powerful, or that one has an exceptional destiny (e.g. a man who requested admission to hospital because he had become convinced that God had granted him 'the greatest possible sort of mind' and that coming into contact with him would cure others of mental illnesses). Occurs in all psychotic illnesses but particularly in manic illnesses.

Grandiosity An exaggerated sense of one's own importance or abilities. Seen in manic illnesses.

Hallucination An internal percept without a corresponding external object. The subjective experience of hallucination is that of experiencing a normal percept in that modality of sensation. A true hallucination will be perceived as in external space, distinct from imagined images, outside conscious control, and as possessing relative permanence. A **pseudo-hallucination** will lack one or all of these characteristics.

Hallucinations are sub-divided according to their modality of sensation and may be auditory, visual, gustatory, tactile, olfactory, or kinaesthetic. Auditory hallucinations, particularly of voices, are characteristic of schizophrenic illness, while visual hallucinations are characteristic of organic states.

Hemiballismus Involuntary, large-scale, 'throwing' movements of one limb or one body side.

Hypersomnia Excessive sleepiness with increased length of nocturnal sleep and daytime napping. Occurs as core feature of narcolepsy and in atypical depressive states.

Hypnagogic hallucination A transient false perception experienced while on the verge of falling asleep (e.g. hearing a voice calling one's name which them startles you back to wakefulness to find no-one there). The same phenomenon experienced when waking up is called **hypnopompic hallucination.** Frequently experienced by healthy people and so not a symptom of mental illness.

Hypnopompic hallucination See **hypnagogic hallucination**.

Hypochondriacal delusions A delusional belief that one has a serious physical illness (e.g. cancer, AIDS). Most common in psychotic depressive illnesses.

Hypochondriasis The belief that one has a particular illness despite evidence to the contrary. Its form may be that of a primary **delusion**, an **overvalued idea**, a **rumination**, or a **mood congruent** feature of depressive illness.

Hypomania Describes a mild degree of mania where there is elevated mood but no significant impairment of the patient's day-to-day functioning.

Illusion A type of false perception in which the perception of a real world object is combined with internal imagery to produce a false internal percept. Three types are recognised: **affect, completion,** and **pareidolic illusions.** In **affect illusion** there is a combination of heightened emotion and misperception (e.g. whilst walking across a lonely park at night, briefly seeing a tree moving in the wind as an attacker). **Completion illusions** rely on our brain's tendency to 'fill-in' presumed missing parts of an object to produce a meaningful percept and are the basis for many types of optical illusion. Both these types of illusions resolve on closer attention. **Pareidolic illusions** are meaningful percepts produced when experiencing a poorly defined stimulus, (e.g. seeing faces in a fire or clouds).

Imperative hallucination A form of **command hallucination** in which the hallucinatory instruction is experienced as irresistible, a combination of **command hallucination**, and **passivity of action**.

Impotence Loss of the ability to consummate sexual relationships. Refers to inability to achieve penile erection in men and lack of genital preparedness in women. It may have a primary medical cause, be related to psychological factors, or can be a side-effect of many psychotropic medications.

Incongruity of affect Refers to the objective impression that the displayed affect is not consistent with the current thoughts or actions, (e.g. laughing while discussing traumatic experiences). Occurs in schizophrenia.

Initial insomnia Difficulty getting off to sleep. Seen as a symptom of primary insomnia as well as in **depressive sleep disturbance.**

Insightlessness See **lack of insight.**

Irritability Diminution in the stressor required to provoke anger or verbal or physical violence. Seen in manic illnesses, organic cognitive impairment, psychotic illnesses, and drug and alcohol intoxication. Can also be a feature of normal personality types and of personality disorder.

Jamais vu The sensation that events or situations are unfamiliar, although they have been experienced before. An everyday experience but also a non-specific symptom of a number of disorders including temporal lobe epilepsy, schizophrenia, and anxiety disorders.

Knight's move thinking Synonym for **derailment**.

Lability of mood Marked variability in the prevailing affect.

Lack of insight Loss of the ability to recognise that one's abnormal experiences are symptoms of psychiatric illness and that they require treatment.

Lilliputian hallucination A type of visual **hallucination** in which the subject sees miniature people or animals. Associated with organic states, particularly delirium tremens.

Logoclonia Symptom of Parkinson's disease where the patient gets 'stuck' on a particular word of a sentence and repeats it.

Logorrhoea Excess speech or 'verbal diarrhoea'. Symptom of mania.

Loosening of associations A symptom of **formal thought disorder** in which there is a lack of meaningful connection between sequential ideas.

Loss of libido Loss of the desire for sexual activity. Common in depressive illness and should be inquired about directly as it is usually not mentioned spontaneously. Should be distinguished from **impotence**.

Magical thinking A belief that certain actions and outcomes are connected although there is no rational basis for establishing a connection (e.g. 'if you step on a crack, your mother will break her back'). Magical thinking is common in normal children and is the basis for most superstitions. A similar type of thinking is seen in psychotic patients.

Malingering Deliberately falsifying the symptoms of illness for a secondary gain (e.g. for compensation, to avoid military service, or to obtain an opiate prescription).

Mania A form of mood disorder initially characterised by **elevated mood**, **insomnia**, loss of appetite, increased libido, and **grandiosity**. More severe forms develop **elation** and **grandiose delusions.**

Mannerism Abnormal and occasionally bizarre performance of a voluntary, goal-directed activity (e.g. a conspicuously dramatic manner of walking. Imagine John Cleese's 'the minister of funny walks').

Mental retardation Diminished intelligence below the second standard deviation (IQ<70). Increasing severity of retardation is associated with decreased ability to learn, to solve problems, and to understand abstract concepts. Subdivided as: mild: 50–69; moderate 35–50; severe 20–49; profound 0–19.

Micrographia Small 'spidery' handwriting seen in patients with Parkinson's disease; a consequence of being unable to control fine movements. This is most easily recognised by comparing their current signature with one from a number of years previously.

Middle insomnia Wakefulness and inability to return to sleep occurring in the middle part of the night.

Mirror sign Lack of recognition of one's own mirror reflection with the perception that the reflection is another individual who is mimicking your actions. Seen in dementia.

Mitgehen An extreme form of **mitmachen** where the patient's limbs can be moved to any position by very slight or fingertip pressure ('anglepoise lamp sign').

Mitmachen A **motor symptom of schizophrenia** where the patient's limbs can be moved without resistance to any position (c.f. **mitgehen**). The limbs return to their resting state once the examiner lets go, in contrast with **catalepsy,** where the limbs remain in their set positions for prolonged periods.

Mood The subjective emotional state over a period of time, in contrast to **affect** which describes the emotional response to a particular situation or event.

Mood congruent A secondary symptom which is understandable in the light of an abnormal mood state (e.g. a severely depressed patient developing a **delusion** that they are in severe debt, or a manic patient developing a **delusion** that they are exceptionally wealthy).

Morbid jealousy Synonym for **delusional jealousy**.

Motor symptoms of schizophrenia Schizophrenic illness is associated with a variety of soft neurological signs and motor abnormalities. In the modern era many motor abnormalities will be attributed to the side-effects of neuroleptic drugs, but all were described in schizophrenic patients prior to the introduction of these drugs in 1952.

Recognised motor symptoms in schizophrenia include: **catatonia, catalepsy, automatic obedience, negativism, ambitendency, mitgehen, mitmachen, mannerism, stereotypy, echopraxia,** and **psychological pillow.**

Muddling A feature of **schizophrenic thought disorder** caused by simultaneous **derailment** and **fusion**. The speech so produced may be very bizarre.

Multiple personality The finding of two or more distinct 'personalities' in one individual. These personalities may answer to different names, exhibit markedly different behaviours, and describe amnesia for periods when other personalities were active. This symptom is most probably an iatrogenic condition produced during exploratory psychotherapy in suggestible individuals.

Mutism Absence of speech without impairment of consciousness.

Negative symptoms (of schizophrenia) The symptoms of schizophrenia which reflect impairment of normal function. They are: lack of volition, lack of drive, apathy, **anhedonia, flattening of affect blunting of affect**, and **alogia**. Believed to be related to cortical cell loss.

Negativism A **motor symptom of schizophrenia** where the patient resists carrying out the examiners' instructions and his attempts to move or direct the limbs.

Neologism A made-up word or normal word used in an idiosyncratic way. Neologisms are found in schizophrenic speech.

Nihilistic delusions A delusional belief that the patient has died or no longer exists or that the world has ended or is no longer real. Nothing matters any longer and continued effort is pointless. A feature of psychotic depressive illness.

Nystagmus Involuntary oscillating eye movements.

Obsession An idea, image, or impulse which is recognised by the patient as their own, but which is experienced as repetitive, intrusive, and distressing. The return of the obsession can be resisted for a time at the expense of mounting **anxiety**. In some situations the anxiety accompanying the obsessional thoughts can be relieved by associated **compulsions**, (e.g. a patient with an obsession that his wife may have come to harm feeling compelled to phone her constantly during the day to check she is still alive).

Othello syndrome A monosymptomatic delusional disorder where the core delusion has the content of **delusional jealousy.**

Overvalued ideas A form of **abnormal belief.** These are ideas which are reasonable and understandable in themselves but which come to unreasonably dominate the patient's life.

Palimpsest Episode of discrete amnesia related to alcohol or drug intoxication. The individual has no recall for a period when, although intoxicated, he appeared to be functioning normally. This is also commonly known as 'blackout', but the term palimpsest is preferable as it avoids confusion with episodes of loss of consciousness.

Panic attack Paroxysmal, severe **anxiety.** May occur in response to a particular stimulus or occur without apparent stimulus.

Paranoid delusion Strictly speaking this describes self-referential delusions (i.e. **grandiose delusions** and **persecutory delusions**). It is however more commonly used as a synonym for **persecutory delusion.**

Paraphasia The substitution of a non-verbal sound in place of a word. Occurs in organic lesions affecting speech.

Passivity phenomena Synonym for **delusions of control**.

Persecutory delusion A delusional belief that one's life is being interfered with in a harmful way.

Perseveration Continuing with a verbal response or action which was initially appropriate after it ceases to be apposite (e.g. 'Do you know where you are?'—'in the hospital'; 'do you know what day it is?'—'in the hospital'. Associated with organic brain disease and is occasionally seen in schizophrenia).

Phobia A particular stimulus, event, or situation which arouses **anxiety** in an individual and is therefore associated with **avoidance**. The concept of 'biological preparedness' is that some fears (e.g. of snakes, fire, heights) had evolutionary advantage and so it is easier to develop phobias for these stimuli than other, more evolutionarily recent threats (e.g. of guns or electric shock).

Phantom mirror image Synonym for **autoscopy.**

Pica The eating of things which are not food or of food items in abnormal quantities.

Positive symptoms (of schizophrenia) The symptoms of schizophrenia which are qualitatively different from normal experience (i.e. **delusions, hallucinations, schizophrenic thought disorder**). Believed to be related to neuro-chemical abnormalities.

Posturing The maintenance of bizarre and uncomfortable limb and body positions. Associated with psychotic illnesses and may have **delusional** significance to the patient.

Pressure of speech The speech pattern consequent upon **pressure of thought.** The speech is rapid, difficult to interrupt, and, with increasing severity of illness, the connection between sequential ideas may become increasingly hard to follow. Occurs in manic illness.

Pressure of thought The subjective experience of one's thoughts occurring rapidly, each thought being associated with a wider range of consequent ideas than normal and with inability to remain on one idea for any length of time. Occurs in manic illness.

Priapism A sustained and painful penile erection, not associated with sexual arousal. A rare side-effect of antidepressant medication. If not relieved can cause permanent penile damage.

Pseudocyesis A false pregnancy. May be hysterical or delusional in nature and can occur in both sexes although more commonly in women. The belief in the false pregnancy may be accompanied by abdominal distension, lumbar lordosis, and amenorrhoea.

Pseudo-hallucination A **false perception** which is perceived as occurring as part of one's internal experience, not as part of the external world. They may be described as having an 'as if' quality or as being seen with the 'mind's eye'. Additionally, hallucinations experienced as true hallucinations during the active phase of a patient's illness may become perceived as pseudo-hallucinations as they recover. They can occur in all modalities of sensation and are described in psychotic, organic, and drug-induced conditions as well as occasionally in normal individuals. (The hallucinations of deceased spouses commonly described by widows and widowers may have the form of a pseudo-hallucination.)

Pseudologica fantastica The production of convincing false accounts, often with apparent sincere conviction. There may be a grandiose or over-exaggerated flavour to the accounts produced. A feature of Munchausen's disease.

Psychic anxiety See **anxiety**.

Psychogenic polydipsia Excessive fluid intake without organic cause.

Psychological dependence See **dependence**.

Psychological pillow A **motor symptom of schizophrenia**. The patient holds their head several inches above the bed while lying and can maintain this uncomfortable position for prolonged periods of time.

Psychomotor agitation A combination of **psychic anxiety** and excess and purposeless motor activity. A symptom common to many mental illnesses and found in normal individuals in response to stress.

Psychomotor retardation Decreased spontaneous movement and slowness in instigating and completing voluntary movement. Usually associated with subjective sense of actions being more of an effort and with subjective retardation of thought. Occurs in moderate to severe depressive illness.

Physiological dependence See **dependence**.

Receptive dysphasia **Dysphasia** affecting the understanding of speech. There is impairment in understanding spoken commands and repeating back speech. There are also significant abnormalities in spontaneous speech with word substitutions, defects in grammar, and syntax and **neologisms**. The abnormal speech so produced is however fluent (cf. **expressive dysphasia**) and the patient may be unconcerned by his deficits.

Reflex hallucination The experience of a real stimulus in one sensory modality triggering a hallucination in another.

Retrograde amnesia The period of **amnesia** between an event (e.g. head injury) and the last continuous memory before the event.

Rumination A **compulsion** to engage in repetitive and pointless consideration of phrases or ideas, usually of a pseudo-philosophical nature. May be resisted for a period with consequent mounting **anxiety.**

'Running commentary' A type of third-person auditory **hallucination** which is a **first-rank symptom** of schizophrenia. The patient hears one or more voices providing a narrative of their current actions, 'he's getting up... now he's going towards the window'.

Russell sign Skin abrasions, small lacerations, and calluses on the dorsum of the hand overlying the metacarpophalangeal and interphalangeal joints found in patients with symptoms of bulimia. Caused by repeated contact between the incisors and the skin of the hand which occurs during self-induced vomiting.

Schizophasia Synonym for **word salad.**

Schizophrenic speech disorder This includes the abnormalities in the form of speech consequent upon **schizophrenic thought disorder**, and those abnormalities in the use of language characteristic of schizophrenia such as use of **neologisms** and **stock words/phrases.**

Schizophrenic thought disorder A group of abnormalities in the subjective description of the form of thought which occur in schizophrenia. They include: **loosening of associations**, **derailment**, **thought blocking**, **fusion**, and **muddling.**

Sensory distortions Changes in the perceived intensity or quality of a real external stimulus. Associated with organic conditions and with drug ingestion or withdrawals. Examples include: hyperacusis (hearing sounds as abnormally loud), micropsia ('wrong end of the telescope effect', perceiving objects which are close as small and far away).

Snapping off Synonym for **thought blocking**.

Somatic anxiety See **anxiety**.

Somatisation The experience of bodily symptoms with no, or no sufficient, physical cause for them, with presumed psychological causation.

Splitting of perception Loss of the ability to simultaneously process complimentary information in two modalities of sensation (e.g. sound and pictures on television). Rare symptom of schizophrenia.

Stereotypy A repetitive and bizarre movement which is not goal directed (in contrast to **mannerism**). The action may have delusional significance to the patient. Seen in schizophrenia.

Stock phrases/stock words Feature of **schizophrenic speech disorder**. The use of particular words and phrases more frequently than in normal speech and with a wider variety of meanings than normal.

Stupor Absence of movement and **mutism** where there is no impairment of consciousness. Functional stupor occurs in a variety of psychiatric illnesses. Organic stupor is caused by lesions in the midbrain (the 'locked-in' syndrome).

Synaesthesia A stimulus in one sensory modality is perceived in a fashion characteristic of an experience in another sensory modality (e.g. 'tasting' sounds or 'hearing' colours). Occurs in hallucinogenic drug intoxication and in epileptic states.

Tangentiality Producing answers which are only very indirectly related to the question asked by the examiner.

Tardive dyskinesia A movement disorder associated with long-term treatment with neuroleptic drugs (although it was described in psychotic patients before the use of these drugs in clinical practice). There is continuous involuntary movement of the tongue and lower face. More severe cases involve the upper face and have choreoathetoid movements of the limbs.

Teleological hallucination Synonym for **command hallucination**.

Terminal insomnia Synonym for **early morning waking**.

Third-person auditory hallucinations Auditory hallucinations characteristic of schizophrenia where voices are heard referring to the patient as 'he' or 'she', rather than 'you'. The **first-rank symptoms** of **'voices heard arguing'** and **'running commentary'** are of this type.

Thought blocking A symptom of **schizophrenic thought disorder**. The patient experiences a sudden break in the chain of thought. It may be explained as due to **thought withdrawal.** In the absence of such **delusional elaboration** it is not a **first-rank symptom**.

Thought broadcasting The delusional belief that one's thoughts are accessible directly to others. A **first-rank symptom** of schizophrenia.

Thought disorder See **formal thought disorder**.

Thought echo The experience of an auditory **hallucination** in which the content is the individual's current thoughts. A **first-rank symptom** of schizophrenia. Also known as **gedankenlautwerden** or **echo de la pensée**.

Thought insertion The delusional belief that thoughts are being placed in the patient's head from outside. A **first-rank symptom** of schizophrenia.

Tic Sudden twitches of a single muscle or muscle group.

Trichotillomania The **compulsion** to pull one's hair out.

Verbigeration Repetition of words or phrase while unable to articulate the 'next' word in the sentence. Seen in **expressive dysphasia.**

Verschmelzung Synonym for **fusion.**

'Voices heard arguing' A type of auditory **hallucination** which is a **first-rank symptom** of schizophrenia. The patient hears two or more voices debating with one another, sometimes about a matter over which the patient is agonising (e.g. 'he should take the medication, it's worked before', 'no, not again, he'll not take it this time').

Vorbeigehen Synonym for **Ganser symptom.**

Vorbeireden Synonym for **Ganser symptom.**

Waxy flexibility Synonym for **catalepsy.**

Wernicke's dysphasia A type of **receptive dysphasia** due to cortical lesions in or near the posterior portion of the left first temporal convolution (superior temporal gyrus)—known as the Wernicke area.

Withdrawals The physical sequelae of abstinence from a drug to which one is **dependent**. These are individual to the drug concerned (e.g. sweating, tachycardia, and tremor for alcohol; dilated pupils, piloerection, abdominal pain, and diarrhoea for opiates).

Word salad The most severe degree of **schizophrenic thought disorder** in which no connection of any kind is understandable between sequential words and phrases the patient uses. Also called **schizophasia**.

Evidence-based psychiatry

What is evidence-based medicine (EBM)?

EBM is the integration of the best research evidence with clinical expertise and patient values.

• Best research evidence means the study most likely to yield an accurate and unbiased answer to a question we have about a particular patient or patient group

• Clinical experience means the skills we have learned during our medical training (e.g. history taking, bedside examination) and also our ability to elicit our patients' preferences and goals

In order to practice EBM we need to first appreciate that we don't always know all the answers to our clinical questions. Once that fact[1] has been appreciated, the following five skills need to be mastered:

1. To be able to ask a clinical question in a way that captures the essence of the 'problem', is structured, and is most likely to yield an answer.
2. To be able to search for an answer ('the evidence') to our question in a way that is most efficient.
3. To be able to critically appraise the evidence.
4. To apply the evidence to the patient.
5. To monitor our own progress.

1 Lawrie S (2000) Evidence-based psychiatry—do psychiatrists want it and can they do it? *Health Bulletin (Edinb)* **58**, 25–33.

Asking clinical questions

There are generally two types of question we ask about patients: those that we ask them (fact-finding questions) and questions about diagnosis, cause (or harm), treatment, and prognosis ('clinical questions'). Consider the following patient scenario:

A 29-year-old woman is admitted to your ward 6 weeks post-partum complaining of hearing voices commenting on her actions and thoughts that her baby is evil. She has never sought help for psychiatric reasons before, although her mother has long-standing bipolar disorder and has had many admissions to your hospital previously. She does not wish to be admitted to hospital.

Examples of fact-finding questions include:
• Does she have any wish to harm her baby?
• Is there anyone at home who could support her?
• Does she have any symptoms of affective disorder?
• Is there a history of drug misuse?

Examples of clinical questions include:
• **Diagnosis**: what is the likelihood that the diagnosis will be schizophrenia given she describes a first-rank symptom of schizophrenia (running commentary)?
• **Cause/harm**: does a family history of bipolar disorder increase the risk of post-partum psychosis in a relative?
• **Treatment**: is it likely that this woman would benefit rapidly from the administration of ECT?
• **Prognosis**: what are the chances that the woman will harm her baby?

The ability to tactfully ask fact-finding questions is something taught to us as medical undergraduates and postgraduates. There is no underlying structure to these questions and searching the literature will not provide an answer.

Structuring good clinical questions Clinical questions, however, follow a standard format which is likely to clarify the question in your own mind, suggest a suitable study type to address the problem, and more likely to yield an answer when you search for one. The general form of a question is as follow (pico format):

P: the patient problem to be addressed. A description of the main characteristics of the patient problem.

I: the intervention or manoeuvre being considered (e.g. the treatment or diagnostic test being contemplated). May also be a harmful exposure (e.g. 10 years of schizophrenia for prognosis, smoking).

C: the comparison intervention (e.g. treatments) are usually compared to placebo or standard therapy; diagnostic tests are usually compared to a 'gold standard' such as post-mortem, although the 'gold standard' test in psychiatry is usually a structured clinical history and examination (e.g. the Structured Clinical Interview for DSM-IV)

O: the outcome of interest (e.g. improvement in symptoms, accurate diagnosis, side-effects).

Examples of questions in the PICO format

	P	I	C	O
Diagnosis	In post-partum mothers with psychosis	Do first-rank symptoms	Compared to full clinical examination and follow-up	Suggest a diagnosis of schizophrenia
Cause/harm	In post-partum mothers	Does a family history of bipolar disorder	Compared to no family history of mental illness	Raise the probability of post partum psychosis
Treatment	In post-partum mothers with psychosis	Does ECT	Compared to antipsychotic drug treatment	Rapidly improve psychotic symptoms
Prognosis	In post-partum mothers with psychosis	After 1 year		What is the chance that the baby will be harmed

Note:
• Prognosis questions often have only three parts to their structure, unless two prognostic factors are being compared.
• It is likely that many of the above questions will be asked by your patient or will occur to you in the course of decision-making (e.g. when contemplating detention under the Mental Health Act, the prognosis is likely to influence your decision).

Searching for the evidence

By formulating a structured clinical question, the nature of an underlying question should now be apparent. The next step is to decide upon the study type best able to answer the question. Taking the example of a therapy question, the study types most likely to answer a question in such a way that minimises bias are ranked as follows:

Hierarchy of evidence (therapy)

- A systematic review of two or more randomised controlled trials (RCTs)
- A single randomised controlled trial
- A quasi-experimental study without randomisation
- Observational studies (e.g. cohort and case control studies)
- Case reports and series
- Expert opinion

Wherever possible, a systematic review of RCTs should be sought because it is less liable to bias than the other studies further down the hierarchy. Many people, when asked 'where would you look for a study to answer your question', will often suggest 'a textbook' or 'Medline'. However, textbooks are likely to be out of date (especially for therapy) and most doctors have not been trained to use Medline to its greatest effect.

Searching Medline (*www.PubMed.org*) Medline can be searched by referring to the PICO structure, and by thinking about the hierarchy of evidence. For example, if we wish to ask our question 'in women with post-partum psychosis, does ECT lead to rapid improvement in symptoms when compared to antipsychotic drug treatment', we might conduct the following search:

1: Post-partum psychosis
2: ECT
3: 1 AND 2
4: random$ (this line will identify most RCTs in any subject)
5: 3 AND 4

Medline is organised by subject headings, but we do not need to know the subject heading to search. Medline will automatically look up a thesaurus and use more effective terms than the ones we specify.

A note on PubMed clinical queries The PubMed website has a feature called 'clinical queries' which searches for articles of a specific design. For example, if you search for 'schizophrenia' AND 'cognitive behaviour therapy' in the clinical queries section of PubMed, you could specify that you are only interested in systematic reviews.

Limitations of Medline Unfortunately, Medline covers only a proportion (<30%) of the psychiatric literature. Embase and PsychINFO cover a greater proportion, but are often not available to health professionals because of their cost. However, many health boards in Scotland and England do have access to both Embase and PsychINFO through Athens (*www.athens.ac.uk*). You should contact your local library for details. Further training on Medline is available on the PubMed website.

Other resources

Fortunately, although Medline is a useful source of research evidence, there are several other resources which can be more efficient:

- **The Cochrane Library** Consists of several sections including the database of systematic reviews and the register of controlled trials. The database of systematic reviews is probably the single most useful source of systematic reviews on the topic of *therapy*, although does not consider other areas of medical practice such as diagnosis, prognosis, etc. The database of controlled trials is also probably the single most useful source of individual RCTs and is easy to use. The Cochrane Library is available free to all doctors in the UK via:
  - The National Electronic Library for Health (*www.nelh.nhs.uk*) in England and Wales.
  - The e-Library (*www.elib.scot.nhs.uk*) in Scotland.
  - Doctors.net (*www.doctors.net.uk*) for all UK doctors.
- **Clinical Evidence** Directory of evidence on the effects of common clinical interventions. It provides a concise account of the current state of knowledge, ignorance, and uncertainty about the prevention and treatment of a wide range of clinical conditions based on thorough searches of the literature. It does not make recommendations but summarises the best available evidence, and where there is no good evidence, it says so. It can be accessed free through *www.nelh.nhs.uk* by all UK doctors.
- **The National Electronic Library for Health and Mental Health** (NELMH) Contains information on all aspects of clinical management in a few given areas. At the time of going to press, the website provided information on schizophrenia, depression, and suicide. More topics are planned in future. The site may be accessed via a web portal at *www.nelmh.org*. The NELMH is part of a larger project called the National Electronic Library for Health (*www.nelh.nhs.uk*).
- **PsychINFO** The American Psychological Association publishes an online database of abstracts of relevance to psychiatry and psychology. Many journals not indexed on either Medline or Embase can be found here. PsychINFO is not provided free of charge in the UK but a subset of PsychINFO called ClinPsych is available free through the *www.doctors.net.uk* website.
- **Evidence Based Mental Health Journal** Provides critically appraised articles meeting pre-specified quality criteria along with a clinical commentary attempting to place them in a meaningful clinical context. The journal is available in print and online (with subscription) though the *BMJ* web site, although many institutions do not purchase online access currently (*http://ebmh.bmjjournals.com/*).
- **Other resources** There are many other web sites that provide either biomedical databases or pre-appraised evidence of relevance to practising clinicians. The tendency for these links to become inactive has prevented us from printing a list of them here, although an up-to-date list is kept on the Centre for Evidence-Based Mental Health website at *www.cebmh.com*.

Critical appraisal

Critical appraisal can help us decide if a paper is likely to be valid (i.e. the results are likely to be true) or important (i.e. contain results important for clinical practice). The decision to use the published evidence also takes into account our patients' preferences and goals. When embarking on the critical appraisal of an article, many people consider this as an invitation to 'trash' the article as vigorously as possible. This approach does little to inform our management of patients and should be replaced with a more considered judgement of validity:

- Is the study performed so badly that it can be of no use whatsoever?
- Is the study flawed and what effects are the flaw(s) likely to have upon the published results?

The critical appraisal of an article addresses two main areas: **validity** and **importance**, irrespective of the study type. However, the questions we should ask ourselves in order to address these two areas depend on the study type.

Questions to assess the validity of a systematic review (p. 112)

- Does the review address a clearly focused question?
- Does the review apply suitable quality criteria?
- Does the review search for all relevant articles?
- Are the results consistent from study to study?

Questions to assess the validity of a RCT (pp. 114–15)

- Were patients randomised to two or more treatments and was the allocation of patients to treatments concealed?
- Were patients and investigators blind to the intervention received?
- Were patients treated equally apart from the intervention of interest?
- Was follow-up sufficiently long and complete?
- Were drop-outs accounted for and included in the final results?

Questions to assess the validity of a harm/aetiology study (see Case-control studies pp. 116–17)

- Was the exposure measured objectively?
- Was the outcome measured objectively and blind to exposure status?
- Was follow-up sufficiently long and complete?
- Did the investigators take into account any potential confounders?

Questions to assess the validity of a diagnostic study (p. 120)

- Were the study patients similar to those on whom the test would be used in clinical practice?
- Were the test and 'gold standard' applied blind to the results of the other?
- Was the test applied irrespective of the results of the gold standard (and vice versa)?

Questions to assess the validity of a prognosis study (see Cohort studies p. 118)

• Was a representative group of patients assembled at a common, preferably early, point in their illness?
• Were patients followed up prospectively for a sufficiently long period?
• Was the outcome assessed objectively?
• Did the investigators correct for the presence of confounding?

Systematic reviews (SRs) of RCTs[1]

Formulation of questions and protocol Questions should be precise. The research designs, characteristics of participants/interventions, and outcomes should be pre-specified. Research designs (e.g. RCT with inadequate concealment) likely to yield biased results should be excluded, or at least noted and the effects examined in detail.

Search for relevant articles Search should be comprehensive and repeatable. Should include more than Medline, as it is more likely to catalogue English language, positive studies whilst ignoring foreign language, negative studies. Consider grey literature (e.g. abstracts, personal communications, and others) and unpublished articles.

Review of abstracts and retrieval of full text Potentially relevant abstracts should be reviewed by 2+reviewers with a mechanism for resolving disagreements. The same applies to retrieved articles. Proformas and pre-specified criteria are likely to improve reliability and repeatability.

Summary of included/excluded studies Reasons for exclusion and inclusion should be given to allow scrutiny/repeatability.

Meta-analysis (statistical summary) Study results should be combined statistically, weighted for precision.

- **Heterogeneity**: results vary from study to study more than expected by chance alone.
- **Fixed effects analysis**: assumes a single treatment effect, which is estimated by each study in an unbiased manner.
- **Random effects analysis**: doesn't assume single effect. Produces an average effect across all studies taking heterogeneity into account in the estimate of treatment effect and its confidence interval.
- **Publication bias**: the tendency for certain studies to be published according to their results. Usually, more positive results are more likely to be published. Measured using a funnel plot (see opposite).
- **Common statistical tests**: χ^2 test for heterogeneity; Q test for heterogeneity; Z test for overall effect.
- **Effect size measurements**: *dichotomous data* (relative, absolute risks, odds ratios—odds ratios/relative risks preferred because of statistical properties. *Continuous data*: Mean difference—for several studies using the same scales; *Standardised effect size* (mean difference/pooled standard deviation)—for several studies using different scales—rescales the results using standard deviation of each scale allowing them to be combined (e.g. 'Cohen's d' and others).

1 Egger M, Davey Smith G, Altman DG (eds.) (2001) *Systematic Reviews in Healthcare: Meta-analysis in Context.* BMJ Books.

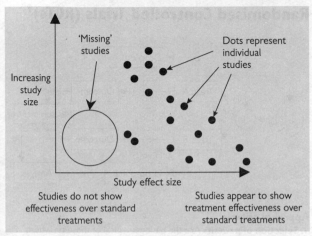

Funnel plot showing how small negative studies appear 'missing'

Randomised Controlled Trials (RCTs)[1]

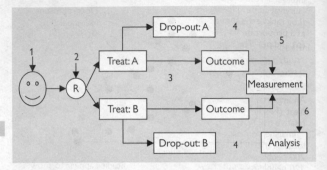

Appraisal criteria

1. **Selection of patients** Are the patients typical of those on whom the drug/therapy will be used in practice? (generalisability/external validity). Do they differ from the average patient in clinical practice such that we would expect (a) the results to not apply at all or (b) there be a smaller/greater effect in clinical practice.

2. **Randomisation** Was the randomisation method adequate? Computer generated randomisation by a third party on a geographically separated site at the point of entry into the trial is probably 'best'. Would it be possible for patients/clinicians to guess, better than chance, the treatment to which they would eventually be allocated (allocation concealment) Has randomisation succeeded in forming two groups with similar baseline characteristics? Methods of ensuring this are: *minimisation* (allocate patients to minimise differences) and *stratification* (stratify randomisation by important prognostic/treatment factor).

3. **Performance of interventions** Were patients/clinicians/investigators/ statisticians 'blind' to the treatment. N.B. There is no universally accepted meaning of blind; authors should explain what they mean.

4. **Drop-out** Was the number of drop-outs in both arms of the trial unequal (differential attrition) or greater than 10–20%? If so, even if the analysis takes this into account, the trial may be biased either to/against the true effect size.

5. **Measurement** Were all patients analysed in the groups to which they were randomised? (Intention to treat analysis). If not, ignoring drop-outs (completer only analysis) may overestimate effects of treatment.

Methods of intention to treat include:
- Last observation carried forward (assume no change in a score).
- Worst/case scenario (assume drop-outs in active arm have negative outcomes and drop-outs in control arm have positive ones).
- Mean imputation (assume drop-out was average for his group).
- Multiple imputations (model mean and variance taking into account characteristics of the drop-out)

6. Analysis (see below) If results are presented as means, typically mean differences are shown, with a t-test or ANOVA and 95% confidence interval. If results are 'time to an event', then a Kaplan Maier curve (survival curve) may be shown with the results of a survival analysis (Log rank test, Cox proportional hazards). Often the results are shown as a proportion of people with a good or bad even in both groups (p1 and p2). The NNT is given by 1/(p1−p2)—see below.

Relative risk, absolute risk, and the number needed to treat

An important value to calculate from RCTs is the number needed to treat (NNT). The NNT arose because of limitations with the terms relative risk (RR) and absolute risk reduction (ARR).

Imagine you have an intervention for schizophrenia 'Nopixol'. You locate a trial in Medline, which finds the following results:
200 people with schizophrenia were randomised to placebo or Nopixol. 120 people received Nopixol, of which 30 relapsed at 6 weeks; 80 were randomised to placebo, of which 60 relapsed over the same time. A '2x2' table helps to clarify the numbers:

	Relapse	No relapse	
Nopixol	30	90	120
Placebo	60	20	80

- The risk or probability of relapse in the Nopixol group is 30/120 or 0.25. This is called the experimental event rate (**EER**).
- The risk or probability of relapse in the placebo group is 60/80 or 0.75. This is called the control event rate (**CER**).
- The relative risk (**RR**) is the EER/CER = 0.25/0.75, which is 0.33. This means the risk of relapse on Nopixol is 0.33 times the risk on placebo. Another way of saying this would be to say that the relative risk of relapse is reduced by 67% on Nopixol. This is sometimes called the relative risk reduction (**RRR**). This is usually not a good measure of clinical usefulness since if relapse was 100x less common in both groups, the RR and RRR would stay the same. This would not reflect the fact that clinically the treatment effect had diminished considerably.
- The absolute risk reduction (**ARR**) is the CER−EER = 0.75−0.25, which is 0.5. This means that for every person treated with Nopixol, the risk of relapse is reduced by about 50%.
- If the risk for each person is reduced by 50% by Nopixol instead of placebo, then it's intuitive that we need to treat two people to prevent, on average, one relapse. This is called the NNT. More generally, the **NNT** is equal to 1/ARR, or 1/0.5. In this case the **NNT = 2**

1 Pocock SJ (1983) *Clinical Trials: A Practical Approach.* John Wiley and Sons Ltd

Case-control studies

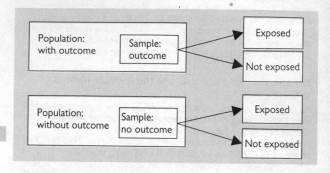

Appraisal criteria

- **Exposure** Case control studies are an alternative to cohort studies when the outcome is rare.
- **Cases** The sample cases (those with the outcome) should 'ideally' be a random sample of all cases from the population. Investigators should say how the sample was selected. You should decide what effect this will have on the sorts of cases included in the study.
- **Controls** The sample controls (those without the outcome) should ideally be a random sample of all controls from the population and be as similar to the cases as possible (except for the exposure of interest). In practice this is difficult.
- **Selection of cases and controls** Ideally should also be independent of exposure. For example, the selection of depressed people from psychiatric hospital and controls from a community newsletter to assess whether child sex abuse is associated with depression may introduce bias since people with childhood sexual abuse are possibly more likely to be admitted to hospital in general.
- **Assessment of exposure** Measurement should be conducted objectively and blind to outcome status. In practice this is often difficult to accomplish since raters may be affected by their expectations and those with the outcome may be more likely to recall an exposure in a 'search for meaning' (recall bias).
- **Confounding** Where the controls and cases differ in important respects (apart from the exposure of interest), correction for this may be made in the statistical analysis. Correction should be made only when differences exist in a characteristic which is associated with the exposure and outcome (e.g. age may confound an association between intravenous drug use and depression).

- **Analysis** It is not possible to calculate absolute and relative risks from a case control study directly since the proportion of people developing the outcome in exposed/non-exposed populations has not been assessed. Odds ratios are often used and may be given, along with a 95% confidence interval. A chi-square test will usually be used. If the investigators have examined to see if increasing levels of exposure are more strongly associated with the outcome, a chi-squared test (for linear trend) or Mantel-Haenszel test may be reported.

Cohort studies

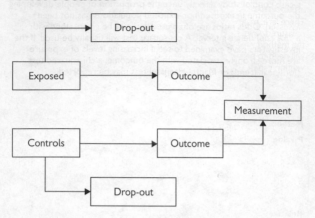

Appraisal criteria

- **Exposure** The exposure should be clearly defined and may be stratified into levels of increasing 'dose'. The controls should not be exposed but be similar to the exposed group. Bias will be introduced if controls differ in many ways apart from the exposure (e.g. drug users differ from non-drug users in many respects: employment, criminal record-etc.)
- **Drop-out** Drop-outs are virtually inevitable. The effects may bias the results, especially if drop-outs >20% or unequal. Some studies minimise attrition by consulting several sources, sending reminders, consulting government statistics (e.g. records of hospital admissions), and other methods of tracking people.
- **Measurement** Should be conducted objectively and blind to exposure status. In practice this is sometimes difficult.
- **Retrospective/prospective** Exposure may be ascertained from case notes (retrospectively) or at interview (prospectively). Cohort studies often have retrospective and prospective components.
- **Analysis** $P_{a,b}$—proportion in group a or b who have the outcome, then: $P_a - P_b$ = absolute risk, p_a/p_b = relative risk, NNH = 1/absolute risk. If results are 'time to an event', then a survival analysis may be conducted. Correction for confounding is usually accomplished using ANCOVA, linear regression (outcomes measured on a scale), or logistic regression (where the outcome is an event).

Comparing ways of measuring the importance of an intervention

There are many ways in which the benefit of an intervention can be measured. Cynically, one might expect the authors of an article to present the method which shows their intervention in the best light, so the reader will need to be aware of the main methods by which the utility of an intervention can be measured and their consequent strengths and limitations.

Treatment benefit

Method	Explanation	Advantages	Disadvantages
P-value	Gives the probability that the observed difference between the treatments is due to chance.	Provides a clear test of an investigator's hypothesis and is provided with all major statistical packages.	Clinically insignificant treatments may still be statistically significant. Gives little indication of precision.
Relative risk	Gives the risk of an event in one group divided by the risk in the other group.	Provides a clear indication of how many times better or worse a treatment is compared to another.	May mislead when outcomes are rare. (e.g. a relative risk of 10 would be unimpressive if the event occurred only once in 10000 patients).
Absolute risk	Gives the risk of an event in one group minus the risk in the other group.	Provides a clearer indication of clinical significance. Takes appropriate account of baseline risk.	The figure in itself may not seem very meaningful either to clinicians or patients.
Number needed to treat (NNT)	States the number of patients required to be treated with the experimental intervention in order to prevent one additional adverse outcome.	Relatively intuitive. Provides a clear indication of how much therapeutic effort is required to bring about one additional 'good' outcome.	In spite of obvious advantages, has not come into universal use. NNTs published in meta-analyses may be misleading unless the patients included in the primary studies are very like your own.

N.B. Confidence intervals are a welcome addition to any published figure about treatment benefit since they convey information about precision and statistical significance.

Diagnostic studies

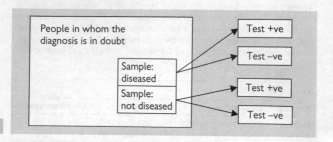

Appraisal criteria
- **Sample** Did the sample consist of people in whom the diagnosis was in doubt and in whom the test would be used in practice?
- **Gold standard** Was a suitable gold standard applied regardless of the test results?
- **Test** Was the test applied blindly without knowledge of the results of the gold standard and vice versa?
- **Reliability** Could the diagnostic test be applied reliably over time or between raters?
- **Diagnostic test performance**
  - What are the sensitivity and specificity? They are portable properties, but less clinically useful than the positive and negative predictive values (PPV and NPV).
  - What are the PPV and NPV? These are useful when you have a test result and you want to know its meaning.
- **Other considerations** Is the test affordable, accurate, and feasible in our setting? What is our patients post-test probability for a PPV?
  - Post-test odds = Likelihood ratio × Pre-test odds
  - And, likelihood ratio (LR) is:

$$LR = \frac{\text{Probability of the test result in someone with the disease}}{\text{Probability of the test result in someone without the diseases}}$$

Ways of measuring diagnostic utility

Method	Explanation	Advantages	Disadvantages
Sensitivity	Measures the proportion of people with a disorder correctly classified by a test. When sensitivity is very high, a negative test will tend to rule out the disorder (SnNOut).	Easily calculated and intuitive. Usually supplied in published papers. Does not depend on prevalence.	Not very useful in clinical practice unless very high.
Specificity	Measures the proportion of people *without* a disorder correctly classified by a test. When specificity is very high, a positive test will tend to *rule in* the disorder (SpPIn).	Easily calculated and intuitive. Usually supplied in published papers. Does not depend on prevalence.	Not very useful in clinical practice unless very high.
Positive predictive value	Measures the proportion of people with a positive test result who actually have the disorder.	Clinically useful. Easy to understand and communicate to colleagues and patients.	Tend to fall as the prevalence of the disorder falls. May mislead if the prevalence of the disorder in your practice is lower than that of the study.
Likelihood ratio for a positive test	A ratio of the probability of a positive test coming from someone with the disorder compared to one without the disorder.	Does not depend on the prevalence. Can be adapted to a variety of other situations.	More difficult to calculate than the above. May not seen intuitively very meaningful

Calculating useful values:

		Target disorder	
Diagnostic test		Present	Absent
	Positive	a	b
	Negative	c	d

Sensitivity = a/(a + c)   Positive predictive value (PPV) = a/(a + c)

Specificity = d/(b + d)   Negative predictive value (NPV) = d/(c + d)

Likelihood ratio for a positive test = Sensitivity/(1 − Specificity)

Likelihood ratio for a negative test = (1 − Sensitivity)/Specificity

N.B.*Further details on how to calculate these values are provided in several texts[1] and on a number of websites[2]*

1 Lawrie SM, McIntosh AM, Rao S (2000) *Critical Appraisal for Psychiatry.* Churchill Livingstone.

2 www.cebm.net

Qualitative studies

Purpose

Qualitative studies are usually used to measure beliefs or attitudes in situations where quantitative research would be less meaningful or impractical. Results are usually presented as text without numbers or figures in a way which is intended to preserve the richness of the data in its rightful context. For example, 'What are the attitudes of patients with borderline PD to their diagnosis?' might be answered better by describing what the patients actually said than by performing a survey and summarising attitudes on a scale with medians and inter-quartile ranges.

Appraisal criteria

- **Clear question** Like all studies, the research should address a clear topic or question. Unlike quantitative research, hypotheses may emerge in the course of the study and be tested out.
- **Patient selection** Unlike quantitative research which should address a representative sample, qualitative researchers often 'purposively sample' patients in order to obtain 'typical' or exemplar cases.
- **Information gathering** The gathering and analysis of information is not standardised. Therefore, the study should describe exactly how this was performed.
- **Material engagement** Did investigators make intense contact with their subject material? Did they check reactions? Did investigators seek non-confirming data?
- **Iteration** Did investigators cyclically develop hypotheses and then test them with their sample?
- **Grounding** Were there systematic ways of linking observations with interpretations?
- **Disclosure of investigators' prejudice** Did investigators examine their own attitudes/beliefs/values/preconceptions as they embarked on the study?
- **Coherence** Are the results coherent? Was the interpretation internally consistent?
- **Testimonial validity** Did the study subjects agree with the investigator's interpretations?
- **Reflexive validity** Did the observations change the investigator's understanding of theory?
- **Catalytic validity** Did the investigator reorient, focus, and energise participants?
- **Triangulation** Was there an attempt to confirm the investigators using another method (e.g. by obtaining another sample or by observation of the same sample using a different method)?

Economic studies

Types of studies

- **Cost analysis** Costs only.
- **Effectiveness analysis** Consequences only.
- **Economic analyses** Costs and consequences of ≥2 interventions.

Types of analyses

- **Consequences equal** Cost minimisation analysis (find cheapest intervention).
- **Consequences unequal** Outcomes measured in same natural units (e.g. rating scales or admission/readmissions) = cost effectiveness analysis.

If consequences unequal, and benefits measured in different units (e.g. comparing CBT for schizophrenia with ECT for depression) then convert consequences:
1) to monetary units = cost-benefit analysis, or
2) to patient preferences = cost-utility analysis

Costs and perspective

Costs should be considered from a broad perspective. Interventions, which appear to be less expensive and equally effective at a hospital level, may shift costs to other areas (e.g. social work, criminal justice system), which were not apparent because of too narrow a perspective.
- **Direct costs** Salaries, drugs, buildings, etc.
- **Indirect costs** Usually gains/losses in productivity.
- **Intangible costs** e.g. cost of improved health.
- **Incremental cost** Cost of each additional unit of production.
- **Opportunity cost** Benefits forgone by using capital to provide one intervention over another (a concept of economic analyses rather than an actual cost).

Discounting

In order to take into account (1) the preference to pay for things later rather than sooner and (2) the devaluation in currency over time, future costs should be discounted so they appear at current prices. Occasionally economists argue that future *consequences* should also be discounted.

Consequences

The consequences of an intervention should be measured alongside the study used to measure costs (usually a clinical trial). The more rigorous the study design (SRs > RCTs > CTs) and the more valid, the more likely the results of the economic analysis are to be true.

Dominance

If one intervention is **more effective and cheaper** than an alternative, then choice is easy. In all other situations, consider the incremental cost-effectiveness ratio:

Incremental cost-effectiveness ratio (ICER) =

$$\frac{\text{Differences in costs}}{\text{Differences in consequences}}$$

For example, an intervention causing 2 extra remissions in schizophrenia at an extra cost of £100 000 has an ICER of £50 000 per additional remission. ICER gives a measure of the extra cost for **each additional unit of benefit**. There's no cut-off; the ICER should help compare different interventions and come to a decision. Non-parametric statistics are used to give p-values and 95% confidence intervals for the ICER (**randomisation tests, Monte-Carlo analyses**).

Sensitivity analysis

Economic analyses make assumptions about costs and consequences of different treatments. To test the robustness of an economic analysis, estimated benefits and costs can be varied one at a time or simultaneously to see if they alter the results of the analysis:

- **One-way** (one variable at a time).
- **Extreme case** (alter a variable to the extremes of its plausible range).
- **Multi-way** (vary 2 or more variables simultaneously).
- **Monte-Carlo analyses** are a way of varying several parameters simultaneously without assuming normality.

Applying the evidence to patients

Having found valid and important new evidence about a particular problem, a couple of further question need to be asked:

- What is the likely benefit for my patient?
- Does my patient actually want it?

Treatment

Chronic intractable conditions and mild and very benign conditions may fail to show the benefits of therapy demonstrated in clinical trials because the patient's baseline risk differs from those patients initially randomised.

In either situation, it is possible simply to 'guess' what the likely benefit for your patient will be, or one of several numerical methods may be used instead. The simplest numerical method involves an educated guess as to how likely your patient is to benefit compared to the average patient in the trial. If your patient is half as likely to benefit, then the NNT from the trial is doubled. Other techniques are available that are both more accurate and more time consuming[1].

Finally, the decision to start a new treatment depends on other things apart from efficacy. Firstly, and most importantly, your patient may actually not want it because of undue side-effects or perhaps the regime (e.g. thrice-daily dosing) may be excessively inconvenient for them.

As well as potential harms, the decision to adopt a treatment or service at a health service level may also take account of economic evaluations.

N.B. **Guard against drug company information!** Although drug representatives will extol the virtues of their medication over the competition, often on the basis of efficacy, little evidence exists to suggest, for example, that one antipsychotic is more effective than another[2]. Although doctors do not feel pharmaceutical representatives influence them, this is in contradiction to the best available evidence on the subject.

Diagnosis

Diagnostic tests shown to be effective in a research setting may be of little utility in your clinical practice for two main reasons. Firstly, the prevalence of the condition may be different in your setting. If the prevalence of the condition is lower in your setting, the PPV will be lower, although a negative result will actually be more likely to indicate an absence of the condition. Secondly, the test itself may be too costly in terms of the financial, staff, and training resources required to administer it.

Patients' values and expectations may also be very important in the context of a disease for which there is no effective intervention (e.g. Huntington's disease) or where the diagnostic test is itself harmful or unpleasant.

Objections to EBM

Case against EBM	Answer to criticism
It denigrates clinical experience.	EBM is the integration of the best available evidence with clinical expertise and patient values. Both are necessary for EBM.
It is 'cook book' medicine.	EBM takes into account our individual patient's likely risk/benefit, goals, and preferences.
It is a cost-cutting tool.	EBM has been used by governments and other organisations to cut costs/resources. In most cases this has nothing to do with the original meaning of EBM which can result in increased costs as well as efficiency savings
It is based on patients in clinical trials who are very unlike patients in practice.	This is true of published clinical research in general. This should prompt us to conduct pragmatic, large trials which mirror actual clinical practice more closely than ever[3].

Evidence-based mental health (EBMH) often attracts an additional criticism:
- Psychiatric patients are unique and their problems cannot be reduced into neat categories.

The truth is all people are unique and we must separate those characteristics patients share with other patients (i.e. diagnoses) from those which are common to all patients and those which are unique to an individual.

Medicine, and psychiatry, can learn nothing without imposing an organisation (e.g. diagnoses or dimensions). However, the practice of psychiatry must take into account individual preferences/goals as much as any other field of medicine.

1 Lawrie SM, McIntosh AM, Rao S (2000) *Critical Appraisal for Psychiatry*. Churchill Livingstone.

2 Geddes J, Freemantle N, Harrison P, Bebbington P (2000) Atypical antipsychotics in the treatment of schizophrenia: systematic overview and meta-regression analysis. *BMJ* **321**, 1371–6.

3 e.g. BALANCE *cebmh.warne.ox.ac.uk/balance/*

Measuring performance and implementing evidence-based practice

In the last few years there has been a proliferation in evidence-based guidelines[1] and attempts to audit our performance against those guidelines[2].

Guidelines

Guidelines can be thought of as a top-down approach to evidence-based practice. They are particularly useful where there is clear evidence that an intervention is effective in a given condition, but for some reason isn't being given. It can also be useful when there are wide national variations in practice, as is often the case in mental health (e.g. ECT, clozapine).

The process of guideline development is a bit like EBM in miniature. Relevant representatives from all groups (patients, doctors, nurses, pharmacists, etc.) ask key questions which will form the basis for a systematic review. A systematic review is then conducted and the articles are appraised by the guideline group. Articles are graded according to their rigour and members use their clinical judgement in assessing how directly relevant they are to clinical practice in the UK. The group then makes recommendations on the evidence, which are then put into a guideline. The adherence to the guideline is then assessed, usually by audit.

Unfortunately, although many good guidelines have been developed, many have not been implemented. This may be because the methodology of guideline development was faulty or, more likely, because the implementation was inadequate.

Strategies for guideline implementation include[3]:

- Educational outreach
- Advertisement
- Local opinion leaders
- Written and computerised reminders
- Reminders at the point of patient care

Audit

Audit is an attempt to measure actual clinical practice against a number of standards of good clinical care. Standards are sometimes drawn from guidelines, where the strength of evidence is overwhelming in a given area. Alternatively, standards of good medical practice are set based on common sense and good medical practice (e.g. we should discuss treatment with patients in a collaborative way).

There is some evidence that audit improves adherence to clinical guidelines and also improves individual patient outcomes. It is a cyclical process, with re-audit every few months/years when standards should be reviewed and changed if necessary.

1 e.g. NICE (www.nice.org) and SIGN (www.sign.ac.uk)

2 e.g. CHI (www.chi.nhs.uk) and CSBS (www.nhshealthquality.org/)

3 see www.york.ac.uk/inst/crd/ehc51.pdf for further details.

Chapter 5

Organic illness

Presentations of organic illness

All psychiatric illnesses are by their nature organic—that is, they involve abnormalities of normal brain structure or function. The term 'organic illness' in modern psychiatric classification, however, refers to those conditions with demonstrable aetiology in CNS pathology. Organic disorders related to substance misuse are dealt with in Chapter 13. This chapter deals with those disorders that are caused by traumatic, inflammatory, degenerative, infective, and metabolic conditions.

Many psychiatric syndromes can have an organic aetiology. For this reason, every patient who presents with psychiatric symptomatology requires a thorough physical examination (in most cases including neurological examination and special investigations) before a diagnosis of functional illness is made. While psychiatrists do not have to be expert neurologists, a sound knowledge of those conditions that bridge neurology and psychiatry is essential. Historically, these disciplines have not always been separated and, in this era of biological psychiatry, they are once again converging as increasing evidence emerges of brain dysfunction underlying most psychiatric disorders. Having said this, it is important to remember that biological, psychological, and social factors interact in a dynamic two-way process in the generation of psychiatric symptoms.

Below are listed common organic causes of psychiatric syndromes (delirium, dementia, and amnestic disorders are discussed later):

Organic causes of psychosis

- Neurological (epilepsy; head injury; brain tumour; dementia; encephalitis e.g. HSV, HIV; neurosyphilis; brain abscess; CVA)
- Endocrine (hyper/hypothyroidism; Cushing's; hyperparathyroidism; Addison's disease)
- Metabolic (uraemia; sodium imbalance; porphyria)
- SLE ('lupus psychosis')
- Medications (steroids; L-dopa; INH; anticholinergics; antihypertensives; anticonvulsants; Ritalin)
- Drugs of abuse (cocaine; LSD; cannabis; PCP; amphetamines; opioids)
- Toxins

Organic causes of depression

- Neurological (CVA; epilepsy; Parkinson's disease; brain tumour; dementia; MS; Huntington's disease; head injury)
- Infectious (HIV; EBV/infectious mononucleosis; brucellosis)
- Endocrine and metabolic (hypothyroidism; Cushing's; Addison's disease; parathyroid disease; vitamin deficiency [B_{12} and folate]; porphyria)
- Cardiac disease (MI; CCF)
- SLE
- Rheumatoid arthritis
- Cancer
- Medications (analgesics; antihypertensives; L-dopa; anticonvulsants; antibiotics; steroids; OCP; cytotoxics; cimetidine; salbutamol)
- Drugs of abuse (alcohol; benzodiazepines; cannabis; cocaine; opioids)
- Toxins

Organic causes of mania
- Neurological (CVA; epilepsy; brain tumour; head injury; MS)
- Endocrine (hyperthyroidism)
- Medications (steroids; antidepressants; mefloquine; INH; cytotoxics)
- Drugs of abuse (cannabis; cocaine; amphetamines)
- Toxins

Organic causes of anxiety
- Neurological (epilepsy; dementia; head injury; CVA; brain tumour; MS; Parkinson's disease)
- Pulmonary (COAD)
- Cardiac (arrhythmias; CCF; angina; mitral valve prolapse)
- Hyperthyroidism
- Medications (antidepressants; antihypertensives; flumazenil; yohimbine; fenfluramine)
- Drugs of abuse (alcohol; benzodiazepines; caffeine; cannabis; cocaine; LSD; ecstasy; amphetamines)

Dementia—general overview

Essence Dementia is a syndrome characterised by progressive, usually irreversible, global cognitive deficits. Often memory impairment is the first symptom with progression to other deficits including dysphasia, agnosia, apraxia, impaired executive function, and personality disintegration. For a diagnosis to be made there must be significant impairment of normal functioning and other possible diagnoses (see **Differential diagnosis** below), particularly delirium or depression, should be excluded.

Common causes Alzheimer's disease (55%); vascular dementia (20%); general medical condition + substance-induced persisting disorders (10%)

Reversible causes (15%): subdural haematoma; NPH; vit B$_{12}$ deficiency; metabolic causes; hypothyroidism

Aetiology

- **Parenchymal/degenerative** Alzheimer's disease; Pick's disease; Parkinson's disease; Huntington's disease; Wilson's disease; MS; MND; Lewy Body disease; progressive supranuclear palsy
- **Intracranial** Tumour; head trauma; subdural haematoma; CVA; normal pressure hydrocephalus (NPH)
- **Infection** Creutzfeldt-Jakob disease (prion disease); neurosyphilis; HIV-associated dementia; TB; SSPE; other
- **Endocrine** Hypothyroidism; hyperparathyroidism; Cushing's and Addison's disease
- **Metabolic** Uraemia; hepatic encephalopathy; hypoglycaemia; calcium imbalance; magnesium imbalance; electrolyte imbalance
- **Vitamin deficiency** B$_{12}$; folate; pellagra (niacin); thiamine
- **Toxins** Prolonged alcohol misuse; heavy metal poisoning

Clinical features (see 'Clinical syndromes' opposite)

- Memory impairment: starts with short-term and progresses to long-term.
- History of personality change, forgetfulness, social withdrawal, lability of affect, disinhibition, 'silliness', diminished self-care, apathy, fatigue, deteriorating executive functioning.
- Other specific cognitive deficits are seen in cortical dementias (see opposite).
- Hallucinations and delusions often paranoid (20–40%) and poorly systematized.
- Anxiety and/or depression in 50%.
- Neurological features (e.g. seizures, focal deficits, primitive reflexes, pseudobulbar palsy, long-tract signs).
- 'Catastrophic reaction', p. 84.
- 'Pathological emotion'—spontaneous lability.
- 'Sundowner syndrome'—as evening approaches confusion increases and falls become common.

Differential diagnosis Delirium; depression ('pseudodementia' p. 478); amnestic syndromes (pp. 148–9); LD; psychotic disorders; normal ageing (p. 472).

Investigations Include: FBC; LFT; U&E; glucose; ESR; TSH; calcium; magnesium; phosphate; VDRL; HIV; vit B_{12} and folate; blood culture; LP; EEG; CXR; ECG; CT ('optima and axial protocol'); MRI; SPECT.

Principles of management

- **Assessment:** diagnostic; functional; and social.
- **Cognitive enhancement:** acetylcholinesterase inhibitors (Tacrine; Donepezil; Rivastigmine); antioxidants (Selegiline, vit E); ? hormonal (oestrogen; HRT).
- **Treat psychosis/agitation:** antipsychotics (novel agents preferable).
- **Treat depression/ insomnia:** SSRIs; hypnotics.
- **Treat medical illness.**
- **Psychological support:** to both patient and care-givers.
- **Functional management:** maximise mobility; encourage independence with self-care, toilet, and feeding; assist with communication.
- **Social management:** accommodation; activities; financial matters; legal matters (power of attorney, wills, and curatorship).

Clinical syndromes of dementia

Dementias may be classified in terms of primary site of pathology. Since site of pathology in the brain correlates with neuropsychiatric symptomatology, this is a useful system of classification.

1. Cortical dementias involve primarily the cortex and are divided into:

- **Fronto-temporal** Pick's disease (20%) (pp. 142–3); NPH and MND (70%) (p. 150). Characterised by prominent 'personality change' which may manifest as a 'frontal lobe syndrome'. A common cause of early-onset dementia, it is often undiagnosed. Language impairments tend to involve reduction in content (semantic anomia). CT shows fronto-temporal atrophy and SPECT shows FT metabolism.
- **Posterior-parietal** Alzheimer's disease (pp. 134–9). Characterised by early memory loss and focal cognitive deficits. 'Personality changes' are later manifestations. Language impairments involve problems with word-finding (lexical anomia). CT ('optima protocol') shows thinning (<12mm) of the cortex of the medial temporal lobe.

2. Subcortical dementias Parkinson's disease (pp. 170–1); Huntington's disease (p. 172); Wilson's disease (p. 173); Binswanger encephalopathy (p. 144); PSNP (p. 169); HIV-associated dementia (p. 165); NPH (p. 150). *Clinical features:* gross psychomotor 'slowing'; depressed mood; movement disorders; mild amnesia; and personality changes.

3. Cortical-subcortical dementias e.g. Lewy Body dementia (pp. 140–1). *Clinical features:* cortical and subcortical symptoms.

4. Multifocal dementias e.g. CJD (p. 146). *Clinical features:* rapid onset and course; involves cerebellum and subcortical structures.

Alzheimer's disease (1)

Also termed '**dementia of the Alzheimer type**' (DAT)[1], this is the most common cause (70%) of dementia in older people. It is a degenerative disease of the brain with prominent cognitive and behavioural impairment that is sufficiently severe to interfere significantly with social and occupational function. It affects approximately 500 000 people in the UK and more than 30 million worldwide. A larger number of people have less severe impairments that usually evolve into the full disorder with time. The percentage of the total population aged over 65 is increasing in the developed world, meaning that the burden of DAT-related health care is likely to increase.

Epidemiology Risk of DAT increases with age: 1% at age 60 yrs; doubles every 5 years; 40% of those aged 85 yrs. ♀:♂ is about 1:4. Other risk factors include: Down's syndrome, previous head injury, or hypothyroidism; family history of Down's syndrome, Parkinson's disease, or DAT.

Possible protective factors Smoking; oestrogen (e.g. HRT); NSAIDs; vit E; higher level of pre-morbid education.

Pathophysiology

- Amyloid plaques—insoluble β-amyloid peptide deposits as senile plaques or 'β-pleated sheets' in the hippocampus, amygdala, and cerebral cortex. Increased density with advanced disease.
- Neurofibrillary tangles (NFTs)—consist of phosphorylated Tau protein and are found in the cortex, hippocampus, and substantia nigra. (NFTs also found in normal aging, Down's syndrome, dementia pugilistica, and progressive supranuclear palsy). However, even low densities of NFTs in the cortices of the medial temporal lobes should be considered abnormal.
- The co-occurrence of amyloid plaques and NFTs was described by Alois Alzheimer in his original description of the disorder and now is accepted universally as a hallmark of the disease.
- Up to 50% loss of neurons and synapses in the cortex and hippocampus.
- **Genetics:** 40% have a positive family history of DAT (esp. early onset: <55yrs)
  - Chromosome 21—the gene for amyloid precursor protein (APP) is found on the long arm. Also implicated in Down's syndrome.
  - Chromosome 19—codes for apolipoprotein E4. Presence of E4 alleles increases risk of DAT.
  - Chromosome 14—codes for presenilin 1 (implicated in β-amyloid peptide).
  - Chromosome 1—codes for presenilin 11 (implicated in β-amyloid peptide).
- **'Cholinergic hypothesis':** the pathological changes lead to degeneration of cholinergic nuclei in the basal forebrain (nucleus basalis of Meynert). This results in ↓cortical acetylcholine (ACh).

Pray, do not mock me: I am a very foolish fond old man, Fourscore and upward, not an hour more or less; And, to deal plainly, I fear I am not in my perfect mind. Methinks I should know you and know this man; Yet I am doubtful: for I am mainly ignorant what place this is, and all the skill I have remembers not these garments; nor I know not where I did lodge last night. Do not laugh at me; For as I am a man, I think this lady to be my child Cordelia.

Shakespeare: King Lear: Act II Scene 7

1 Kuljis RO (2002) www.emedicine.com

Alzheimer's disease (2)

Clinical features[1] Symptoms usually start insidiously but first presentation may be related to an identifiable life event.

- **Early symptoms** include increasing forgetfulness, deterioration in self-care, and changes in behaviour such as wandering and irritability. By the time the patient presents to clinicians, cognitive deficits are usually apparent.
- **Amnesia** is universal and is mainly for recent events.
- **Disorientation** is common, especially for time.
- **Aphasia** follows later and typically involves both receptive and expressive problems. The patient may exhibit **lexical anomia** (word-finding difficulty). Other focal cognitive deficits include **apraxia**, (evidenced by awkwardness with the sequence of dressing) and **agnosia** (inability to recognise parts of the body). Occasionally, a patient may present with Gerstmann syndrome (p. 68), indicating right parietal disease, characterised by finger agnosia, R/L disorientation, acalculia, and dysgraphia. Impaired **visuospatial skills** and **executive function** are common, while **spastic paraparesis** is a late and unusual feature.
- **Psychiatric symptoms** Delusions (15%)—usually of a paranoid nature. Auditory and/or visual hallucinations (10–15%)—which may be simple misidentification, and indicate rapid cognitive decline. Depression is common, requiring treatment in up to 20% of patients.
- **Behavioural disturbances** include aggression, wandering, explosive temper, sexual disinhibition, incontinence, excessive eating, and searching behaviour.
- **Personality change** often reflects an exaggeration of premorbid traits with coarsening of affect and egocentricity.

Clinical subtypes and course Mayeux (1985) described 4 groups:

- The most common presentation is a gradual and progressive decline without distinguishing features.
- A group with early onset (<65), more aphasia and apraxia, a rapid course with severe intellectual decline, and poor survival rate.
- A group with extrapyramidal signs, severe functional impairment, and associated psychotic symptoms.
- A benign group with little or no progression over a 4-year follow-up.

Factors associated with poor prognosis

- Being male
- Onset <65 years
- Parietal lobe damage
- Prominent behavioural problems
- Severe focal cognitive deficits such as apraxia
- Observed depression
- Absence of misidentification syndrome

Assessment

- **Mental state examination** Noting any clouding of consciousness (delirium), symptoms of depression, psychosis, etc.
- **Cognitive testing** is essential and may begin with a mini-mental state examination (MMSE) (p. 66), but later involve specific neuropsychological testing.
- **Physical examination** To detect presence or absence of focal signs, reflexes, and plantar responses, as well as gait disturbance and signs of Parkinson's disease.
- **Blood tests** (p. 74).
- **EEG** useful to exclude delirium, CJD, etc.
- **Brain imaging:** CT—cortical atrophy, esp. over parietal and temporal lobes and ventricular enlargement. MRI—(optima protocol) atrophy of grey matter (hippocampus, amygdala, and medial temporal lobe). SPET—reduced rCBF in temporal and posterior parietal lobes (also frontal lobes in advanced disease). PET—20–30% reduction in oxygen and glucose metabolism in temporal and posterior parietal lobes. MRS—↓N-acetylaspartate.

National Institute of Neurological and Communicative Disorders and Stroke (NINCDS) and Alzheimer's Disease and Related Disorders Association (ADRDA) criteria[2]

Probable Alzheimer's disease

- Criteria include: the presence of dementia, deficits in at least two areas of cognition, progressive deterioration, no clouding of consciousness, age between 40 and 90, absence of systemic disorders.
- Diagnosis is supported by: progressive deterioration of individual cognitive function, impaired activities of daily living, family history of dementia, normal lumbar puncture, electroencephalogram, and evidence of atrophy (or progression) on CT scan.
- Features consistent with the diagnosis: plateaus in the course of the disease, associated psychiatric symptoms, neurological signs, seizures, normal CT scan.
- Diagnosis unlikely if: sudden onset, focal neurological signs, seizures or gait disturbance early in the disease.

Possible Alzheimer's Disease

- Diagnosis can be made in the presence of atypical features; in the presence of a systemic disease (not considered to be the cause of dementia); in the presence of a single progressive cognitive deficit.

Definite Alzheimer's Disease

- Criteria are the clinical criteria for probable Alzheimer's Disease plus histological evidence of the disorder.

---

1 Burns A and Forstl H (1998) Alzheimer disease. In: *Seminars in Old Age Psychiatry* Eds. Butler R and Pitt B. Gaskell, London.

2 McKhann G, Drachman D, Folstein M, *et al.* (1984) Clinical diagnosis of Alzheimer's disease: report of the NINCDS-ADRDA Work Group under the auspices of Department of Health and Human Services Task Force on Alzheimer's Disease. *Neurology* **34**, 939–44.

Alzheimer's disease (3)— pharmacological treatments[1]

Acetylcholinesterase inhibitors (AChEIs) were the first drugs to be licensed for the treatment of DAT. They act by enhancing ACh at cholinergic synapses in the CNS, and in this way may slow progression of the disease, reducing time spent in full nursing care. They have beneficial effects on cognitive, functional, and behavioural symptoms of the disease and are recommended as 1st-line agents in the treatment of mild-moderate DAT. (See NICE guidelines opposite.)

1st generation AChEIs

- **Tacrine** Developed in the 1980s; easily absorbed with a short ½ life; liver metabolism; non-linear kinetics; non-selective (also acts at parasympathetic receptors outside the CNS). *Problems:* GI side-effects; ↑liver enzymes/hepatotoxicity; wide dose range, therefore unpredictable kinetics; 4x daily dosage.

2nd generation AChEIs

Similar efficacy over 6 months; long-term efficacy unknown. Switching between agents is acceptable.

- **Donepezil** Piperidine derivative, developed in 1996; GIT absorbed with liver metabolism; long ½ life (70hrs); highly selective (acts centrally only); linear kinetics. *Problems:* GIT side-effects at high dose; bradycardia; GIT bleed (rare); contraindicated in asthma. *Benefits:* selective therefore ↓side-effects; no liver toxicity; predictable kinetics; narrow dose range; 1x daily dosage. *Dose:* 5–10mg/day.
- **Rivastigmine** Developed in 1998; short ½ life (12hrs); inhibits AChE and butyrylcholinesterase in CNS. *Problems:* GIT side-effects; 2x daily dosage. *Benefits:* safe in asthma and COAD. *Dose:* start with 1.5mg BD; increase to 3–6mg BD.
- **Galantamine** Selectively inhibits AChE and acts as an allosteric ligand at nicotinic ACh receptors; metabolised in liver; short ½ life (5hrs); selective. *Problems:* 2x daily dosage. *Dose:* 4–12mg BD.

NMDA-receptor partial antagonist The NMDA receptor binds excitatory glutamate in the CNS and has a role in LTP and learning/memory function.

- **Memantine** In Feb 2002, this new agent was approved in Europe for the treatment of moderately severe to severe DAT (MMSE 3–14). It is a non-competitive, PCP-site, NMDA antagonist that may protect neurons from glutamate-mediated excitotoxicity. Trials show benefits of memantine augmentation of donepezil. Cochrane review indicates use in DAT, vascular, and mixed dementia.

Other (possible) treatment strategies Although only at experimental stages, there is some evidence for other approaches to DAT. These include: anti-oxidants (vit E; selegiline); anti-inflammatories; secretase inhibitors; metal chelators; amyloid-β-peptide vaccination; cholesterol-lowering drugs; red wine (!).

NICE guidance on drug treatment for Alzheimer's disease—donepezil, rivastigmine, and galantamine (N0 19)

The three drugs-donepezil, rivastigmine, and galantamine-should be made available in the NHS as one component of the management of those people with mild and moderate Alzheimer's disease (AD) whose MMSE score is above 12 points, under the following conditions:

- Diagnosis that the form of dementia is AD must be made in a specialist clinic according to standard diagnostic criteria.
- Assessment in a specialist clinic, including tests of cognitive, global, and behavioural functioning and of activities of daily living, should be made before the drug is prescribed.
- Clinicians should also exercise judgement about the likelihood of compliance; in general, a carer or care-worker who is in sufficient contact with the patient to ensure compliance should be a minimum requirement.
- Only specialists (including old age psychiatrists, neurologists, and care of the elderly physicians) should initiate treatment. Carers' views of the patient's condition at baseline and follow-up should be sought. If GPs are to take over prescribing, it is recommended that they should do so under an agreed shared-care protocol with clear treatment end points.
- A further assessment should be made, usually 2–4 months after reaching maintenance dose of the drug. Following this assessment, the drug should be continued only where there has been an improvement or no deterioration in MMSE score, together with evidence of global improvement on the basis of behavioural and/or functional assessment.
- Patients who continue on the drug should be reviewed by MMSE score and global, functional, and behavioural assessment every 6 months.
  - The drug should normally only be continued while their MMSE score remains above 12 points, and their global, functional, and behavioural condition remains at a level where the drug is considered to be having a worthwhile effect.
  - When the MMSE score falls below 12 points, patients should not normally be prescribed any of these three drugs.
  - Any review involving MMSE assessment should be undertaken by an appropriate specialist team, unless there are locally agreed protocols for shared care.

1 Scarpini E, Scheltens P, and Feldman H (2003) Treatment of Alzheimer's disease: current status and new perspectives. *Lancet (Neurology)* **2**, 539–47.

Dementia with Lewy bodies (DLB)

Common form of senile dementia (~15–20% of cases in hospital[1] and community-based samples[2]) that shares clinical and pathological features of both DAT and Parkinson's disease.

Epidemiology Age of onset: 50–83y. Age at death: 68–92y. ♂>♀.

Clinical features Dementia (relative sparing of STM); parkinsonism (~70%: bradykinesia, limb rigidity, gait disorder); fluctuating cognitive performance and level of consciousness; complex hallucinations—visual (~60%): often people and animals, auditory (~20%)—with associated emotional responses; significant depressive episode (~40%); recurrent falls/ syncope (~30%: due to autonomic dysfunction), transient disturbances of consciousness (mute and unresponsive for several minutes); antipsychotic sensitivity (~60%.) The mean survival time/rate of cognitive decline is similar to Alzheimer's disease (but rapid deterioration over 1–2y does occur). Worsening of parkinsonism is similar in rate to Parkinson's disease (10% decline per year.)

Pathological features Typically 'mixed' picture[2]. **Lewy bodies** eosinophilic intracytoplasmic neuronal inclusions of abnormally phospho-rylated neurofilament proteins aggregated with ubiquitin and α-synuclein, found in brain-stem nuclei (esp. basal ganglia) and neocortical structures. Associated neuronal loss (esp brain-stem and basal forebrain cholinergic projection neurones—with associated ↓ACh transmission in neocortex.) **Lewy neurites** distinctive pattern of ubiquitin and α-synuclein immunoreactive neuritic degeneration—in substantia nigra, hippocampal region (CA2/3), dorsal vagal nucleus, basal nucleus basilis of Meynert, and transtentorial cortex (may be more relevant to neuropsychi-atric symptom formation than cortical Lewy bodies[3]). **Alzheimer-type changes** senile plaques present in a similar density and distribution, fewer neurofibrillary tangles, less tau pathology. **Vascular disease** occurs in ~30% with unknown clinical significance.

Differential diagnosis Other dementia syndromes (esp DAT), delirium, neurological causes (e.g. Parkinson's disease, progressive supranuclear palsy, multi-system atrophy, CJD), psychiatric disorders (e.g. late-onset delusional disorder, depressive psychosis, mania).

Investigations

- **CT/MRI:** relative sparing of medial temporal lobes in most cases. Moderate increases in deep white-matter lesions, frequent peri-ventricular lucencies on MRI.
- **SPECT HMPAO scan (blood flow):** global↓ (esp occipital), medial temporal lobes relatively preserved. **SPECT FP-CIT (presynaptic dopamine transporter):** reduced in putamen (like Parkinson's disease).
- **ApoE genotype:** ↑frequency of ε4 allele.

Management

- **Antipsychotics** Avoid/use with great caution: severe sensitivity reactions (40–50%)—e.g. irreversible parkinsonism, ↑impairment of consciousness, NMS-like autonomic disturbances—with 2–3 fold-increase in mortality.

- **AChEls** Not yet recommended by National Guidelines, substantial provisional evidence suggests AChEls effective in some DLB cases (↑cognitive function, ↓apathy/psychosis/agitation[4]).
- **Other** No clear evidence for antidepressants, anticonvulsants, or BDZs for psychiatric and behavioural symptoms. Clonazepam may be useful for sleep disturbance (vivid dreams, muscle atonia, excessive jerking, and other complex movements.) Antiparkinsonian medication—use cautiously for clinically significant motor symptoms (risk of exacerbating psychotic symptoms).

Consensus criteria for the clinical diagnosis of probable and possible dementia with Lewy bodies[5]

- The central feature required for a diagnosis of DLB is progressive cognitive decline of sufficient magnitude to interfere with normal social or occupational function. Prominent or persistent memory impairment may not necessarily occur in the early stages but is usually evident with progression. Deficits on tests of attention and of fronto-subcortical skills and visuospatial ability may be especially prominent.
- Two of the following core features are essential for a diagnosis of probable DLB; one is essential for possible DLB.
  - Fluctuating cognition with pronounced variations in attention and alertness.
  - Recurrent visual hallucinations, which are typically well formed and detailed.
  - Spontaneous motor features of parkinsonism.
- Features supportive of the diagnosis are:
  - Repeated falls; syncope; transient loss of consciousness; neuroleptic sensitivity; systematised delusions; hallucinations in other modalities.
- A diagnosis of DLB is less likely in the presence of:
  - Stroke, evident as focal neurological signs or on brain imaging.
  - Evidence on physical examination and investigation of any physical illness, or other brain disorder, sufficient to account for the clinical picture.

1 Weiner M (1999) Dementia associated with Lewy bodies: dilemmas and directions. *Archives of Neurology* **56**, 1441.

2 Holmes C, Cairns N, Lantos P, Mann A (1999) Validity of current clinical criteria for Alzheimer's disease, vascular dementia and dementia with Lewy bodies. *Br J Psych* **174**, 45–50.

3 Gómez-Tortosa E, Newell K, Irizarry MC, *et al.* (1999) Clinical and quantitative pathologic correlates of dementia with Lewy bodies. *Neurology* **53**, 1284–91.

4 McKeith I, Del Ser T, Spano P, *et al.* (2000) Efficacy of rivastigmine in dementia with Lewy bodies: a randomised, double-blind, placebo-controlled international study. *Lancet* **356**, 2031–6.

5 McKeith IG, Galasko D, Kosaka K, *et al.* (1996) Consensus guidelines for the clinical and pathologic diagnosis of dementia with Lewy bodies (DLB): report of the consortium on DLB international workshop. *Neurology* **47**, 1113–24.

Fronto-temporal dementia (FTD) (Pick's disease)[1,2]

A form of dementia, characterised by preferential atrophy of fronto-temporal regions, with usually early onset (accounts for ~20% of presenile cases). Early symptoms include personality change and social disinhibition, preceding memory, or other cognitive impairment.

Clinical features Profound alteration in character/social conduct, relative preservation of perception, spatial skills, praxis, memory. **Decline/impaired regulation of social conduct**: (e.g. breaches of etiquette, tactlessness, disinhibition, changes in usual behaviour, passivity, inertia, overactivity, pacing, and wandering). **Emotional blunting**: e.g. primary emotions (happiness, sadness, fear) and social emotions (embarrassment, sympathy, empathy). **Impaired insight**: of symptoms and expression of distress. **Dietary changes**: overeating, preference for sweet foods. **Perseverative behaviours** (e.g. drinking from an empty cup). **Speech**: echolalia, perseveration, verbal stereotypies, mutism. **Cognitive**: frontal lobe dysfunction: impaired attention, ineffective retrieval strategies, poor organisation, lack of self-monitoring and concern for accuracy. **Neurological**: no early signs; primitive reflexes and parkinsonism (with progression); MND signs (in a minority.)

Onset usually 45–65y, can occur before age 30 and in the over 65s. ♂=♀. Mean time to death 8y (range 2–20y). FHx in 50%.

Clinical subtypes Disinhibited form: orbito-medial frontal and anterior temporal regional pathology. **Apathetic form**: extensive frontal (esp. dorsolateral) lobe pathology. **Stereotypic form**: marked striatal/variable cortical involvement (often temporal>frontal.) N.B. changes in social behaviour often related to right-hemispheric pathology. Repetitive/compulsive behaviours may be associated with striatal pathology and the disinhibited form, suggesting temporal lobe pathology (unlike OCD, anxiety is not experienced).

Pathological features Macroscopic: bilateral atrophy of frontal and anterior temporal lobes, degeneration of the striatum. **Microscopic:** 3 subtypes (similar distribution of changes within frontal/temporal lobes): Common *(microvacuolar) type* (60%)—loss of large cortical nerve cells, spongiform degeneration (microvacuolation) of the superficial neurophil, minimal gliosis, and no swellings or inclusions in remaining nerve cells; *Pick type* (25%)—loss of large cortical nerve cells, widespread gliosis, minimal or no spongiform (microvacuolar) change, swollen neurones and inclusions positive for tau and ubiquitin (in most cases); limbic system and striatum more seriously damaged; *Associated with MND* (15%) demonstrating microvacuolar (rarely Pick type) histological features like MND.

Differential diagnosis DAT, cerebrovascular dementia, rare forms of fronto-temporal lobar degeneration (e.g. 'semantic' dementia, progressive non-fluent aphasia, progressive apraxia).

Investigations Neuropsychology: Impaired frontal lobe function, relatively spared memory, speech, and perceptuospatial functions. **EEG:** usually normal. **CT/MRI:** bilateral (asymmetrical) abnormalities of frontal/temporal lobes. **SPECT:** frontal and/or temporal lobe abnormalities. **Genetics:** associations with: 17q21–22 (familial inheritance) and mutations in the tau gene; 3; 9q21–22 (familial amyotrophic lateral sclerosis.)

Management Currently, no specific treatments. **AChEIs:** unlikely to be beneficial (no specific abnormality of the cholinergic system). **SSRIs:** of limited benefit for behavioural symptoms (disinhibition, overeating, and compulsions).

Behavioural features of FTD specified in diagnostic criteria

Core features
- Insidious onset and gradual progression.
- Early decline in social interpersonal conduct.
- Early impairment in regulation of personal conduct.
- Early emotional blunting.
- Early loss of insight.

Supportive features
- Behavioural disorder
  - Decline in personal hygiene and grooming.
  - Mental rigidity and inflexibility.
  - Distractibility and impersistence.
  - Hyperorality and dietary changes.
  - Perseverative and stereotyped behaviour.
  - Utilisation behaviour.
- Speech and language
  - Altered speech output (aspontaneity and economy of speech/ pressured speech).
  - Stereotypy of speech.
  - Echolalia.
  - Perseveration.
  - Mutism.
- Physical signs
  - Primitive reflexes.
  - Incontinence.
  - Akinesia, rigidity, and tremor.
  - Low and labile blood pressure.
- Investigations
  - **Neuropsychological:** significant impairment on frontal lobe tests; absence of severe amnesia, aphasia, or perceptuospatial disorder.
  - **EEG:** normal on conventional EEG, despite clinically evident dementia.
  - **Brain imaging** (structural and/or functional): predominant frontal and/or temporal abnormality.

1 Neary D, Snowden JS, Gustafson L, et al. (1998) Frontotemporal lobar degeneration: a consensus on clinical diagnostic criteria. Neurology **51**, 1546–54.

2 Snowden JS, Neary D, Mann DM (2002) Frontotemporal dementia. BJP **180**, 140–3.

Vascular dementia

Vascular dementia is the second most common cause of dementia after DAT, accounting for 20% of cases. It can coexist with DAT and results from thromboembolic or hypertensive infarction of small and medium size vessels. Features that suggest vascular dementia include: sudden onset; stepwise deterioration; and risk factors for cardiovascular disease. Its presentation is variable and three syndromes are commonly recognised[1]:

1. *Cognitive deficits following a single stroke* Not all strokes result in cognitive impairment, but when they do the deficits depend upon the site of the infarct. Cognitive deficits tend to be particularly severe with certain midbrain and thalamic strokes. Cognitive deficits may remain fixed or recover, either partially or completely.

2. *Multi-infarct dementia (MID)* Multiple strokes lead to stepwise deterioration in cognitive function. Between strokes there are periods of relative stability. There are often risk factors for cardiovascular disease.

3. *Progressive small-vessel disease (Binswanger disease)* Multiple microvascular infarcts of perforating vessels leads to progressive lacunae formation and white matter leukoariosis on MRI. This is a subcortical dementia with a clinical course characterised by gradual intellectual decline, generalised slowing, and motor problems (e.g. gait disturbance and dysarthria). Depression and pseudobulbar palsy are not uncommon.

Epidemiology Most common in the 60–70y age group. ♂>♀. Other risk factors include: family or personal history of cardiovascular disease, smoking, diabetes mellitus, hypertension, hyperlipidaemia, polycythaemia, coagulopathies, sickle cell anaemia, valvular disease, atrial myxoma, and carotid artery disease. There are rare familial cases with onset in the 40s—cerebral autosomal dominant arteriopathy with subcortical infarcts and leukoencephalopathy (CADASIL).

Clinical features[2] Onset may follow a CVA and is more acute than DAT. **Emotional and personality changes** are typically early, followed by **cognitive deficits** (including memory deficits) that are often fluctuating in severity. **Depression** with episodes of **affective lability** and **confusion** are common, especially at night. **Behavioural slowing, anxiety**, and occasional **episodes of cerebral ischaemia** occur frequently. Physical signs include features of arteriovascular disease together with neurological impairments (e.g. rigidity, akinesia, brisk reflexes, pseudobulbar palsy). 10% have **seizures** at some point. Course is stepwise, with periods of intervening stability Prognosis is poorer than in DAT with average life-span of 5y from onset. Cause of death is usually ischaemic heart disease (50%), CVA, or renal failure.

Investigations

• Routine 'dementia screen' (p. 74).
• Serum cholesterol, clotting screen, vasculitis screen (ESR; CRP; complement; ANF; rheumatoid factor; anti-DNA antibodies; antiphospholipid antibodies; etc.), and syphilis serology are additional tests in unusual cases (e.g. 'young strokes').

- ECG, CXR, CT, and MRI are essential.
- Other investigations may include:echocardiography (for cardiac/valvular defects or disease); carotid artery Doppler ultrasound.

Management
- Establish causative factors.
- Medical or surgical diseases that are contributory need to be treated early.
- Daily aspirin may delay course of disease.
- General health interventions include changing diet, stopping smoking, managing hypertension, optimising diabetic control, and increasing exercise.

1 Rossor M and Brown J (1998) Vascular and other dementias In: *Seminars in Old Age Psychiatry* Eds. Butler R and Pitt B. Gaskell, London.

2 Gelder M, Gath D, Mayou R, Cowen P (1996) *Oxford Textbook of Psychiatry*, 3rd Edition, Oxford University Press, Oxford.

Prion diseases

Prion diseases are rapid, aggressive, dementing illnesses caused by deposits of prion proteins throughout the brain. They are rare and are best considered as 'slow virus infections'. Prions spread throughout the brain by causing irreversible change in neighbouring tissue. The typical pathological finding is a 'spongy encephalopathy', and in terms of the nosology of the dementias, prion disease is considered a 'multifocal dementia'. While prion diseases tend to respect the species barrier (e.g. 'scrapie' is a prion disease limited to sheep), there is emerging evidence that this is not always the case (e.g. vCJD). Three diseases are recognised in humans:

Creutzfeldt-Jakob disease (CJD)

A rare disease (approximately 50 cases/year in UK) of 50–70y-olds with equal sex distribution. 85% cases are spontaneous or sporadic; 10% result from genetic mutation; 5% result from iatrogenic transmission during transplant surgery of dura, corneal grafts, and pituitary growth hormone. The clinical picture is one of rapidly deteriorating dementia, cerebellar and extrapyramidal signs, myoclonus, and death within a year. EEG shows 'periodic complexes'. CT atrophy of cortex and cerebellum.

New variant CJD (vCJD): BSE

The rise of vCJD followed an epidemic of bovine spongiform encephalopathy (BSE) in cattle. BSE is a prion disease of cows that is thought to have been caused by cattle feeds that contained CNS material from infected cows. The disease in humans affects mainly young men in their 20s and is characterised by early anxiety and depressive symptoms, followed by personality changes, and finally a progressive dementia. Ataxia and myoclonus are prominent and the typical course is 1–2 yrs until death. EEG and CT changes are similar to CJD.

Kuru

This was a rare disease of New Guinea cannibals who ate the brains of their deceased relatives. The incubation period was prolonged—up to 40yrs before disease onset, which was then rapid and fatal.

Recent research reveals 'cannibalism genotype'

Researchers at University College London have recently suggested that cannibalism was common and widespread in human ancestors. They analyzed DNA from 30 elderly Fore women from Papua New Guinea who had participated in many cannibalistic feasts before they were banned by the Australian government in the 1950s. It was the practice of the Fore for women and children to consume the brains of dead kin in the belief that this act would 'recycle' the spirit of the dead within the living. At the peak of the epidemic (1920–1950) Kuru killed 1% of the population annually. Most of the women survivors tested by researchers had a particular genotype that was much less common in the younger population, indicating that it conferred substantial protection against the disease. Interestingly, none of the patients who have to date contracted new variant CJD in Britain carry the protective genotype. This suggests that this genotype is protective against prion diseases in humans. The researchers then examined DNA from various ethnic groups around the world and found that all, except the Japanese, carried the protective genotype to a similar degree. Genetic tests showed that this gene could not be there by chance, but was a result of natural selection. This implies that ancestral human populations were exposed to some form of prion disease. They conclude that frequent epidemics of prion disease caused by cannibalism in human ancestors would explain the worldwide existence of the protective genotype in modern humans.

From Mead S, Stumpf MP, Whitfield J, et al. (2003) Balancing selection at the prion protein gene consistent with prehistoric kurulike epidemics. *Science* **300**, 640–3.

Amnestic disorders

The amnestic disorders are syndromes characterised by memory impairment (anterograde and/or retrograde amnesia), which are caused by a general medical condition or use substance, and where delirium and dementia have been excluded as causative of the amnesia. Amnestic disorders may be transient or chronic (< or > 1mth). Amnestic conditions usually involve some or all of the following neuroanatomical structures: frontal cortex; hippocampus and amygdala; dorsomedial thalamus; mamillary bodies; and the periaqueductal grey matter (PAG). In terms of neurochemistry, glutamate transmission at the NMDA receptor is often implicated in amnesia, mainly due to its role in memory storage in the limbic system (LTP). A number of amnestic disorders are recognised:

Wernicke's encephalopathy (p. 530)

An acute syndrome, with a classic tetrad of symptoms (ataxia, ophthalmoplegia, nystagmus, and acute confusional state), caused by thiamine depletion, usually related to alcohol abuse, and associated with pathological lesions in the mamillary bodies, PAG, thalamic nuclei, and the walls of the 3rd ventricle.

Korsakoff psychosis (pp. 530–1)

Amnesia and confabulation associated with atrophy of the mamillary bodies, usually following Wernicke's encephalopathy (rarer causes include: head injury; hypoxia brain injury; basal/temporal lobe encephalitis; and vascular insult).

Vascular disease

Insults to the hippocampus (especially involving the posterior cerebral artery or basilar artery) may result in an amnestic disorder. Other regions implicated include: parietal-occipital junction; bilateral medio-dorsal thalamus; basal forebrain nuclei (e.g. aneurysm of the anterior communicating artery).

Head injury

An open or closed head injury involving acceleration or deceleration forces may result in injury to the anterior temporal poles (as this structure collides with the temporal bone). Anterograde or post-traumatic amnesia (PTA) is prominent with retrograde amnesia relatively absent. Prognosis is related to length of PTA-better prognosis associated with PTA of less than 1wk.

HSV encephalitis

Affects medial temporal lobes and results in deficits in STM storage.

Temporal lobe surgery

Bilateral damage or surgery to the medial temporal lobes results in an inability to store new short-term memories (e.g. 'patient HM') (see box opposite).

Hypoxic brain damage

Hypoxia following asphyxia from CO poisoning, near drowning, etc, may damage sensitive CA1 and CA3 neurons in the hippocampus. This results in problems with STM storage.

MS

40% of patients have some amnesia due to plaques in the temporal lobes and diencephalon resulting in difficulty with recall.

Alcohol blackouts ('palimpsest')

Significant alcohol intoxication may lead to amnesia for the period of intoxication. This usually only occurs in the context of chronic alcohol misuse.

ECT

There may be a period of mild anterograde and/or retrograde amnesia for several hours following administration of ECT. More rarely there may be ongoing patchy memory loss for up to 6–9 mths.

Transient global amnesia (TGA)

This is a syndrome of amnesia lasting 6–24 hrs caused by transient ischaemia of the temporal lobes and/or diencephalon. It is more common over 50 yrs and may occur in the context of hypertension or migraine. Differential diagnosis includes dissociative disorders and malingering, and diagnosis is often unclear.

Other causes of amnesia

Substances (benzodiazepines, anticholinergics); space occupying lesions (e.g. tumours); hypoglycaemia.

'Patient HM'

On 23 August 1953, patient HM underwent a bilateral medial temporal lobe resection in an attempt to control his epileptic seizures. This resulted in a severe anterograde memory impairment that has made HM one of the most studied patients in the history of cognitive psychology.

HM's syndrome is surprisingly isolated, with impairment mostly limited to his inability to register new facts into long-term memory, despite immediate memory being preserved for both verbal and non-verbal tasks. Although his operation was performed when he was 27, his memories are intact until age 16, with an 11-year retrograde amnesia.

His IQ is above average, with almost normal language production and comprehension—he can understand and produce complex verbal material (but is impaired on tests of semantic and symbolic verbal fluency). His perceptual abilities are normal except for his sense of smell (2° to damage of the olfactory tracts). Despite the fact that some of his spatial abilities are compromised, he does not have any attentional deficit.

Normal pressure hydrocephalus (NPH)

Essence A syndrome where there is dilatation of cerebral ventricles (especially 3rd ventricle) and normal CSF pressure at lumbar puncture. It typically presents with the triad of: **dementia, gait ataxia**, and **urinary incontinence**. Importantly, the dementia is potentially reversible if NPH is treated promptly.

Aetiology 50% cases are idiopathic. 50% are secondary to mechanical obstruction of CSF flow across the meninges (e.g. meningitis; subarachnoid haemorrhage; trauma; radiotherapy).

Clinical features There is progressive slowing of cognitive and motor functioning consistent with a pattern of subcortical dementia. Ataxia is due to pyramidal upper motor neuron paraparesis. Urinary incontinence is a late symptom.

Investigations CT scan shows ↑size of the lateral ventricles and thinning of the cortex. 24-hour intracranial pressure monitoring shows typical 'β' pattern.

Treatment Those cases where NPH is 2° to an identified cause are the best candidates for ventriculo-peritoneal shunt.

Chronic subdural haematoma (SDH)

Essence An insidious and fluctuating organic syndrome may result from an undetected chronic subdural haematoma. A SDH results from rupture of the bridging veins between the dura and arachnoid mater and tends to occur over the frontal and/or parietal cortices. In 30% of cases there is bilateral SDH. SDH should be suspected where there is a changing pattern in cognitive function, especially if **risk factors for SDH** exist: post trauma; elderly after a fall; infancy; cerebral atrophy (e.g. chronic alcoholism); clotting disorders.

Clinical features A SDH may only manifest with symptoms months after it develops., therefore there may be no history of recent trauma. Headache, altered level of consciousness, and amnesia may all occur, often with fluctuations in severity. Typically, the mental state may be variable on different occasions and there may be periods of unusual drowsiness as well as both cognitive and physical slowness and sluggishness. Minor focal signs are sometimes detected. The general trend is towards a dementia picture, which is characteristic of a subcortical nature.

Investigations CT scan during the first 3 weeks may not show the SDH as it is isodense during the early phase. Therefore, contrast should be used. Later on, as the SDH liquefies, a low-density convexity may be detected over the fronto-parietal cortex.

Treatment Surgical drainage of SDH via burr holes. Steroids for conservative treatment.

Psychiatric sequelae of CVA

A range of psychiatric problems may occur following stroke[1]. These include:

Cognitive disorders
- Vascular dementia (see pp. 144–5)
- Subcortical dementia (see p. 133)
- Amnestic disorder (see pp. 148–9)

Personality changes
These tend to involve a constriction in the range of interests and a loss of intellectual flexibility. Irritability is common and 'catastrophic reactions' may occur in response to stress or change in routine. Emotional flexibility may be reduced and affective responses often become shallow and stereotyped.

'Pathological emotionalism'
May occur 4–6 weeks post-CVA, especially following left frontal infarcts. Presentation involves outbursts of unprovoked and uncontrollable emotion and distress, with disinhibition a major feature.

Post-stroke depression
Depressive illness after stroke is extremely common, occurring in up to 60% of cases. Its onset is usually between 3 and 24 months following the stroke. It was a neglected phenomenon until recently and many cases are mis- or under-diagnosed with symptoms being attributed to the cognitive insult.

Aetiology *Biological factors*—direct physiological effects of the brain injury, with location (e.g. left anterior frontal), large size, increased age and female gender being risk factors. *Psychological factors*—sudden dependency; disability; premorbid personality traits (especially neurotic or highly independent individuals). *Social risk factors*—being alone; lack of social support; financial worries.

Treatment Antidepressants: SSRIs and mianserin are considered safe following stroke but some evidence suggests that TCAs are more efficacious.

Psychoses
Manic, hypomanic, and paranoid psychoses may result from a CVA, especially right hemisphere infarcts. **'Peduncular hallucinosis'** is an uncommon psychosis characterised by visual and auditory hallucinations and is associated with infarcts involving the pons and midbrain.

Korsakoff psychosis (pp. 530–1)
A rare chronic complication of subarachnoid haemorrhage.

---

1 Lishman WA (1997) *Organic Psychiatry*. Blackwell Science (UK).

Psychiatric aspects of head injury (1)[1,2]

Head injuries are unfortunately common in a world characterised by mass use of motor vehicles and widely misused alcohol. The peak incidence of head injury is between the ages of 15 and 24 years and improved medical care has resulted in large numbers of individuals surviving with neuropsychiatric consequences. Most head injury survivors who present to psychiatric services have emotional symptoms and personality changes ranging from subtle to severe. A smaller number manifest serious and lasting cognitive sequelae, such as apathy, disinhibition, and amnesia. There are also important acute psychiatric effects of head injury.

Acute psychological effects of head injury

Most significant head injuries are closed and involve a period of loss of consciousness (which may extend from brief concussion to prolonged coma). On recovery of consciousness there are often memory deficits. Amnesia is classified in terms of:

- **Post-traumatic amnesia (PTA)** includes the period of injury and the period following injury (until normal memory resumes). Apparently normal behaviour often occurs during this period. PTA may end abruptly.
- **Retrograde amnesia (RA)** includes the period between the last clearly recalled memory prior to the injury and the injury itself. It is usually a dense amnesia that is brief, lasting seconds or minutes, and shrinks with time.

Acute post-traumatic delirium (PTD)

A state that may follow severe head injury and occurs as the individual begins to regain consciousness. This is sometimes also called 'post-traumatic psychosis' and is characterised by prolonged and variable confusion, with or without behavioural symptoms, anxiety, affective lability, paranoia, delusional misinterpretation, and hallucinations.

Factors associated with increased psychiatric morbidity following head injury

- Increased duration of loss of consciousness
- Increased duration of PTA
- Increased duration of PTD
- Increased age, arteriosclerosis, and alcoholism
- Increased area of damage
- Increased neurological sequelae (focal deficits, epilepsy, etc.)
- Dominant or bilateral hemisphere involvement

1 Lishman WA (1997) *Organic Psychiatry*. Blackwell Science (UK).

2 Rao V and Lyketsos C (2000) Neuropsychiatric sequelae of traumatic brain injury. *Psychosomatics* **41**, 95–103.

Psychiatric aspects of head injury (2)

Chronic psychiatric syndromes following head injury

A number of chronic syndromes are recognised following head injury:

- **Cognitive impairment** Especially after closed head injuries with PTA lasting >24 hours. There may be focal cognitive deficits such as amnesia, or diffuse problems including slowing, apathy, affective blunting, decreased concentration, executive difficulties, amnesia, and affective lability. 'Catastrophic reactions' and emotional incontinence may occur. In its severest form the cognitive impairment may present as a dementia ('post-traumatic dementia'). If symptoms are severe, it is particularly important to exclude NPH, SDH, or coexisting DAT. *Treatment*: antipsychotics; stimulants.
- **Personality/behavioural changes** Personality changes are most likely after head injury to the orbito-frontal lobe or anterior temporal lobe. 'Frontal lobe syndrome' (p. 68) is characterised by disinhibition, impulsivity, irritability, and aggressive outbursts. *Treatment* may include ß-blockers (e.g. atenolol), carbamazepine.
- **Psychoses** A schizophrenia-like psychosis with prominent paranoia is associated with left temporal injury, while affective psychoses (esp. mania in 9% patients) are associated with right temporal or orbito-frontal injury. There is also an increased prevalence of schizophrenia post head injury (~2.5% develop the disorder). *Treatment* Cautious use of antipsychotics (risk of seizure), anticonvulsants.
- **Neurotic disorders** Depressive illness is most common but anxiety states (including PTSD) are common sequelae. Persistent depression and anxiety occur in roughly ¼ of head injury survivors. Suicide risk is also higher post head injury. *Treatment:* SSRIs; ECT.
- **'Post-traumatic syndrome'** Also called 'post-concussional syndrome'. This is a common phenomenon after head injury. The main symptoms are: headache; dizziness; insomnia; irritability; emotional lability; increased sensitivity to noise, light, etc; fatigue; poor concentration; anxiety; and depression. Although this syndrome was previously thought to be a purely psychological phenomenon (since in many cases the injury was minor), it is now recognised that it probably involves a complex interplay of both organic and non-organic factors.

Factors influencing psychiatric disability and prognosis

- Mental constitution—i.e. vulnerability due to genetics, temperament (premorbid personality: increased risk in histrionic, hypochondriacal and dependent personalities), IQ ('cerebral reserve'), age.
- Emotional impact of injury—i.e. extent of psychological trauma.
- Setting, circumstances, and repercussions of injury.
- Iatrogenic factors.
- Home and social environment (including 2° gain issues).
- Compensation and litigation issues (including 2° gain issues).
- Post-traumatic epilepsy (PTE)—occurs in 5% closed and 30% open head injuries (usually during first year) and worsens prognosis.
- Size and location of brain damage: frontal, temporal, dominant side worse.

Sequelae in children

Less psychopathology after head injury due to increased brain plasticity. Recovery may continue for up to 5 years after injury (as opposed to 2 years in adults). Problems are generally behavioural in nature and include aggression, delinquency and ADHD-like syndromes.

'Punch-drunk syndrome'

Boxers may develop diffuse injury to the cortex, basal ganglia, and cerebellum, giving rise to extra-pyramidal symptoms or a subcortical dementia. Pathology shows cerebral atrophy and neuro-fibrillary tangles.

Psychiatric aspects of epilepsy (1)

The lifetime prevalence of experiencing a 'seizure' is approximately 5%, while the prevalence of epilepsy (recurrent seizures) is 0.5–1%. Most (~60%) cases of epilepsy have unknown aetiology. Seizures may be *generalized* or *focal*. Generalised seizures involve the whole cortex and lead to loss of consciousness (LOC). Focal seizures begin in one area of the cortex and may become *secondarily generalized*. Focal seizures are subclassified as *simple partial* (i.e. localised motor/sensory features without LOC or memory loss); *complex partial* (i.e. with or without aura/automatism, and associated changes in conscious level). Between 10% and 50% of patients with epilepsy have psychiatric symptoms.

Psychiatric aspects of epilepsy may be related to:
- Psychosocial consequences of diagnosis (e.g. unemployment, stigma and ostracism, restricted activities, dependency).
- Psychiatric syndromes directly attributed to epilepsy.
- Neuropsychiatric effects of medication.

Psychiatric syndromes attributed to epilepsy are best considered by their temporal relationship to seizures (**pre-ictal, ictal, post-ictal, inter-ictal**.)

Pre-ictal
- Patients may experience a variety of vague symptoms during the days and hours leading up to the seizure. These are termed **prodromal symptoms** and include feelings of tension, dysphoria, and insomnia.
- An **aura** may occur immediately prior to seizure onset. This is most common in complex partial seizures (CPSs)—temporal lobe epilepsy or extra-temporal epilepsy (e.g. frontal CPSs). Auras are typically stereotyped e.g. autonomic or visceral aura (epigastric sensation); derealisation and depersonalisation experiences; cognitive symptoms (dysphasia, 'forced thinking', ideomotor aura, déjà vu, jamais vu, fugue and twilight states); affective symptoms (anxiety, euphoria); perceptual experiences (auditory, visual, sensory, and olfactory hallucinations or illusions).

Ictal
- **Automatisms** May occur during the seizure and suggest a focal origin for the seizure such as medial temporal lobe. There is LOC during the ictus and amnesia for the automatism, which usually lasts < 5 minutes. There are simple or complex stereotyped movements that tend to be disorganised and purposeless (although complex actions may be carried out). At this time the individual seems 'out of touch' Automatisms may be the basis of twilight and fugue states (EEG may aid differential diagnosis.)
- **Epilepsy partialis continuans (EPC)** A condition of prolonged CPSs, lasting hours-days (may be confused with delirium or psychosis) (e.g. temporal, frontal, or cingulate seizures). There are variable behavioural, cognitive, and perceptual symptoms and periods of amnesia.
- **Bizarre aggressive behaviour**

Post-ictal

- **Post-ictal delirium** A very common (10%) confusional state following a seizure with disorientation, inattention, variable levels of consciousness, and sometimes paranoia. Tends to last hours to days and shows a trend towards improvement and normal consciousness. If prolonged, suspect EPC.
- **Post-ictal psychosis**[1] Usually follows a cluster of seizures or an increase in the frequency of seizures; may follow withdrawal of anticonvulsant therapy. Thought to result from sub-threshold kindling activity. It usually only occurs in individuals with epilepsy for >10 yrs (particularly associated with a left temporal lobe focus). Clinically, there is an initial non-psychotic interval (lasting hours to weeks) following a seizure. Thereafter, the individual develops a brief psychotic episode with variable psychotic and affective symptoms. The episode resolves after a period of days to 1 month. It may recur 2 or 3 times in a year. EEG shows marked changes during the psychotic episode.

Inter-ictal[2]

- **Brief inter-ictal psychosis** occurs unrelated to a seizure, when there is good control of epilepsy. In this way seizures are antagonistic to the psychosis in that the EEG normalises during the psychosis. This is called '*forced normalisation*'. A seizure may end the psychotic episode. This form of psychosis has been termed '*alternating psychosis*' (i.e. there is an inverse relationship between severity of epilepsy and severity of psychosis). There may be premonitory symptoms such as anxiety and insomnia while the psychosis is characterised by hallucinations and paranoia. Notably the antagonistic relationship between seizures and psychosis is demonstrated where anticonvulsants may aggravate psychosis, and where antipsychotics may reduce the seizure threshold.
- **Chronic inter-ictal 'schizophrenia-like' psychosis** A chronic schizophrenia-like psychotic illness is 6–12 times more common in epileptics than in the general population. It is particularly associated with left temporal lobe epilepsy and is more common in early onset severe epilepsy and in women with epilepsy. There is often a period of 10–15 years that elapses between diagnosis of epilepsy and onset of the psychotic illness. Clinically the illness is very similar to 'idiopathic' schizophrenia although there tends to be a prominent affective component. The chronic course is likewise similar. There is typically no family history of schizophrenia and an absence of premorbid schizotypal traits. Pathologically, it may represent the cumulative effects of chronic kindling due to a temporal lobe focus (e.g. in TLE).

1 Sachdev P (1998) Schizophrenia-like psychosis and epilepsy: the status of the association. *AJP* **155**, 325–36.
2 Lishman WA (1997) *Organic Psychiatry*. Blackwell Science (UK).

Psychiatric aspects of epilepsy (2)

Other presentations

Cognitive deterioration is a common outcome of chronic epilepsy and is caused by a number of factors including repeated seizures with cerebral hypoxia as well as the neurological effects of chronic anti-convulsant therapy.

Neuroses Epilepsy is associated with a 50% risk of a major depressive episode. Suicide risk is also increased x25 over non-epileptics. There is an increased prevalence of conversion disorder in epileptics, including an increased risk of 'pseudoseizures'.

Mania Flor-Henry first described the association between right-side TLE and manic illness.

Epileptic personality syndrome Also named the Waxman-Geshwind syndrome, this is a controversial phenomenon traditionally associated with chronic TLE. The classic traits include: religiosity; hyposexuality; hypergraphia; and 'viscosity of personality'.

Violence Also a controversial issue. There does seem to be an increased risk of violence and aggression in people with TLE or frontal lobe epilepsy. 'Episodic dyscontrol' is believed to be the result of sub-threshold kindling in these regions of the brain and anti-convulsants are often effective in reducing aggressive outbursts.

The ecstatic seizures of Prince Myshkin

He was thinking, incidentally, that there was a moment or two in his epileptic condition almost before the fit itself (if it occurred in waking hours) when suddenly amid the sadness, spiritual darkness and depression, his brain seemed to catch fire at brief moments…. His sensation of being alive and his awareness increased tenfold at those moments which flashed by like lightning. His mind and heart were flooded by a dazzling light. All his agitation, doubts and worries, seemed composed in a twinkling, culminating in a great calm, full of understanding…but these moments, these glimmerings were still but a premonition of that final second (never more than a second) with which the seizure itself began. That second was, of course, unbearable.

Dostoevsky: *The Idiot*

HIV/AIDS and psychiatry (1)

The HIV/AIDS epidemic means that, increasingly, psychiatrists are encountering individuals with psychological and neuropsychiatric complications of HIV infection. In some developing countries, rates of infection are as high as 20–30% (with rates in hospitals as high as 70–80%). Both diagnosis with the disease and the mortality associated with it has major consequences for the psychological and social functioning of individuals and their communities. In areas where large numbers of young adults are dying from the disease, there are even larger numbers of children becoming orphans, with all the developmental, emotional, and social problems associated with the loss of parental care and support. In other communities people with HIV/AIDS are subject to stresses related to their lifestyle choices (e.g. prejudice related to sexual orientation or directed at those with addictions). Stigma also contributes to the psychological burden of infected individuals and their families.

Improved outcome for patients on anti-retroviral therapy brings additional stresses related to living with uncertainty about the future. The responsibility of carers working with patients with HIV/AIDS goes far beyond treating immediate physical problems. Holistic practice requires the health care professional to adopt a true biopsychosocial approach with appreciation of the emotional state of the patient as well as the host of social, economic, spiritual, and ethical challenges accompanying diagnosis with the disease.

Contexts in which psychiatric problems may arise

There are a number of contexts in which psychiatric problems may arise in relation to HIV/AIDS:

- The 'worried well' (i.e. HIV-ve people may be concerned about being infected due to contact with HIV+ve sources/individuals).
- Pre-test anxiety.
- Post-test stress may precipitate a psychiatric illness such as adjustment disorder, major depressive episode, and suicidality.
- Living with HIV/AIDS often results in stressful life events (e.g. losing a job, becoming economically disadvantaged, experiencing social alienation).
- In some cases individuals with psychiatric needs (e.g. victims of abuse; LD patients) may be more vulnerable to becoming infected with the virus.
- HIV directly infects neurons in the brain causing neuropsychiatric symptoms.
- HIV+ve individuals are susceptible to 2° opportunistic infections and/or tumours of the CNS, which may manifest as neuropsychiatric symptoms.
- Anti-retroviral medications may cause psychiatric symptoms (e.g. AZT may precipitate a major depressive episode, while isoniazid prophylaxis has been known to precipitate a psychotic illness).

Counselling HIV/AIDS patients

- **Pre-test counselling** Consider: meaning of a +ve result; what actions the individual will take; confidentiality issues; fears of individual; high

risk behaviours; reactions to stress; social and other implications of +ve result.
- **Post-test counselling** Clarify distortions; assess emotions; decide who to tell; discuss prevention of transmission; offer support to individual and family.

Ethical issues

- **HIV testing**: issues of informed consent; only test without consent if a test result will significantly alter clinical management.
- **Confidentiality**: encourage individual to tell sexual partner and other medical personnel; if individual refuses, one may be obliged to inform without consent.
- **Resource allocation**: e.g. availability of anti-retroviral drugs.

HIV/AIDS and psychiatry (2)—clinical presentations

Depression

At least 30–50% of individuals with the disease become depressed (MDE) at some time following diagnosis. Clearly depression in this context has multiple causes and the challenge is to identify all the contributory factors. Depressive illness should be differentiated from physical effects of HIV (weight loss, loss of energy, etc.) as well as from HIV-associated dementia. *Treatment*: SSRIs, but problems of weight loss and headache; newer compounds such as Nefazodone and Venlafaxine may be indicated.

Suicide

There is a 30x increased risk of suicide in individuals who are HIV+ve. High-risk times include: at diagnosis; at the death of an HIV+ve friend; as the individual experiences deterioration in physical health.

Mania

Manic symptoms may develop in the context of HIV psychosis or as a result of treatment with anti-retroviral agents such as AZT. *Treatment*: Lithium is preferable (beware risk of toxicity) since there is some evidence suggesting that sodium valproate may increase viral replication and reduce WCC.

Anxiety

Infection with the virus is associated with increased risk of GAD, panic disorder, PTSD, and OCD.

Chronic pain

Up to 80% of patients experience chronic pain at some point, in particular chronic headache. This may lead some individuals to self-medicate, putting them at risk of substance dependence.

Delirium

Delirium occurs in up to 30% of infected patients and is sometimes irreversible. It is caused either by direct infection of the brain by the virus or by 2° infections and/or tumours. Delirium may be the initial manifestation of HIV-associated dementia.

Psychosis

A psychotic illness characterised by fluctuating symptoms that may alter over hours to days may occur in the context of HIV infection. Atypical bizarre psychotic symptoms may give way to prominent mixed affective symptoms, which in turn may change to a withdrawn apathetic state.

Aetiological factors include the effects of stress, medications, and 2° infections/tumours superimposed on the effects of direct infection of the brain by the virus. Thus psychosis is a common early manifestation of subsequent HIV-associated dementia and it is likely that mild cognitive deficits coexist with the psychotic illness.

Preferred treatment includes low-dose haloperidol or an atypical (e.g. olanzapine, quetiapine)—due to increased sensitivity to extrapyramidal side-effects. Anti-retroviral agents such as AZT may also reduce psychotic symptoms.

HIV-associated dementia (HAD)
Previously termed 'AIDS dementia', HAD is a relatively common outcome in full-blown AIDS.

Epidemiology 90% of AIDS patients have CNS changes post-mortem. 70–80% develop a cognitive disorder. 30% develop HAD. Mean survival after diagnosis with HAD is 6 months.

Pathology
(a) *Direct CNS infection*: HIV is neurotropic, entering the brain through endothelial gaps; the virus attaches to group 120 on CD4 +ve sites of microglial cells; a cascade opens calcium channels leading to glutamate and nitrous oxide excitotoxicity; this results in neuronal death and increased apoptosis. Sites include basal ganglia and sub-cortical and limbic white matter.
(b) *Opportunistic infections/tumours*: toxoplasmosis, papovavirus, CMV, HSV, non-Hodgkin's lymphoma, and Kaposi sarcoma give rise to variable neuropathology including encephalitis and focal necrosis.

Clinical presentation
- *Early 'minor' cognitive disorder*: asymptomatic HIV+ve patients may have very early CNS infection that is often discounted as 'stress'. Symptoms include cognitive slowing and memory deficits as well as motor slowing and subtle incoordination.
- *HIV-associated dementia (HAD)*: with worsening of symptoms, the clinical picture constitutes a dementia syndrome and is an AIDS-defining disorder. Clinical features are classified as cognitive (subcortical dementia, focal cognitive deficits, amnesia, mutism), motor (movement disorders e.g. tremor, ataxia, choreo-athetosis, spasticity, myoclonus), and affective (depression, apathy, agitation, disinhibition, mania). Cognitive decline can be assessed using the *HIV Dementia Scale* and the *Global Deterioration Scale of Reisberg* (functional measure).

Investigations CT/MRI: atrophy, ↑T2 signal. CSF: opportunistic infection, cytology, ELISA+ve. EEG: generalised slowing.

Treatment Reverse transcriptase inhibitors (AZT) delay HAD progression, while protease inhibitors reduce HIV load.

Neuropsychiatric aspects of CNS infections

Viral encephalitis

- **Mumps, varicella-zoster, arbovirus, rubella**—may result in behavioural problems, learning difficulties, and ADHD-like symptoms in children.
- **HSV 1**—involves inferior frontal and anterior temporal lobes, resulting in the acute phase, in delirium, hallucinations, and TLE. Chronic outcomes include Korsakoff's psychosis, dementia, and Kluver-Bucy syndrome. *EEG*: slowing with bursts of increased slow-wave in the temporal region.
- **Influenza**—a rare chronic outcome is *Encephalitis Lethargica* (see p. 169), characterised by parkinsonism, oculogyric crises, and psychosis.
- **Ebstein-Barr virus/infectious mononucleosis**—may result in myalgic encephalitis or chronic fatigue syndrome.
- **Measles**—rarely gives rise to subacute sclerosing panencephalitis, a 'slow virus infection'. *Features* include: behavioural problems, deteriorating intellectual function, movement disorders (ataxia, myoclonus), seizures, and, finally, dementia in a child. *Pathology*: white and grey matter changes to occiput, cerebellum and basal ganglia. *EEG*: 'periodic complexes'.

Tuberculosis

- **TB meningitis**—especially in children and young adults; caseating exudate covers the base of the skull leading to vascular infarcts and hydrocephalus; cranial nerves may become involved. *Psychiatric symptoms* include: apathy; withdrawal; insidious personality changes; delirium; hallucinations; chronic behavioural problems.
- **Tuberculoma**—presents with focal signs, seizures, raised ICP.

Neurosyphilis

Historically known as '**General Paresis of the Insane**' or '**Cupid's disease**', neurosyphilis is a chronic outcome of direct spirochaetal infection of the brain parenchyma. It manifests more commonly in men in their 40s-50s, roughly 15–20 years after infection. The spirochaetes have a predilection for frontal and parietal lobes and the disease typically presents as a progressive frontal dementia.

Classic symptoms Grandiosity, euphoria, and mania with mood-congruent delusions. Disinhibition, personality change, and memory impairment are also common.

Neurological features Argyll-Robinson pupils; 'trombone tongue'; tremor; ataxia; dysarthria; myoclonus; hyperreflexia; spasticity; and extra-pyramidal signs.

'Megalomania in General Paralysis'

Gentlemen,—You have before you today a merchant, aged forty-three, who sits down with a polite greeting, and answers questions fluently and easily…His illness began about two years ago. He became absent-minded and forgetful, to such an extent at last that he was dismissed by the firm for whom he had worked. Then, a year ago, he became excited, made extensive purchases and plans, weeping now and then in the deepest despair, so that he had to be taken into the hospital. On admission, he felt full of energy…and intended to write verses here, where he was particularly comfortable. He could write better than Goethe, Schiller, and Heine. The most fabulous megalomania quickly developed. He proposed to invent an enormous number of new machines, rebuild the hospital, build a cathedral higher than that at Cologne, and put a glass case over the asylum. He was a genius, spoke all the languages in the world, would cast a church of cast-steel, get us the highest order of merit from the Emperor, find a means of taming the madmen, and present the asylum library with 1000 volumes, principally philosophical works. He had quite godly thoughts… When at its height, the disease may present a great resemblance to maniacal states, but the physical examination and proof of the defective memory will save us from confusing it with them. So also will the senseless nature of the plans and the possibility of influencing them, and the feebleness and yielding character of the manifestations of the will, which are all greater in general paralysis.

Kraepelin E (1913) *Lectures on Clinical Psychiatry*,
3rd English Ed. Bailliére, Tindall and Cox: London.

Autoimmune disorders and psychiatry

Systemic lupus erythematosis (SLE)

This multi-system autoimmune vasculitis is most common in women in their 30s and neuropsychiatric symptoms occur in 75% of individuals with the disease. CNS changes include microvasculitis with infarction, inflammation, and coagulopathy. Seizures, cranial nerve palsies, peripheral neuropathy, 'spinal stroke', and other focal signs may occur in addition to dermatological, rheumatological, haematological, and cardiovascular complications of the disorder. Importantly, drugs used to treat the condition may have psychiatric side-effects (e.g. steroids; Isoniazid; Hydralazine). Psychiatric symptoms occur in 60% of cases and syndromes include:

- **'Lupus psychosis'**—transient psychotic episodes with a recurrent and fluctuating course. Relapses are frequent and symptoms are variable with auditory and visual hallucinations as well as paranoia, affective instability, and disturbed sensorium characteristic of the illness. Severe and prolonged psychosis due to SLE may result in vascular dementia.
- **Depression**—up to 30% of SLE patients experience clinically significant depressive illness.
- **Schizophrenia-like psychosis**—a rare finding in SLE.

Poly-arteritis nodosa (PAN)

Most common in young men, PAN is an immune-mediated necrotising vasculitis characterised by saccular aneurysms and infarction. Neuropsychiatric findings include: stroke; focal signs; seizures; 'spinal stroke'; delirium; auditory and visual hallucinations.

Movement disorders in psychiatry

Movement disorders occur in three contexts within psychiatry:
- **Extra-pyramidal diseases with psychiatric symptoms** (e.g. Parkinson's disease)
- **Psychiatric disorders with abnormal movements** (e.g. stereotypies; tics)
- **Medication-induced movement disorders** (e.g. EPSEs)

Pathophysiology Movement disorders commonly involve a disequilibrium of neurotransmitters such as dopamine (DA), acetylcholine (ACh), and GABA within the circuits of the basal ganglia. Levels of DA and ACh tend to be inversely related. For example, in parkinsonism, there is ↓DA with ↑ACh; conversely, chorea is characterised by ↑DA and ↓ACh.

Core symptoms in extra-pyramidal disease:
- **Negative symptoms**—bradykinesia, postural abnormalities, etc.
- **Positive symptoms**—rigidity and involuntary movements (resting tremor, chorea, athetosis, hemiballismus, dystonia)

'Parkinsonism' This is a syndrome characterised by 4 core symptoms: slow "pill-rolling" tremor (4Hz); rigidity; bradykinesia; postural abnormalities.
Aetiology includes:
- Degenerative diseases—idiopathic Parkinson's disease (PD) (85% cases); progressive supranuclear palsy (PSNP); multiple system atrophy (MSA); corticobasal degeneration (CBD); ALS-dementia-Parkinson complex of Guam (ADPG)
- Medication—neuroleptics; antidepressants
- Toxins—cobalt; manganese; magnesium; organophosphates
- Infections—Encephalitis lethargica (post-influenza); CJD
- Miscellaneous—CVA of the basal ganglia; trauma of the basal ganglia; NPH; neoplasia of the basal ganglia; dementia pugilistica ('punch drunk' syndrome); Lewy body dementia

Multiple system atrophy (MSA) 3 syndromes: striatonigral degeneration; Shy-Drager syndrome; olivopontocerebellar degeneration. Characterised by: parkinsonism; ataxia; vertical gaze palsies; pyramidal signs; autonomic abnormalities.

Progressive supranuclear palsy (PSNP) Also known as Steele-Richardson-Olzewski syndrome, PSNP has its onset in the 50s and 60s and is characterised by a tetrad of clinical findings: subcortical dementia; pseudobulbar palsy; supranuclear palsy; dystonia (of the head and neck).

Encephalitis lethargica Roughly 20 years after the great influenza epidemic of the 1920s, large numbers of patients who had suffered influenza encephalitis during the epidemic, developed this disorder (also called '**post-encephalitic parkinsonism**'). **Clinical findings** were: parkinsonism; oculogyric crises; pupillary abnormalities; psychosis). The disorder was the subject of the book (and film) by Oliver Sacks entitled Awakenings.*

---

* Recent examination of archived brain material from the epidemic has failed to demonstrate influenza RNA. It is now thought to be autoimmune mediated—see Dale RC, Church AJ, Surtees RA, et al. (2004) Brain **127**, 21–33.

Parkinson's disease (PD) and psychiatry

Parkinson's disease results in progressive impairment of voluntary initiation of movement, associated with a dementia of variable severity, as well as psychiatric morbidity. It is caused by gradual loss of dopaminergic neurons in the substantia nigra (pars compacta). This results in reduced DA and increased ACh in the basal ganglia. The remaining cells of the substantia nigra contain Lewy bodies.

Epidemiology Occurs in 20:100 000 people; typically has its onset in the 50s and peaks during the 70s; ♂:♀ = 3:2; 5% of cases are familial; 25% patients are disabled or die within 5 years and ~60% within 10 years; rare survival ~20 years.

Symptoms and signs of PD

- **Tremor**—resting, 'pill-rolling' tremor of 4Hz; this is an early sign that may start unilaterally and may be asymmetrical in intensity; tremor increases with excitement or fatigue and diminishes during sleep.
- **Rigidity**—'lead-pipe' or 'cog-wheel' rigidity, especially in flexor muscles.
- **Bradykinesia**—slowness; difficulty initiating movement; reduced facial expression and blinking; 'mask facies'; reduced arm swing; 'festinating gait'; reduced voluntary speech; micrographia; 'freezing' episodes.
- **Postural abnormalities**—flexed posture; postural instability with frequent falls.
- **Autonomic instability**—postural hypotension; constipation; urinary retention; sweaty, greasy, seborrheic skin; hypersalivation with drooling.
- **Fatiguability**.
- **+ve glabellar tap**.
- **'Air pillow sign'**.

Dementia in PD

20–30% of patients develop some cognitive deterioration. Risk of dementia in patients with PD is increased 2–3 fold. Risk of dementia increases with increasing age, increasing severity of symptoms, and coexistent cardiovascular disease.

   Clinically usually a subcortical dementia with slowing, impaired executive function, personality change, and memory impairment. Some patients merely develop 'subtle cognitive deficits' (difficulties with shifting and sequence).

   Pathology due to reduced DA in the frontal lobes; there is some evidence of overlap with LBD, while some patients have coexisting DAT.

Depression in PD

Very common finding with 40–70% patients affected. While depression may be partly 'reactive' to receiving the diagnosis or experiencing a worsening of PD symptoms, the depressive illness may be due to the actual disease process itself. Specifically, reduced levels of monoamines (DA, NA, and 5HT) may lead to depression. Mood fluctuations are often noted in association with changes in plasma DA levels. Depression in PD is more common in women and in left-sided disease and is often atypical in nature.

Treatment: SSRIs; ECT (improves the depressive illness but can precipitate delirium).

Psychosis/delirium in PD

Psychotic depression is most common. Psychosis is commonly due to medications used in PD such as:

- **Anticholinergics**—delirium; agitation; hallucinations; etc.
- **L-Dopa and DA agonists**—10–50% have psychiatric complications including delirium, psychosis, and mania.

Treatment Use 'atypical' antipsychotics with a lower risk of EPSEs.

Huntington's disease (HD)

A genetic disease characterised by a combination of progressive dementia and worsening chorea. There is autosomal dominant inheritance with 100% penetrance; thus 50% of a patient's offspring will be affected. Onset of symptoms and diagnosis is usually after the patient has reproduced. A diagnostic test has become available which allows presymptomatic diagnosis, but as no treatment is available, there are major ethical issues surrounding screening.

Pathology The genetic defect is a trinucleotide repeat of CAG—between 37 and 120 repeats on chromosome 4. ↓↓GABA neurons in the basal ganglia; this leads to increased stimulation of the thalamus and cortex by the globus pallidus. Also increase in DA transmission.

Clinical features Classic triad of chorea, dementia, and a family history of HD. Chorea is a movement disorder characterised by initial jerks, tics, gross involuntary movements of all parts of the body, grimacing, and dysarthria. There is increased tone with rigidity and stiffness, positive primitive reflexes, and abnormal eye movements. **Clinical course**: onset usually during 30s and 40s; a small number of 'juvenile onset' cases; deteriorating course to death within 10–12 years.

Psychiatric syndromes Occur in 60–75% of patients with HD.
• Anxiety and depression are common
• Psychosis occurs early and paranoia is common—'schizophrenia-like'
• Aggression and violence
• Subcortical dementia—slowing, apathy and amnesia

Investigations *EEG*: slowing. *CT/MRI*: atrophy of basal ganglia with 'boxing' of the caudate and dilation of ventricles. *PET*: ↓metabolism in the basal ganglia.

Treatment No treatment arrests the course of the disease. However haloperidol (or other antipsychotics) may help reduce abnormal movements.

Wilson's disease (WD)

A rare genetic disease mapped to the long arm of chromosome 13 that involves an abnormality of copper metabolism. Copper deposits in the liver cause cirrhosis and in the basal ganglia, resulting in degeneration of the lentiform nucleus ('hepato-lenticular degeneration').

Clinical features Onset in childhood/adolescence or early adulthood. Liver cirrhosis. E/P signs include: tremor; dystonia; increased tone; 'flapping tremor' of wrists; 'wing beating tremor' of shoulders; 'risus sardonicus' of face; bulbar signs (dysphagia, dysarthria); Kayser-Fleisher rings (green-brown corneal deposits).

Psychiatric syndromes
- Mood disturbances—common
- Subcortical dementia—25%
- Psychosis—rare

Investigations ↑serum/urine copper; ↓caeruloplasmin.

Treatment Penicillamine.

Other movement disorders

Tics

Tics are spontaneous, stereotyped movements that can be motor or vocal and usually involve ↑DA in the basal ganglia. Tics are classified as 1° or 2°.

1° tics A spectrum with genetic overlap with each other and with ADHD and OCD (p. 602):
- Tourette syndrome
- Transient tic disorder
- Chronic motor or vocal tic disorder

2° tics
- Infection—CJD; Sydenham's chorea; encephalitis
- Drugs—L-dopa; Ritalin; cocaine; amphetamines
- Other—toxic (CO); CVA; trauma

Tremor
- **Exaggerated physiological tremor**—(8–12Hz); occurs at rest and with action; causes: stress; anxiety; caffeine; medications.
- **Essential tremor**—(6–12Hz); at rest, with action and postural; most noticeable symmetrically in upper limbs.
- **Extrapyramidal tremor**—(4Hz); resting tremor; e.g. parkinsonism.
- **Cerebellar, midbrain, or red nucleus**—(4–6Hz); intention tremor; causes: trauma; vascular; MS; neoplasia; etc.

Catatonia (see pp. 898–9)
A motor syndrome that has several causes and is diagnosed (DSM-IV) by the presence of 2 or more of the following:
- Motor immobility—catalepsy ('waxy flexibility'); stupor
- Motor excitement
- Negativism or mutism
- Posturing, stereotypies, or mannerisms
- Echolalia or echopraxia

Schizophrenia and related psychoses

Introduction

The term 'psychosis' has a number of different meanings. It is sometimes used simply as a synonym for 'severe mental disorder'. It can also be used as a qualifier to distinguish this group of disorders from the 'neurotic disorders' which tend to be defined by exaggerated or quantitatively abnormal responses (e.g. exaggerated anxiety, fear of certain stimuli, exaggerated grief) rather than symptoms which are *qualitatively* different from normal experience (e.g. hallucinations/delusions, formal thought disorder). The 'true' meaning of psychosis[1] is, however, simply the presence of hallucinations and/or delusions. The presence of these symptoms without conspicuous mood symptoms is what many people would conceptualise as 'the essence' of schizophrenia.

Schizophrenia is one of a group of psychiatric disorders traditionally called the 'functional psychoses'. The functional[2] psychoses include psychotic depression, bipolar disorder, schizoaffective disorder, delusional disorder and others, as well as schizophrenia.

The symptoms of schizophrenia are conventionally divided into positive (new symptoms or signs) and negative (loss of a previous function):

- **Positive symptoms** Delusions (commonly persecutory, thought interference, or passivity) and hallucinations (usually auditory hallucinations commenting on the subject or referring to them in third person e.g. 'he looks like a fool').
- **Negative symptoms** Loss of the normal level of motivation or drive, loss of awareness of socially appropriate behaviour, flattening of mood, and difficulty in abstract thinking.
- **Other symptoms** Formal thought disorder (a loss of the normal flow of thinking usually shown in the subject's speech or writing), agitation, depression, poor concentration, poor sleep, 'soft' non-localising neurological signs, cognitive impairment.

Schizophrenia strikes individuals in their late adolescence or early adulthood and has a devastating effect on their subsequent lives and the lives of their families. The presence of this chronic and debilitating disease severely impairs the individual's quality of life and their prospects for employment, marriage, and parenthood. In addition to this personal tragedy, schizophrenia creates a substantial public health burden due to the cost of lifelong health care needs and lost productivity. Fortunately, there are effective interventions that can benefit individuals and help them to lead more normal lives. Current research is directed towards establishing the cause(s) of schizophrenia and investigating the possibility of *early* interventions in those identified at high risk for the disorder or with prodromal symptoms.

---

1 This is the modern meaning of 'psychosis' as used in ICD-10 and DSM-IV.

2 The term functional was used to distinguish them from disorders where there was a demonstrated lesion.

Why are there so few famous people with schizophrenia?

Often there is a history of declining social and educational function which precludes significant achievements (sometimes in spite of early promise). The chronic course of the condition and the major disruptions caused by periods of more severe symptoms also makes it less likely that a person with schizophrenia will achieve as much as their peers. Until relatively recently there have been few specific treatments for the disorder, and even today prognosis is at best guarded (see p. 196).

Nonetheless, there are notable exceptions to the rule: people who have battled with the disorder and achieved greatness in their chosen fields—in the arts, Vaslov Fomich Nijinski (1891–1950), the 'God of the Dance', whose personal account is to be found in his autobiography 'The Diary of Vaslov Nijinksy' (1999); in sport, Lionel Aldridge (1941–1998), a member of Vince Lombardi's legendary 'Green Bay Packers' of the 1960s, who played in two Super Bowls, and, until his death, gave inspirational talks on his battle against paranoid schizophrenia; and, in popular music, Roger (Syd) Barrett (1946–) of Pink Floyd and Peter Green (1946–) of Fleetwood Mac. Perhaps the most famous, due to a recent academy award-winning dramatisation of his life, is the mathematician John Forbes Nash Jr. (1928–), who was awarded (jointly with Harsanyi and Selten) the 1994 Nobel Prize in Economic Science for his work on game theory. His life story (upon which the film was based) is recorded by Sylvia Nasar in the book A Beautiful Mind (1998).

Background (1)—historical overview

In 1856, Morel coined the term 'démence précoce' to describe a once bright and active adolescent patient who had gradually become silent and withdrawn. Other clinical descriptions included Kahlbaum's 'Katatonie' (1868), Griesinger's (1868) 'primare Verrücktheit' (insanity that developed in the absence of mood disturbance), Hecker's 'Hebephrenie' (1869), and Sommer's inclusion of deteriorating paranoid syndromes in the concept of dementia (1894). It was Emil Kraepelin, who in the 5th edition of his textbook of psychiatry (1896) separated, on the basis of different symptoms, and validated by differences in prospective outcome data, two major forms of insanity. The first, manic-depressive insanity, had a relapsing and remitting course, with full recovery after each episode. The second grouped together catatonia, hebephrenia, and the deteriorating paranoid psychoses under the term 'dementia praecox', which had a progressive deteriorating course, where any improvement was only partial.

Over the next two decades (and further revisions of his textbook), Kraepelin's ideas were gradually accepted, although the influence of Freud's psychoanalytical ideas shifted the focus from Kraepelin's 'disease of the brain' to a 'splitting of the mind' (schizophrenia), as proposed by Eugen Bleuler in his book *Dementia Praecox or the Group of Schizophrenias*(1911). He believed the disorder to be due to a 'loosening of associations' between psychic functions, with fundamental symptoms being thought disorder, blunting/incongruity of affect, autism, and ambivalence. He added 'simple schizophrenia' to Kraepelin's subtypes and did not consider hallucinations, delusions, and catatonic symptoms to be necessary for the diagnosis. This view of schizophrenia was to have a profound influence on clinical practice, particularly in the USA, and led to blurring of the boundaries of what actually constituted schizophrenia, when it could be diagnosed without the presence of psychotic symptoms.

European psychiatrists, particularly in Germany, still regarded schizophrenia as a disease of the brain. Detailed classification systems were developed based on symptomatology, culminating in the teachings of Kurt Schneider, who described 'symptoms of first rank' in the acute phase of the illness (see opposite page) and 'second rank symptoms' which, although highly suggestive of schizophrenia (in the absence of organic brain disease), could also occur in other psychoses (e.g. emotional blunting, perplexity, and other kinds of delusions and hallucinations).

The differences in diagnostic practices were highlighted in the 1970s. In 1972, Cooper found identical symptomatology in psychiatric admissions in New York and London, but higher rates of schizophrenia diagnosed in NY. Similarly, in 1973, the WHO's *International Pilot Study of Schizophrenia* found the incidence of schizophrenia, using agreed diagnostic criteria, to be 0.7–1.4 per 10 000 aged 15–54 across all countries studied, but with much higher rates of diagnosis evident in Washington and Moscow. This was explained by broader syndrome definition, related in the US to considering many milder abnormalities as part of the schizophrenia spectrum, and in the USSR to the political pressure to declare dissidents 'insane'.

This led to a international push towards operationally defined criteria (based on symptoms and course), with various systems proposed. The St Louis Criteria (Feighner *et al.* 1972) require the patient to have been continuously ill for 6 months, with no prominent affective symptoms, the presence of delusions, hallucinations, or thought disorder, and for personal and family history to be taken into account (marital status, age under 40, premorbid social adjustment). Other systems adopt the Schneiderian concept of schizophrenia, including Catego (Wing et al., 1974)—a computer programme that uses the PSE to generate diagnoses (without accounting for symptom duration/presence of affective symptoms); Spitzer et al.'s (1975) research diagnostic criteria (RDC)—requiring at least 2 week's duration, lack of affective symptoms, presence of thought disorder, and hallucinations and delusions similar to Schneiderian first-rank symptoms; as well as our current versions of the ICD-10 (WHO 1992) and the American Psychiatric Association's DSM-IV (1994) criteria (see p. 186).

Schneider's 'symptoms of first rank' (1959)

- *Auditory hallucinations* taking the form of one of the following:
  - Voices repeating the subject's thoughts out loud ('Gedankenlautwerden', 'écho de la pensée') or anticipating their thoughts.
  - Two or more hallucinatory voices discussing the subject or arguing about them in the third person.
  - Voices commenting on the subject's thoughts or behaviour, often in the form of a running commentary.
- The sensation of alien thoughts being put into the subject's mind by some external agency (**thought insertion**) or of their own thoughts being taken away (**thought withdrawal**).
- The sensation that the subject's thinking is no longer confined to their own mind, but is instead shared by, or accessible to, others (**thought broadcasting**).
- The sensation of feelings, impulses, or acts being experienced or carried out under external control, so that the subject feels as if they were being hypnotised or had become a robot (**passivity of affect, impulse, or volition**)
- The experience of being a passive and reluctant recipient of bodily sensations imposed by some external agency (**somatic passivity**)
- **Delusional perception**—a delusion arising fully fledged on the basis of a genuine perception which others would regard as commonplace and unrelated

Background (2)—pathophysiological hypotheses

More recent attempts have been made to categorize schizophrenia on the basis of symptomatology, course, treatment responsiveness, outcome, and structural or functional brain abnormalities. Examples of these include:

Crow's (1980) two syndrome hypothesis of schizophrenia[1]

Type 1 Predominant positive symptoms, acute onset, good premorbid adjustment, good treatment response, normal cognition and brain structure, reversible neurochemical disturbance.

Type 2 Predominant negative symptoms, insidious onset, poor premorbid adjustment, poor treatment response, impaired cognition, structural brain abnormalities (ventricular enlargement), underlying irreversible neuronal loss.

Andreasen's (1982) positive and negative symptoms of schizophrenia[2]

Schizophrenic symptoms can be seen to represent either an excess or a distortion of normal functioning (so-called positive symptoms) or a decrease or loss of functioning (negative symptoms). Even as early as 1931, Hughlings-Jackson considered positive symptoms to be 'release phenomena' occuring in healthy tissue and attributed negative symptoms to neuronal loss. Andreasen and Olsen (1982) validated this concept using factor analysis, and subsequently developed scales for assessing positive and negative symptoms (SAPS and SANS).

Positive symptoms Formal thought disorder, disorganised behaviour, inappropriate affect, delusions, and hallucinations.

Negative symptoms Poverty of thought and speech, impaired volition, blunted affect and anhedonia, and social withdrawal.

Liddle's (1987; 1992) three syndrome hypothesis of schizophrenia[3,4]

Using both examination of symptomatology and functional brain imaging Liddle et al. identified three syndromes in schizophrenia disease processes with associated perfusion patterns.

Psychomotor poverty syndrome Poverty of speech, flattened affect, and decreased spontaneous movement; hypoperfusion of left dorsal prefrontal cortex, extending to the medial prefrontal cortex and the cingulate cortex and hypoperfusion in the head of caudate; reduced ability to generate action.

Disorganisation syndrome Disorders of form of thought and inappropriate affect; hypoperfusion of right ventral prefrontal cortex and increased activity in anterior cingulate and dorsomedial thalamic nuclei projecting to the prefrontal cortex; relative hypoperfusion of Broca's area and bilateral hypoperfusion of parietal association cortex; reduced ability to inhibit inappropriate mental activity.

Reality Distortion Syndrome Delusions and hallucinations; increased activity in left parahippocampal region and left striatum; disorder of internal monitoring.

Weinberger's (1987) neurodevelopmental model[5]

Based on the findings of non-specific histopathological changes in the limbic system, diencephalon, and prefrontal cortex of patients with a diagnosis of schizophrenia. This pathology (a form of fixed 'lesion') occurs early in development, and interacts with normal brain maturational events that occur much later. It is proposed that the appearance of diagnostic symptoms is linked to the normal maturation of brain areas affected by the early developmental pathology, particularly the dorsolateral prefrontal cortex. The course of the illness and the importance of stress may be related to normal maturational aspects of dopaminergic neural systems, particularly those innervating prefrontal cortex.

1 Crow TJ (1980) Molecular pathology of schizophrenia: more than one disease process? *BMJ* **280**, 66–8.

2 Andreasen NC and Olsen S (1982) Negative v positive schizophrenia. Definition and validation. *Arch Gen Psychiatry* **39**, 789–94.

3 Liddle PF (1987) The symptoms of chronic schizophrenia. A re-examination of the positive-negative dichotomy. *BJP* **151**, 145–51.

4 Liddle PF, Friston KJ, Frith CD, *et al.* (1992) Patterns of cerebral blood flow in schizophrenia. *BJP* **160**, 179–86.

5 Weinberger DR (1987) Implications of normal brain development for the pathogenesis of schizophrenia. *Arch Gen Psychiatry* **44**, 660–9.

Background (3)—neurotransmitter theories

It is unlikely that the aetiology of schizophrenia, with its multi-faceted clinical presentations, could be fully explained by a single neurotransmitter abnormality (although there are precedents, notably Parkinson's disease). Indeed, in the study of models for psychosis, particularly with the 'psychotomimetic' (psychosis-mimicking) effects of certain drugs, there is evidence for the involvement of multiple neurotransmitters in the genesis of psychotic symptoms. Nonetheless, the dopamine (DA) theory of psychosis remains the most widely accepted theory of neurotransmitter abnormalities (and DA hyperactivity may be a final common pathway for various psychotomimetics). Some of the evidence implicating different neurotransmitters is outlined below:

Dopaminergic overactivity

- The fact that all known effective antipsychotics are DA antagonists.
- Demonstrated positive correlation between the antipsychotic efficacy of a drug and its potency as a DA receptor antagonist.
- Induction of psychotic symptoms by dopaminergic agents (e.g. amphetamine, cocaine, phencyclidine (PCP), L-dopa, bromocriptine).
- Evidence of a correlation between the DA metabolite homovanillic acid (HVA) plasma levels and both severity of psychotic symptoms and treatment response to antipsychotics.

Glutaminergic hypoactivity

- NMDA receptor antagonists, (e.g. ketamine) have been shown to induce both positive and negative symptoms of schizophrenia in healthy volunteers (possibly via modulation of the DA system).
- The effects of ketamine (in both animals and humans) are attenuated by antipsychotic medication (notably clozapine).

Serotonergic (5-HT) overactivity

- The primary mode of action of LSD is through partial 5-HT agonism, associated with sensory distortions and hallucinations.
- The superior efficacy of clozapine in treatment-resistant cases of schizophrenia is thought to be due to its combined dopaminergic and serotonergic antagonism.

α_1-adrenergic overactivity

- Some antipsychotics also have clear adrenergic antagonism.
- Increased levels of noradrenaline (NA) have been found in the CSF of patients with acute psychotic symptoms.
- Chronic treatment with antipsychotic drugs leads to decreased firing rates in the locus coeruleus (the origin of the noradrenergic system).

γ-aminobutyric acid (GABA) hypoactivity

- Loss of GABA inhibition has been shown to lead to overactivity in other neurotransmitter systems (e.g. DA, 5-HT, NA).

- There is some evidence to support loss of GABAergic neurones in the hippocampus of patients with schizophrenia.
- Use of benzodiazepines may augment the therapeutic effects of antipsychotic, by their GABA facilitation.

Diagnosis (1)—symptoms and categories

The diagnosis of schizophrenia is made on the basis of symptoms and, to date, no confirmatory test is available. For this and other reasons, several concepts of schizophrenia exist and patients meeting criteria in one diagnostic system may not satisfy the criteria in another[1]. DSM-IIIR (and its successor DSM-IV) and ICD-10 were the first to set out operational criteria against which a clinical diagnosis could be confirmed (see table) and both give greater weight to certain delusions or hallucinations formerly referred to as 'first rank'.

N.B. It is possible to satisfy both sets of criteria without ever displaying one of these symptoms. DSM-IV criteria for schizophrenia include that symptoms must have been present for at least 6 months, in contrast to ICD-10, which dictates symptoms should have been present for only 1 month. This means that DSM criteria are somewhat narrower than those used by ICD-10, and some would argue renders the ICD-10 cut-off more valid.

Diagnostic hierarchy

In the past it was customary to make a diagnosis of schizophrenia when patients showed certain hallucinations or delusions, regardless of whether criteria for depression or mania were also met. However, DSM-IV and ICD-10 both classify schizophrenia and affective disorders at the same level and a diagnosis of schizophrenia should not be made where the criteria for mania or depression are also met, except where the symptoms of schizophrenia clearly predate the affective symptoms.

1 McGuffin P, Farmer A, Harvey I (1991) A polydiagnostic application of operational criteria in studies of psychotic illness. Development and reliability of the OPCRIT system. *Arch Gen Psychiatry* **48**, 764–70.

Categories

Schizophrenia has been sub-classified on the basis of symptoms into the following syndromes or subtypes:

ICD-10	DSM-IV	Key symptoms
Paranoid schizophrenia	Paranoid Type	Delusions and hallucinations
Hebephrenic schizophrenia	Disorganised type	Disorganised speech behaviour (often silly/shallow) and flat or inappropriate affect
Catatonic schizphrenia	Catatonic type	Psychomotor disturbance (see pp. 898–9)
Undifferentiated schizophrenia	Undifferentiated type	Meeting general criteria, but no specific symptom subtype predominates
Post-schizophrenic depression		Some residual symptoms, but depressive picture predominates
Residual schizophrenia	Residual type	Previous 'positive symptoms' less marked; prominent 'negative' symptoms
Simple schizophrenia		No delusions or hallucinations—a 'defect state' (negative symptoms) gradually arises without an acute episode.

Note:
- Although these sub-types are listed in both ICD-10 and DSM-IV, their nosological status remains uncertain (however, note similarity between Liddle's three syndromes and simple, hebephrenic and paranoid subtypes—see pp. 180–1).
- Hebephrenia and simple schizophrenia are believed to have the worst prognosis, although this observation may be confounded by negative symptoms, which appear to independently confer a worse prognosis whatever symptoms characterise the acute episodes.

Diagnosis (2)—ICD-10/DSM-IV criteria

DSM-IV schizophrenia

A. Characteristics of symptoms: two or more of the following, each present for a significant portion of time during a 1-month period (or less if successfully treated):

- Delusions
- Hallucinations
- Disorganised speech
- Grossly disorganised or catatonic behaviour
- Negative symptoms (i.e. affective flattening, alogia, or avolition)

N.B. only one 'A' symptom is required if delusions are bizarre or hallucinations consist of a voice keeping up a running commentary on the person's behaviour or thoughts, or two more voices conversing with each other.

B. Social/occupational dysfunction

C. Duration: continuous signs of the disturbance persist for at least 6-months. This 6-month period must include at least one month of symptoms that meet criterion A.

N.B. DSM-IV also allows for course specifiers: 'episodic'—with (no) inter-episode residual symptoms (with negative symptoms); 'continuous' (with prominent negative symptoms); 'single episode in partial remission' (with prominent negative symptoms); 'single episode in full remission'; 'other or unspecified pattern'.

ICD-10 schizophrenia

1. At least one of the following:

- Thought echo, insertion, withdrawal, or broadcasting.
- Delusions of control, influence, or passivity; clearly referred to body or limb movements or specific thoughts, actions, or sensations; and delusional perception.
- Hallucinatory voices giving a running commentary on the patient's behaviour or discussing him/her between themselves, or other types of hallucinatory voices coming from some part of the body.
- Persistent delusions of other kinds that are culturally inappropriate or implausible, (e.g. religious/political identity, superhuman powers and ability).

2. Or, at least two of the following:

- Persistent hallucinations in any modality, when accompanied by fleeting or half-formed delusions without clear affective content, persistent over-valued ideas, or occurring every day for weeks or months on end.
- Breaks of interpolations in the train of thought, resulting in incoherence or irrelevant speech or neologisms.
- Catatonic behaviour such as excitement, posturing, or waxy flexibility, negativism, mutism, and stupor.
- Negative symptoms such as marked apathy, paucity of speech, and blunting or incongruity of emotional responses.

- A significant and consistent change in the overall quality of some aspects of personal behaviour, manifest as loss of interest, aimlessness, idleness, a self-absorbed attitude, and social withdrawal.

3. Duration of ≥ 1 mth.

Other clinical presentations

Schizophrenia may occasionally present with symptoms more typically characteristic of another disorder (e.g. depression, mania, OCD, panic disorder). Occasionally the diagnosis may take months/years to become clear.

Catatonia

True incidence unknown but probably in decline. Catatonia is considered to be a variant of schizophrenia and is included as such in both ICD-10 and DSM-IV (i.e. catatonic schizophrenia/schizophrenia—catatonic type). Some authors argue for its reinstatement as a disorder in its own right, or that catatonic symptoms may be features of a variety of primary psychiatric diagnoses (not just schizophrenia)[1].

Clinical features Stupor, waxy flexibility, mannerisms, stereotypy, ambitendency, mitgehen/mitmachen, and automatic obedience.

Differential diagnosis (see p. 899) Depression, manic stupor, organic disorders, other drug-related causes (e.g. NMS—pp. 868–9).

Management Parenteral lorazepam and ECT may be helpful in addition to antipsychotic treatment.

Water intoxication

Occurs particularly in patients with chronic schizophrenia. Cause(s) unknown although many have been suggested[2].

Clinical features Presents with polyuria, hyponatraemia, and polydipsia. May cause confusion, seizures, cerebral and peripheral oedema. May be fatal.

Differential diagnosis Renal failure, syndrome of inappropriate ADH secretion, IDDM/NIDDM

Investigations U&E and plasma osmolality, glucose, haematocrit, 24hr creatinine clearance, renal USS, and specialist referral where appropriate (severe, recurrent, or life-threatening)

Management Restrict oral fluids, review and/or optimise antipsychotic medication.

---

1 Taylor MA and Fink M (2003) Catatonia in psychiatric classification: a home of its own. *AJP* **160**,1233–41.

2 Ferrier IN (1985) Water intoxication in patients with psychiatric illness. *BMJ* **291**,1594–6.

Epidemiology

Epidemiology

Incidence The incidence of schizophrenia worldwide is relatively similar when restricted, operational diagnostic criteria are used to establish the diagnosis. The incidence in the UK and US is around 15 new cases per 100 000 population. $\male = \female$, although males tend to have an earlier onset than females (23y vs. 26y) and develop more severe illnesses. A few studies have reported a falling incidence over time, although this may be due to changing diagnostic practices/criteria.

Prevalence The lifetime risk of schizophrenia is between 7 and 13 per 1000 population. The point prevalence is between 2 and 5 per 1000. There are some differences between countries, although these differences are minimised when a restrictive definition of schizophrenia based on first-rank symptoms is used.

Mortality Suicide is the most common cause of premature death in schizophrenia. It accounts for 10–38% of all deaths in schizophrenia. Risk is probably highest in the year after first presentation[1].

Genetic factors Genetic factors account for the majority of liability to schizophrenia. Heritability estimates range from 60–80%. The liability to schizophrenia depending on which relative(s) are affected is shown in the table.

Environmental factors The following have been associated with an increased risk of schizophrenia:
- Complications of pregnancy, delivery, and the neonatal period
- Delayed walking and neurodevelopmental difficulties
- Early social services contact and disturbed childhood behaviour
- Maternal influenza in pregnancy and winter births
- Degree of urbanisation at birth

Social theories In the 1960s social theories of schizophrenia (e.g. schizophrenogenic mother, marital skew and schism) were common. They are now of historical interest only, having not withstood scientific scrutiny.

Schizophrenia liability based on affected relatives

Family member(s) affected	Risk (approximate)
Identical twin	46%
One sibling/fraternal twin	12–15%
Both parents	40%
One parent	12–15%
One grandparent	6%
No relatives affected	0.5–1%

1 Mortensen PB and Juel K (1993) Mortality and causes of death in first admitted schizophrenic patients. *BJP* **163**, 183–9.

Integrated aetiological theories

A number of integrated aetiological theories have been developed to explain the disparate findings:

The neurodevelopmental hypothesis

Some authors hypothesise that schizophrenia may be a disorder of neurodevelopment based on the following:

- There is an excess of obstetric complications in those who develop the disorder.
- Affected subjects have motor and cognitive problems which precede the onset of illness.
- Schizophrenic subjects have abnormalities of cerebral structure at 1st presentation.
- Schizophrenic subjects have dermatoglyphic and dysmorphic features.
- Although the brain is abnormal, gliosis is absent—suggesting that differences are possibly acquired in utero.

The disconnection hypothesis

Neuropsychological, neuroanatomical, and functional investigations (SPET, PET, fMRI) have revealed:

- Widespread reductions in grey matter in schizophrenia (particularly temporal lobe).
- Disorders of memory and frontal lobe function occurring in a background of widespread cognitive abnormalities.
- Reduced correlation between frontal and temporal blood flow on specific cognitive tasks.
- A reduction in white matter integrity in tracts connecting the frontal and temporal lobes.

These findings have led to speculation that frontal-temporal/parietal connectivity may be the final common pathway for the development of schizophrenia

Neurodegenerative theories

A number of studies have suggested that the brain changes found in first-episode schizophrenic subjects progress over time. This has led some to speculate that schizophrenia is at least partially acquired during adolescence/early adulthood[1].

Other theories

A number of other theories exist, including those which postulate that schizophrenia is an abnormality of:

- Information processing[2]
- Meta-representation/'theory of mind'[3]
- Working memory
- Neuronal migration
- Language[4]

A note on formulation

Even in the absence of a specific cause, the aetiology of schizophrenia is predominantly influenced by factors affecting the brain. However, the following areas might be considered as a guide to the assessment of predisposing, precipitating, and perpetuating factors:

- **Biological** Consider family history of psychiatric illness, recent substance misuse, drug non-compliance, history of obstetric complications, brain injury, and comorbid medical illness.
- **Psychosocial** Consider recent stressful life events, family cohesion/friction, living conditions, attitude and knowledge of illness.

1 See: Weinberger DR, McClure RK (2002) Neurotoxicity, neuroplasticity, and magnetic resonance imaging morphometry: what is happening in the schizophrenic brain? *Arch Gen Psych* **59**, 553–8 for review and critique.

2 Braff DL (1993) Information processing and attention dysfunctions in schizophrenia. *Schizophr Bull.* **19**, 233–59.

3 Pickup GJ and Frith CD (2001) Theory of mind impairments in schizophrenia: symptomatology, severity and specificity. *Psychol Med.* **31**, 207–20.

4 Berlim MT, Mattevi BS, Belmonte-de-Abreu P, Crow TJ (2003)The etiology of schizophrenia and the origin of language: overview of a theory. Compr Psychiatry **44**, 7–14.

Differential diagnosis

Common differentials Acute/transient psychotic disorder, delusional disorder, paranoid personality disorder, bipolar disorder, depressive episode with psychotic symptoms, manic episode with psychotic symptoms, drug intoxication or withdrawal, drug-induced psychosis, alcohol withdrawal. Negative symptoms may also be mimicked by the effects of medication (extrapyramidal side-effects, sedation) or by depression coexisting or following an acute episode of illness.

Uncommon differentials Agoraphobia, generalised anxiety disorder, panic disorder, and obsessive-compulsive disorder. Schizophrenia-like symptoms may also be the expression of underlying 'organic' brain disease (tumour, TLE, post-epileptic states, vCJD) metabolic (hypernatraemia, hypocalcaemia) or endocrine disturbance (hyperthyroidism, Cushing's syndrome). Rarely, psychotic symptoms are feigned in factitious disorder (pp. 752–3).

Physical examination

Neurological Full neurological examination is the most important 'investigation' of all. Particularly: fundoscopy; gait inspection; examination of four limbs for weakness/altered sensation; examination of hand-eye coordination; and cranial nerve examination are all mandatory.

Cognitive examination Orientation, attention/concentration, and anterograde/retrograde memory (minimum). Consider underlying neurological condition when disorientation present (even in acute episode) or if memory problems are severe or persistent in spite of adequate treatment.

Investigations

Blood tests *Routine*: U + E, LFT, calcium, FBC, glucose. *When suggested by history/examination*: VDRLs, TFTs, PTH, cortisol, tumour markers.

Radiological CT or MRI only in the presence of suggested neurological abnormality or persistent cognitive impairment. CXR only where examination/history suggests comorbid respiratory/cardiovascular condition.

Urine Urine drugs screen (particularly stimulants and cannabis), microscopy and culture (where history suggestive).

Other EEG rarely necessary unless history of seizure or symptoms suggest TLE.

Special investigations 24hr collection for cortisol (if Cushing's disease suggested from history/examination). 24hr catecholamine/5-HIAA collection for suspected phaeochromocytoma/carcinoid syndrome respectively.

Course and prognosis

There is usually a large degree of uncertainty regarding the course and prognosis in first-episode patients, regardless of their presenting symptoms or demographic/personal history.

Approximate guide to course and prognosis at 13 years' follow-up[1]:

- Approximately 15–20% of first episodes will not recur.
- Few people will remain in employment.
- 52% are without psychotic symptoms in the last two years.
- 52% are without negative symptoms.
- 55% show good/fair social functioning.

Prognostic factors in schizophrenia

Poor prognostic indicators Poor premorbid adjustment; insidious onset; early onset in childhood/adolescence; cognitive impairment; enlarged ventricles; symptoms fulfil more restrictive criteria (e.g. DSM-IV).

Good prognostic factors Marked mood disturbance, especially elation, during initial presentation; family history of affective disorder; female sex; living in a developing country.

---

1 Mason P, Harrison G, Glazebrook C, et al. (1995) Characteristics of outcome in schizophrenia at 13 years. *BJP* **167**, 596-603.

Patients presenting with acute psychotic symptoms

Initial assessment

In view of the range and variety of presentations and the broad differential (p. 194), it is difficult to be prescriptive in dealing with a patient who presents with psychotic symptoms (i.e. hallucinations and delusions). Symptoms may range from mild paranoid ideas to severe systematised delusions with associated auditory hallucinations. Often it is difficult to establish a clear history initially, and assessment is focused on the immediate concerns:

• The risk they currently pose to themselves—not just the possibility of acts of self-harm (p. 730) or suicide (p. 731), but also because of other aspects of their behaviour (e.g. police becoming involved, family relationships, work, continued driving, etc.)
• Risk of violence—the nature of risk (pp. 646–7) and any association with current symptoms (e.g. delusions about a specific person or group of individuals; what the 'voices' are telling them to do).
• The degree of insight retained by the patient and the likelihood of them cooperating with medical management.
• Whether their current behaviour is so disturbed as to require urgent treatment (p. 200)—to allow further assessment, including physical examination and other routine investigations (p. 195).
• Whether hospital admission or transfer to a psychiatric ward is warranted to assess and manage the acute symptoms (with or without the use of the MHA).
• The person's current social circumstances and the level of support available to them (partner, relatives, friends, CPN, etc.) that may allow some flexibility in management (as well as being a source of 3rd party information).

When there is a good account of the history of the presenting complaint(s), it may be possible to establish the most likely diagnosis and proceed accordingly (e.g. drug-or alcohol-related disorder (pp. 542–3, p. 560), acute confusional state (pp. 734–5), first episode of schizophrenia (p. 202), relapse of known schizophrenia (p. 203), delusional disorder (pp. 230–5), acute psychotic disorder (pp. 202–3)).

The initial assessment is also a critical time, particularly with *unmedicated* patients, to record (verbatim if possible) specific aspects of the patient's psychopathology (nature and content of delusions and hallucinations), before they become modified by the necessary use of medication. This information is important as it will influence later decisions regarding, for example, assessment of treatment response and need for continued use of MHA.

Points to note

• When available, any records of past or current contact with services will be invaluable in determining the best course of action, when confronted with urgent and difficult situations.

- Comorbidity is high for drug and alcohol problems in patients with schizophrenia—addressing immediate concerns (see above) is more important than debating the causal link when faced with a patient who is acutely psychotic.
- The greatest influence on your course of action will be the reason why the person has been referred in the first place (e.g. brought up by a concerned relative, no longer able to be managed at home, breach of the peace, self-referral because of own concerns, attempted suicide).

Hospital admission

As noted above, certain clinical features and situations will determine whether hospital admission (or transfer to psychiatric ward) is necessary:
- High risk of suicide or homicide.
- Other illness-related behaviour that endangers relationships, reputation, or assets.
- Severe psychotic symptoms.
- Severe depressive symptoms.
- Catatonic symptoms.
- Lack of capacity to cooperate with treatment.
- Lack or loss of appropriate psychosocial supports.
- Failure of outpatient treatment.
- Non-compliance with treatment plan (e.g. depot medication) for patients detained under the MHA (recall to hospital as part of CPA, 'aftercare under supervision', or community treatment order).
- Significant changes in medication for patient at high risk of relapse (including clozapine 'red' result—p. 220).
- Need to address comorbid conditions (e.g. inpatient detoxication, physical problems, serious medication side-effects).

Suitability of the ward environment

For a patient experiencing significant acute psychotic symptoms, a busy psychiatric ward may not be a perfect environment. As far as possible the person should be nursed in calm surroundings (a single room, if possible), with little stimulation (e.g. unfamiliar people, TV, radio). When managing risk, a balance ought to be struck between the necessity of regular observation and the likelihood that this may reinforce persecutory delusions. If behaviour becomes unmanageable despite regular medication, it may be necessary to consider referral of the patient to a more secure environment.

Early review

Regular review is critical in the first 72 hrs in order to assess any improvement in mental state, response to medication, level of observation needed, and to carry out statutory duties under the MHA (including the need for continued detention, if emergency powers have been used). This is also a time for information gathering from friends, family, GP, other agencies, etc. and organising any investigations, including physical examination and routine blood tests that may not have been possible initially.

Treating psychotic symptoms

Emergency treatment

Follow guidance as detailed for the management of acute behavioural disturbance (pp. 896–7).

Points to note

- Attempts to diffuse the situation (e.g. careful observation from a distance) should be attempted, whenever possible.
- Reassurance and the offer of voluntary oral/intramuscular medication is often successful.
- The content of delusions and hallucinations is of poor diagnostic value, but may better predict violence/behavioural disturbance.
- Act decisively and with sufficient support to ensure restraint and forcible administration of medication proceeds without unnecessary delay or undue risk to the patient or staff.
- Do not attempt to manage severe violence on an open ward when secure facilities with appropriately trained staff are available elsewhere.

Non-urgent treatment

In the treatment of psychotic symptoms, antipsychotic medication has the strongest evidence base. Although little evidence exists to support the choice of one drug over the other (see p. 126), the following may be used as a guide to treatment.

Option 1[1]

- Commence atypical antipsychotic(amisulpride, risperidone, olanzapine, quetiapine, or zotepine) at an effective dose (see BNF).
- Use long-acting benzodiazepine (e.g. diazepam) to control non-acute anxiety/behavioural disturbance.

Option 2

- Prescribe a low potency antipsychotic (such as chlorpromazine), initially in the range 100–200 mg/day in divided doses for a first episode.
- Increase the dose according to clinical effect and the need for sedation.
- Previous episodes and the response/side-effects experienced should inform the management of subsequent episodes.
- No additional antipsychotic benefit is likely when doses of 400–600 mg chlorpromazine (or equivalent) are exceeded, However, sedation may be a useful effect of increasing the dose above this level.

Extrapyramidal side-effects (EPSEs)

- EPSEs are less likely with option 1, although the tolerability of both options overall is approximately equal[2].
- Prescribe procyclidine (or alternative) orally as required for parkinsonian side-effects.
- Review regularly, since requirement for procyclidine may diminish over time and the drug may contribute to non-response and tardive dyskinesia.

Psychological
- There is some evidence that CBT, family therapy, and psychoeducation may be helpful during acute episodes.
- However, there is often a long waiting list, or no provision at all, for these interventions.

Social
- Liaison with family and carers; and provide information on diagnosis and progress.
- Refer to a social worker for resolution of housing or other difficulties as they arise.

1 www.nice.org.uk

2 Geddes J, Freemantle N, Harrison P, Bebbington P (2000) Atypical antipsychotics in the treatment of schizophrenia: systematic overview and meta-regression analysis. *BMJ* **321**, 1371–6.

Considerations in the management of schizophrenia[1]

The management of schizophrenia should include, wherever possible, the usual features of good medical practice, including:
- Involving patients and their relatives in decisions about medical care.
- Undertaking a comprehensive assessment of medical, social, and psychological needs.
- Providing patients and carers with clear verbal and, if necessary, written information.
- Obtaining consent from the patient for any procedures or treatments.

Prodromal interventions

Before an individual fulfils DSM-IV/ICD-10 criteria for schizophrenia, there may be an intervening period of disturbed behaviour and partial psychotic symptoms that suggest, especially in the presence of other risk factors, that schizophrenia is imminent and inevitable. This observation has led some to propose early interventions for schizophrenia which aim to prevent a schizophrenic episode by treating these 'prodromal' symptoms. However, since many people with partial symptoms and behaviour disturbance never develop schizophrenia, the efficacy of these interventions must be addressed using RCTs.

While some evidence has emerged that 'prodromal' treatment may prevent, or at least delay onset of schizophrenia[2], the research has been widely criticised for several reasons. It is possible that evidence supporting or refuting these early interventions will emerge in the lifetime of this text.

The first schizophrenic episode

The first episode of schizophrenia is often a time of diagnostic uncertainty. Frequently, the clinical picture includes comorbid substance misuse, personality difficulties, recent stressful life events, or a combination of all three.
- It is usually necessary to admit people suspected of first schizophrenic episodes in order to assess the extent of their psychopathology, to provide a time for education of both the patient and their family, and to provide pharmacological and psychological treatments in an environment where compliance can be carefully assessed.
- Inpatient admission is <u>always</u> necessary where the patient poses a significant danger to themselves or others.
- In practice, stringent admission criteria are difficult to establish since in the individual patient risk is difficult to assess and there are few well-designed prospective studies which can be used to guide clinical practice.

Acute presentations

There are many possible presentations of schizophrenia. Many people experiencing their first episode will have no personal or family experience to draw upon and will find their symptoms particularly distressing. It is

common for acute, particularly first episodes, to present in crisis. The following presentations (or their variants) are commonly seen:
- A spouse or relative noticing withdrawn or bizarre behaviour.
- Not achieving educational potential—referred by school or student health services.
- Complaining to GP about various symptoms.
- Presentation to criminal justice system (see section on schizophrenia and offending, p. 644).
- Deliberate self harm.
- Complaining to council/police etc. on basis of delusional symptoms (e.g. hearing voices of neighbours throughout the night).

Management

Principles of assessment and management are as for patients presenting with psychotic symptoms (pp. 198–9). Once the acute symptoms have settled, a more considered view of management may be taken, with the aims of establishing compliance with medication, minimising side-effects, and addressing residual problems (e.g. persistent psychotic symptoms, social/family interventions, psychological treatments), with the ultimate aims of successful discharge (pp. 204–5) and outpatient follow-up (p. 208).

Treatment continuation
- After the symptoms of an acute episode subside, it is important not to reduce the dose of antipsychotic medication prematurely, since early relapse is a frequent consequence.
- In general the treatment dose which has been successful in abolishing symptoms in the acute episode should be continued as the prophylactic dose in the medium term (i.e. up to 2 years).

Subsequent episodes

Subsequent presentations may be similar to those mentioned above, but are probably more likely to include negative symptoms. Examples include:
- Complaints to GP about depression[*] or negative symptoms.
- Long-term unemployment/rising debts.
- Social isolation (e.g. homelessness).
- Complaints about medication side-ffects, especially EPSEs.
- Non-compliance with medication.

Management
- The treatment decisions taken at later episodes will depend on several factors including: compliance with medication, therapeutic response, side-ffects, and 'treatment resistance' (p. 206).
- The usual goal is to commence, reinstate,or continue antipsychotic treatment.
- There is little evidence of benefit from high dose or polypharmacy and clozapine is the only intervention for treatment-resistant schizophrenia for which there is good evidence.

[*] Post-schizophrenic depression is a common differential diagnosis.

1 www.nice.org.uk

2 www.pace-clinic.org

Discharge planning

Good communication between members of the multidisciplinary team (psychiatry, community nurse, GP, social worker, etc.) is essential for good overall care. This may be formalised using the care programme approach (CPA), when patients are detained under the MHA, although many of the components are useful in everyday practice:

Components of CPA (as implemented in Edinburgh):
- Assess clinical and other needs.
- Formulate a care plan.
- Arrange discharge planning meeting where patient, carer(s), and key clinical staff are invited.
- Appoint a care manager who should be contacted in case of concern.
- Maintain contact with the patient.
- Decide on criteria for recall and/or other interventions.
- Document the people involved in the care package and their responsibilites.
- Arrange to meet again as a group.

For further discussion of CPA and 'aftercare under supervision' see Mental health legislation—England & Wales (pp. 806–7).

Relapse prevention

Medication Continue antipsychotic medication at minimum necessary dose. Possible regimes include:
- An atypical antipsychotic (amisulpride, olanzapine, risperidone, quetiapine, zotepine).
- A preferably non-sedating, conventional antipsychotic (e.g. trifluoperazine, flupenthixol, haloperidol).
- Depot antipsychotic medication, particularly where use of oral medication has resulted in relapse due to non-compliance. Depot medication is slightly more effective[1] than oral antipsychotic treatment.

Psychological[2]
- Family therapy and psychoeducation are effective in reducing relapse.
- Less convincing evidence also exists for CBT.
- Compliance therapy may be helpful.

Social/community
- Social work and housing involvement are often necessary.
- Community psychiatric nurses (CPNs) may help to provide information/education and monitor for early signs of relapse.
- For patients on depot, non-attendance at GP surgery/CPN appointment may act as an 'early warning' system.

Service provision

- Community mental health teams provide effective treatment.
- Assertive community treatment may provide additional benefits.
- CPA may reduce the risk of losing contact.
- Day hospitals can provide an alternative to inpatient care in some situations.

1 Adams CE, Fenton MK, Quraishi S, David AS (2001) Systematic meta-review of depot antipsychotic drugs for people with schizophrenia. *BJP* 179,290-9.

2 Nadeem Z, McIntosh A, Lawrie S (2003) Schizophrenia. *Clinical Evidence* **Jun(9)**, 1103–33

An approach to treatment-resistant schizophrenia (TRS)

Definition

Treatment resistance is the failure to respond to 2 or more antipsychotic medications given in therapeutic doses for 6 weeks or more.

Patients with refractory symptoms have severe functional impairments and are more likely to have abnormalities of cerebral structure and neuropsychology.

Prevalence

Approximately 30% of patients respond poorly and the number of people who show 'total non-response' is ~7%.

Aetiology

The aetiology is uncertain. However, the following factors may be important:

- 'Neurodevelopmental' factors: soft signs, history of obstetric complications, cognitive impairment.
- Drug non-compliance.
- Lack of adequate treatment: poor drug administration/absorption. However over-treatment (>12 mg haloperidol or equivalent) may also lead to poor tolerability/response.
- Aggravating factors *despite* adequate treatment: concurrent drug misuse, anticholinergic effects of anti-parkinsonian medication or antidepressants.

Management

- **Clarify diagnosis** The clinical history and presentation should always be re-inspected to ensure the correct diagnosis has been reached.
- **Address comorbidity and non-compliance** Comorbid substance misuse is common in schizophrenia, but is nevertheless treatable. Consider interventions such as psychoeducation, compliance therapy, or family therapy to improve compliance with prescribed medication.
- **Pharmacological interventions** Clozapine is the intervention most strongly supported by the evidence. However, there is also evidence that depot antipsychotic medication may convey a small advantage over the same compound given orally.
- **Rehabilitation** When conventional pharmacological/psychological interventions fail, behavioural, social work, and non-evidence based pharmacological interventions may help a few individuals. Interventions of possible benefit include: pindolol supplementation of existing antipsychotic treatment and augmentation of clozapine with amisulpride.

Outpatient treatment and follow-up

Medical

- Conduct a MSE at every appointment.
- Enquire about side-effects and attitude to medication.
- Record any recent life events or current stresses.
- Enquire about suicidal ideas and, if appropriate, homicidal ideas.
- When symptoms appear unresponsive to treatment, review the history and provide additional investigations/interventions as appropriate (e.g. clozapine).
- Conduct appropriate investigations where complications of illness or its treatment arise (e.g. LFT, FBC, U&E, glucose), or where monitoring is indicated (e.g. high-dose guidelines p. 216, ECG—when cardiac complication are common).

Psychological

- Above all, try to provide supportive and collaborative treatment wherever possible.
- Provide education about schizophrenia and its treatment.
- Do not dismiss concerns, even if apparently based on delusional content[1].
- Offer to meet family members or carers where appropriate.
- Be aware that following an acute episode, post-psychotic depression is particularly common but also treatable[2].

Social

- Remember statutory obligations (e.g. review of compulsory powers).
- Consider referral to social work where there are housing, benefit, or other problems.
- Drop-in community centres and other support provided by non-statutory or voluntary organisations are often helpful.
- Consider interventions offered by other professions (e.g. occupational therapy, physiotherapy) when particular problems arise (e.g. poor sleep, hygiene, anxiety management, etc).
- Some patients and their carers find user organisations helpful (e.g. SANE or Rethink—see useful addresses pp. 916–18).

1 McCabe R, Heath C, Burns T, Priebe S (2002) Engagement of patients with psychosis in the consultation: conversation analytic study. *BMJ* **325**, 1148–51.

2 Whitehead C, Moss S, Cardno A, Lewis G (2003) Antidepressants for the treatment of depression in people with schizophrenia: a systematic review. *Psychol Med.* **33**, 589–99.

General approach to prescribing

Efficacy There is some evidence than depot antipsychotic medication offers a slight advantage over antipsychotic medication given orally[1]. In TRS there is good evidence that clozapine may be more effective than other drugs.

Tolerability No single antipsychotic is substantially better tolerated than another at doses of <12 mg haloperidol or equivalent. However, conventional antipsychotics prescribed above this range are less well tolerated and probably also less effective than atypical drugs. The choice of antipsychotic therefore depends substantially on the profile of side-effects and which ones are more important to avoid.

- **Sedation** Avoid chlorpromazine/promazine. *Prescribe* high-potency antipsychotics (e.g. haloperidol) or non-sedating atypical (risperidone, amisulpride).
- **Weight gain** *Avoid* phenothiazines, olanzapine and clozapine. *Prescribe* haloperidol, fluphenazine
- **EPSEs** *Avoid* high-dose conventional antipsychotics. *Prescribe* atypical.
- **Postural hypotension** *Avoid* phenothiazines. *Prescribe* haloperidol, amisulpride, trifluoperazine.

Dosing High-potency conventional antipsychotics, (trifluoperazine, haloperidol), depot antipsychotics, and olanzapine may be given once daily. This may be an advantage in non-compliant, institutionalised, or cognitively impaired patients. In patients with complicated drug regimes, cognitive impairment, or dubious compliance, consider a compliance aid such as a ©Dosette box.

---

1 Adams CE, Fenton MK, Quraishi S, David AS (2001) Systematic meta-review of depot antipsychotic drugs for people with schizophrenia. *BJP* **179**, 290–9.

Side-effect profiles of conventional antipsychotics

Side-effects of conventional antipsychotic medication tend to fall into certain categories (antimuscarinic, antiadrenergic, antihistaminic). The following provides a guide to the side-effects of commonly used antipsychotic medication.

Group 1: 'Chlorpromazine-like' (promazine, zuclopenthixol)
- Antiadrenergic and antihistaminic side-effects predominate.

Group 2: 'Thioridazine-like' (thioridazine, fluphenazine)
- Antimuscarinic side-effects predominate.

Group 3: 'Trifluoperazine-like' (haloperidol, benperidol, droperidol)
- EPSEs predominate.

EPSEs (for assessment, see pp. 214–15)
- **Acute dystonia** Contraction of muscle group to maximal limit, typically sternocleidomastoid and tongue, although can be widespread (e.g. opisthoclonus); eye muscle involvement (e.g. oculogyric crisis) may occur. Virtually always distressing and preceded by increasing agitation. *Treatment* Parenteral antimuscarinic (e.g. procyclidine 10mg i.v.)—see p. 866 for more detail.
- **Parkinsonism** Tremor, rigidity, and bradykinesia occurring >1 week after administration. *Treatment* Consider dose reduction/use of oral antimuscarinic (e.g. procyclidine 5mg tds)—see p. 860 for more detail.
- **Akathisia** Restlessness, usually of lower limbs, and a drive to move. Occurs usually >1 month after initiation of antipsychotic drug. *Treatment* Propranolol and benzodiazepines may be helpful. Symptoms can be notoriously difficult to treat—see pp. 862–3 for more detail.
- **Tardive dyskinesia** Continuous slow writhing movements (i.e. athetosis) and sudden involuntary movements, typically of the oral-lingual region (chorea). Symptoms of TD tend to be irreversible. *Treatment*[1] Although a consequence of antipsychotic treatment, there is little evidence that a reduction in the dose of antipsychotic improves symptoms in the short or long term. Vitamin E may prevent deterioration but does not improve established symptoms—see pp. 864–5 for more detail.

Anticholinergic side-effects Dry mouth, blurred vision, difficulty passing urine, urinary retention, constipation, rarely-ileus, glaucoma.

Antiadrenergic side-effects Postural hypotension, tachycardia (sometimes bradycardia), sexual dysfunction (particularly erectile dysfunction—see p. 856).

Antihistaminic side-effects Sedation, weight gain (although precise mechanism unclear—see p. 852).

Idiosyncratic Cholestatic jaundice, altered glucose tolerance, hypersensitivity reactions, skin photosensitivity (sun block important in sunny weather), yellow pigmentation to skin (chlorpromazine), neuroleptic malignant syndrome (rigidity, fluctuating consciousness, and pyrexia)—may be fatal, requires immediate transfer to general medical care and usually ICU/anaesthetic support/dantrolene may be helpful—see pp. 868–9 for more detail.

1 Soares-Weiser KV and Joy C (2003) Miscellaneous treatments for neuroleptic-induced tardive dyskinesia. *Cochrane Database Syst Rev.* **3**, CD000208.

Side-effect profiles of atypical antipsychotics

All atypical antipsychotics (amisulpride, clozapine, olanzapine, quetiapine, risperidone, zotepine) are less likely to cause EPSEs compared to conventional drugs. Side-effects are listed for each drug[1]. Clozapine is covered separately in a subsequent section (pp. 222–3).

Amisulpride Drowsiness/ insomnia, weight gain, anxiety, agitation, EPSEs, anticholinergic effects (e.g. dry mouth, constipation), increased prolactin (breast changes, sexual problems, menstrual irregularities).

Olanzapine Drowsiness and weight gain are particularly common. Also: dizziness, postural hypotension, peripheral oedema, anticholinergic side-effects, EPSEs, increases in liver enzymes (AST and ALT).

Risperidone Insomnia, agitation, anxiety, headache, EPSEs, postural hypotension, drowsiness, dizziness, impaired concentration, gastric discomfort, weight gain, blurred vision, sexual disturbances, and rash.

Quetiapine Drowsiness, dyspepsia, constipation, dry mouth, rhinitis, hypertension, tachycardia, anxiety, fever, myalgia, ear pain, rash, blood dyscrasias, elevated plasma lipids, possible QT prolongation, oedema, priapism.

Zotepine Constipation, dyspepsia, dry mouth, tachycardia, QT interval prolongation, rhinitis, agitation, anxiety, depression, asthenia, headache, increased salivation, blood dyscrasias, blurred vision, sweating, sexual dysfunction. N.B. ECG monitoring is recommended initially and at each dose increment.

Diabetes and atypical antipsychotics

At the time of writing, there had been case reports and some epidemiological evidence that risperidone and olanzapine may be linked to the onset of diabetes mellitus. It remains unclear whether this is a risk associated with all atypicals.

Cardiac effects (see pp. 880–1)

Many antipsychotics are associated with QT prolongation and sudden deaths have been associated with many compounds from different chemical classes.

- Thioridazine and droperidol are not recommended for general use because of the risk of cardiac problems.
- Many antipsychotics may cause cardiac problems in overdose. Specialist referral is suggested in all cases of overdose.
- Cardiac monitoring is always necessary for clozapine and zotepine.
- Physical examination is essential in all patients commencing on an antipsychotic. ECG examination may also be helpful, particularly in the elderly or in those with a personal or close family history of cardiac disease.

Interactions

- **Decreased breakdown:** e.g. with SSRIs and P450 inhibitors (cimetidine)
- **Increased antimuscarinic side-effects** e.g. TCAs, procyclidine
- **Decreased anticonvulsant efficacy:** carbamazepine, valproate, and others
- **Increased sedation:** TCAs, benzodiazepines, alcohol, and other CNS depressants
- **Neurotoxicity:** idiosyncratic interaction reported between haloperidol and lithium, particularly in overdose

1 See *www.bnf.org* for comprehensive information on side-effects.

Examining for abnormal involuntary movements

The Abnormal Involuntary Movements Scale (**AIMS**)[1]: is a useful tool for examining and monitoring (e.g. every 6 mths), the occurrence of EPSEs in patients on antipsychotic medication.

AIMS—examination procedure

- Either before or after completing the examination procedure, observe the patient unobtrusively at rest (e.g. in the waiting room).
- The chair to be used in this examination should be a hard, firm one without arms.
  1. Ask the patient whether there is anything in his or her mouth (such as gum or candy) and, if so, to remove it.
  2. Ask about the *current* condition of the patient's teeth. Ask if he or she wears dentures. Ask whether teeth or dentures bother the patient *now*.
  3. Ask whether the patient notices any movements in his or her mouth, face, hands, or feet. If yes, ask the patient to describe them and to indicate to what extent they *currently* bother the patient or interfere with activities.
  4. Have the patient sit in a chair with hands on knees, legs slightly apart, and feet flat on floor. (Look at the entire body for movements while the patient is in this position.)
  5. Ask the patient to sit with hands hanging unsupported—if male, between his legs; if female and wearing a dress, hanging over her knees. (Observe hands and other body areas.)
  6. Ask the patient to open his or her mouth. (Observe the tongue at rest within the mouth.) Do this twice.
  7. Ask the patient to protrude his or her tongue. (Observe abnormalities of tongue movement.) Do this twice.
  8. Ask the patient to tap his or her thumb with each finger as rapidly as possible for 10 to 15 seconds, first with right hand, then with left hand. (Observe facial and leg movements.) [± activated]
  9. Flex and extend the patient's left and right arms, one at a time.
  10. Ask the patient to stand up. (Observe the patient in profile. Observe all body areas again, hips included.)
  11. Ask the patient to extend both arms out in front, palms down. (Observe trunk, legs, and mouth.) [± activated]
  12. Have the patient walk a few paces, turn, and walk back to the chair. (Observe hands and gait.) Do this twice. [± activated]

AIMS—scoring procedure

- Complete the examination procedure before making ratings.
- For the movement ratings (the first 3 categories below), rate the highest severity observed:
  0 = none
  1 = minimal (may be extreme normal)
  2 = mild
  3 = moderate
  4 = severe

- According to the original AIMS instructions, one point is subtracted if movements are seen **only on activation**, but not all investigators follow that convention.

1. Facial and oral movements
- Muscles of facial expression (e.g. movements of forehead, eyebrows, periorbital area, cheeks frowning, blinking, grimacing).
- Lips and perioral area (e.g. puckering, pouting, smacking).
- Jaw (e.g. biting, clenching, chewing, mouth opening, lateral movement).
- Tongue. Rate only increase in movement both in and out of mouth, **not** inability to sustain movement.

2. Extremity movements
- Upper (arms, wrists, hands, fingers). Include movements that are choreic (rapid, objectively purposeless, irregular, spontaneous) or athetoid (slow, irregular, complex, serpentine). Do **not** include tremor (repetitive, regular, rhythmic movements).
- Lower (legs, knees, ankles, toes) (e.g. lateral knee movement, foot tapping, heel dropping, foot squirming, inversion and eversion of foot).

3. Trunk movements
- Neck, shoulders, hips (e.g. rocking, twisting, squirming, pelvic gyrations). Include diaphragmatic movements.

4. Global judgements
- Severity of abnormal movements. 0 1 2 3 4 (based on the highest single score on the above items.)
- Incapacitation due to abnormal movements. 0 = none, normal; 1 = minimal; 2 = mild; 3 = moderate; 4 = severe
- Patient's awareness of abnormal movements. 0 = no awareness; 1 = aware, no distress; 2 = aware, mild distress; 3 = aware, moderate distress; 4 = aware, severe distress

5. Dental Status
- Current problems with teeth and/or dentures. 0 = no; 1 = yes
- Does patient usually wear dentures? 0 = no; 1 = yes

1 AIMS was originally described by Ecdeu GW (1976) in the *Assessment Manual for Psychopharmacology*, revised ed. (Washington, DC, US Department of Health, Education, and Welfare). A more recent discussion can be found in: Munetz MR and Benjamin S (1988) How to examine patients using the Abnormal Involuntary Movement Scale. *Hospital and Community Psychiatry* **39**, 1172–7.

Guidelines for the use of high-dose antipsychotics

- High-dose antipsychotic prescribing (>1 g chlorpromazine or equivalent) should be avoided wherever possible.
- Where patients receive one or more antipsychotics at high dose, regular physical examination, ECG, LFTs, U&E, FBC should be performed.
- A local protocol should exist for the purpose of informing good medical practice.
- *There is no* evidence that high-dose prescribing confers any therapeutic advantage.

Royal College of Psychiatrists guidelines for high-dose prescribing

- Consider alternative approaches including adjuvant therapy and newer or atypical antipsychotics such as clozapine.
- Bear in mind risk factors, including obesity—particular caution is indicated in older patients, especially those over 70.
- Consider potential for drug interactions.
- Carry out ECG to exclude abnormalities such as prolonged QT interval; repeat ECG periodically and reduce dose if prolonged QT interval or other adverse abnormality develops.
- Increase dose slowly and not more often than weekly.
- Carry out regular pulse, blood pressure, and temperature checks; ensure that patient maintains adequate fluid intake.
- Consider high-dose therapy to be for limited period and review regularly; abandon if no improvement after 3 months (return to standard dosage).

Chlorpromazine equivalents for commonly prescribed conventional antipsychotics

Drug	Equivalent dose (mg)
ORAL MEDICATION	
Chlorpromazine	100
Thioridazine	100
Fluphenazine	2
Trifluoperazine	5
Flupenthixol	3
Zuclopenthixol	25
Haloperidol	2
Sulpiride	200
Pimozide	2
Loxapine	10
Risperidone	2
Olanzapine	5
Quetiapine	75
Ziprasidone	60
Aripiprazole	7.5
INJECTABLE MEDICATION	
Fluphenazine decanoate	10 every 2 weeks
Pipothiazine palmitate	40 every 4 weeks
Flupenthixol decanoate	10 every week
Zuclopenthixol decanoate	100 every week
Haloperidol decanoate	5 every 4 weeks

Clozapine (clozaril) (1)—guidelines

Clozapine is an atypical antipsychotic, which was withdrawn from use because of several episodes of fatal agranulocytosis in patients on treatment. It was thought to have special efficacy in treatment-resistant schizophrenia, and this clinical belief was supported by an important trial by Kane *et al* (1988), leading to its reintroduction in psychiatric practice, albeit with strict limitations to its prescription. Patients on clozapine must be registered with a central monitoring agency and have regular, initially weekly, full blood counts-with discontinuation of the drug where there is evidence of neutropenia.

Evidence from a Cochrane systematic review[1] has shown clozapine to be more effective than conventional antipsychotic medication in the management of acute schizophrenia (NNT 6) in both the short and long term and of even greater benefit in those patients resistant to typical antipsychotics (NNT 5). Clozapine is also more acceptable in long-term treatment than conventional antipsychotic drugs (usually haloperidol or chlorpromazine NNT 6).

NICE guidelines

NICE recommends that clozapine should be used in treatment-resistant schizophrenia where there has been a lack of a satisfactory clinical improvement 'despite the sequential use of the recommended doses for 6 to 8 weeks of at least two antipsychotics at least one of which should be an atypical'.[2]

Mode of action

Clozapine mainly blocks D_1 and D_4 receptors; its effects on D_2 receptors are relatively less than traditional antipsychotics. The lower affinity of clozapine for D_2 receptors may partially explain its lack of EPSEs and hyperprolactinaemia.

The superior efficacy of clozapine in treating resistant schizophrenic patients may be due to its additional blockade of $5HT_2$ receptors. Antipsychotic activity also may be due to an increased turnover of GABA in the nucleus accumbens, which inhibits dopaminergic neurons.

Pharmacokinetics Rapidly absorbed when taken orally (unaffected by food). Extensive first-pass metabolism means only 27–50% of a dose reaches the systemic circulation unchanged, with wide inter-individual variations in the resulting plasma concentrations (influenced by factors such as smoking, hepatic metabolism, gastric absorption, age, and possibly gender). Steady-state plasma concentrations take 7–10 days of treatment. Mean terminal elimination half-life ranges from 6–33 hours. Onset of antipsychotic effect may take several weeks, but maximal effects can require several months (and improvement may continue for up to 2 yrs).

Interactions See opposite for summary.

Contraindications Previous/current neutropenia or other blood dyscrasias, previous myocarditis, pericarditis and cardiomyopathy, severe renal or cardiac disorders, active liver disease, progressive liver disease, hepatic failure. See BNF for a complete list.

Abrupt discontinuation of clozapine is not recommended, unless required by the patient's medical condition (e.g. leukopenia). Otherwise discontinuation should usually occur via a gradual 1-2 week reduction in dosage. Patients should be carefully observed for the recurrence of psychotic symptoms during drug discontinuation. Symptoms related to cholinergic rebound, such as profuse sweating, headache, nausea, vomiting and diarrhoea may also occur.

Clozapine interactions

Effect	Examples
Increased drowsiness, sedation, dizziness, and the possibility of respiratory depression	Ethanol, H_1-blockers, opiate agonists, anxiolytics, sedatives/hypnotics, tramadol, and TCAs
Increased possibility of developing myelosuppressive effects	Concomitant use of clozapine with other drugs known to cause bone marrow depression (e.g. chemotherapy agents)
Drugs known to induce CYP1A2 activity may reduce clozapine efficacy	Carbamazepine, phenobarbital, phenytoin, rifabutin, and rifampicin
Drugs known to inhibit the activity of CYP1A2 may increase clozapine serum levels	Cimetidine, clarithromycin, ciprofloxacin, diltiazem, enoxacin, erythromycin, or fluvoxamine
Drugs known to inhibit the activity of CYP2D6 may increase clozapine serum levels	Amiodarone, cimetidine, clomipramine, desipramine, fluoxetine, fluphenazine, haloperidol, paroxetine, quinidine, ritonavir, sertraline, and thioridazine
Highly protein-bound drugs (may increase serum concentrations)	Digoxin, heparin, phenytoin, or warfarin
Worsening of anticholinergic effects	H_1-blockers; phenothiazines; TCAs; and other drugs with antimuscarinic properties
Increased risk of hypotension	Antihypertensive agents

Other specific interactions
- Lithium can increase the risk of developing seizures, confusion, dyskinesia, and possibly, neuroleptic malignant syndrome (NMS).
- May interfere with the action of AChEIs (e.g. donepezil and tacrine).
- Smoking cigarettes (tobacco) increases the clearance of clozapine and may result in a substantial reduction in clozapine plasma concentrations (higher doses of clozapine may be necessary).
- Because the plasma concentration of clozapine is increased by caffeine intake and decreased by nearly 50% following a 5-day caffeine-free period, dosage changes of clozapine may be necessary when there is a change in caffeine-drinking habit.

1 Wahlbeck K, Cheine M, Essali MA (2003) Clozapine versus typical neuroleptic medication for schizophrenia. *Cochrane Database Syst Rev.* **3**, CD000059.

Clozapine (2)

Initiation of treatment and monitoring

This is best done as either an inpatient or where appropriate facilities exist for monitoring, (e.g. at a day-patient facility). All patients must be registered with the Clozaril Patient Monitoring Service (CPMS[1])—see useful addresses,—p. 920). A normal leukocyte (WBC > 3500/mm^3, neutrophils > 2000/mm^3) count must precede treatment initiation. Full blood counts must be repeated (and sent to CPMS) at weekly intervals for 18 weeks and then fortnightly until 1 year. Blood monitoring should continue monthly indefinitely thereafter.

Dose (see opposite)

- Starting regime: 12.5 mg once or twice on first day, then 25–50 mg on second day, then increased gradually (if well tolerated) in steps of 25–50 mg daily over 14–21 days up to 300 mg daily in divided doses (larger dose at night; up to 200 mg daily may be taken as a single dose at bedtime).
- May be further increased in steps of 50–100 mg once or twice weekly.
- Usual dose 200–450 mg daily (max. 900 mg daily).
- Note: increase in seizure frequency occurs above 600 mg/day.

CPMS 'traffic light' notification

Each time a blood sample is sent to the CPMS, the results will be telephoned through to you if urgent, or will be posted in the form of a typed report, if routine. Examples of possible outcomes are listed below:

Telephone

- *No sample received* CPMS will probably suggest you send another sample to CPMS and also to your local haematology laboratory so that the next supply of medication may be dispensed.
- *Sample non-suitable for analysis* As for 'no sample received'.
- *Abnormal haematological results (e.g. neutrophil count)* CPMS may advise you to repeat the blood count or may instruct you to STOP clozapine and will advise further monitoring.

Written reports

- *Green light* Normal—clozapine may be administered to the patient
- *Amber light* Caution—further sampling advised by CPMS. If either WCC falls to 3000–3500/mm^3 or the absolute neutrophil count falls to 1500–2000/mm^3, blood monitoring must be performed at least twice weekly until the WCC and absolute neutrophil count stabilise within the range 3000–3500/mm^3 and 1500–2000/mm^3 respectively, or higher.
- *Red light* STOP clozapine immediately. This will have been preceded by a telephone call from CPMS and/or your hospital pharmacy. If either the WCC < 3000/mm^3 or the absolute neutrophil count >1500/mm^3, treatment with clozapine has to be discontinued. Blood samples must be taken daily until the abnormality is resolved. Specialist advice may be sought from a haematologist. Patients should be monitored closely for symptoms suggestive of infection and should not routinely be administered other antipsychotic drugs.

Clozapine dosing guidelines

Day	Morning dose (mg)	Night-time dose (mg)
1	—	12.5
2	12.5	12.5
3	25	25
4	25	25
5	25	50
6	25	50
7	50	50
8	50	75
9	75	75
10	75	100
11	100	100
12	100	125
13	125	125
14	125	150
15	150	150
18	150	200
21	200	200
28	200	250

* Gradually increase* by 50–100 mg/wk (max dose should not exceed 900 mg/d).
* If adverse effects are noted, reduce dose until side-effects settle, then increase again more slowly.
* Lower doses may be required for elderly, female, or non-smoking patients, and if the patient is on other medication that may affect the metabolism of clozapine.
* Where there has been a break in treatment of more than 48 hours, treatment should be re-initiated with 12.5 mg once or twice on the first day, and re-escalated.

* Routine blood level monitoring is not recommended; however, increasing dose until plasma level of 350 mcg/L is achieved is sometimes recommended.

1 Generic brands of clozapine are expected by 2004. CPMS may no longer be the sole monitoring authority

Clozapine (3)—side-effects

(See opposite for management)

Common side-effects
- **Anticholinergic** Constipation, dry mouth, blurred vision, difficulty passing urine.
- **Anti-adrenergic** Hypotension, sexual dysfunction
- **Other** Sedation, weight gain, nausea, vomiting, ECG changes, headache, fatigue, hypersalivation, tachycardia, hypertension, drowsiness dizziness.

Less common
- Fainting spells
- Gastric discomfort
- Small involuntary muscle contractions
- Periodic catalepsy (reduced responsiveness and prolonged lack of movement)
- Enuresis

Rarer or potentially life-threatening
- Impaired temperature regulation, fever, hepatitis, cholestatic jaundice, pancreatitis.
- Agranulocytosis: leucopenia, eosinophilia, leucocytosis. (N.B. the risk of **fatal agranulocytosis*** is estimated to be 1:4250 patients treated.)
- Thrombocytopenia (discontinuation of clozapine is recommended if platelet count falls below 50 000/mm^3).
- Dysphagia.
- Circulatory collapse, arrhythmias, myocarditis, cardiomyopathy, pericarditis, pericardial effusion, thromboembolism. Discontinue if persistent tachycardia occurs in the first two months of treatment. (N.B. The risk of **fatal myocarditis** or **cardiomyopathy** is estimated to be up to 1:1300 patients treated, although there is wide variation in data, (e.g. USA—1:67 000 patients treated)).
- Pulmonary embolism (N.B. The risk of **fatal pulmonary embolism** is estimated to be 1:4500 patients treated.)
- Confusion, delirium, restlessness, agitation.
- Diabetes mellitus, hypertriglyceridaemia, intestinal obstruction, paralytic ileus, enlarged parotid gland, fulminant hepatic necrosis.
- Interstitial nephritis, priapism, skin reactions.
- Neuroleptic malignant syndrome.

Of note: clozapine actually *reduces* mortality in schizophrenia, mainly due to a lower risk of suicide.

---

* A report of data from the Clozaril® National Registry revealed that agranulocytosis occurred in 400 (0.6%) of 67 600 patients during the period of 1990–95. 12 of these 400 patients died; 340 of these 400 developed agranulocytosis in the first 6 months of therapy. The incidence rate of 0.6% is similar to earlier data published in 1993. The risk of developing agranulocytosis increased with age and was higher in women.

Dealing with clozapine side-effects

Problem	Possible solution
Constipation	Encourage high-fibre diet, adequate fluid intake, use of aperients if persistent
Fever	Symptomatic relief, check FBC and look for sources of infection
Hypersalivation	Consider use of hyoscine hydrobromide (up to 300mcg tds), pirenzepine (up to 50mg tds)
Hypertension	Monitor closely, slow rate or halt dose increase, if persistent consider use of hypotensive agent (e.g. atenolol)
Hypotension	Advise caution when getting up quickly, monitor closely, slow or halt dose increase
Nausea	Consider use of anti-emetic (avoid metoclopramide and prochlorperazine if previous problems with EPSEs)
Neutropenia/ agranulocytosis	Stop clozapine, if outpatient admit to hospital
Nocturnal enuresis	Avoid fluids in the evening, alter dose scheduling, if severe consider use of desmopressin
Sedation	Reschedule dosing to give smaller morning or total dose
Seizures	Withhold clozapine for 24hrs, recommence at lower dose, consider prophylactic anticonvulsant (e.g. valproate)
Weight gain	Dietary and exercise counselling (see p. 852)

Antipsychotic depot injections

Antipsychotics may be given as a long-acting depot injection (the active drug in an oily suspension) injected into a large muscle (usually gluteus maximus), allowing for sustained release over 1–4 weeks. Previously, only conventional antipsychotics were available, but now a number of atypical preparations, with a variety of slow-release systems, have been developed and are finding their place in clinical practice. Dose for dose, the efficacy of these preparations is not greater than oral medication, but they do increase likelihood of compliance.

Indications Poor compliance with oral treatment, failure to respond to oral medication, memory problems or other factors interfering with ability to take medication regularly, clinical need to ensure patient compliance (e.g. due to treatment order for patients detained on MHA or CPA legislation).

Administration Patients should first be given a small test dose as undesirable side-effects can be prolonged. In general not more than 2–3 mL of oily injection should be administered at any one site; correct injection technique (including the use of z-track technique) and rotation of injection sites are essential. If the dose needs to be reduced to alleviate side-effects, it is important to recognise that the plasma-drug concentration may not fall for some time after reducing the dose, therefore it may be a month or longer before side-effects subside.

Dosing schedules (see opposite)

Specific side-effects Pain/swelling at injection site, rarely abscesses, nerve palsies. Side-effects as for oral medication but may take 2–3 days to emerge and may persist for weeks after discontinuation. May be more likely to cause EPSEs, although good evidence for this is lacking.

Cautions As for oral antipsychotic medication. Also: previous neuroleptic malignant syndrome or any condition where the drug may need to be withdrawn rapidly.

Dose equivalents

These equivalences are intended only as an approximate guide; individual dosage instructions should also be checked; patients should be carefully monitored after any change in medication.

⚠ **Do not extrapolate beyond the maximum dose for the drug.**

Flupenthixol decanoate 40mg/2wks
    = Fluphenazine decanoate 25mg/2wks
    = Haloperidol decanoate 100mg/4wks
    = Pipothiazine palmitate 50mg/4wks
    = Zuclopenthixol decanoate 200mg/2wks
Risperidone 25mg/2wks DEPOT is equivalent to approx. 4mg/d ORAL

Dosing schedules for depot antipsychotics

Generic name	Brand name	Test dose	Interval between test & treatment	Usual starting dose	Usual between-dose interval	Max. dose	Usual dose range
Flupenthixol decanoate	Depixol® (Lundbeck)	20mg	7 days	20-40mg	2– wks	400mg/wk	50mg/4 wks–300mg/2 wks
Fluphenazine decanoate	Modecate® (Sanofi-Synthelabo)	12.5mg	4–7 days	12.5-100mg	14–35 days		
Haloperidol decanoate	Haldol® (Janssen-Cilag)	50mg	4 wks	50-300mg	4 wks	300mg/4 wks	50mg/4 wks–300mg/4 wks
Pipothiazine palmitate	Piportil® (JHC)	25mg	4–7 days	25-50mg	4 wks	200mg/4 wks	50mg/4wks–100mg/4 wks
Zuclopenthixol decanoate	Clopixal® (Lundbeck)	100mg	7 days	200-500mg	1–4 wks	600mg/wk	
Risperidone	Risperdal Consta® (Janssen/Organon)	25mg	2 wks	25-37.5mg	2 wks	50mg/2 wks	25–50mg/2 wks

Schizotypal disorder

Schizotypal disorder is classified along with schizophrenia and related disorders in ICD-10, but along with cluster A/'odd-eccentric' personality disorders in DSM-IV. It is thought to be related to schizophrenia because:

• MZ twin studies have shown an increased risk of schizotypy in the 'unaffected' relative.
• Schizotypy is more common in the other first-degree relatives of schizophrenic subjects than in the general population.
• Relatives for schizotypal subjects have an increased risk of schizophrenia.
• Schizotypy shares some of the clinical features of schizophrenia, but not the delusions or hallucinations.

DSM-IV criteria

• Ideas of reference.
• Excessive social anxiety.
• Odd beliefs or magical thinking.
• Unusual perceptions (e.g. illusions).
• Odd/eccentric behaviour or appearance.
• No close friends/confidants.
• Odd speech.
• Inappropriate or constricted affect.
• Suspiciousness or paranoid ideas.

Epidemiology Approximately 3% of the general population and approximately 4.1% of psychiatric inpatients. The disorder tends to run a stable course.

Differential diagnosis Autism, Asperger syndrome, expressive/mixed receptive-expressive language disorder chronic substance misuse, other personality disorders (especially borderline, schizoid and paranoid)

Treatment Risperidone (≤2mg/day)[1] has some support from a RCT. Other antipsychotics may also be helpful.

---

1 Koenigsberg HW, Reynolds D, Goodman M, et al. (2003) Risperidone in the treatment of schizo-typal personality disorder. *J Clin Psychiatry* **64**, 628-34.

Schizophreniform disorder (DSM-IV)

(Included under 'other schizophrenia' in ICD-10)

Original term refers to patients with schizophrenic symptoms with a good prognosis[1]. Now refers to a schizophrenia-like psychosis that fails to fulfil duration criterion for schizophrenia in DSM-IV. Treatment is the same as for an acute episode of schizophrenia.

Good prognostic signs Psychotic symptoms appear early in illness, confusion/perplexity, good premorbid personality, absence of blunted/flat affect.

1 Langfeldt G (1982) Definition of "schizophreniform psychoses". *AJP* **139**, 703.

Schizoaffective disorder

Schizophrenia is a disorder in which the symptoms of affective disorder and schizophrenia are present in approximately equal proportion. Its nosological status is uncertain since some believe it to be a variant of schizophrenia, others, bipolar disorder, and some believe it represents a point on a continuum of 'unitary psychosis' lying quantitatively between schizophrenic and mood symptoms[1].

ICD-10

- Schizophrenic and affective symptoms simultaneously present and both are equally prominent.
- Excludes patients with separate episodes of schizophrenia and affective disorders.

DSM-IV

- Major depressive, manic, or mixed episode concurrent with symptoms that meet criterion A for schizophrenia.
- ≥2 weeks of delusions and/or hallucinations without prominent mood symptoms.
- Symptoms meeting criteria for a mood episode are present for a substantial portion of the active and residual periods.

Causes The aetiology is assumed to be intermediate to that of schizophrenia and affective disorder.

Treatment As for schizophrenia but treat manic or depressive symptoms as outlined in bipolar disorder (see pp. 318–19; pp. 320–1).

Prognosis Depressive symptoms are more likely to signal a chronic course compared to manic presentations. Good/poor prognostic factors are the same as for schizophrenia.

1 Mellor C. (1998) Chapter 11 In: Stein G and Wilkinson G (eds.) *Seminars in general adult psychiatry.* Gaskell, London.

Delusional disorder (1)

Essence Delusional disorder is an uncommon condition in which patients present with circumscribed symptoms of non-bizarre delusions, but with absence of prominent hallucinations and no thought disorder, mood disorder, or significant flattening of affect. Symptoms should have been present for at least 1 month (DSM-IV). ICD-10 specifies at least 3 months for *delusional disorder* but, if it less than this, allows diagnosis under *other persistent delusional disorder*. DSM-IV specifies particular subtypes (see opposite).

Points to note

- Patients rarely present directly to psychiatrists. More often they may be seen by other physicians due to somatic complaints, lawyers due to paranoid ideas, or the police when they act on, or complain about their delusions.
- Careful assessment and diagnosis is vital, because delusions are the final common pathway of many illnesses (see p. 232). When delusional disorder is discovered, treatment can be fraught with difficulty because of the reticent nature of such patients. With persistence, a combination of biopsychosocial treatments can be effective.

Diagnosing pathological delusions—key points[1]

Clinical judgement is necessary to distinguish delusions from overvalued ideas, particularly when the ideas expressed are not necessarily bizarre or culturally abnormal (and may actually have some basis in reality). Such judgements may be informed by:

- The degree of plausibility.
- Evidence of systemisation, complexity, and persistence.
- The impact of the beliefs on behaviour.
- Allowing for the possibility that they might be culturally sanctioned beliefs different from one's own.
- Observation of associated characteristics, including hallucinations.
- History of 'morbid change'.
- Evidence of other risk factors (see below).

Clinical features Level of consciousness is unimpaired; observed behaviour, speech, and mood may be affected by the emotional tone of delusional content (e.g. hyperalertness with persecutory delusions); thought process is generally unimpaired, but thought content reflects preoccupation with circumscribed (usually single theme), non-bizarre delusions; hallucinations may occur, but generally are not prominent and reflect delusional ideas (more commonly olfactory/tactile than visual/auditory); cognition and memory are generally intact; insight and judgement are impaired to the degree that the delusions influence thought and behaviour; risk should be formally assessed (e.g. potential for violence to self and others and past history of previous behaviour influence by delusions)—persistent anger and fear are risk factors for aggressive 'acting-out' behaviours.

Epidemiology Relatively uncommon, but not rare—prevalence estimated at 0.025-0.03% (may account for 1–2% of hospital admissions); age range

18–90yrs (mean 40–49yrs); ♂ = ♀ but delusional jealousy more common in men and erotomania more common in women; 50% of patients are in employment; 80% are married.

Risk factors Advanced age, social isolation, group delusions, low socio-economic status, premorbid personality disorder, sensory impairment (particularly deafness), recent immigration, family history, and history of head injury or substance abuse disorders.

Course and prognosis Onset may be acute or insidious. Course is very variable-with treatment: remission (33–50%), improvement (10%), persisting symptoms (33–50%). Better prognosis in acute subtypes, where stress is a factor, and for jealous or persecutory subtypes. If symptoms have persisted for >6mths outcome is worse.

DSM-IV subtypes

- **Erotomanic (de Clérambault syndrome-see p. 86)** Patients present with the belief that some important person is secretly in love with them. Clinical samples are often female and forensic samples contain a preponderance of males. Patients may make efforts to contact this person, and some cases are associated with dangerous or assaultive behaviour.

- **Grandiose** Patients believe they fill some special role, have some special relationship, or possess some special ability(ies). They may be involved with social or religious organisations.

- **Jealous[2] (Othello syndrome—see p. 87)** Patients possess the fixed belief that their spouse or partner has been unfaithful. Often patients try to collect evidence and/or attempt to restrict their partner's activities. This type of delusional disorder has been associated with forensic cases involving murder.

- **Persecutory** This is the most common presentation of delusional disorder. Patients are convinced that others are attempting to do them harm. Often they attempt to obtain legal recourse, and they sometimes may resort to violence.

- **Somatic** Varying presentation, from those who have repeat contact with physicians requesting various forms of medical or surgical treatment to patients who are delusionally concerned with bodily infestation, deformity (see *dysmorphophobia*—p. 739), or odour.

- **Mixed** Presence of one or more of the above themes; no single theme predominating.

- **Unspecified** The theme cannot be determined or does not fit the listed categories.

1 Manschreck, T (1996) Delusional disorder: the recognition and management of paranoia. *Journal of Clinical Psychiatry,* **57**(suppl 3): 32–8.

2 Shepherd M (1961) Morbid jealousy: some clinical and social aspects of a psychiatric symptom. *Journal of Mental Science* 107, 607–753. (The 'classic' paper)

Delusional disorder (2)—differential diagnosis and aetiology

Differential diagnoses

- **Substance-induced delusional disorders** (e.g. alcohol, stimulants, hallucinogens, steroids, antihistamines, sympathomimetics). Careful history taking may reveal onset, persistence, and cessation of symptoms to be related to drug use.
- **Other physical disorders** Focused history, examination, and investigations should help exclude other disorders (e.g. head injury, CNS infection, epilepsy).
- **Mood disorders with delusions (manic and depressive types)** Mood and related biological symptoms are usually more severe and *precede* delusions.
- **Schizophrenia** Presence of psychotic symptoms other than relatively circumscribed delusions, greater functional impairment.
- **Dementia and delirium** Evidence of cognitive impairment or altered/fluctuating level of consciousness.
- **Elderly patients (late paraphrenia)** Thought to be distinct from delusional disorder (see p. 480) and schizophrenia, associated with social isolation, aging, medical problems/treatments, and sensory loss.
- **Dysmorphophobia/body dysmorphic disorder** (see p. 739) Significant overlap with delusional disorder, few significant differentiating factors exist.
- **Obsessive-compulsive disorder** (see p. 358) Significant overlap with delusional disorder and, if reality testing regarding obsessions or compulsions is lost, delusional disorder often is diagnosed.
- **Hypochondriasis** (see p. 748) Health concerns generally are more amenable to reality testing and are less fixed than in delusional disorder.
- **Paranoid personality disorder** (see p. 447) Absence of clearly circumscribed delusions, presence of a pervasive, stable pattern of suspiciousness or distrust.
- **Misidentification syndromes** (see p. 239) Easily confused with delusional disorder, may be associated with other CNS abnormalities.
- **Induced/shared psychotic disorder** (see p. 238) Evidence that relatives/close friends share similar delusional beliefs.

Aetiology

Delusional disorders represent a heterogeneous group of conditions that appear distinct from mood disorders and schizophrenia, although there is significant diagnostic (and genetic) overlap with paranoid personality traits/disorder. Data suggest that among patients diagnosed with delusional disorder, less than 3–22% are later reclassified as schizophrenic and less than 10% are later diagnosed with a mood disorder.

Biological

- Delusions can be a feature of a number of biological conditions, suggesting possible biologic underpinnings for the disorder.
- Most commonly, neurological lesions associated with the temporal lobe, limbic system, and basal ganglia are implicated in delusional syndromes.
- Neurological observations indicate that delusional content is influenced by the extent and location of brain injury.
- Prominent cortical damage often leads to simple, poorly formed, persecutory delusions.
- Lesions of the basal ganglia elicit less cognitive disturbance and more complex delusional content.
- Excessive dopaminergic and reduced acetyl cholinergic activity have been linked to the formation of delusional symptoms.

Psychological/psychodynamic

- Freud proposed that delusions served a defensive function, protecting the patient from intrapsychically unacceptable impulses through reaction formation, projection, and denial.
- Cognitive delusions are seen as the result of cognitive defects where patients accept ideas with too little evidence for their conclusions; delusions as the result of attempting to find a rational basis for abnormal perceptual experiences.

Social/other

Certain social situations may increase the chances of developing delusional disorder e.g.:
- distrust and suspicion
- social isolation
- jealousy
- lowered self-esteem
- people seeing their own defects in others
- rumination over meaning and motivation

Delusional disorder (3)—assessment and management

Assessment

Patients with delusional disorder are exceptionally difficult to assess. At interview they may be evasive, guarded, and suspicious. Often they become irritated, angry, or hostile. They may be overly sensitive to some lines of questioning, even to the point of threatening legal action. Assessment should include:

- A thorough history and MSE.
- Information gathering (3rd party and other sources).
- Exclusion of underlying causation (including physical investigations) to rule out other conditions that commonly present with delusions (see *differential diagnosis*-p. 232).
- Clearly documented risk assessment (especially aggression/ self harm).

Where there is significant risk to another person/partner, duty of care may override patient confidentiality and allow warning of that individual and/or informing the police (see pp. 826–7).

Management

Typical obstacles to the treatment of delusional disorder:

- The patient's denial of the illness which causes difficulties in establishing a therapeutic alliance.
- The patient's experiences of significant social and interpersonal problems (which may confirm their firmly held beliefs).
- The fact that antipsychotic medication is often of limited efficacy.

Admission to hospital ought to be considered if there is a clear risk of harm to self or violence towards others. Otherwise, outpatient treatment is preferred. Approaches to management include:

- **Separation** From source or focus of delusional ideas (if possible).
- **Pharmacological**
  - Data for the pharmacotherapy are limited to case reports or small open-label interventions.
  - Given the symptomatic overlap with psychotic disorders, antipsychotics (typical and atypical) have some utility.
  - A recent review[1] suggested there was evidence to support the widely-held anecdotal view for the preferential use of pimozide (68.5% efficacy) above other antipsychotics (moderate benefits have been found for chlorpromazine, thioridazine, haloperidol, clozapine, and risperidone).
  - Other sources favour the use of SSRIs[2] given the overlap with obsessive-compulsive disorder, body dysmorphic disorder, and mood disorder.
  - Benzodiazepine may be useful when there are marked anxiety symptoms.
  - Data for the use of anticonvulsant agents and mood stabilisers are even more limited.

- **Psychological/psychotherapeutic**
  - *Individual therapy* requires persistence in establishing a therapeutic alliance without validating or overtly confronting the patient's delusional system.
  - *Supportive therapy* may help with isolation and distress stemming from the delusional beliefs (reframing problems due to delusional beliefs as symptoms).
  - Cognitive techniques; reality testing and reframing. *Insight-orientated therapy* to develop a sense of 'creative doubt' in the internal perception of the world through empathy with the patient's defensive position.
  - *Educational and social interventions* Social skills training (e.g. not discussing delusional beliefs in social settings) and minimising risk factors (e.g. sensory impairment, isolation, stress, and precipitants of violence).

1 Munro A and Mok H (1995) An overview of treatment in paranoia/delusional disorder. *Can J Psychiatry* **40**, 616–22.

2 Manschreck TC (1996) Delusional disorder: the recognition and management of paranoia. *J Clin Psychiatry* **57**, Suppl. 3, 32–8.

Acute and transient psychotic disorders

(Brief psychotic disorder-DSM-IV)

Clinical features Sudden onset, variable presentation (including perplexity, inattention, formal thought disorder, delusions or hallucinations, disorganised or catatonic behaviour), usually resolving within less than 1 mth (DSM-IV) or 3 mths (ICD-10).

Aetiology Sometimes these disorders occur in the context of an acute stressor (both ICD-10 and DSM-IV allow for specifying 'with or without' marked stressor(s)/acute stress) e.g. life events such as bereavement, marriage, unemployment, imprisonment, accident, childbirth, or migration and social isolation (with language and cultural factors).

Epidemiology Associated with certain personality types (e.g. paranoid, borderline, histrionic); more prevalent in developing nations where, there is a strong emphasis on traditional values (may demonstrate 'culture-specific' features—see p. 836).

Differential diagnosis

- Organic disorders—dementia/delirium
- BAD/depression—delusions of guilt and persecution
- Drug and alcohol disorders
- Personality disorder—paranoid/borderline/histrionic
- Culture specific disorders (see p. 840)
- Factitious disorder/malingering
- Schizophrenia (if goes on to last for more than 1 month)

Management (cf. pp. 198–201)

- Assessment is vital to make the appropriate diagnosis.
- Short-term admission may be necessary to provide support, nursing care, and specific assistance with psychosocial stressors.
- Where medication is considered, short-term use of antipsychotics/benzodiazepines may be helpful.
- Antidepressants/mood stabilisers may be useful to prevent relapse/further episodes.

Course and prognosis

- By definition these disorders are brief and resolve within days, weeks, or months.
- Prognosis is better if there is a short interval between onset and full-blown symptoms (DSM-IV: within 4wks, confusion and perplexity, good premorbid social and occupational functioning, absence of blunted or flat affect).
- Outcome is better than schizophrenia (both socially and symptomatically).
- Relapse is common, with increased mortality and suicide rates compared to the general population.

ICD-10 subtypes

ICD-10 allows for these disorders to occur with or without the presence of an acute stressor, and outlines the following subtypes:

- **Acute polymorphic psychotic disorder with or without symptoms of schizophrenia**
  - Variable and changeable psychotic symptoms (from day to day, or hour to hour) with frequent intense emotional turmoil.
  - Includes Perris' (1974) 'cycloid psychosis' after Karl Leonard's description for which the treatment of choice is lithium (Perris, 1978).
  - Also 'bouffee delirante' (Magnan), the concept of which was reviewed by Allodi (1982) who stressed the avoidance of long-term medication, highlighting socio-cultural factors, especially migration and language.
- **Acute schizophrenia-like psychotic disorder** Also referred to as 'brief schizophreniform psychosis' or 'schizophrenic reaction' where the psychotic symptoms are relatively stable but have not lasted more than a month (ICD-10, DSM-IV brief psychotic disorder), or have lasted between 1 mth and 6 mths (DSM-IV Schizophreniform disorder).
- **Other acute predominantly delusional psychotic disorder**
  - Onset is acute (2 wks or less), delusions or hallucinations present most of the time. If delusions persist for longer than 3 mths, then the diagnosis is that of *persistent delusional disorder* (see p. 230).
  - Includes the Scandinavian concept of 'psychogenic/reactive psychosis' for which the prognosis is good and the treatment of choice is supportive psychotherapy and the short-term use of medication (Stromgren, 1989).
  - 'Hysterical psychosis' (Hirsch and Hollander 1969) which includes 3 subtypes: culturally sanctioned behaviour (like culture specific disorders); appropriation of psychotic behaviour (conversion process); true psychosis ('failure of repression when faced with acute stress in a vulnerable ego', in e.g. histrionic personality)—in USA this is used as a diagnostic label for 'reactive psychosis'.
  - 'Ganser syndrome' (p. 93)-characterised by approximate answers, disorientation, clouding of consciousness, hallucinations, motor disturbance, anxiety or apathy, normal ADLs, sudden resolution with amnesia for the period of illness. Proposed mechanisms read much like the differential diagnosis for acute and transient psychotic disorders (see opposite): hysterical conversion, organic confusion, psychosis, or malingering.

Induced (ICD-10) or shared (DSM-IV) delusional disorder

Also known as **'folie à deux'** (or even **'folie à trois'** or **'folie à familie'**!), this disorder was recognised and described by Harvey as early as 1651, and recently reviewed as a concept by Howard in 1994. Silveira and Seeman (1995) also reviewed the literature and found equal sex ratio; broad range of ages; 90% couples, siblings, or parent/child; comorbidity with depression, dementia, and mental retardation; 2/3 socially isolated; and a common association with hallucinations.

Subtypes

1. *Folie imposée*—primary psychotic illness in one adopted by another.
2. *Folie simultanée*—primary psychotic illness in both with identical delusions.
3. *Folie communiqué*—primary psychotic illness in both at different times with delusions shared or passed on.
4. *Folie induite*—pre-existing primary psychosis in one patient, adopts fellow patient's delusions.

Aetiology

Psychodynamic Theories include: the fear of losing important relationship in an otherwise isolated individual with little scope for reality testing; or the passive acceptor has repressed oedipal fantasies that are released by the psychotic partner causing identification of dominant partner with a parent.

Learning theory Suggests that psychotic thinking is learned through 'observational learning'.

Management

- Separation—may lead to complete remission in up to 40% of cases.
- Psychological—aimed at giving up delusional beliefs (equivalent to rejecting a close relationship).
- Pharmacological—for the active *not* the passive partner.

Delusional misidentification syndromes

Usually manifest as symptoms of an underlying disorder (e.g. schizophrenia, mood disorder, delusional disorder, organic disorder), these syndromes rarely occur in isolation. Recently, interest has been focused on these rare (and bizarre) symptoms because of the insight they may give into the normal functioning of the brain (a 'lesion' paradigm). Examples include:

Capgras delusion (l'illusion de sosies) see p. 84—the patient believes others have been replaced by identical or near identical imposters. Can apply to animals and other objects, and often associated with aggressive behaviour.

Frégoli delusion (l'illusion de Frégoli) see p. 92—an individual, most often unknown to the patient, is actually someone they know 'in disguise'. Usually the individual is thought to be pursuing or persecuting the patient in some way.

Intermetamorphosis delusion—the patient believes they can see others change (usually temporarily) into someone else (both external appearance and internal personality).

Subjective doubles delusion—the patient believes there is a double ('dopplegänger') who exists and functions independently.

Autoscopic syndrome—the patient sees a double of themselves projected onto other people or objects nearby.

Reverse subjective double syndrome—the patient believes that they are an imposter in the process of being physically and psychologically replaced.

Reverse Frégoli syndrome—the patient believes others have completely misidentified them.

Aetiology

Psychodynamic Views include seeing these syndromes as the extremes of normal misidentification due to intense focusing on particular details; the effects of beliefs/emotions on perception; the effects of vivid imagination in a person experiencing a disorder of mood, judgement, and coenaesthesia; manifestations of the defence mechanisms of projection, splitting, or regression with loss of identity and flawed reconstruction.

Biological There may be evidence of underlying right hemisphere dysfunction, anterior cortical atrophy, temporal lobe pathology, bifrontal disconnectivity-with resultant impaired facial recognition and/or information processing.

Management

• Full physical and psychiatric assessment.
• Interventions should be directed towards any underlying problem.

Depressive illness

Introduction

Depressive disorders are common, with a prevalence of 5–10% in primary care settings. They rank fourth as causes of disability worldwide, and it has been projected that they may rank second by the year 2020. The prevalence of *depressive symptoms* may be as high as 30% in the general population with women being twice as likely to be affected as men.

Although effective treatments are available, depression often goes undiagnosed and undertreated. Symptoms often are regarded by both patients and physicians as *understandable* given current social circumstances and/or background. Although in many cases this may be true, people should not be denied interventions that may help relieve some of the disabling symptoms of the disorder, allowing them to cope better with any current social problems.

It should be borne in mind that depressive disorder has significant potential morbidity and mortality. Suicide is the second leading cause of death in persons aged 20–35 yrs and depressive disorder is a major factor in around 50% of these deaths. The death rate amongst people with a mood disorder may be as high as 15%. Depressive disorder also contributes to higher morbidity and mortality when associated with other physical disorders (e.g. myocardial infarction) and its successful diagnosis and treatment has been shown to improve both medical and surgical outcomes. It is also associated with high rates of comorbid alcohol and substance misuse, and has a considerable social impact on relationships, families, and productivity (through time off work).

The majority of patients will present to primary care, often with problems other than low mood (see 'Other clinical presentations' p. 250). Physicians ought to remain alert to this possibility as early interventions may be critical in the prevention of major morbidity and comorbidity.

There remains an innate reluctance to consider *pharmacological* interventions for *emotional* problems, despite overwhelming evidence of efficacy. There is also a widespread concern that drugs which improve mood *must* be addictive, despite evidence to the contrary. While medication is not the only possible treatment for mild to moderate depression, when antidepressants are prescribed the onus is on the physician to give a *therapeutic* dose for an *adequate* length of time. Treatment failure is often due to patient non-compliance, particularly when the patient feels that their problems have not been taken seriously and they have been 'fobbed off'. In a group of patients who generally have feelings of low self-worth or guilt, it is critical that they understand the rationale behind any treatment, and that their progress is regularly reviewed, at least in the early stages.

Depression amongst the famous

As depression is common it is not surprising that many famous people have had a depressive illness. However, there still remains a stigma attached to psychiatric illness and it is only recently that people have become more willing to publicly discuss their illnesses. A recent study examined the lives of almost 300 world famous men and found that over 40% had experienced some type of depression during their lives[1]. Highest rates (72%) were found in writers, but the incidence was also high in artists (42%), politicians (41%), intellectuals (36%), composers (35%), and scientists (33%).

Famous people who have publicly stated they have had a depressive illness include:

Alanis Morissette, musician, composer
Anthony Hopkins, actor
Barbara Bush, former First Lady (U.S.)
Billy Joel, musician, composer
Courtney Love, musician, actor
Donny Osmond, musician
Ellen DeGeneres, comedienne, actor
Elton John, musician, composer
Germaine Greer, writer
Halle Berry, actress
Harrison Ford, actor
Janet Jackson, musician
Jessica Lange, actress
Jim Carrey, actor, comedian
Joan Rivers, comedienne, TV host
John Cleese, comedian, actor, writer

Leonard Cohen, musician, writer
Lou Reed, musician
Marie Osmond, musician
Marlon Brando, actor
Monica Seles, athlete (tennis)
Ozzy Osbourne, musician
Paul Gascoigne, professional footballer
Paul Merton, comedian
Paul Simon, composer, musician
Roseanne, actress, writer, comedienne
Sheryl Crow, musician
Sinead O'Connor, musician
S.P. Morrissey, musician
Stephen Hawking, scientist, writer
Winona Ryder, actress
Yves Saint Laurent, fashion designer

Other famous people (deceased) known to have had a depressive illness:
Samuel Becket, Menachem Begin, Kurt Cobain, Michel Foucault, Judy Garland, Ernest Hemingway, Audrey Hepburn, William James, Franz Kafka, Claude Monet, Richard M. Nixon, Laurence Olivier, Wilfred Owen, George S. Patton, Sylvia Plath, Jackson Pollock, Cole Porter, Mark Rothko, Dmitri Shostakovich, Tennessee Williams.

1 Post F (1994) Creativity and psychopathology. A study of 291 world-famous men. *BJP* **165**, 22–34.

Historical perspective*

The changing face of 'depression'

Our current ideas of what constitutes depression date from the mid-eighteenth century. Before this, old notions of 'melancholia', steeped in classical humoral theories (melancholia derived from the Greek *melaina kole*—black bile), reflected 'intensity of idea' (Haslam, 1809)—i.e. the presence of few, rather than many, delusions. Sadness or low mood were not primary symptoms. The 'melancholic' symptoms we regard today as part of depressive disorder would have been called 'vapours', 'hypochondria', or 'neuroses'. 'Depression', a term used to mean 'reduced functioning' in other medical disciplines, came to be associated with 'mental depression'. It was adopted because it implied a 'physiological' change, and was defined as 'a condition characterised by a sinking of the spirits, lack of courage or initiative, and a tendency to gloomy thoughts' (Jastrow, 1901).

The concept was enlarged and legitimised by Kraepelin (1921) who used the term 'depressive states' in his description of the unitary concept of 'manic-depressive illness', encompassing melancholia simplex and gravis, stupor, fantastical melancholia, delirious melancholia, and involutional melancholia. A number of assumptions surrounded the affective disorders at that time: they involved primary pathology of affect, had stable psychopathology, had brain pathology, were periodic in nature, had a genetic basis, occurred in persons with certain personality traits, and were 'endogenous' (not related to precipitants).

In 1917 Freud published *Mourning and melancholia* influencing more than a generation in emphasising cognitive and intra-psychic factors in the aetiology of depressive disorders, and shifting the focus of clinical descriptions from *objective* behavioural signs to *subjective* symptoms.

Over the intervening years there has been much debate as to whether a 'biological' type of depression exists separate from a 'neurotic' type. Terminology has fluctuated around 'endogenous', 'vital', 'autonomous', 'endomorphic', and 'melancholic' depression, characterised by distinctive symptoms and signs, a genetic basis, and running an independent course unrelated to psychosocial factors. In contrast, 'neurotic' or 'reactive' depression could manifest in multiple forms, showed clear responsiveness to the environment, and ran a more variable course. Both ICD-10 and DSM-IV 'fudge' the issue somewhat by using severity specifiers (i.e. mild, moderate, severe) as well as 'symptom' specifiers (i.e. somatic symptoms, psychotic symptoms).

The advent of the 'antidepressants' in the 1950s introduced a further complication into the mix. Although ECT was widely accepted as a treatment for 'vital' depression, the idea of a drug treatment for 'reactive' depressive disorders ran counter to the received wisdom of the psychological basis to these conditions and the need for psychological treatment.

The antidepressants and beyond

The antidepressant effects of isoniazid were first observed in 1952 by Lurie and Salzer in patients being treated for TB . Similar effects were noted by Shepherd and Davies for reserpine. They even conducted the first RCT in psychiatry, clearly demonstrating efficacy in anxious-depression in 1955. The psychiatric community was initially reluctant to accept the idea of chemical 'cures' for mental disorders, and it was not until iproniazid was promoted by Kline in 1957 as a 'psychic energiser', capable of treating 'nervous' conditions, that the tide began to turn.

In 1956, Kuhn demonstrated the antidepressant effects of imipramine, the TCA, which was marketed worldwide in 1958, closely followed by amitriptyline in 1960. Around the same time new 'anxiolytics' were also emerging, with meprobamate in 1955, and the first benzodiazepine— chlordiazepoxide—in 1960. The search for greater dissociation of anxiolytic and sedative properties led to the introduction of diazepam in 1963.

The downside of this new psychopharmacology was the overprescription in the 1960s and 70s of these drugs to help with 'the problems of living' and evidence of dependence, particularly in the case of the benzodiazepines. As a result, *non-pharmacological* treatments flourished, in the form of the 're-branded' psychotherapies.

Behind the scenes, biological psychiatrists and psychopharmacologists developed monoamine theories of depression, based upon the discovery of the neuropharmacological action of the antidepressants. This would lead to the development of more *selective* antidepressants—in the first instance, the SSRIs, with zimelidine patented in 1971, and indalpine marketed in 1978.

The emphasis on safety and side-effect issues when comparing the SSRIs to the TCAs, and the fall from grace of the benzodiazepines, opened the floodgates in the 1980s and 1990s for the promotion of SSRIs not only in the treatment of depression, but also for anxiety disorders (see p. 341). Advances in monoamine theories also allowed for the development of 'dual-action' agents (e.g. SNRIs—venlafaxine; NaSSAs—nefazodone/mirtazepine; DNRIs—bupropion) and other *selective* agents (e.g. NARIs—reboxetine).

Current theories of depression attempt to integrate biological models of 'stress' (and the involvement of the HPA axis) with evidence from biological psychology, genetics, neuropharmacology, and functional neuropathology. In this way a multifactorial 'biopsychosocial model' (see p. 255) emerges which may help to unite the apparently divergent ideas of depression.

Clinical symptoms and signs are seen as the final common pathway in a complex interaction between genes and the environment in determining *predisposition* or *biological vulnerability*, which may (or may not) subsequently lead to *biological variations* in functioning necessary for behavioural and emotional change. This may be due to further psychosocial stressors or genetically predetermined factors which give rise to alterations in *brain functioning*. Research into these interdependent factors may well lead to greater understanding of the aetiology of depressive disorder, as well as allowing the development of diagnostic tests and *individualised* treatments.

---

* For an exhaustive critique of conceptual ideas see: Jackson SW (1987) *Melancholia and depression: from Hippocratic times to modern times.* New Haven, Yale University Press.

Diagnosis (1)—symptoms

Although the terminology is slightly different between ICD-10 and DSM-IV (see opposite), the core symptoms are almost identical and should fulfil the following criteria:

• Present for at least 2 weeks and represent a change from normal.
• Are not secondary to the effects of drug/alcohol misuse, medication, a medical disorder, or bereavement (see p. 366).
• May cause significant distress and/or impairment of social, occupational, or general functioning.

Core symptoms

• *Depressed mood* present most of the day, nearly every day, with little variation, and often lack of responsiveness to changes in circumstances. There may be diurnal variation in mood with mood worse in the morning and improving as the day goes on.
• *Anhedonia* Markedly diminished interest or pleasure in all, or almost all, activities most of the day, nearly every day (as indicated by either sub-jective account or observation made by others).
• *Weight change* Loss of weight when not dieting or weight gain (e.g. a change of more than 5% of body weight in a month), associated with decreased or increased appetite.
• *Disturbed sleep*—*insomnia* (with early morning wakening 2–3 hrs sooner than usual) or *hypersomnia* (esp. in atypical depression, see p. 268).
• *Psychomotor agitation* or retardation observable by others, not just sub-jective feelings of restlessness or being slowed down.
• Fatigue or *loss of energy*.
• *Reduced libido*.
• Feelings *of worthlessness* or *excessive or inappropriate guilt* (which may be delusional); not just self-reproach or guilt about being ill.
• Diminished ability *to think or concentrate* or *indecisiveness*.
• Recurrent thoughts of death or suicide (not 'fear of dying') which may or may not have been acted upon.

'Somatic symptoms'

Also called 'biological', 'melancholic' (DSM-IV), or 'vital', include:

• Loss of emotional reactivity
• Diurnal mood variation
• Anhedonia
• Early morning wakening
• Psychomotor agitation or retardation
• Loss of appetite and weight
• Loss of libido

Psychotic symptoms/features

• Delusions e.g. poverty; personal inadequacy; guilt over presumed mis-deeds; responsibility for world events: accidents, natural disasters, war; deserving of punishment; other nihilistic delusions.

- Hallucinations e.g. auditory: defamatory or accusatory voices, cries for help or screaming; olfactory: bad smells such as rotting food, faeces, decomposing flesh; visual: tormentors, demons, the Devil, dead bodies, scenes of death or torture.

N.B. These examples are *mood-congruent*. However, other *mood-incongruent* psychotic symptoms are also possible (i.e. persecutory delusions, thought insertion/withdrawal, delusions of control—not of a clearly depressive nature).

- Catatonic symptoms or *marked psychomotor retardation* ('depressive stupor').

ICD-10 and DSM-IV Terminology

ICD-10	DSM-IV
Depressive episode	*Depressive disorders*
Mild depressive episode	Major depressive disorder, single
—without somatic symptoms	episode
—with somatic symptoms	Major depressive disorder, recurrent
Moderate depressive episode	*Severity specifiers:*
—without somatic symptoms	—mild, moderate, severe (with or
—with somatic symptoms	without psychotic features)
Severe depressive episode	—in partial or full remission
—without psychotic symptoms	*Special syndrome specifiers:*
—with psychotic symptoms	—with catatonic, melancholic, or
Other depressive episode	atypical features
Depressive episode unspecified	—with postpartum onset
	Longitudinal course specifiers:
Recurrent depressive episode	—with/without full interepisode recovery
	—with seasonal pattern
	—with rapid cycling
	Depressive disorder, not otherwise stated
	—premenstrual dysphoric disorder
	—minor depressive disorder
	—recurrent brief depressive disorder
	—post-psychotic depressive disorder of schizophrenia
	—major depressive disorder superimposed on delusional disorder, psychotic disorder NOS, active phase of schizophrenia
	—uncertain aetiology
	Dysthymic disorder

Diagnosis (2)—'caseness' and subtypes

Clinically significant depressive episode (minimum criteria)

- ICD-10 specifies the presence of at least 2 *typical symptoms* (depressed mood, anhedonia, or fatigue), *plus* at least 2 others from the **core symptoms** list.
- DSM-IV requires the presence of 5 or more symptoms from the *core symptoms* list (at least one of which must be **depressed mood** or **anhedonia**).

Severity criteria

Both ICD-10 and DSM-IV distinguish **mild**, **moderate**, and **severe episodes** on the basis of symptomatology (see opposite).

Subtypes

- **'Non-melancholic' (DSM-IV) or 'without somatic symptoms' (ICD-10).** Essentially, defined as absence of psychotic or marked somatic symptoms, this subtype captures the clinical picture historically described by 'neurotic depression' (in those with certain premorbid personality traits and/or high levels of anxiety) and 'reactive depression' (due to a severely stressful life event—see **'Adjustment disorder'** p. 364). Counter-intuitively, there is little need to subdivide on the basis of there being a clear precipitant. Life events appear to be provoking factors, but only in those with a predisposition to depression, and treatment should focus on the underlying disorder as well as 'coming to terms with' any significant provoking factors. Recent research[1] also supports the long-held clinical impression of two different presentations:
  - 'Irritable/hostile' depression—younger, anxiety expressed as irritability, history of 'acting out' behaviours in response to stress (e.g. yelling, smashing things up, recklessness, impulsiveness, DSH). Poor response to antidepressants.
  - 'Anxious' depression—shy and withdrawn, highly anxious ('always a worrier'), usually early onset depression, with a recurrent, persistent course, increased likelihood of drug/alcohol dependency, and frequent DSH/attempted suicide. Better response to antidepressants (SSRIs).
- **'Melancholic' (DSM-IV) or 'with somatic symptoms'** (ICD-10) The presence of 'somatic symptoms' (see p. 246) defines what is regarded as a more 'biological' or 'endogenous' depressive episode, which is more severe (and more amenable to antidepressant treatment). DSM-IV also includes 'excessive or inappropriate guilt', although this may often be difficult to distinguish from delusional guilt. In clinical studies, the best distinguishing factor from 'non-melancholic' disorders is actually the presence of psychomotor disturbance (an *objective sign* manifest by motor retardation, periodic agitation, and reduced/slowed cognitive functioning).

- **With psychotic symptoms (ICD-10)** or **features (DSM-IV)**—see
  pp. 246–7. Usually there is pervasive depressed mood (no reactivity)
  and marked psychomotor disturbance (sometimes to the point of
  'depressive stupor'/catatonia) accompanying delusions (commonly)
  and hallucinations (10–20%). Constipation is often a feature (~30%),
  unrelated to medication, and may have a delusional interpretation
  (e.g. presence of cancer, bowels have been sewn up).

Severity criteria

	ICD-10	DSM-IV
Mild	2 typical symptoms + 2 other core symptoms	5 core symptoms + minor social/ occupational impairment
Moderate	2 typical symptoms + 3+ other core symptoms	5+ core symptoms + variable degree of social/occupational impairment
Severe	3 typical symptoms + 4+ other core symptoms	5+ core symptoms + significant social/ occupational impairment

1 Parker G, Hadzi-Pavlovic D, Roussos J, et al. (1998) Non-melancholic depression: the contribution
of personality, anxiety and life events to subclassification. *Psychological Medicine* **28**, 1209–19.

Diagnosis (3)—other clinical presentations

There may be marked individual variation in the clinical presentation. Sometimes anxiety may also be prominent (**Mixed anxiety and depressive disorder**—ICD-10). Patients with a depressive disorder may not present complaining of low mood, but may consult with other primary problems. The possibility of a depressive disorder should be borne in mind, particularly in the primary care setting, where many of these patients first seek treatment.

Indirect presentations may include:

- Insomnia, fatigue, or other somatic complaints (e.g. headache, GI upset, change in weight). On further questioning patients may describe irritability or anhedonia, but attribute this as secondary to what they regard as the primary problem (see **insomnia** pp. 392–7, **symptoms of chronic fatigue** pp. 754–5, **somatisation disorder** pp. 742–3).
- Elderly persons presenting with agitation, confusion, or a decline in normal functioning ('pseudodementia')—see p. 478.
- Children presenting with symptoms such as irritability, decline in school performance, or social withdrawal—see p. 604.
- Persons from a different cultural background presenting with 'culture-specific' symptoms—see p. 836.

Other symptoms that may hinder diagnosis

- Presence of a physical disorder whose secondary symptoms (e.g. anorexia, fatigue, insomnia) may mask symptoms of depression.
- Histrionic behaviour (making assessment of severity difficult).
- Exacerbation of other underlying disorders (phobias, OCD—especially when there are depressive ruminations).
- Hypochondriacal ideas (which may have been longstanding).
- The presence of self-harming behaviours (e.g. cutting, frequent overdose) which may represent underlying borderline traits (usually individuals will say they have never felt happy, or describe chronic feelings of 'emptiness').
- Cognitive impairment or LD (which may mask depressive symptoms, or appear more severe because of depression and hence improve with antidepressants).
- Alcohol and drug misuse (primary or secondary).

Other subtypes of depressive disorder

are formally recognised in DSM-IV, but are subsumed under the ther depressive episodes' in ICD-10. They include:
- Se_pression (p. 268)
- pre__ression (p. 756)
- __e disorder (p. 270)
- __ric disorder (p. 435)

As a description of the experience of the symptoms of depression, the following has never been bettered:

I have of late but wherefore I know not lost all my mirth, forgone all custom of exercises; and indeed it goes so heavily with my disposition that this goodly frame, the earth, seems to me a sterile promontory, this most excellent canopy, the air, look you, this brave o'erhanging firmament, this majestical roof fretted with golden fire, why, it appears no other thing to me than a foul and pestilent congregation of vapours. What a piece of work is a man! how noble in reason! how infinite in faculty! in form and moving how express and admirable! in action how like an angel! in apprehension how like a god! the beauty of the world! the paragon of animals! And yet, to me, what is this quintessence of dust? man delights not me: no, nor woman neither.

Shakespeare: *Hamlet* (Act II Scene 2)

Epidemiology

Prevalence 2–5% (derived from multiple sources for general population).
Lifetime rates 10–20% (but very variable across populations).
Sex ratio ♂:♀ = 1:2.
Risk factors:

- *Genetic* Heritability estimates range from 40–70% and families also have high rates of anxiety disorders and neuroticism.
- *Childhood experiences* Loss of a parent, lack of parental care, parental alcoholism / antisocial traits, childhood sexual abuse.
- *Personality traits* Neuroticism / anxiety, impulsivity, obsessionality.
- *Social circumstances*
  - Marital status (men—low rates associated with marriage, high rates with separation or divorce; women—probably similar, but less clear-cut).
  - Brown and Harris[1] found that, for women, having 3 or more children under the age of 11, lack of paid employment, and lack of a confiding relationship were associated with increased risk of depression (recent studies support the *lack of a confiding relationship*, but not the other factors).
  - Adverse life *events*—particularly 'loss' events (increased risk 2–3 months after event) in vulnerable individuals.
- *Physical illness* Especially if chronic, severe, or painful. Neurological disorders (e.g. Parkinson's disease, MS, stroke, epilepsy) have higher risk (perhaps due to 'shared' pathology). Higher rates also noted in post-MI, diabetic, and cancer patients, although family or personal history of depression are important determinants of occurrence.

Comorbidity About two-thirds of patients will also meet criteria for another psychiatric disorder (e.g. anxiety disorders, substance misuse, alcohol dependency, personality disorders).

1 Brown GW and Harris TO (1978) *Social origins of depression: a study of psychiatric disorders in women.* Tavistock Publications, London.

Aetiology

Neurobiological factors

Aetiology

The aetiology of depression has yet to be fully understood, however it is likely to be due to the interplay of biological, psychological, and social factors in the life-span of an individual. Psychosocial stressors may play a role both as *precipitants* and *perpetuating factors*, increasing the risk of chronicity and recurrence; while individuals with established depression are at higher risk of further stressors of many kinds. One attempt to integrate these factors is the biopsychosocial model (see opposite).

Neurobiological factors

Structural brain changes In chronic cases—esp. left hippocampus, left parietal, and frontal association cortices.

Functional brain changes Hypoperfusion in frontal, temporal, and parietal areas (esp. older patients); increased perfusion in frontal and cingulate cortex (in younger patients, associated with good treatment response).

Neurotransmitter abnormalities The discovery that all antidepressants increase monoamine (i.e. 5HT, NA, DA) release and/or reduce their reuptake in the synaptic cleft, led to the development of the *monoamine theory of depression*, which suggests that reduced monoamine function may cause depression. Blunted neuroendocrine responses and symptom induction by tryptophan depletion (5HT precursor) suggest an important role for 5HT.

Endocrine changes Blunted prolactin and growth hormone (GH) responses to tryptophan/citalopram (5HT system), blunted GH responses to clonidine (NA system) and apomorphine (DA system), increased GH response to physostigmine (ACh system) suggest reduced monoamine functioning and increased cholinergic functioning in depression. Increased cortisol seen in ~50% of patients (particularly 'endogenous' subtype), associated with adrenal hypertrophy, and dexamethasone non-suppression of cortisol (also in other psychiatric conditions, hence not a sensitive test, despite apparent specificity of ~96%).

Changes in sleep pattern Reduced total SWS and shortened REM latency (secondary to increased cholinergic and/or reduced serotonergic/noradrenergic drive).

Genetic factors appear to influence the risk of depression by altering individual sensitivity to the effects of life stressors. Linkage analysis suggests an association between the serotonin transporter gene (17q11.1–12), depression, treatment response, and, possibly, suicidal behaviour.

Personality/temperament factors These are enduring traits with a biological basis, influenced over the life-span by inherited factors, experience, and maturation. They mediate the level and nature of response to sensory experience, regulated by context, and manifest as subjective emotions and objective behaviours. Certain temperaments (e.g. 'neuroticism') may increase vulnerability to depression perhaps due to the presence of autonomic hyperarousal (heightened responses to emotional stimuli) or lability (unpredictable responses to emotional stimuli).

Psychological factors Disruption of normal social, marital, parental, or familial relationships is correlated with high rates of depression, and are risk factors to recurrence. An aetiological role has yet to be demonstrated, but

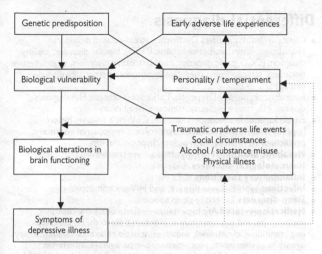

The biopsychosocial model of depression

adverse childhood experiences/chronic stressors may influence the sensitivity of individuals to later stressful events. Low self-esteem (negative view of self, the past, current events, and the future) is proposed as a vulnerability factor—it remains debatable whether this is a *causal* factor or merely a *symptom* of depression.

Gender Although the increased prevalence of depression in women is a robust finding, explanations of why this may be so are various. These include: restricting social and occupational roles, being over- or under-occupied, ruminative response styles, and endocrine factors (suggested by increased risk of depression in the premenstrual and post-partum periods). There is little supportive evidence for these theories. One popular hypothesis is that women are more likely to admit to depressive symptoms, whereas men are not and tend to express their symptoms differently (e.g. through alcohol abuse and antisocial behaviour).

Social factors In explaining why people of low socio-economic status (i.e. low levels of income, employment, and education) are at demonstrably higher risk of depression, two main arguments exist: *social causation*—stress associated with such problems leads to depression (i.e. an 'environmental' argument); and *social selection*—predisposed individuals 'drift' down to lower social positions, or fail to rise from them (i.e. a 'genetic' argument).

N.B. There is stronger evidence for the social causation argument, as *social isolation* has been shown to be a key risk factor.

Differential diagnosis

- *Other psychiatric disorders* Dysthymia, stress-related disorders (adjustment disorders/bereavement, PTSD), bipolar disorder, anxiety disorders (OCD, panic disorder, phobias), eating disorders, schizoaffective disorders, schizophrenia (negative symptoms), personality disorders (esp. BPD).
- *Neurological disorders* Dementia, Parkinson's disease, Huntington's disease, MS, stroke, epilepsy, tumours, head injury.
- *Endocrine disorders* Addison's disease, Cushing's disease, hyper/hypothyroidism, perimenstrual syndromes, menopausal symptoms, prolactinoma, hyperparathyroidism, hypopituitarism.
- **Metabolic disorders** Hypoglycaemia, hypercalcaemia, porphyria.
- **Haematological disorders** Anaemia.
- **Inflammatory conditions** SLE.
- **Infections** Syphilis, Lyme disease, and HIV encephalopathy.
- **Sleep disorders** Especially sleep apnoea.
- **Medication-related** Antihypertensives (beta-blockers, reserpine, methyldopa, and calcium channel blockers); steroids; H_2 blockers (e.g., ranitidine, cimetidine); sedatives; muscle relaxants; chemotherapy agents (e.g., vincristine, procarbazine, L-asparaginase, interferon, amphotericin B, vinblastine); medications that affect sex hormones (oestrogen, progesterone, testosterone, gonadotropin-releasing hormone [GnRH] antagonists); and psychiatric medication (esp. antipsychotics)
- *Substance misuse* Alcohol, benzodiazepines, opiates, marijuana, cocaine, amphetamines and derivatives.

Investigations

There are no specific tests for depression. Investigations focus on the exclusion of treatable causes (see above), or other secondary problems (e.g. loss of appetite, alcohol misuse).

- **Standard tests** FBC, ESR, B_{12}/folate, U&Es, LFTs, TFTs, glucose, Ca^{2+}
- **Focused investigations** (if indicated by history or physical signs)
  - Urine toxicology
  - Thyroid antibodies
  - Antinuclear antibody
  - Syphilis serology
  - CT/MRI, EEG, LP (VDRL, Lyme antibody, cell count, chemistry, protein electrophoresis)
  - HIV testing
  - Dexamethasone suppression test (Cushing's disease)
  - Cosyntropin stimulation test (Addison's disease)

Course and prognosis

Points to note

Mortality

Prognostic factors

Course and prognosis

Points to note

- Depression may occur at any age, although late onset depression may be milder, more chronic, more likely to be associated with life events, and more likely to have a sub-clinical prodrome.
- Depressive episodes vary from 4–30 wks for mild-moderate cases, to an average of about 6 mths for severe cases (25% will last up to 1 yr).
- Episodes of recurrent depression tend to be shorter (4–16 wks).
- 10–20% of patients will have a chronic course, with persistent symptoms lasting over 2 yrs.
- The majority of patients experiencing a depressive episode will have further episodes later in life (risk of recurrence is ~30% at 10 yrs, ~60% at 20 yrs), but inter-individual variation makes it impossible to predict the likely period of time before future episodes, although, as with bipolar disorder, the greater the number of recurrences, the shorter the time between episodes.
- Risk of recurrence is greater when there are residual symptoms after remission (about a third of cases)—e.g. low mood, anxiety, sleep disturbance, reduced libido, and physical symptoms (headache, fatigue, GI upset).
- There is good evidence that modern antidepressant treatments impact significantly upon all these quoted figures, reducing the length of depressive episodes; and if treatment is given long term, the incidence of residual symptoms is less, there are fewer recurrent episodes, and chronicity may be as low as 4%.

Mortality

- Suicide rates for severe depressive episodes vary but may be up to 13% (i.e. up to 20 times more likely than the general population), with a slightly higher rate for those who have required hospital admission (12–19%). For less severe episodes the rates are much lower.
- The overall death rate for patients with depression is higher than the general population (SMR 1.37–2.49) with the cause of death usually due to suicide, drug and alcohol problems, accidents, cardiovascular disease, respiratory infections, and thyroid disorders.

Prognostic factors

- **Good outcome** Acute onset, 'endogenous' depression, earlier age of onset.
- **Poor outcome** Insidious onset, 'neurotic' depression, elderly, residual symptoms, neuroticism, low self-confidence, comorbidity (alcohol or drug problems, personality disorders, physical illness), lack of social supports.

Management principles and outpatient treatment

Initial assessment

- **History** Key areas of enquiry include: any clear psychosocial precipitants, current social situation, use of drugs / alcohol, past history of previous mood symptoms (including 'subclinical' periods of low or elevated mood, previous DSH / suicide attempts), previous effective treatments, premorbid personality, family history of mood disorder, physical illnesses, current medication.
- **MSE** (see p. 44) Focused enquiry about subjective mood symptoms, somatic symptoms, psychotic symptoms, symptoms of anxiety, thoughts of suicide. Objective assessment of psychomotor retardation/agitation, evidence of DSH, cognitive functioning (MMSE).
- **Physical examination** Focused on possible differential diagnoses (see p. 256).
- **Baseline investigations** (see p. 256).

Initiating treatment

Once a positive diagnosis has been made, possible treatments should be discussed with the patient. There is a wide range of effective treatments, both psychological (e.g. CBT, IPT—see pp. 786–95) and pharmacological (see pp. 274–85).

- **Use of psychological therapies** is influenced by the severity of the depressive episode (usually for mild-moderate cases), local availability, and patient preference. Medication alone can effectively relieve symptoms. However, a combined approach may provide the quickest and most sustained response (in mild-moderate episodes).
- **Pharmacological treatment** of mild-moderate depressive episodes can be initiated on an outpatient basis.
  - Choice of antidepressant is guided by anticipated safety and tolerability, physician familiarity (which allows for better patient education in anticipation of adverse effects), presenting symptoms, and history of prior treatments (see *Choosing an antidepressant* p. 262).
  - Initially follow-up will usually be fairly frequent (1–4 wks) to monitor treatment response and assess for any unwanted side-effects (see *Outpatient follow-up* p. 261).
  - Once treatment is established (and is effective) the time between appointments may be increased (see *Treating depressive illness* p. 263 and p. 264 for further guidance).

Hospital admission

Sometimes acute episodes of depressive disorder are severe enough to require hospital admission (which may be on a compulsory basis). As for all psychiatric disorders, issues of safety and the provision of effective treatment will govern the decisions about whether a patient can remain in the community.

Points to note

- Due to symptoms of low self-esteem or guilt, some patients may refuse admission to hospital because they feel 'unworthy' or they are 'using up a valuable bed'. Sympathetic reassurance that this is not the case and that the clinician believes they are sufficiently unwell to benefit from hospital admission may avoid unnecessary detention.
- Some patients (or relatives) may 'demand' admission to hospital. Although this usually is due to personality factors, it may also be due to (sometimes erroneous) ideas of what may be reasonably achieved in a hospital setting (e.g. 'intensive' psychotherapy for one specific issue), or reflect undisclosed factors which have created a social crisis. A non-confrontational approach in eliciting the reasons behind such demands may reveal other important issues that may help the decision-making process (including those which may be dealt with by other agencies— e.g. emergency accommodation/refuge).

Common reasons for hospital admission

- Serious risk of suicide(see p. 45—for assessment of suicide risk)
- Serious risk of harm to others (esp. children—see PND p. 756)
- Significant self-neglect (esp. weight loss)
- Severe depressive symptoms
- Severe psychotic symptoms
- Lack or breakdown of social supports
- Initiation of ECT
- Treatment-resistant depression (where inpatient monitoring may be helpful)
- A need to address comorbid conditions (e.g. physical problems, other psychiatric conditions, inpatient detoxification)

Suitable environment?

Where there is significant risk of harm to self (or others), admission should be to a ward where close observation and monitoring are possible. Observation levels ought to be regularly reviewed. The ward environment is often not the quiet 'sanctuary' patients hope for and this may lead to difficult decisions in balancing the risk of self-harm against the use of compulsory admission. Careful assessment of a patient's insight into their illness, issues of comorbid substance misuse, and clear evidence of their ability to seek additional support when symptoms are worse, may allow for a more flexible approach in permitting 'time out' from the ward environment (perhaps in the company of a responsible relative or friend).

Outpatient follow-up

Following hospital discharge, or for outpatients started on antidepressant treatment, initial follow-up should be regular (2–4 wks) to monitor progress, ensure treatment response is maintained, and to allow time for other supports (e.g. CPN services, day hospitals, specific psychotherapies) to become established.

⚠ **Risk of suicide is increased at this time** as energy and motivation improve and the patient struggles with the consequences of being unwell.

Key aims for follow-up

- Establishing and maintaining a therapeutic alliance.
- Monitoring the patient's psychiatric status.
- Providing education regarding depressive disorder and the treatment options.
- Enhancing treatment compliance.
- Monitoring side-effects of medication.
- Identifying and addressing any significant comorbidity (see p. 252).
- Promoting regular patterns of activity (e.g. regular exercise) and rest.
- Identifying unmet needs for specific (practical) support, counselling, (bereavement, stress management) or psychotherapy.
- Promoting understanding of and adaption to the psychosocial effects of symptoms.
- Identifying new episodes early.
- Reducing the morbidity and sequelae of depressive disorder.

The ultimate aim is a return to normal activities (academic, employment, home life, social activities), usually in a graded way as the resolution of symptoms allows, using a collaborative approach.

Maintenance treatment (see p. 263 and p. 264) will usually be monitored in the primary care setting, with specific advice about continuation of medication and what to do should symptoms recur.

Treating depressive illness (without psychotic features)

First-line treatment

Antidepressant drugs are effective in 65–75% of patients[1]. For mild-moderate episodes, or where antidepressants are contraindicated (e.g. recent MI) CBT or other psychotherapies may have a role (see pp. 786–95). The combination of psychological approaches and pharmacotherapy may be synergistic, but in severe cases treatment is almost exclusively pharmacological or physical (e.g. ECT).

Choosing an antidepressant

The decision about *which* antidepressant to choose will depend upon:
- **Patient factors** Age, sex, comorbid physical illness (cardiac, renal, liver, neurological)—see prescribing in different patient groups (pp. 876–87), previous response to antidepressants.
- **Issues of tolerability** See 'Side-effect profiles of the antidepressants' (pp. 274–85).
- **Symptomatology** Sleep problems (more sedative agent), lack of energy/hypersomnia (more adrenergic/stimulatory agent), 'mixed' (e.g. with anxiety/panic (SSRI/imipramine)), OCD symptoms (clomipramine/SSRI), risk of suicide (avoid TCAs).

Adequate trial

Generally an adequate trial of an antidepressant is defined as at least 6 wks of the highest tolerated dose (up to BNF maximum).

⚠ Suicide risk

The risk of suicide may actually be *increased* in the early stages of antidepressant treatment. Often patients with previous marked psychomotor retardation have been unable to act upon their thoughts of self-harm. Partial treatment response may 'free' them to do this, hence careful monitoring is critical (and admission to hospital may be indicated).

'Treatment failure'—second-line treatment

Failure of an adequate trial of an antidepressant may occur in ~25% of cases. A similar number of patients will experience unacceptable side-effects, leading to the withdrawal of the agent without completing an adequate trial. For these patients, second-line treatment is with an alternative agent usually from a different class of antidepressant, or from the same class but with a different side-effect profile.

Partial responders

~50% of patients who have only partially responded to a TCA, SSRI, or MAOI may benefit from the addition of *lithium* (usual dose 600–900mg/d). Treatment response is generally observed within 2 wks. Alternative 'augmentative' strategies include the use of triiodothyronine (T_3), L-tryptophan, or pindolol.

ECT[2] (see p. 286)

ECT may be considered as a first-line therapy when there are severe bio-logical features (e.g. significant weight loss/reduced appetite) or marked psychomotor retardation. It is sometimes used when the patient is at high risk of harming themselves or others (where there is clear evidence of repeated suicide attempts or significantly aggressive behaviour) or where psychotic features are prominent (see p. 264). Under these circumstances issues of consent to treatment must be considered (see pp. 820–3). It may also be considered as a second- or third-line treatment for non-responders to pharmacotherapy.

Maintenance therapy

First episode

- A collaborative approach with the patient should emphasise compliance (even when feeling 'better') with advice to continue the effective treatment for 6 mths to 1 yr after remission (particularly if there are residual symptoms).
- Discontinuation should be gradual and if there is recurrence of symptoms revert to effective dose with further attempt at withdrawal after at least a further 4–6 mths.
- Often patients wish to continue medication indefinitely (particularly after a severe episode) and reassurance should be given that there is no evidence of any specific long-term problems with such a course of action.

Recurrent episodes

- If period between episodes is less than 3 yrs, or with severe episodes (esp. with marked suicidal thought/actions) prophylactic treatment should be maintained for at least 5 yrs (often indefinitely—risk of relapse if medication stopped is 70–90% within 5 yrs).
- Otherwise treat as for *first episode* (see above).

ECT

- If ECT has been used as a first-line therapy, and remission maintained with medication, treat as above.
- If ECT has been used successfully as second- or third-line treatment, consider *maintenance* ECT as an option (N.B. *Not* recommended in recent NICE guidelines—see p. 287) where there is evidence that ECT effectively treats relapse of symptoms. There is some evidence that ECT every 2-wks may be an effective prophylactic (this does not pre-clude further trials of pharmacotherapy).

---

1 It should be noted that many patients do spontaneously improve without active antidepressant treatment. The Medical Research Council Clinical Psychiatry Committee 1965 clinical trial of the treatment of depressive illness found that outcomes (patients with no or only slight symptoms) for different treatments were: ECT (71%), imipramine (52%), phenelzine (30%), and **placebo (39%)**.

2 Recently published NICE guidelines (see p. 287) do not allow for some of these uses of ECT. However, NICE guidance does not override the individual responsibility of health professionals to make decisions appropriate to the circumstances of a specific patient (such action should be discussed, documented in the notes, and, where appropriate, validated by a second opinion).

Treating depressive illness (with psychotic features)

ECT (see p. 286)

For depression with psychotic features, ECT should be considered as first-line therapy, as evidence supports the superior efficacy of ECT to pharmacotherapy in this patient group, with significant benefit in 80–90% of cases (N.B. *Current NICE guidelines do not support this practice—see p. 287*). However, often issues of consent or relative contraindications may preclude the immediate use of ECT and its role is often that of a second-line treatment after partial response or failure of pharmacotherapy.

Combination treatment (antidepressant *plus* antipsychotic)

It is usual to commence treatment with an antipsychotic agent (as for an acute psychotic episode see p. 200) for a few days before commencing an antidepressant. This allows for a period of assessment (to exclude a primary *psychotic* disorder), may improve compliance (when psychotic symptoms are seen to improve with medication), avoids potential *worsening* of psychotic symptoms with an antidepressant (in some predisposed individuals), and may help identify the 30–50% of patients who do respond to an antipsychotic alone. There is no clear evidence for any *particular* combination of medication being more efficacious, but this approach is effective in 70–80% of patients.

Points to note include:

- Symptoms ought to be carefully monitored, as antipsychotic side-effects may mask improvement in depressive symptoms—hence use of lowest effective dose is advocated (e.g. around 2–4mg haloperidol or equivalent).
- Combinations of antidepressant / antipsychotic may worsen side-effects common to both (e.g. sedation, anticholinergic effects) and careful dose titration is necessary.
- Once acute psychotic symptoms have resolved, a lower dose of antipsychotic (or withdrawal) may be indicated, particularly when patients begin to manifest side-effects (which were not seen in the acute stages, even with higher doses)—with careful monitoring for recurrence of psychotic symptoms.

Dual-action agents

There is some evidence that single agents with dual actions, such as **amoxapine** (a tetracyclic antidepressant with significant D_2 antagonism), or antipsychotics, such as **olanzapine**, may be effective in treating both aspects of depression with psychotic symptoms. To date, evidence does not exist to support use of these agents for *long-term* treatment:, where there are issues of compliance/tolerability the utility of using a *single* agent is attractive, but should be considered carefully.

Maintenance therapy

- When ECT has been used, maintenance usually involves the treatment of the underlying depressive symptoms with an antidepressant (as in episodes *without* psychotic symptoms—see p. 262).

- When combination treatment has been successful, maintenance often involves a clinically effective antidepressant with the lowest effective antipsychotic dose. As for dual-action agents, evidence is lacking with regards to long-term treatment and this tends to be pragmatic, on the basis of continued symptomatology.
- In view of the severity of the disorder, prophylactic use of an antidepressant and/or antipsychotic is prudent (often indefinitely, as for recurrent depressive episodes—see p. 263).

An approach to treatment-resistant depression

Commonly defined as 'failure to respond to adequate (dose and duration—i.e. max. BNF dose for at least 6 weeks) courses of 2 antidepressants, or 1 antidepressant and ECT'. The consequences of resistant depression include reduced quality of life, excessive strain on relationships (which may lead to break-up of families), significant personal economic impact, increased physical comorbidity (e.g. malignancy, cardiovascular disease, even premature death), increased risk of suicide, therapeutic alienation (making further interventions difficult due to difficulties forming a therapeutic alliance), and high use of psychiatric services (without clear benefit).

Differentiating 'treatment resistance'

It is important to distinguish actual treatment resistance from chronicity of symptoms. *Apparent* treatment failure may also occur due to: incorrect initial diagnosis (i.e. *not* depressive disorder in the first place), inadequate initial treatment, poor compliance, incomplete formulation (esp. role of maintaining factors), and issues of comorbidity (both physical and other psychiatric disorders).

Risk factors for treatment resistance

Concurrent physical illness, drug/alcohol abuse, personality disorder, delayed treatment, high premorbid neuroticism.

Management

- **Review diagnostic formulation** Is diagnosis correct? Are there any unaddressed maintaining factors (e.g. social, physical, psychological)?
- **Check patient understanding and compliance** (serum levels may help).
- **Continue monotherapy at maximum tolerable dose** May mean exceeding BNF guidelines (esp. if there has been partial benefit).
- **Consider change in antidepressant** Try a different class of antidepressant.
- **Consider augmentation with a mood stabiliser** (e.g. lithium).
- **Consider additional augmentative agents** (e.g. L-tryptophan, T$_3$).
- **Consider combining antidepressants from different classes** Caution is advised, due to possible serious adverse reactions (e.g. serotonin syndrome pp. 870–1).
- **Consider use of ECT**—see p. 286 (esp. if severe biological features or psychotic symptoms).
- **Consider possibility of psychosurgery** (see p. 294).

Points to note

- There is little *definitive* evidence to support any *specific* augmentative regime.
- Spontaneous remission is possible: 'regression to the mean' suggests that symptoms will improve; bear in mind that the natural life of depression is 6–18 mths, even when untreated.
- Psychological and social interventions, particularly when psychosocial factors appear paramount, may be important (often overlooked or undisclosed) aspects of management.

Atypical depressive episode

Regarded as a subtype of depressive disorder, rather than a separate entity. Atypical features coded in DSM-IV as an 'episode specifier', (like melancholic, postpartum, catatonic). Included in 'other depressive episodes' in ICD-10.

Clinical features

- Mood is depressed but remains reactive (able to enjoy certain experiences but not to 'normal' levels).
- Hypersomnia (sleeping more than 10 hrs/day, at least 3 days/wk, for at least 3 mths).
- Hyperphagia (excessive eating with weight gain of over 3kg in 3 mths).
- 'Leaden paralysis' (feeling of heaviness in the limbs, present for at least 1 hr/day, 3 days/wk, for at least 3 mths).
- Over-sensitivity to perceived rejection[1].
- Other infrequent symptoms may include: initial insomnia rather than EMW; reversed diurnal mood variation (better in the morning); severe motor retardation; absence of feelings of guilt.

Epidemiology Onset usually in late teens and early twenties, often (up to 30%) family history of affective disorders.

Comorbidity Higher rates of anxiety (esp. panic disorder and social phobia), somatisation disorder (see pp. 742–3), alcohol and drug misuse than in other depressive disorders.

Management

- Best evidence is for the use of phenelzine (15mg/d increased gradually to 60–90mg/d—continue for 8–12 wks to assess benefit) or another MAOI (see p. 278 for guidance on prescribing/dietary advice). RIMAs theoretically ought to be as effective and safer (but evidence is lacking).
- Alternatives include SSRIs (e.g. fluoxetine or sertraline), or possibly an NARI (e.g. reboxetine).
- TCAs have traditionally been regarded as less effective. However, some individuals may respond well, and the best evidence is for the use of imipramine.
- Where there is failure to respond to an adequate trial of an antidepressant, follow management principles outlined for **Treating depressive illness** (p. 262) and **An approach to treatment-resistant depression** (p. 266).

1 'Rejection sensitivity' (to both *real* and *imagined* rejection) adds to the difficulty of managing atypical depression, as the patient may have had adverse experiences with doctors in the past, been labelled as 'personality disordered', and may find the idea of a therapeutic alliance alien.

Seasonal affective disorder (SAD)

Clinical features

Aetiology

Epidemiology

Management

Seasonal affective disorder (SAD)

Somewhat controversial concept, both in terms of diagnosis (see below) and treatment using light therapy (see p. 296). In DSM-IV **seasonal pattern** is included in specifiers describing the course of recurrent depressive episodes of both depressive and bipolar disorder. Included under 'recurrent depressive disorder' in ICD-10.

Clinical features There may be a clear seasonal pattern to recurrent depressive episodes (i.e. they have occurred at the same time of year each time). In the northern hemisphere this is said to be usually around January/February ('winter depression'). Symptoms are generally mild to moderate with low self-esteem, hypersomnia, fatigue, increased appetite (including carbohydrate craving) and weight gain, and decreased social and occupational functioning.

Aetiology It is unclear whether this constitutes a separate subtype of depressive disorder, or whether it is simply a manifestation of atypical depression (see p. 268). The speculated mechanism involving melatonin synthesis has not been confirmed in controlled studies, and some authors suggest that seasonal psychosocial factors may be more important in determining the timing of recurrent depressive episodes (e.g. increased work demands over the Christmas and New Year periods for shopworkers).

Epidemiology In the US, prevalence of SAD is estimated at ~5%, ♂:♀ = 1:5.

Management

- *Light therapy* (see p. 296) Initially 2 hrs of 2500lux (or equivalent) on waking (response seen within 5 days and full response in 1–2 wks). Maintenance therapy should be given all winter (30 mins of 2500lux every 1–2 days). Patients should avoid exposure to bright light during night-time. *Good prognostic factors* Patients with clear hypersomnia, carbohydrate craving, reduced energy in the afternoon..
- *Pharmacological* Best evidence for fluoxetine (but no reason why other antidepressants would not be as effective); propranolol (either alone or in combination with an antidepressant) may also have some efficacy (assumed mode of action: suppression of melatonin).

Dysthymia (ICD-10)/dysthymic disorder (DSM-IV)

Clinical features

Epidemiology

Management

Prognosis

Dysthymia (ICD-10)/dysthymic disorder (DSM-IV)

Previously considered a subtype of personality disorder, dysthymia is essentially the presence of chronic, low-grade depressive symptoms. These may be longstanding; however, careful history taking does reveal a time when the person *did* feel 'well'. It is possible to have superimposed depressive episodes ('double depression'), when care is needed in assessing treatment response, as baseline may be dysthymic rather than euthymic.

Clinical features
- Depressed mood (<2yrs)
- Reduced/increased appetite
- Insomnia/hypersomnia
- Reduced energy/fatigue
- Low self-esteem
- Poor concentration
- Difficulties making decisions
- Thoughts of hopelessness.

Epidemiology Prevalence ~5%, ♂:♀ = 1:2

Course Less severe, but more chronic than depression—community studies show a low spontaneous remission rate (2–20yrs, median 5yrs).

Management
- **Pharmacological** Best evidence exists for the use of phenelzine, but response rates vary (30–70%). Alternatives include an SSRI (e.g. fluoxetine, sertraline) or a TCA (e.g. desipramine, imipramine, amitriptyline).
- **Psychological** Although evidence is lacking, CBT may be useful (often in combination with an antidepressant).

Prognosis
Variable: Only 10–20% of patients achieve complete remission within a year of treatment; ~25% suffer chronic symptoms.

Antidepressants

Assumed mode of action All currently available antidepressants appear to exert their antidepressant action by increasing the availability of monoamines (5HT, NA and DA) via one or more of the following:

- Presynaptic inhibition of reuptake of 5HT, NA, or DA.
- Antagonist activity at presynaptic inhibitory 5HT or NA receptor sites, which enhances neurotransmitter release.
- Inhibition of monoamine oxidase, reducing neurotransmitter breakdown.
- Increasing the availability of neurotransmitter precursors.

Although this net increase happens almost immediately following administration, initial resolution of depressive symptoms generally takes 10–20 days, implying therapeutic effect involves 2° mechanisms possibly related to receptor regulation over time/changes in intracellular signalling.

Selectivity vs. specificity Although the newer antidepressants are more **selective** than the TCAs and MAOIs in their pharmacological effects, this should not be confused with them being more **specific** for any particular type of depressive symptoms. All antidepressants have unwanted and often unpleasant side-effects. A balance needs to be struck between efficacy in treating psychiatric symptoms and the possibility of iatrogenic problems. Patients may not be able to tolerate the anticholinergic side-effects of TCAs, or will be unable to achieve a therapeutic level because of side-effects. Similarly, nausea or GI upset may limit the usefulness of SSRIs in some individuals. Sometimes side-effects may be useful (e.g. sedation for patients with insomnia) or combinations of antidepressants may be more efficacious than one alone (or may offset side-effects) (e.g. mirtazepine + SSRIs/SNRIs for sexual side-effects; SSRI + trazodone combination for those troubled by insomnia, but who have responded well to the antidepressant effects of the SSRI).

Cautionary notes Particular caution is necessary in prescribing for certain patient groups (see pp. 876–87) such as those with renal or hepatic impairment, cardiac problems, epilepsy; pregnant or breast-feeding women; the elderly; children; and those on other medications which may interact with antidepressants. There are also well-recognised problems such as weight gain (p. 852), hyponatraemia (p. 874), sexual dysfunction (pp. 856–7), and withdrawal syndromes (pp. 872–3).

Combining/switching antidepressants (see opposite) An adequate 'washout' period is required when switching to or from the MAOIs, whereas it is usual to *cross-taper* between other antidepressants (i.e. gradually reducing the dose of one, whilst slowly increasing the dose of the other). During this process, or when combining antidepressants, side-effects may be enhanced (due to pharmacokinetic effects) and it is possible to induce the **serotonin syndrome** (see pp. 870–1).

The following pages outline the main groups of antidepressants. This information should be used as a guide and the clinician is always advised to consult manufacturers' data sheets, or more detailed formularies, for less common problems or specific details of administration.

Switching antidepressants (adapted from Bazirre (2000) Psychotropic Drug Directory, Fivepin Publishing Ltd.)

FROM \ TO	MAOIs		TCAs	SSRIs					Trazodone	Tryptophan	Moclobemide	Venlafaxine	Mirtazepine	Viloxazine & Mianserin	Reboxetine
	Hydrazines	Tranyl-cypromine		Citalopram/ Escitalopram	Fluvoxamine	Fluoxetine	Sertraline	Paroxetine							
MAOIs Hydrazines	■	2wks	1-2wks	2wks	2wks	2wks	2wks	2wks	2wks	2wks Care	1day Care	2wks	2wks	2wks	2wks
Tranylcypromine	2wks	■	2wks	2wks	2wks	2wks	2wks	2wks	2wks	1day	1wk Care	2wks	2wks	2wks	2wks
TCAs	1wk	1wk	■	Care	Great Care	Great Care	Care	Great Care	NRP	NRP	NRP	Variable	NRP	NRP	NRP
SSRIs Citalopram/Escitalopram	1wk	1wk	Care	■	SS	SS	SS	SS	Care	Care	1wk	Care	NRP	NRP	NRP
Fluvoxamine	4d	1wk	Great care	SS	■	SS	SS	SS	Care	Care	4-5d	Care	NRP	NRP	NRP
Fluoxetine	5wks	5wks	Great care	SS	SS	■	SS	SS	Care	Care	4-5d	Care	NRP	NRP	NRP
Sertraline	1wk	1-2wks	Care	SS	SS	SS	■	SS	Care	Care	4-13d	Care	NRP	NRP	NRP
Paroxetine	2wks	2wks	Great care	Care	Care	SS	SS	■	Care	Care	4-5d	Care	NRP	NRP	NRP
Trazodone	1wk	1wk	OccP	Care	Care	Care	Care	Care	■	NRP	NRP	NRP	NRP	NRP	NRP
Tryptophan	2wks Care	1-2wks Care	NRP	Care	Care	Care	Care	Care	NRP	■	NRP	NRP	NRP	NRP	NRP
Moclobemide	NRP	NRP	OccP	NRP	NRP	2wks	NRP	NRP	NRP	NRP	■	NRP	NRP	NRP	NRP
Venlafaxine	1wk	1wk	NRP	Care	Care	Care	Care	Care	Care	NRP	NRP	■	NRP	NRP	NRP
Mirtazepine	2wks	2wks	NRP	NRP	NRP	NRP	NRP	NRP	NRP	NRP	NRP	NRP	■	NRP	NRP
Viloxazine & Mianserin	2wks	2wks	NRP	NRP	NRP	NRP	NRP	NRP	NRP	NRP	NRP	NRP	NRP	■	NRP
Reboxetine	1wk	1wk	NRP	NRP	NRP	NRP	NRP	NRP	NRP	NRP	NRP	NRP	NRP	NRP	■

Key: NRP no reported problems; OccP occasional problems; SS possible serotonin syndrome

Tricyclic antidepressants (TCAs)

Common mode of action and effects/side-effects

• **Serotonin/noradrenaline (and dopamine) reuptake inhibition**
Antidepressant effects.

• **Anticholinergic (antimuscarinic—M$_1$)**
Dry mouth, blurred vision, constipation, urinary retention, drowsiness, confusion/memory problems (particularly in the elderly), palpitations/tachycardia.

• **Adrenergic antagonism (α_1)**
Drowsiness, postural hypotension (occasionally syncope), tachycardia, sexual dysfunction.

• **5HT$_2$ antagonism**
Anxiolytic, reduced sexual dysfunction, sedation.

• **Antihistaminergic (H$_1$)**
Drowsiness, weight gain.

Advantages Well-established efficacy and large literature (in all varieties of patient groups); possibly more effective in severe depression; low cost.

Disadvantages Toxicity in overdose; may be less well tolerated than SSRIs; all TCAs may slow cardiac conduction and lower seizure threshold.

Contraindications Acute MI, heart block, arrhythmias, IHD, severe liver disease, pregnancy and lactation (see pp. 876–83).

Cautions (also see 'Cautionary notes' p. 274) Cardiovascular, liver, renal disease; endocrine disorders (hyperthyroidism, adrenal tumours, diabetes); urinary retention/prostatic hypertrophy; constipation; glaucoma; epilepsy; psychotic disorders; patients with thoughts of suicide; elderly (use lower doses).

Significant interactions (variable for different agents—always check data sheets) Alcohol, anticoagulants, anticonvulsants, antihypertensives, antipsychotics, barbiturates, benzodiazepines (rare), cimetidine, digoxin, MAOIs (rare), methylphenidate, morphine, SSRIs, smoking.

Monitoring It is good practice to monitor cardiac and liver function, U&Es, and FBC during long-term therapy.

Tricyclic antidepressants (TCAs)

Drug	Half life (hrs)	Formulations	Usual starting dose	Usual maintenance dose	Max. daily dose	Notes	Indications
Amitriptyline	8–24	T 10/25/50mg C 25/50mg S25 or 50mg/5ml	75mg/d (divided or just at night)	100–150mg	150mg	Metabolised to nortriptyline	Depression, nocturnal enuresis, chronic pain, migraine, insomnia
Amoxapine	8	T 50/100mg	100–150mg/d	150–250mg/d	300mg		Depression
Clomipramine	17–28	T 10/25/50mg SR 75mg Inj 12.5mg/ml	10mg/d	30–150mg/d (divided or just at night)	250mg	Most SSRI-like of the TCAs Can be given IV/IM	Depression, OCD & phobic disorders, adjunctive treatment of cataplexy (in narcolepsy)
Dothiepin	14–40	C/T 25mg	75–150mg/d	75–150mg/d	225mg (hospital)		Depression (with anxiety)
Doxepin	8–24	C 10/25/50/75mg	75mg/d	Up to 300mg/d (divided if <100mg/d)	300mg		Depression (esp. if sedation needed)
Imipramine	4–18	T 10/25mg S25mg/5ml	25mg up to tds	50–100mg/d	200mg	Metabolised to desipramine	Depression, nocturnal enuresis
Lofepramine	1.6–5	T 70mg S 70mg/5ml	70mg/d	70–210mg/d	210mg	May be safer in overdose Least proconvulsant Metabolised to desipramine	Depression
Nortriptyline	18–96	T 10/25mg	25mg tds	75–100mg/d	150mg	Manufacturer recommends plasma monitoring in does < 100mg/d ('therapeutic window' 50–150 ng/ml)	Depression, nocturnal enuresis
Trimipramine	7–23	T 10/25mg C 50mg	75mg/d	150–300mg/d	300mg	May be very sedating	Depression (with anxiety)

Key: T = tablets; C = capsules; S = oral suspension/solution; SR = modified release capsules; Inj = injectable form

Monoamine oxidase inhibitors (MAOIs) and reversible monoamine oxidase inhibitors (RIMAs)

Mode of action
- **MAOIs** Irreversible inhibition of MAO-A (acts on NA, DA, 5HT, and tyramine) and MAO-B (acts on DA, tyramine, phenylethylamine, benzylamine), leading to accumulation of monoamines in synaptic cleft.
- **RIMAs** Act by reversible inhibition of MAO-A.

Side-effects
- **Risk of hypertensive crisis** due to inhibition of peripheral pressor amines (hence foods high in tyramine and certain medications should be avoided):
  - *Sources of dietary tyramine* Cheese (except cottage and cream cheese), meat extracts and yeast extracts (including Bovril®, Marmite®, Oxo®, and other fermented soya bean extracts), alcohol—including low-alcohol drinks (especially chianti and fortified wines and beers), non-fresh fish, non-fresh poultry, offal, avocado, banana skins, broad-bean pods, caviar, herring (pickled or smoked).
  - *Medications* Indirect sympathomimetics (amphetamine, fenfluramine, ephedrine, phenylephrine, phenylpropanolamine), cough mixtures containing sympathomimetics, nasal decongestants with sympathomimetics, L-dopa, pethidine, TCAs.
  - These effects may be less with RIMAs. However, large amounts of tyramine-rich food should be avoided.
- **Other side-effects** Antimuscarinic actions, hepatotoxicity, insomnia, anxiety, appetite suppression, weight gain, postural hypotension ankle oedema, sexual dysfunction, possible dependency.

Indications Usually used as second-line therapy for treatment-resistant depression (particularly atypical symptoms)/anxiety disorders (with or without panic attacks).

Cautions Avoid MAOIs in cardiac/hepatic failure, porphyria.

Advantages Well-established efficacy in a broad range of affective and anxiety disorders.

Disadvantages Dietary restrictions and drug interactions (less so with RIMAs).

Other significant drug interactions (**variable for MAOIs vs. RIMAs—always check data sheets**) Antidiabetics, antiepileptics, antihypertensives, antipsychotics, barbiturates, benzodiazepines, β-blockers, buspirone, cimetidine, dopaminergics (selegiline), dextromethorphan, mazinol, pethidine, morphine, SSRIs, $5HT_1$ agonists (rizatriptan, sumatriptan), tetrabenazine.

MAOIs and RIMAs

Drug	Class	Half Life (hrs)	Formulations	Usual starting dose	Usual maintenance dose	Max. daily dose	Notes
Isocarboxazid	MAOI	36	T 10mg	30mg/d (divided or single daily dose)	10–40mg/d	60mg/d	Hydrazine derivative—less stimulating
Moclobemide	RIMA	1–2	T 150mg	150mg od	150–600mg/d	600mg/d	May be used for social phobia. Possible hyponatraemia. 'Cheese reaction' least likely.
Phenelizine	MAOI	1.5	T 15mg	15mg tds	15mg every other day to 15mg qds	90mg/d	Hydrazine derivative—less stimulating.
Tranylcypromine	MAOI	2.5	T 10mg	10mg bd	10mg/d	30mg/d (or greater if supervised)	Most stimulant of MAOIs (am-phetamine-related). Do not give after 3pm. Increased risk of significant interactions.

Key: T = tablets

Selective serotonin reuptake inhibitors (SSRIs)

Common mode of action and effects/side-effects

- **Serotonin reuptake inhibition** (leads to ↑5HT in the synaptic cleft)
  - 5HT$_{1A}$ agonism
    Antidepressant, anxiolytic, anti-obsessive, anti-bulimic effects.
  - 5HT$_2$ agonism
    Agitation, akathisia, anxiety/panic, insomnia, sexual dysfunction.
  - 5HT$_3$ agonism
    Nausea, GI upset, diarrhoea, headache.

Advantages Ease of dosing; may be better tolerated than TCAs—less cardiotoxic; fewer anticholinergic side-effects; low toxicity in overdose.

Disadvantages Commonly cause nausea and GI upset, headache, restlessness, and insomnia; may be less effective for severe depressive episodes; problems on discontinuation (see pp. 872–3).

Contraindications Manic episode, concomitant use of MAOIs.

Cautions (also see **Cautionary notes** p. 274) Variable and significant inhibitory effects on hepatic P450 (particularly CYP2D6) enzymes (with exception of citalopram/escitalopram). Hence take care when co-prescribing with drugs that undergo extensive liver metabolism and have a narrow therapeutic range.

Significant interactions (**variable for different agents—always check data sheets**) Alcohol, anticoagulants, anticonvulsants, antipsychotics, benzodiazepines, β-blockers, bupropion, buspirone, cimetidine, cyproheptadine, hypoglycaemics, lithium, methadone, MAOIs, morphine, smoking, TCAs, theophylline, warfarin.

Selective serotonin reuptake inhibitors (SSRIs)

Drug	Half Life (hrs)	Formulations	Usual starting dose	Usual maintenance dose	Max. daily dose	Notes	Indications
Citalopram	33	T 10/20/40mg S 40mg/ml	20mg od (10mg for panic, increase slowly)	20–60mg od	60mg	Least likely to interact with other drugs. Less likely to reduce seizure threshold (caution).	Depression, panic disorder (with or without agoraphobia)
Escitalopram	33	T 10mg	10mg od (5mg for panic, increase slowly)	10–20mg od	20mg		Depression (with or without anxiety symptoms), OCD, bulimia nervosa, PMDD
Fluoxetine	24–140	C 20/60mg S 20mg/5ml	20mg od	20–60mg od	80mg	Most alerting May cause weight loss	Depression, OCD
Fluvoxamine	15–22	T 50/100mg	50–100mg od	100–300mg (if <150mg, in divided doses)	300mg	Moderately sedating	Depression (with or without anxiety), OCD, panic disorder (with or without agoraphobia), social phobia, PTSD, GAD
Paroxetine	10–21	T 20/30mg S 20mg/10ml	20mg od (10mg for panic, increase slowly)	20–60mg od	60mg	Most anticholinergic Withdrawal syndrome may be more frequent May be sedating	Depression (with or without anxiety), OCD, PTSD
Sertraline	26	T 50/100mg	50mg (25mg for PTSD, increase slowly)	50–200mg od	200mg	Moderately alerting Fewer drug interactions, but caution still necessary	

Key: T = tablets; C = capsules; S = oral suspension/solution

Other antidepressants (1)

Tetracyclic antidepressants (TeCAs)

Mode of action Similar to TCAs, but with less anticholinergic S/Es.
Indications Depression, particularly if sedation required.
Advantages Better side-effect profile than some TCAs (e.g. cardiotoxicity), sedating (which may be a desirable effect).
Disadvantages Idiosyncratic adverse effects.

Mianserin

Common adverse effects As for TCAs, but less cardiovascular problems, blood dyscrasias more common (esp. elderly—FBC recommended 4 wkly for 1st 3 mths of treatment, therafter 3–6mthly; stop treatment and check FBC if *fever, sore throat, stomatitis,* or other signs of infection develop), jaundice, arthritis, arthralgia.
Usual dose 30–40mg (elderly 30mg) daily in divided doses or as a single night-time dose, increased gradually as necessary; usual range 30–90mg/d.

Maprotiline

Common adverse effects As for TCAs, but rash more common and increased risk of seizure induction at high doses.
Usual dose 25–75mg (elderly 30mg) daily in 3 divided doses or as a single night-time dose, increased gradually as necessary to max. 150mg daily.

Serotonin/noradrenaline reuptake inhibitors (SNRIs)—venlafaxine

Mode of action At low doses, acts like an SSRI; at moderate doses acts as a combined 5HT and NA reuptake inhibitor; and at high doses also inhibits DA reuptake.
Common adverse effects Nausea, GI upset, agitation, insomnia, sexual dysfunction, headache, hypertension.
Indications Depression, generalised anxiety disorder (GAD).
Usual dose 37.5mg bd (or 75mg od of controlled release [XL] form), increased after several weeks to 75mg bd (or 150mg of XL). For severe depression, begin at 150mg/d, increasing by 75mg every few days to max. dose 375mg/d. For GAD 75mg od, discontinue if no response after 8wks.
Advantages Variable pharmacological profile over dose range; possibly more rapid onset of action than other antidepressants; available in controlled release form allowing once-daily administration.
Disadvantages Moderate to high doses less well tolerated; need to monitor BP at doses over 200mg; troublesome side-effects; withdrawal effects common.

Noradrenaline reuptake inhibitors (NARIs)—reboxetine

Mode of action NA reuptake inhibition.
Common adverse effects Insomnia, sweating, postural hypotension/dizziness, tachycardia, sexual dysfunction, dysuria, urinary retention, dry mouth, constipation, may↑ serum K^+ if used long term in the elderly.
Indications Depression (particularly with atypical features).
Usual dose 4mg bd, increased after 3–4wks to 10mg/d if necessary (max. 12mg/d).

Advantages Novel mode of action; alerting effects may be useful for patients with symptoms of fatigue or hypersomnia; may improve social functioning; relatively safe in overdose.
Disadvantages Mainly due to adverse effects.

Serotonin antagonist/reuptake inhibitors (SARIs)—trazodone

Mode of action 5HT reuptake inhibition, $5HT_2$ antagonist (more sedating/anxiolytic, less sexual dysfunction), α_1 antagonist (reduces NA effects), antihistamine (H_1: sedation and weight gain).
Common adverse effects Priapism (see p. 858), sedation, fatigue, otherwise similar to TCAs—but less antimuscarinic and cardiotoxic.
Indications Depression (esp. with insomnia), anxiety disorders.
Usual dose 150mg/d (as divided dose or just at night), increased to 300mg/d (max. dose 600mg—in hospital). For anxiety, start at 75mg/d.
Advantages Sedation (may be used in low doses as an adjunct to other less sedating antidepressants or to counter sexual dysfunction), safer in epilepsy than TCAs.
Disadvantages The higher doses necessary for antidepressant effects may not be tolerated.

Noradrenergic and specific serotonergic antidepressant (NaSSA)—mirtazapine

Mode of action α_2 antagonist (increased 5HT and NA release—antidepressant), $5HT_2$ antagonist (more sedating/anxiolytic, less sexual dysfunction), $5HT_3$ antagonist (reduced nausea/GI upset), antihistamine (H_1: sedation and weight gain).
Common adverse effects Sedation, increased appetite/weight gain; less common: jaundice/LFT changes, oedema, postural hypotension, tremor, myoclonus, blood dyscrasias.
Indications Depression (with anxiety/panic, agitation, insomnia, weight loss); as an adjunct to SSRIs/venlafaxine to improve sexual dysfunction, nausea, GI upset, insomnia.
Usual dose 15mg nocte, increased if necessary to max. 45mg/d (divided dose or just at night).
Advantages Low toxicity in overdose, less sexual dysfunction and GI upset.
Disadvantages Weight gain, sedating effects may be lost at higher doses (may be used to advantage).

Other antidepressants (2)

Noradrenergic and dopaminergic reuptake inhibitor (NDRI)—bupropion (Wellbutrin, Zyban)

Mode of action NA and DA reuptake inhibition.

Indications Depression (with marked psychomotor retardation or hypersomnia); treatment of nicotine dependence (and possibly withdrawal from other stimulants); may be useful in adult/child ADHD.

Usual dose 150mg od, increased after 6d to 150mg bd (max. duration of treatment for nicotine dependence 7–9wks).

Common adverse effects Agitation/insomnia, dry mouth, GI upset (nausea, vomiting, abdominal pain, constipation), hypertension (esp. if concomitant use of nicotine patches), risk of seizures (0.4%), disturbance of taste.

Advantages Unusual mode of action, alerting effects may be useful for patients with symptoms of fatigue or hypersomnia, may help treat impulse disorders and addictions as a secondary benefit when used as an antidepressant.

Disadvantages Possible seizure induction, hypersensitivity reactions (rare, but may be severe)

L-tryptophan

Mode of action Precursor for serotonin.

Indications Restricted specialist use as an adjunct for treatment-resistant depression (lasting more than 2 years).

Usual dose 1g tds, increased to max. 6g/d.

Common adverse effects Drowsiness, headache, nausea, dizziness, eosinophilia-myalgia syndrome (rare—but monitoring of FBC necessary).

St. John's wort (*Hypericum perforatum*)

Considered a first-line antidepressant in many European countries (and recently becoming popular in the US); not yet in the UK. May be effective for mild-moderate depressive symptoms.

Mode of action Recent research suggests it may act as a weak SSRI.

Usual dose 300mg tds (with food to prevent GI upset).

Notable interactions Anticoagulants (esp. warfarin), antidepressants (risk of SS—see pp. 870–1), antiepileptics, antivirals, barbiturates, cyclosporin, digoxin, $5HT_1$ agonists (rizatriptan, sumatriptan), oral contraceptives, theophylline.

ECT (1)—background and indications

Electroconvulsive therapy (ECT) is a highly effective (if controversial) treatment for depression (particularly with psychotic symptoms), which may act more rapidly than antidepressant medication. Advances in brief anaesthesia and neuromuscular paralysis have led to improved safety and tolerability. Decline in the use of ECT reflects the influence of non-evidence based factors on the choice of treatment modalities rather than being an indicator of its efficacy[*]. A systematic review of 153 studies (~6000 patients)[1] found the treatment response of ECT to be superior to other modes of treatment: ECT (72%), TCAs (65%), MAOIs (50%), placebo (23%).

Mode of action Specific mode of action is unknown. ECT does cause a wide range of effects on neurotransmitters with net functional increases in monoamine systems (NA, 5HT, DA), GABA, ACh, endogenous opioids (increase/altered binding of met-enkephalin and beta-endorphin), and adenosine (A_1 purinoceptors). Also profound effects on the neuroendocrine system, with release of hypothalamic, pituitary, and adrenal hormones.

Indications (see also opposite)

- **Depressive episode:** severe episodes, need for rapid antidepressant response (e.g. due to failure to eat or drink in depressive stupor; high suicide risk), failure of drug treatments, patients who are unable to tolerate side-effects of drug treatment (e.g. puerperal depressive disorder—see p. 757), previous history of good response to ECT, patient preference.
- **Other indications:** treatment-resistant psychosis and mania (50–60% effective), schizoaffective disorder (see p. 228), catatonia (see p. 899), neuroleptic malignant syndrome (see pp. 868–9), neurological crises (e.g. extreme Parkinsonian symptoms: on-off phenomena), intractable seizure disorders (acts to raise seizure threshold).

Contraindications There are no **absolute** contraindications. Where possible, use of ECT should be limited for patients with cerebral aneurysm, recent MI, cardiac arrhythmias, intracerebral haemorrhage, acute/impending retinal detachment, phaeochromocytoma, high anaesthetic risk, and unstable vascular aneurysm or malformation.

---

[*] In the last 15yrs, there have been 6 studies on ECT effectiveness, demonstrating the efficacy of ECT over and above any placebo effect in 5/6 studies (the one study showing a negative result had small numbers and used unilateral brief pulse stimulus).

1 Wechsler H, Grosser GH, Greenblatt M (1965) Research evaluating antidepressant medications on hospitalized mental patients: a survey of published reports during a five-year period. *Journal of Nervous and Mental Disease* **141** 231–9.

ECT—an historical perspective

The use of convulsive treatments for psychiatric disorders has at its origin the clinical observation of apparent antagonism between schizophrenia (then *dementia praecox*) and epilepsy. It appeared that patients who had a seizure were relieved of their psychotic symptoms and Meduna noted increased glial cells in the brains of patients with epilepsy compared to reduced number in those with schizophrenia. In 1934 he induced a seizure with an injection of campor-in-oil in a patient with catatonic schizophrenia, and continued this treatment every 3 days. After the fifth seizure the patient was able to talk spontaneously and began to eat and care for himself for the first time in 4 years, making a full recovery with 3 further treatments. Chemically-induced convulsive treatments using camphor or metrazol (pentylenetetrazol) became accepted for the treatment of schizophrenia, but were not without problems. Cerletti and Bini introduced the use of 'electric shock' to induce seizures in 1938, and soon this method became the standard. Initially ECT was 'unmodified' (i.e. without anaesthetic or muscle relaxant), but because of frequent injury, and advances in brief anaesthesia, the current procedure is the more 'humane' modified ECT. *Indications* have also changed, with the majority of patients receiving ECT due to severe depressive illness, although it is also effective in other conditions (see opposite).

NICE Technology Appraisal 59

Guidance on the Use of Electroconvulsive Therapy (May 2003)
'ECT is used only to achieve rapid and short-term improvement of severe symptoms after an adequate trial of other treatment options has proven ineffective and/or when the condition is considered to be life-threatening, in individuals with **severe depressive illness, catatonia, prolonged or severe manic episode** ... The current state of the evidence did not allow the general use of ECT in the management of schizophrenia to be recommended ... ECT is **not recommended as a maintenance therapy in depressive illness** because the longer-term benefits and risks of ECT have not been clearly established ... The decision as to whether ECT is clinically indicated should be based on a documented assessment of the risks and potential benefits to the individual, including: the risks associated with the anaesthetic, contemporaneous comorbidities, anticipated adverse events, particularly cognitive impairment, and the risks of not having the treatment.'

ECT (2)—problems and treatment course

Limitations Time-limited action (tends to dissipate after a couple of weeks, hence need for follow-up medication, or **maintenance treatment**, issues of consent to treatment (see pp. 820–3).

Side-effects
- *Early* Some loss of short-term memory: retrograde amnesia—usually resolves completely (64%), headache (48%—if recurrent, use simple analgesia), temporary confusion (27%), nausea/vomiting (9%), clumsiness (5%), muscular aches.
- *Late* Loss of long-term memory (rare—see opposite).
- *Mortality* No greater than for general anaesthesia in minor surgery (2:100 000)—usually due to cardiac complications in patients with known cardiac disease (hence need for close monitoring).

A course of ECT
- Rarely will a single treatment be effective to relieve the underlying disorder (but this does occasionally occur).
- ECT is usually given 3 times a week , reduced to twice a week or once a week once symptoms begin to respond. This limits cognitive problems, and there is no evidence that treatments of greater frequency enhance treatment response.
- Treatment of depression usually consists of 6–12 treatments; treatment-resistant psychosis and mania up to (or sometimes more than) 20 treatments; and catatonia usually resolves in 3–5 treatments.

Maintenance or continuation ECT
- Although evidence is limited (N.B. Not recommended in NICE guidelines—see p. 287), many psychiatrists recommend maintenance ECT (e.g. once a week, or every 2 weeks, for 4 months or more—N.B. Not often as an outpatient procedure) when a patient has responded well to ECT, and when drug treatments have been ineffective prior to ECT.
- Usually patients are aware of how effective ECT has been for them and a collaborative approach can be established (balancing frequency of ECT against return of symptoms and side-effects, esp. memory problems).

Does ECT cause brain damage?

ECT is not the devastating purveyor of wholesale brain damage that some of its detractors claim. For the typical individual receiving ECT, no detectable correlates of irreversible brain damage appear to occur. Still, there remains the possibility that either subtle, objectively undetectable persistent defects, particularly in the area of autobiographical memory function, occur, or that a rarely occurring syndrome of more pervasive persistent deficits related to ECT use may be present.

From Devanand DP, Dwork AJ, Hutchinson ER, *et al.* (1994)
Does ECT alter brain structure? *AJP* **151**, 957–70.

ECT (3)—'work-up' and administration

ECT 'work-up'
- Ensure full medical history and current medication noted on ECT recording sheet.
- Also note any relevant findings from physical examination.
- Ensure recent routine blood results available (FBC, U&Es, any other relevant investigations).
- If indicated, arrange pre-ECT CXR and/or ECG.
- Ensure consent form has been signed.
- Ensure ECT prescribed correctly.
- Inform anaesthetic team of proposed ECT.
- Inform ECT service of proposed ECT.
- Ensure patient is aware of the usual procedure and when treatment is scheduled.

Pre-ECT checks
- Check patient's identity.
- Check patient is fasted (for 8hrs) and has emptied their bowels and bladder prior to coming to treatment room.
- Check patient is not wearing restrictive clothing and jewellery/dentures have been removed.
- Consult ECT record of previous treatments (including anaesthetic problems).
- Ensure consent form is signed appropriately.
- Check no medication that might increase or reduce seizure threshold has been recently given.
- Check ECT machine is functioning correctly.
- Ensure dose settings are correct for specific patient (see **Energy dosing**).

Administration of anaesthetic
- Establish IV access.
- Attach monitoring (HR, BP, EEG/EMG).
- Ventilate patient with pure oxygen via face mask.
- Give muscle relaxant, followed by short-acting anaesthetic.
- (Hyperventilation with oxygen is sometimes used to augment seizure activity.)
- Insert bite-block between patient's teeth to protect tongue and teeth from jaw clenching (due to direct stimulation of masseter muscles).

Administration of ECT
- Apply electrodes to scalp (see opposite for positioning).
- Test for adequate contact between the electrodes and the scalp prior to treatment ('self-test' function on the ECT machine).
- Administer dose.
- Monitor length of seizure (see **Effective treatment**).
- Record dose, seizure duration, and any problems on ECT record (and ensure anaesthetic administration also recorded).
- Transfer patient to recovery.

Recovery
- Ensure that there is an adequate airway.
- Monitor the patient's pulse and blood pressure until stable.
- There should be continuous nursing presence and observation until the patient is fully orientated.
- Maintain IV access until able to leave recovery.

ECT Electrode placement

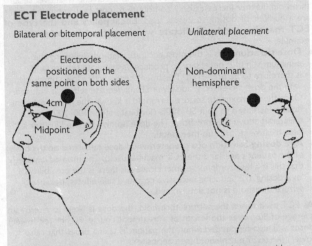

Bilateral or bitemporal placement

Unilateral placement

Electrodes positioned on the same point on both sides

4cm

Midpoint

Non-dominant hemisphere

Notes: The choice of bilateral or unilateral electrode placement remains controversial, although the balance of the evidence points to bilateral electrode placement being preferable in terms of speed of action and effectiveness. There is no doubt that unilateral ECT is associated with substantially less memory impairment, however modern brief pulse, low energy stimuli have reduced the memory impairment commonly associated with the old sine wave stimulation. There may well be regional differences in ECT policy, but the usual reasons for using unilateral/bilateral electrode placement are summarised below:

Electrode Placement	Bilateral	Unilateral (Non-dominant hemisphere)
When to use:	Speed of response a priority.	Speed of response less important.
	Failure of unilateral ECT.	Previous good response to unilateral ECT.
	Previous good response to bilateral ECT without significant memory problems.	Where minimising memory impairment is critical (e.g. evidence of cognitive impairment, outpatient treatment).
	Where determination of cerebral dominance is difficult.	

ECT (4)—notes on treatment

▶ *Ensure adequate training and supervision before administering ECT*

Energy dosing

Because the higher the stimulus used, the greater the likelihood of transient cognitive disturbance, and because once the current is above seizure threshold, further increases only contribute to post-ECT confusion, there are a number of dosing strategies used. **Local policy and the type of ECT machine used will dictate which method is preferred.** For example,

- **Dose titration** This is the most accurate method, delivering the minimum stimulus necessary to produce an adequate seizure, and is therefore to be preferred. Treatment begins with a low stimulus, with the dose increased gradually until an adequate seizure is induced. Once the approximate seizure threshold is known, the next treatment dose is increased to abut 50–100% (for bilateral) or 100–200% (for unilateral) above the threshold. The dose is only increased further if later treatments are sub-therapeutic.
- **Age dosing** Selection of a predetermined dose calculated on the basis of the patient's age (and the ECT machine used). The main advantage is that this is a less complex regime. However, there is the possibility of 'overdosing' (i.e. inducing excessive cognitive side-effects) because seizure threshold is not determined.

As ECT itself raises the seizure threshold, the dose is likely to rise by an average of 80% over the length of a treatment course. Higher (or lower) doses will also be needed when the patient is taking drugs that raise (or lower) the seizure threshold (see opposite).

Effective treatment

It used to be thought that *any* seizure length was therapeutic; however, that is no longer considered to be the case.

EEG monitoring is the *gold standard* with a typical ictal EEG having 4 phases: build-up of energies; 'spike and wave' activity (mixed high voltage spike activity with high voltage 3–6Hz slow waves); trains of lower voltage slow waves; and an abrupt end to activity followed by electrical 'silence'. This will usually last 35–130s, with motor seizure ~720% shorter in duration.

Timing of convulsion Where EEG monitoring is not used, the less reliable measure of length of observable motor seizure is used, with an effective treatment defined as a motor seizure lasting at least 20s (from end of ECT dose to end of observable motor activity).

Cuff technique Often underused technique involving isolation of a forearm or leg from the effects of muscle relaxant, by inflation of a blood pressure cuff to above systolic pressure. As the isolated limb does not become paralysed, the seizure can be more easily observed.

When a sub-therapeutic treatment is judged to have occurred, the treatment is repeated at different energy settings (see **Energy dosing**).

Specific problems
- **Persistent ineffective seizures** Check use of drugs that may raise seizure threshold, consider use of IV caffeine or theophylline.
- **Prolonged seizures** (i.e. over 150–180s) Administer IV diazemuls (5mg) repeated every 30s until seizure stops (alternative—midazolam). Lower energy dosing for next treatment.
- **Post-seizure confusion** (occurs in ~10% of treatments, usually early in a course) Reassurance, nurse in a calm environment, ensure safety of patient, if necessary consider sedation (e.g. diazemuls/midazolam). If a recurrent problem, use a low dose of a benzodiazepine prophylactically during recovery, immediately after ECT.

Psychiatric drugs and ECT

N.B. Ensure anaesthetist is fully informed of *all* medication the patient is currently taking.

Drugs that raise seizure threshold:
- **Benzodiazepines/barbiturates**
  Best avoided during ECT, or reduced to the lowest dose possible.
- **Anticonvulsants**
  Continue during ECT, but higher ECT stimulus will usually be needed.

Drugs that lower seizure threshold:
- **Antipsychotics**
  Continue if clinically indicated.
  Increased risk of hypotension and post-ECT confusion.
  Clozapine should be suspended 24hrs before ECT.
- **Antidepressants**
  TCAs, SSRIs, MAOIs—continue if clinically indicated.
  Increased risk of hypotension and post-ECT confusion (esp. TCAs).
  Moclobemide should be suspended 24hrs before ECT.
- **Lithium**
  Best avoided as may increase cognitive side-effects and increase likelihood of neurotoxic effects of lithium.

Psychosurgery/neurosurgery for mental disorder (NMD)

Despite the controversial nature of irreversible ('barbaric') surgery for mental disorders, it is surprising that patients rather than psychiatrists often raise the issue of neurosurgery, particularly when they retain insight into the chronic, intractable nature of their illness. This phenomenon is also seen in patients with treatment-resistant epilepsy for whom neurosurgery may seem like a 'holy grail'. Neurosurgery is only performed in exceptional cases when all other treatments have failed. It is still possible, however, to encounter patients who have had surgical procedures performed in the past, and this may complicate the diagnosis of current problems (e.g. depression, OCD, dementia—esp. frontal lobe symptoms) when there is demonstrable damage to key brain structures on CT/MRI.

Current criteria for NMD
- Severe mood disorder or obsessive-compulsive disorder (OCD).
- The patient must want the operation.
- All other reasonable treatments have repeatedly failed
  (i.e. pharmacological, ECT, psychological).
- The patient remains ill but competent to provide informed consent.

Current surgical techniques
These employ stereotactic methods, using pre-operative MRI to establish target coordinates and a fixed stereotactic frame (or new 'frameless' stereotactic instruments utilising infrared positioning). Lesioning may be effected by implantation of yttrium rods or radio-frequency lesioning. Lesions are localised to the orbito-frontal and anterior cingulate loop (the 'limbic' loop) which is strongly implicated in the regulation of emotion and mood[1] e.g.:
- Stereotactic subcaudate tractotomy (SST).
- Anterior cingulotomy.
- Stereotactic limbic leucotomy (SLL) (combining subcaudate tractotomy and anterior cingulotomy).
- Anterior capsulotomy.

Adverse effects Older techniques were associated with severe amotivational syndromes (up to 4%), marked personality change (up to 60%), and epilepsy (up to 15%). Stereotactic techniques report minimal post-operative problems with personality change and social functioning (2–8%) or cognitive functioning.

Outcome Given the treatment-resistant nature of the patients receiving surgery, reports of good outcome are surprisingly high (e.g. depression: 34–68%; OCD: 27–67%), although results should be cautiously interpreted in view of the obvious lack of any control data. Anterior capsulotomy and SLL appear better for OCD, and SST is the treatment of choice for severe mood disorder.

Psychosurgery—an historical perspective

In 1935, Egas Moniz and Almeida Lima carried out the first 'prefrontal leucotomy' (based on the work of Fulton and Jacobsen in bilateral ablation of prefrontal cortices in chimpanzees, 1934.) At the time this was viewed with great enthusiasm (culminating in Moniz being awarded a Nobel prize for his work in 1949) and other practitioners adapted the early procedures, with Freeman and Watts introducing the standard 'prefrontal leucotomy' (the notorious 'lobotomy') in 1936, publishing a standard textbook *Psychosurgery* in 1942, and Freeman pioneering 'transorbital leucotomy' in 1946.

The impact of surgical treatment at a time when there were few other physical treatments should not be underestimated, and around 12 000 procedures were performed between 1936 and 1961 in the UK alone (over 40 000 in the US). Techniques were refined (e.g. open cingulotomy, bimedial leucotomy, orbital undercut) from earlier blind, freehand procedures. However, the advent of effective psychopharmacological treatments and changes in the social climate led to a marked decline in practice from the 1960s onwards.

Nowadays, psychosurgery is rarely used, has specific indications (see opposite), and utilises modern imaging and neurosurgical techniques, with clearly defined lesion sites. Between 1984 and 1994 there were a total of only 20 operations per year performed in the UK[2], and since then the number has diminished further.

1 Alexander GE, Crutcher MD, DeLong MR (1990) Basal ganglia-thalamocortical circuits: parallel substrates for motor, oculomotor, "prefrontal" and "limbic" functions. *Progress in Brain Research* **85**, 119–46.

2 CRAG Working Group (1996) *Neurosurgery for Mental Disorder* HMSO Scotland (J2318 7/96).

Other physical treatments

Light therapy (phototherapy)

First introduced for the treatment of SAD (a proposed new syndrome at the time) by Rosenthal[1], on the basis that bright light therapy might ameliorate symptoms of winter depression, due to effects on circadian and seasonal rhythms mediated by melatonin. Recent research has suggested that the effects of phototherapy may be independent of melatonin and produce a 'phase advance' in circadian rhythms (hence treatment may be best given first thing in the morning). It is usually administered by use of a light box (alternatives include light visors) producing 2500–10 000 lux. Treatment duration is for 2hrs (with 2500 lux) or 30mins (with 10 000 lux) a day, with a course lasting 1–2wks (treatment response is noticeable within 5 days).

Adverse effects Particularly with 10 000 lux: headache, visual problems e.g. (eye strain, blurred vision—usually settle; if persistent reduce duration or intensity of exposure), increased irritability. Rarely, manic episodes, increased thoughts of suicide (possibly due to alerting effect and increased energy).

Indications SAD (see p. 270), circadian rhythm disorders (see p. 410), possibly other depressive disorders.

Contraindications Marked agitation, insomnia, history of hypomania/mania.

Repetitive transcranial magnetic stimulation (rTMS)

Currently being researched. However, the difference in stimulation parameters used across reported studies make comparisons difficult[2]. The rationale for treatment is either to increase activity in the left dorsolateral prefrontal cortex (using high-frequency stimulation e.g. 20Hz) or to reduce activity in the right dorsolateral prefrontal cortex (using low-frequency stimulation e.g. 1Hz). Initial results in treatment-resistant depression ought to be viewed with caution, although this mode of therapy presents an attractive alternative to ECT, without the accompanying risks and adverse effects.

Adverse effects Minimal, but patients often report headache.

Indications Experimental treatment for treatment-resistant depression; possible use in treatment of treatment-resistant auditory hallucinations; negative symptoms of schizophrenia.

Contraindications Epilepsy.

Magneto-convulsive therapy (MCT)

Another experimental treatment that utilises the potential problem of seizure induction by rTMS. A varying magnetic field is used to induce seizures in a more controlled way than is possible with ECT. The potential advantages include targeting of brain structures essential for treatment response, and reduction in side-effects (particularly memory impairment)[3].

Vagus nerve stimulation (VNS)

Also being researched. Vagus stimulation by implanted pacemaker (used as a treatment for epilepsy) has been tested as a treatment of depression. Stimulation is of the left cervical vagus nerve using bipolar electrodes, attached below the cardiac branch (usually 0.5 ms pulse-width, at 20–30Hz, with 30s stimulation periods alternating with 5min breaks). Response rates of 40% have been quoted for treatment-resistant depressive disorder[4].

Adverse effects May include voice alteration (e.g. hoarseness), pain, coughing, and dysphagia.

1 Rosenthal NE, Sack DA, Gillin JC, et al. (1984) Seasonal affective disorder. A description of the syndrome and preliminary findings with light therapy. *Archives of General Psychiatry* **41**, 72–80.

2 Holtzheimer PE III, Russo J, Avery DH (2002) A meta-analysis of repetitive transcranial magnetic stimulation in the treatment of depression. *Psychopharmacology Bulletin* **35**, 149–69.

3 Lisanby SH, Schlaepfer TE, Fisch HU, Sackeim HA (2001) Magnetic seizure therapy of major depression. *Archives of General Psychiatry* **58**, 303–5.

4 George MS, Sackeim HA, Rush AJ, et al. (2000) Vagus nerve stimulation: a new tool for brain research and therapy. *Biol Psychiatry* **47**, 287–95.

Vagus nerve stimulation (VNS)

Bipolar illness

Introduction

Bipolar affective disorder (commonly known as manic depression) is one of the most common, severe, and persistent psychiatric illnesses. In the public mind it is associated with notions of 'creative madness', and indeed it has affected many creative people—both past and present (see opposite). Appealing as such notions are, most people who battle with the effects of the disorder would rather live a 'normal' life, free from the unpredictability of mood swings, which most of us take for granted.

Chameleon-like in its presentation, the symptoms may vary from one patient to the next, and from one episode to the next within the same patient. The variety of presentations make this one of the most difficult conditions to diagnose. More than any other psychiatric disorder, the clinician needs to pay attention to the life history of the patient, and to third-party information from family and friends.

Classically, periods of prolonged and profound depression alternate with periods of excessively elevated and/or irritable mood, known as mania. The symptoms of mania characteristically include a decreased need for sleep, pressured speech, increased libido, reckless behaviour without regard for consequences, and grandiosity (see **Mania/manic episode** p. 304). In severe cases there may be severe thought disturbances and even psychotic symptoms. Between these 'highs and lows', patients usually experience periods of full remission.

This classic presentation appears, however, to be one pole of a spectrum of mood disorders (see **Bipolar (affective) disorder (1)—classification** p. 308). A milder form of mania (hypomania), associated with episodes of depression, may also occur (see **Hypomania/hypomanic episode** p. 306). There is also a subclinical presentation—cyclothymia—in which an individual may experience oscillating high and low moods, without ever having a significant manic or depressive episode (see **Cyclothymia** p. 326). Equally, it may be difficult to distinguish a manic episode with psychotic symptoms from schizoaffective disorder (see p. 228) on the basis of a single episode.

Full assessment ought to take account of issues including the number of previous episodes (which may have been subclinical), the average length of episodes, the average time between episodes, the level of psychosocial functioning between episodes, previous responses to treatment (especially treatment of early depressive episodes), family history of psychiatric problems, and current (and past) use of alcohol and drugs.

Although at the present time there is no cure for bipolar disorder, for most cases effective treatment is possible and can substantially decrease the associated morbidity and mortality (the suicide rate is high). Some patients do develop severe or chronic impairments and may need specific rehabilitative services. In general, however, the specific aims of treatment are to decrease the frequency, severity, and psychosocial consequences of episodes and to improve psychosocial functioning between episodes.

Famous people who have publicly stated they have bipolar disorder

Buzz Aldrin, astronaut
Tim Burton, artist, movie director
Francis Ford Coppola, director
Patricia Cornwell, writer
Ray Davies, musician
Robert Downey, Jr., actor
Carrie Fisher, writer, actor
Larry Flynt, magazine publisher
Connie Francis, actor, musician
Stephen Fry, actor, author, comedian
Stuart Goddard (Adam Ant), musician
Linda Hamilton, actor
Kay Redfield Jamison, psychologist, writer
Ilie Nastase, athlete (tennis), politician
Axl Rose, musician
Ben Stiller, actor, comedian
Gordon Sumner (Sting), musician, composer
Jean-Claude Van Damme, athlete (martial arts), actor
Tom Waits, musician, composer
Brian Wilson, musician, composer, arranger

Famous people (deceased) who had a confirmed diagnosis of bipolar disorder

Louis Althusser, 1918–1990, philosopher, writer
Clifford Beers, 1876–1943, humanitarian
Neal Cassady, 1926–1968, writer
Graham Greene, 1904–1991, writer
Frances Lear, 1923–1996, writer, editor, women's rights activist
Vivien Leigh, 1913–1967, actor
Robert Lowell, 1917–1977, poet
Burgess Meredith, 1908–1997, actor, director
Spike Milligan, 1919–2002, comic actor, writer
Theodore Roethke, 1908–1963, writer
Don Simpson, 1944–1996, movie producer
David Strickland, 1970–1999, actor
Joseph Vasquez, 1963–1996, writer, movie director
Mary Jane Ward, 1905–1981, writer
Virginia Woolf, 1882–1941, writer

Other famous people who are thought to have had bipolar disorder

William Blake, Napoleon Bonaparte, Agatha Christie, Winston Churchill, TS Eliot, F Scott Fitzgerald, Cary Grant, Victor Hugo, Robert E Lee, Abraham Lincoln, Samuel Johnson, Marilyn Monroe, Wolfgang Amadeus Mozart, Isaac Newton, Plato (according to Aristotle), Edgar Allen Poe, St Francis, St John, St Theresa, Rod Steiger, Robert Louis Stevenson, Mark Twain, Alfred, Lord Tennyson, Vincent van Gogh, Walt Whitman, Tennessee Williams.

Historical perspective

Bipolar affective disorder has been known since ancient times. Hippocrates described patients as 'amic' and 'melancholic', and clear connections between melancholia and mania date back to the descriptions of the two syndromes by Aretaius of Cappadocia (c.150 BC) and Paul of Aegina (625–690). Thinking at that time reflected 'humoral' theories, with melancholia caused by excess of 'black bile' and mania by excess of 'yellow bile'.

Despite the view of some clinicians in the 18th Century that melancholia and mania were interconnected (e.g. Robert James, 1705–1776), it took to the middle of the 19th Century before this was more widely accepted. In 1854 Jules Baillarger (1809–1890) published a paper in the Bulletin of the Imperial Academy of Medicine describing *la folie à double forme*, closely followed two weeks later by a paper in the same journal by Jean-Pierre Falret (1794–1870), who claimed that he had been teaching students at the Salpetrière about *la folie circulaire* for 10 years. Although the two men were to continue arguing about who originated the idea, they at least agreed that the illness was characterised by alternating periods of melancholia and mania, often separated by periods of normal mood. In 1899, Emil Kraepelin comprehensively described 'manic-depressive insanity' in the 6th edition of his textbook *Psychiatrie: Ein Lehrbuch für Studirende und Ärzte*. In the 5th edition he had already divided severe mental illnesses into those with a 'deteriorating' course (i.e. schizophrenia and related psychoses) and those with a 'periodic' course (i.e. the mood disorders). It was his view that the, mood disorders 'represented manifestations of a single morbid process'.

At the turn of the 20th Century, hopes were high that understanding of the pathophysiology of mental illness might be within reach. In 1906, the German microbiologist August Wassermann discovered a method of detecting syphilitic infection in the CNS, and in the same year an effective treatment was developed by Paul Ehrlich using arsenic compounds. Syphilis was, at that time, one of the most common causes of severe (often mania-like) psychiatric symptoms ('general paralysis of the insane'). Reliably diagnosing and treating such a condition was a huge step forward. In cases of manic-depressive illness, however, neuropathologists failed to find any structural brain abnormalities. Although some still maintained it was a physical illness, caused by disruptions in biological *functioning*, the pervasive 'new' psychodynamic theories regarded *functional* illnesses (i.e. schizophrenia and manic-depressive illness) as illnesses of the *mind*, not the *brain*. The idea that they could be understood and treated only if the traumatic childhood events, repressed sexual feelings, or interpersonal conflicts were uncovered, influenced psychiatric thinking for over half a century.

It was not until *specific* drug treatments for these 'functional illnesses' were found, that psychiatry came full circle again, and new life was breathed into the old search for *biological* mechanisms. In 1949 John Cade published a report on the use of lithium salts in manic patients, but it took nearly three decades, and the work of many psychiatrists, including Morgens Schou in Denmark and Ronald Fieve in the US, before lithium would become the mainstay of treatment for manic-depressive illness. Equally significant was the observation by Ronald Kuhn that when patients with 'manic-depressive psychosis' were treated with imipramine they could switch from depression to mania. That this did not occur in *all* patients with depression suggested that there was a different biological mechanism underlying depressive illness compared to manic-depressive illness. With different pharmacological agents treating different psychiatric disorders, the stage was set for classifying psychiatric disorders in line with their presumed differing aetiologies. The quest had begun to understand the biological mechanisms and, in doing so, to develop better treatments.

Mania/manic episode

Essence A distinct period of abnormally and persistently elevated, expansive, or irritable mood, with 3 (or more) characteristic symptoms of mania (see below). Both DSM-IV and ICD-10 specify the episode should last at least 1 week, or less if admission to hospital is necessary. By definition, the disturbance is sufficiently severe to impair occupational and social functioning. Psychotic features may be present.

Clinical features

- Elevated mood (usually out of keeping with circumstances)
- Increased energy, which may manifest as:
  - Overactivity
  - Pressured speech ('flight of ideas')
  - Racing thoughts
  - Reduced need for sleep
- Increased self-esteem, evident as:
  - Overoptimistic ideation
  - Grandiosity
  - Reduced social inhibitions
  - Overfamiliarity (which may be overly amorous)
  - Facetiousness
- Reduced attention/increased distractibility
- Tendency to engage in behaviour that could have serious consequences:
  - Preoccupation with extravagant, impracticable schemes
  - Spending recklessly
  - Inappropriate sexual encounters
- Other behavioural manifestations:
  - Excitement
  - Irritability
  - Aggressiveness
  - Suspiciousness
- Marked disruption of work, usual social activities, and family life

Psychotic symptoms

In its more severe form, mania may be associated with psychotic symptoms (usually mood-congruent, but may also be incongruent):
- Grandiose ideas may be delusional, related to identity or role (with 'special powers' or religious content).
- Suspiciousness may develop into well-formed persecutory delusions.
- Pressured speech may become so great that clear associations are lost and speech becomes incomprehensible.
- Irritability and aggression may lead to violent behaviour.
- Preoccupation with thoughts and schemes may lead to self-neglect, to the point of not eating or drinking, and poor living conditions.
- Catatonic behaviour—also termed 'manic stupor'.
- Total loss of insight.

Differential diagnosis

- Schizophrenia, schizoaffective disorder, delusional disorder, other psychotic disorders

- Anxiety disorders/PTSD
- Circadian rhythm disorders (see pp. 408–11)
- ADHD/conduct disorder
- Alcohol or drug misuse (e.g. stimulants, hallucinogens, opiates)
- Physical illness (e.g. hyper/hypothyroidism, Cushing's syndrome, SLE, MS, head injury, brain tumour, epilepsy, HIV and other encephalopathies, neurosyphilis, Fahr's disease)
- Other antidepressant treatment or drug-related causes (see below)

Management
- Exclusion of other causes and appropriate investigations (p. 310)
- Address any specific psychosocial stressors
- For specific management, see pp. 318–19

Medications that may induce symptoms of hypomania/mania

Antidepressants Drug-induced mania is described with most antidepressants (or withdrawal from antidepressants p. 872), perhaps less so with SSRIs and bupropion (also seen with ECT and light therapy).

Other psychotropic medication *Benzodiazepines* May be confused with 'paradoxical' reactions (p. 875). *Antipsychotics* Olanzapine, risperidone. *Lithium* Toxicity, and when combined with TCAs. *Anticonvulsants (rare)* Carbamazepine (and withdrawal), valproate, gabapentin. *Psychostimulants* Fenfluramine, amphetamine, dexamphetamine, methylphenidate. *Other* Disulfiram.

Anti-parkinsonian medication Amantadine, bromocriptine, levodopa, procyclidine.

Cardiovascular drugs Captopril, clonidine, digoxin, diltiazem, hydralazine, methyldopa withdrawal, procainamide, propranolol (and withdrawal), reserpine.

Respiratory drugs Aminophylline, ephedrine, salbutamol, terfenadine, psuedoephedrine.

Anti-infection Anti-TB medication, chloroquine, clarithromycin, dapsone, isoniazid, zidovudine.

Analgesics Buprenorphine, codeine, indomethacin, nefopam (IM), pentazocine, tramadol.

Gastrointestinal drugs Cimetidine, metoclopramide, ranitidine.

Steroids ACTH, beclomethasone, corticosteroids, cortisone, dexamethasone, DHEA, hydrocortisone, prednisolone, testosterone.

Other Baclofen (and withdrawal), cyclizine, cyclosporin, interferon.

Hypomania/hypomanic episode

Essence 3 or more characteristic symptoms (see below) last at least 4 days (DSM-IV), and are clearly different from 'normal' mood (third-party corroboration). By definition, not severe enough to interfere with social or occupational functioning, require admission to hospital, or include psychotic features.

Clinical features Hypomania shares symptoms with mania, but these are evident to a lesser degree and do not significantly disrupt work or lead to social rejection, e.g.:
- Mildly elevated, expansive, or irritable mood
- Increased energy and activity
- Marked feelings of well-being, physical, and mental efficiency
- Increased self-esteem
- Sociability
- Talkativeness
- Overfamiliarity
- Increased sex drive
- Reduced need for sleep
- Difficulty in focusing on one task alone (tasks often started but not finished)

Differential diagnosis
- Agitated depression
- OCD/other anxiety disorders
- Circadian rhythm disorders (see pp. 408–11)
- Substance misuse/physical illness/medication-related (as for *Mania*—see p. 305)

Management
- Exclusion of other possible causes with appropriate investigations (see p. 310)
- Address any specific psycho-social stressors
- If sleep disturbance is a problem, consider use of an hypnotic
- If episode is prolonged, discuss medication possibilities (as for *Mania*)

'Bipolar spectrum disorder'

One view of the affective disorders is that they consist of a continuum (see below).

Proposed clinical features

'Bipolar spectrum disorder' is characterised by[1]:
- At least one major depressive episode.
- No spontaneous hypomanic or manic episodes.

And a history including some of the following:
- A family history of bipolar disorder in a first-degree relative.
- Antidepressant-induced mania or hypomania.
- Hyperthymic personality[2] (at baseline, non-depressed state).
- Recurrent major depressive episodes (>3).
- Brief major depressive episodes (on average, < 3 months).
- Atypical depressive symptoms (DSM-IV criteria).
- Psychotic major depressive episodes.
- Early age of onset of major depressive episode (< age 25).
- Postpartum depression.
- Antidepressant 'wear-off' (acute but not prophylactic response).
- Lack of response to up to 3 antidepressant treatment trials.

Management

Patients with features of bipolar spectrum disorder may represent a subset of patients who do not respond well to antidepressants (often precipitating a switch to a hypomanic or manic episode) and for whom an anticonvulsant may be the drug of choice (e.g. valproate—see p. 332).

The 'affective continuum'

Dysthymia
Unipolar depression
Atypical depression
Psychotic depression   } Unipolar spectrum disorder
Recurrent depression
Bipolar spectrum disorder
Bipolar II
Bipolar I

---

1 Ghaemi SN, Ko JY, Goodwin FK (2002) 'Cade's disease' and beyond: misdiagnosis, antidepressant use, and a proposed definition for bipolar spectrum disorder. *Can J Psychiatry* **47**, 125 –34.

2 Characterised by cheerful, optimistic personality style, tendency to become easily irritated, extroverted and sociable, and requiring little sleep (less than 6 hours/night).

Bipolar (affective) disorder (1)—classification

Diagnostic classification (see opposite)
ICD-10
Requires at least 2 episodes, one of which must be hypomanic, manic, or mixed, with recovery usually complete between episodes. Criteria for depressive episodes are the same as unipolar depression (see p. 246). Separate category (*Manic episode*) for hypomania or mania (with or without psychotic symptoms) without history of depressive episodes. Cyclothymia included with dysthymia in *persistent mood disorders* section.

DSM-IV
Allows a single manic episode and cyclothymic disorder to be considered as part of bipolar disorder, and defines two sybtypes (with additional specifiers):

Bipolar I disorder—the occurrence of one or more manic episodes or mixed episodes, with or without a history of one or more depressive episodes.

Bipolar II disorder—the occurrence of one or more depressive episodes accompanied by at least one hypomanic episode.

Severity specifiers Mild, moderate, severe (with or without psychotic features); in partial or full remission.

Special syndrome specifiers With catatonic, melancholic, or atypical features; with postpartum onset.

Longitudinal course specifiers With or without full inter-episode recovery; with seasonal pattern; with rapid cycling.

Mixed episodes (DSM-IV and ICD-10)
- The occurrence of both manic/hypomanic and depressive symptoms in a single episode, present every day for at least 1 week (DSM-IV) or 2 weeks (ICD-10).
- Typical presentations include:
  - Depression *plus* overactivity/pressure of speech
  - Mania *plus* agitation and reduced energy/libido
  - Dysphoria *plus* manic symptoms (with exception of elevated mood)
  - Rapid cycling (fluctuating between mania and depression—4 or more episodes/yr) N.B. 'Ultra-rapid' cycling refers to the situation when fluctuations are over days or even hours.

The clinical reality of manic-depressive illness is far more lethal and infinitely more complex than the current psychiatric nomenclature, bipolar disorder, would suggest. Cycles of fluctuating moods and energy levels serve as a background to constantly changing thoughts, behaviors, and feelings. The illness encompasses the extremes of human experience. Thinking can range from florid psychosis, or 'madness', to patterns of unusually clear, fast and creative associations, to retardation so profound that no meaningful mental activity can occur. Behavior can be frenzied, expansive, bizarre, and seductive, or it can be seclusive, sluggish, and dangerously suicidal. Moods may swing erratically between euphoria and despair or irritability and desperation. The rapid oscillations and combinations of such extremes result in an intricately textured clinical picture. Manic patients, for example, are depressed and irritable as often as they are euphoric; the highs associated with mania are generally only pleasant and productive during the earlier, milder stages.

Dr Kay Redfield Jamison (1993) *Touched With Fire: Manic-Depressive Illness and the Artistic Temperament* The Free Press, Macmillan, New York, pp 47–48.

ICD-10 Bipolar affective disorder.

Current episode, hypomanic
Current episode, manic without psychotic symptoms
Current episode, manic with psychotic symptoms
Current episode, mild or moderate depression
Current episode, severe depression without psychotic symptoms
Current episode, severe depression with psychotic symptoms
Current episode, mixed
Currently in remission
Other bipolar affective disorders: Bipolar affective disorder, unspecified

DSM-IV Bipolar Disorder

Bipolar I disorder	*Bipolar II disorder*
Single manic episode	Most recent episode, hypomanic
Most recent episode, hypomanic	Most recent episode, depressed
Most recent episode, manic	
Most recent episode, mixed	*Cyclothymic disorder*
Most recent episode, depressed	
Most recent episode, unspecified	*Bipolar disorder not otherwise specified*

Bipolar (affective) disorder (2)

Aetiology (see opposite) Factors identified as important include:

Genetic 1st-degree relatives are 7x more likely to develop the condition than the general population (i.e. 10–15% risk). Children of a parent with bipolar disorder have a 50% chance of developing a psychiatric disorder (genetic liability appears shared for schizophrenia, schizoaffective, and bipolar affective disorder). MZ twins: 33–90% concordance; DZ twins: ~23%.

Neurotransmitters NA, DA, 5HT, and glutamine have all been implicated.

HPA axis Given the effects of environmental stressors, and of exogenous steroids, a role has also been suggested for glucocorticoids and other stress-related hormonal responses.

Epidemiology Lifetime prevalence 0.3–1.5% (0.8% bipolar I; 0.5% bipolar II); $\male = \female$ (bipolar II and rapid cycling more common in $\female$; 1st episodes:$\male$ tend to be manic, $\female$ depressive); no significant racial differences; age range 15–50+yrs (peaks at 15–19yrs and 20–24yrs; mean 21yrs).

Course Extremely variable. 1st episodes may be hypomanic, manic, mixed, or depressive. This may be followed by many years (5 or more) without a further episode, but the length of time between subsequent episodes may begin to narrow. There is often a 5–10yr interval between age at onset of illness and age at first treatment or first admission to hospital. Often patients with recurrent depression have a first manic episode in later life (>50yrs). It is known that *untreated* patients may have more than 10 episodes in a lifetime, and that the duration and period of time between episodes stabilises after the 4th or 5th episode. Although the prognosis is better for *treated* patients, there still remains a high degree of unpredictability.

Morbidity/mortality Morbidity and mortality rates are high, in terms of lost work, lost productivity, effects on marriage (increased divorce rates) and the family, with attempted suicide in 25–50%, and completed suicide in ~10% ($\male > \female$ usually during a depressive episode). Often significant comorbidity—esp. drug/alcohol misuse and anxiety disorders (both increase risk of suicide).

Differential diagnosis Depends upon the nature of the presenting episode (See **Mania/manic episode** pp. 304–5, **Hypomania/hypomanic episode** p. 306, and **Depressive illness** p. 256).

Investigations As for depression; full physical and routine blood tests to exclude any treatable cause, including FBC, ESR, glucose, U&Es, Ca^{2+}, TFTs, LFTs, drug screen. Less routine tests: urinary copper (to exclude Wilson's disease [rare]), ANF (SLE), infection screen (VDRL, HIV test). CT/MRI brain (to exclude tumour, infarction, haemorrhage, MS)—may show hyperintense subcortical structures (esp temporal lobes), ventricular enlargement and sulcal prominence; EEG (baseline and to rule out epilepsy). Other baseline tests prior to treatment should include ECG and creatinine clearance.

Management See specific sections (pp. 312–25) for management principles, other issues, treatment of acute manic episodes, depressive episodes, prophylaxis, and psychotherapeutic interventions.

Prognosis Within the first 2 years of 1st episode, 40–50% of patients experience another manic episode. 50–60% of patients on lithium gain control of their symptoms (7% no recurrence; 45% some future episodes; 40% persistent recurrence). Often, the cycling between depression and mania accelerates with age. *Poor prognostic factors:* poor employment history; alcohol abuse; psychotic features; depressive features between periods of mania and depression; evidence of depression; male sex, treatment non-compliance. *Good prognostic factors:* manic episodes of short duration; later age of onset; few thoughts of suicide; few psychotic symptoms; few comorbid physical problems, good treatment response and compliance.

Aetiological theories

Abnormal 'programmed cell death'

Animal studies have recently shown that antidepressants, lithium and valproate indirectly regulate a number of factors involved in cell survival pathways, (e.g. CREB, BDNF, Bcl-2, and MAP kinases) perhaps explaining their delayed long-term beneficial effects (via under-appreciated neurotrophic effects, esp. in the frontal cortex and the hippocampus[1]). Neuroimaging studies also indicate of cell loss in these same brain regions. This suggests that bipolar affective disorder may be the result of abnormal programmed cell death (apoptosis) in critical neural networks involved in the regulation of emotion. Mood stabilisers and antidepressants may act to stimulate cell survival pathways and increase levels of neurotrophic factors that improve cellular resilience.

'Kindling'

An older hypothesis[2], also drawing on animal models, that suggests a role for neuronal injury, through a mechanism involving electrophysiological kindling and behavioural sensitisation. A genetically predisposed individual experiences an increasing number of minor neurological insults (e.g. due to drugs of abuse, excessive glucocorticoid stimulation, to acute or chronic stress, or other factors), which eventually result in mania. After the 1st episode, sufficient neuronal damage may persist, allowing for recurrence with or without minor environmental or behavioural stressors (much like epilepsy), which may in turn result in further injury. This view provides an explanation for later episodes becoming more frequent, why anticonvulsants may be useful in preventing recurrent episodes, and suggests that treatment should be as early as possible and long-term.

1 Manji HK and Duman RS (2001) Impairments of neuroplasticity and cellular resilience in severe mood disorders: implications for the development of novel therapeutics. *Psychopharmacology Bulletin* **35**, 5–49.

2 Post RM and Weiss SR (1989) Sensitization, kindling, and anticonvulsants in mania. *J Clin Psychiatry* **50**, Suppl: 23–30.

Bipolar affective disorder (3)— management principles

Acute episodes

This will depend upon the nature of the presenting episode (See **Treatment of acute manic episodes** pp. 318–19, **Hypomania/hypomanic episode** p. 306, and **Treatment of depressive illness** pp. 320–1). Often the episode is of a nature and degree that hospital admission will be necessary (for criteria and considerations see **Hospital admission** p. 316). Special consideration should also be given to certain specific issues related to the clinical presentation, the presence of concurrent medical problems, and particular patient groups, both in terms of setting and choice of treatment (see **Other issues affecting management decisions** pp. 314–15). Issues of prophylaxis (see **Prophylaxis** p. 322) should be considered, and this may sometimes involve not only pharmacological, but also psychotherapeutic interventions (see **Psychotherapeutic interventions** p. 324).

Outpatient follow-up

Once the diagnosis has been clearly established, possible physical causes excluded, and the presenting episode effectively treated, follow-up has a number of key aims:

- Establishing and maintaining a therapeutic alliance.
- Monitoring the patient's psychiatric status.
- Providing education regarding bipolar disorder.
- Enhancing treatment compliance.
- Monitoring side-effects of medication and ensuring therapeutic levels of any mood stabiliser.
- Identifying and addressing any significant comorbid conditions (p. 314).
- Promoting regular patterns of activity and wakefulness.
- Promoting understanding of and adaption to the psychosocial effects of bipolar disorder.
- Identifying new episodes early.
- Reducing the morbidity and sequelae of bipolar disorder.

Relapse prevention

A key part of psychiatric management—helping patients to identify precipitants or early manifestations of illness, so that treatment can be initiated early. This may be done as part of the 'usual' psychiatric follow-up, or form part of a specific psychotherapeutic intervention (see **Psychotherapeutic interventions** p. 324), (e.g. **insomnia** may often be either a precipitant, or an early indicator, of mania or depression—education about the importance of regular sleep habits and occasional use of an hypnotic (see p. 398) to promote normal sleep patterns may be useful in preventing the development of a manic episode). Other early or subtle signs of mania may be treated with the short-term use of benzodiazepines or antipsychotics. A good therapeutic alliance is critical, and the patient, who often has good insight, ought to feel that they can contact their clinician as soon as they are aware of these 'early warning signs'.

Other issues affecting management decisions

Specific clinical features

Other issues affecting management decisions

Specific clinical features

Certain clinical features will strongly influence the choice of treatment. For issues of substance misuse or other psychiatric morbidity these should be addressed directly (see specific sections).

- **Psychotic symptoms** It is not uncommon for patients to experience delusions and/or hallucinations during episodes of mania or depression. *Management* Mood stabiliser with/without an antipsychotic, consider ECT, if severe consider admission to hospital.
- **Catatonic symptoms** During a manic episode ('manic stupor'). *Management* Admit to hospital, exclude medical problem, clarify psychiatric diagnosis, if diagnosis clear treat with ECT and/or benzodiazepine.
- **Risk of suicide** Assess nature of risk (see p. 45), note association with rapid cycling mood. If significant risk, or unacceptable uncertainty, admit to hospital (or if in hospital, increase level of observation), consider ECT.
- **Risk of violence** Assess nature of risk (see pp. 646–7). Note increased risk with rapid mood cycling, paranoid delusions, agitation, and dysphoria. Admit to hospital, consider need for secure setting.
- **Substance-related disorders**. Comorbidity is high, often confusing the clinical picture. Substance misuse may lead to relapse both directly and indirectly (by reducing compliance). Equally, alcohol consumption may increase when on lithium. *Management* Address issues of misuse, if detoxification considered, admit to hospital as risk of suicide may be increased.
- **Other comorbidities** Personality disorders, anxiety disorder, ADHD, conduct disorder.

Concurrent medical problems

The presence of other medical problems may affect the management either by exacerbating the course or severity of the disorder or by complicating drug treatment (i.e. issues of tolerability and drug interactions).

- **Cardiovascular/renal/hepatic disorders** May restrict the choice of drug therapy or increase the need for closer monitoring (see pp. 880–5).
- **Endocrine disorders** e.g. hypo/hyperthyoidism.
- **Infectious diseases** e.g. HIV-infected patients may be more sensitive to CNS side-effects of mood stabilisers.
- **Use of steroids** e.g. for treatment of asthma/inflammatory bowel disease.

Special patient groups

- *Children and adolescents* (see p. 620) Lithium has been shown to be effective, but long-term effects on development have not been fully studied. Lithium may be excreted more quickly, allowing more rapid dose adjustments, but therapeutic levels are the same as for adults. Risks associated with other adjunctive agents (e.g. antipsychotics, antidepressants, benzodiazepines) should be considered separately. ECT is rarely used, but may be effective. Education, support, and other specific psychosocial interventions should be considered (usually involving family, teachers, etc.)

- *The elderly* (see p. 486) When a first manic episode occurs in a patient after age 60, there is usually evidence of previous depressive episodes in their 40s and 50s. Full physical examination is necessary to exclude medical causes (esp. CNS disorders). Older patients may be more sensitive to the side-effects of lithium (particularly neurological) and may require lower therapeutic levels (i.e. below 0.7mmol/L).
- *Pregnancy and lactation* (see pp. 876–9). Consider ECT as first-line for treatment of significant manic, depressed, or psychotically depressed episodes.

Hospital admission

Frequently acute episodes of bipolar disorder are severe enough to require hospital admission (often on a compulsory basis). Issues of safety and the provision of effective treatment will govern the decisions about whether a patient can remain in the community.

Points to note

- Patients with symptoms of mania/hypomania or depression often have impaired judgement (sometimes related to psychotic symptoms), which may interfere with their ability to make reasoned decisions about the need for treatment.
- Risk assessment includes not only behaviours that may cause direct harm (e.g. suicide attempts or homicidal behaviour), but also those that may be indirectly harmful (e.g. overspending, sexual promiscuity, excessive use of drugs/alcohol, driving whilst unwell).
- The relapsing/remitting nature of the disorder makes it possible to work with the patient (when well) and their family/carers to anticipate future acute episodes and agree a treatment plan should they occur.

Clinical features and situations where admission may be necessary

- High risk of suicide or homicide.
- Illness-related behaviour that endangers relationships, reputation, or assets.
- Lack of capacity to cooperate with treatment (e.g. directly due to illness, or secondary to availability of social supports/outpatient resources).
- Lack (or loss) of psychosocial supports.
- Severe psychotic symptoms.
- Severe depressive symptoms.
- Severe mixed states or rapid cycling (days/hours).
- Catatonic symptoms.
- Failure of outpatient treatment.
- A need to address comorbid conditions (e.g. physical problems, other psychiatric conditions, inpatient detoxification).

Suitable environment?

During an acute manic episode, a routine, calm environment is desirable (but not always possible). A balance should be struck between avoidance of over-stimulation (e.g. from outside events, TV, radio, lively conversations.) and provision of sufficient space to walk or exercise in order to use up excess energy. Where possible, access to alcohol and drugs should be restricted. Patients may find regular observations by staff overly intrusive, feel uncomfortable in a busy ward, and make requests of staff that may well be 'reasonable' but not practical. The psychiatrist needs to adopt a pragmatic approach, listening to concerns, and balancing risks. Sometimes this may result in a difficult decision about whether to detain a patient to a hospital environment, which although far from ideal, is the 'least worst' option.

Treatment of acute manic episodes

First-line treatment

Lithium (see pp. 328–31) Lithium remains the first-line treatment for acute mania, with a response rate of around 80%. *Note:* Up to 2 weeks of treatment may be necessary to reach maximal effectiveness for manic patients. Due to this delayed effect, esp. for severe mania or psychotic symptoms, with associated acute behavioural disturbance, addition of an antipsychotic or a benzodiazepine is usually required (see below).

Predictors of good response Previous response to lithium, compliance with medication, >3 previous episodes, FHx of mood disorder, euphoria (not dysphoria), lack of psychotic symptoms or suicidal behaviour.

Antipsychotics As in acute behavioural disturbance (see p. 896), antipsychotics (e.g. haloperidol, chlorpromazine) are useful in the rapid control of severely agitated or psychotic patients with bipolar disorder[1]. Despite widespread use, the high frequency of EPSEs has led to caution, particularly because of the risk of TD with long-term treatment. There is also evidence that antipsychotic medication, far from helping patients with depressive episodes, may in fact lengthen or exacerbate the next depressive episode. Hence 'novel' antipsychotics have been advocated and evidence is accumulating for treating acute mania with olanzapine (licensed in UK), risperidone, or clozapine[2].

Benzodiazepines Another approach to reduce the need for antipsychotics is the adjunctive use of benzodiazepines. Clonazepam and lorazepam are the most widely studied compounds, either alone or in combination with lithium, and are effective, in place of, or in conjunction with, an antipsychotic, to sedate the acutely agitated manic patient whilst waiting for the effects of other primary mood-stabilising agents. The fact that lorazepam is well absorbed after intra-muscular injection (unlike other benzodiazepines) has made it particularly useful for some very agitated patients.

ECT has been shown to be one of the best treatment options in acute mania[3]. Current practice reserves ECT for clinical situations where pharmacological treatments may not be possible, such as pregnancy or severe cardiac disease, or when the patient's illness is refractory to drug treatments.

Use of anticonvulsants (second-line/augmentation or 'bipolar spectrum')

Carbamazepine (see p. 334) or its derivative, oxcarbazepine, may be effective, either alone or in combination with lithium or antipsychotics.[4] It may be better tolerated in patients with comorbid drug or alcohol problems, obesity, or for women of child-bearing age.

Predictors of good response Previous response to carbamazepine, poor compliance (due to wide therapeutic window), absence of psychotic symptoms, secondary mania (e.g. drug-induced, neurological disorder, brain injury), dysphoria, 'mixed' episode, rapid cycling, episode part of schizoaffective disorder.

Valproate (see p. 332) may also be effective in the treatment of acute mania, although evidence is less convincing. Valproate is well tolerated and has very few drug interactions, making it more suitable for combined treatment regimes.

Predictors of good response May be more effective in particular patients e.g. 'rapid cycling'—where some consider it 'first-line', dysphoric mania, mixed episodes, stable or decreasing frequency of manic episodes, or less severe forms of bipolar spectrum disorders.

Other There is no current evidence to recommend use of gabapentin in bipolar disorder (mania or hypomania). The strongest evidence is for lamotrigine, but in depressive episodes, not mania or hypomania. Topiramate has shown some promise in both depressed and manic bipolar patients, with the added benefit of promoting weight loss. Overall, however, the evidence is still very limited.

1 Gelenberg AJ and Hopkins HS (1996) Antipsychotics in bipolar disorder. *Journal of Clinical Psychiatry* **57**(Suppl.), 49–52.

2 Yatham LN (2002) The role of novel antipsychotics in bipolar disorders. *Journal of Clinical Psychiatry* **63** (Suppl. 3), 10–14.

3 Mukherjee S, Sackeim HA, Schnur DB (1994) Electroconvulsive therapy of acute manic episodes: a review of 50 years' experience. *AJP* **151**, 169–76.

4 McElroy SL and Keck PE Jr. (2000) Pharmacologic agents for the treatment of acute bipolar mania. *Biol Psychiatry* **48**, 539–57.

Treatment of depressive episodes

The pharmacological treatment of depressive episodes in bipolar disorder represents a particular challenge. Although almost all of the antidepressants used in the treatment of unipolar depression are effective in the treatment of bipolar depression, the response rates are lower and there is the risk of precipitating a manic episode or inducing/accelerating rapid cycling[1,2]. When symptoms are mild-moderate, it may be worth considering combining pharmacological and psychological interventions (as in unipolar depression, p. 259).

Initial management

- If severely depressed, suicidal, or where urgent treatment necessary, consider *ECT* (see below).
- If patient currently 'drug-free' consider initiation of either a mood stabiliser (e.g. lithium) or an antidepressant.
- If patient already on prophylaxis, optimise (ensure compliance), check serum levels, exclude/treat associated problems (e.g. hypothyroidism).
- If taking an antipsychotic, consider careful withdrawal.
- If depressive symptoms persist, then consider addition of an antidepressant or an additional mood stabiliser.

Choice of antidepressant

Although evidence is scarce, recent studies have suggested that the (SSRIs) may be better tolerated, work more quickly, and have a lower associated risk of inducing mania or rapid cycling compared to tricyclic antidepressants[3]. In general, choice will depend on issues of previous response, side-effects (both desired and undesired), and tolerability issues (see p. 262). As second-line treatment, an antidepressant may be better tolerated than a second mood stabiliser.

Additional mood stabiliser

Although controlled clinical trials comparing standard treatments for depression in patients with bipolar disorder are lacking, it is a widely accepted practice to add a 2nd mood stabilizer to the treatment regimens of patients with bipolar disorder (e.g. carbamazepine or valproate). N.B. Be alert for evidence of lithium toxicity, even at "normal" serum levels (see p. 331). Recent evidence suggests monotherapy with lamotrigine may have utility in the treatment of refractory bipolar depression[4].

ECT

- Although well established for treatment of unipolar depressive disorder, ECT in bipolar disorder has not been fully researched, but should not be overlooked (esp in severe cases). Take care if the patient is on prophylaxis.
- ECT has been reported to cause memory impairment, acute confusion, and other neurological problems in patients on lithium; hence lithium should be withdrawn prior to treatment.
- Anticonvulsants oppose the desired convulsant effects of ECT and should also be withdrawn prior to treatment.

Alternative strategies/treatment resistance

Other suggested strategies include: the use of adjunctive triiodothyronine (T_3)—even if there is no evidence of (sub)clinical hypothyroidism[5]; and the novel use of inositol[6]. For treatment—resistant depressive episodes, principles of management are as for unipolar depression (see p. 266).

1 Compton MT and Nemeroff CB (2000) The treatment of bipolar depression. *Journal of Clinical Psychiatry* **61** (Suppl.), 57–67.

2 Sachs GS, Koslow CL, Ghaemi SN (2000) The treatment of bipolar depression. *Bipolar Disorders* **2**, 256–60.

3 Nemeroff CB, Evans DL, Gyulai L, *et al.* (2001) Double-blind, placebo-controlled comparison of imipramine and paroxetine in the treatment of bipolar depression. *AJP* **158**, 906–12.

4 Calabrese JR, Vieta E, Shelton MD (2003) Latest maintenance data on lamotrigine in bipolar disorder. *Eur Neuropsychopharmacol.* **13** Suppl 2, S57–66.

5 Bauer M, Berghofer A, Bschor T, *et al.* (2002) Supraphysiological doses of L-thyroxine in the maintenance treatment of prophylaxis-resistant affective disorders. *Neuropsychopharmacology* **27**, 620–8.

6 Chengappa KN, Levine J, Gershon S, *et al.* (2000) Inositol as an add-on treatment for bipolar depression. *Bipolar Disorders* **2**, 47–55.

Prophylaxis

Primary aim

Prevention of recurrent episodes (either mania or depression.)

Indications

Any patient who has had at least 2 episodes in 5 years (APA Guidelines 1994[1]).

First-line treatment

Lithium (see p. 328) To date, lithium remains the first-line choice for maintenance treatment in patients with a 'classical' course of illness. Some subtypes of what has become known as the 'bipolar spectrum' may not respond as well to lithium. These include patients with 'mixed mania' (i.e. depressive symptoms during manic episodes) and patients with 'rapid cycling' mania. Emerging evidence would seem to suggest a role for anticonvulsants in these patients.

Second-line treatments

Carbamazepine Appears to be effective in the long-term treatment of bipolar disorder, with an overall response rate of 63%[2]. Although it does not have worldwide approval as yet, carbamazepine may be more effective in the treatment of bipolar spectrum than classical bipolar disorder.

Sodium valproate/divalproex Has demonstrated efficacy in rapid cycling bipolar disorder and controlled studies on the prophylactic benefits of valproate are beginning to emerge.

Other anticonvulsants There have been promising reports on the efficacy of newer anticonvulsants, such as lamotrigine, gabapentin, and topiramate. Until evidence from controlled studies is available, it remains prudent to reserve these drugs for refractory cases.

Alternative/augmentative agents

Alternatives treatment strategies, or potential augmentative agents, include a number of other compounds which may have some clinical utility, but for which the evidence remains weak. These include: calcium channel antagonists such as verapamil, nifedipine, and nimodipine; thyroid hormones; clozapine and some of the newer antipsychotics, (e.g. risperidone and olanzapine).

Risks of discontinuation

With long-term treatment it is essential that patients are well informed about the risks and implications of stopping medication. Substantial evidence exists that abrupt discontinuation of lithium is associated with an increased risk of relapse. The risk, particularly of mania, may be minimised by gradually reducing the lithium dose. Although comparable studies are not available for the anticonvulsants, a similarly cautious approach would seem advisable.

Suicide prevention

Since patients with bipolar disorder represent a group at high risk of suicide, it is reasonable to ask whether the above treatment strategies reduce the occurrence of suicidal acts. Retrospective and prospective studies do suggest that long-term lithium therapy reduces the risk of suicide, and may even reduce the known associated risk of cardiovascular disease. At present there is still little data available on the anti-suicidal effects of the anticonvulsants in bipolar disorder. Prospective studies looking at the issue of outcome in bipolar disorder suggest that lithium may be significantly superior to carbamazepine in this regard.

1 American Psychiatric Association. Practice guideline for the treatment of patients with bipolar disorder. (1994) *American Journal of Psychiatry* **151** (Suppl.), 1–36.

2 Dunn RT, Frye MS, Kimbrell TA, *et al.* (1998) The efficacy and use of anticonvulsants in mood disorders. *Clinical Neuropharmacology* **21**, 215–35.

Psychotherapeutic interventions

Most patients will struggle with some of the following issues:

- Emotional consequences of significant periods of illness and receiving the diagnosis of a chronic psychiatric disorder.
- Developmental deviations and delays caused by past episodes.
- Problems associated with stigmatisation.
- Problems related to self-esteem.
- Fear of recurrence and the consequent inhibition of normal psychosocial functioning.
- Interpersonal difficulties.
- Issues related to marriage, family, childbearing, and parenting.
- Academic and occupational problems.
- Other legal, social, and emotional problems that arise from illness-related behaviours.

For some patients, a specific psychotherapeutic intervention (in addition to usual psychiatric management and social support) will be needed to address these issues. Approaches include: psychodynamic, interpersonal, behavioural, and cognitive therapies. In addition, couple therapy, family therapy, and group therapy may be indicated for some patients. The selection of appropriate interventions is influenced by the local availability of such treatments, as well as the patient's needs and preferences.

Key elements of selected interventions

CBT Time-limited, with specific aims: educate the patient about bipolar disorder and its treatment, teach cognitive behavioural skills for coping with psychosocial stressors and associated problems, facilitate compliance with treatment, and monitor the occurrence and severity of symptoms.

Interpersonal and social rhythm therapy To reduce lability of mood by maintaining a regular pattern of daily activities (e.g. sleeping, eating, physical activity, and emotional stimulation).

Family therapies Usually brief, include psychoeducation (of patient and family members) with specific aims: accepting the reality of the illness, identifying precipitating stresses and likely future stresses inside and outside the family, elucidating family interactions that produce stress on the patient, planning strategies for managing and/or minimising future stresses, and bringing about the patient's family's acceptance of the need for continued treatment.

Support groups These may provide useful information about bipolar disorder and its treatment. Patients may benefit from hearing the experiences of others, struggling with similar issues. This may help them to see their problems as not being unique, understand the need for medication, and access advice and assistance with other practical issues. In the UK, groups such as the Manic Depression Fellowship, MIND, and SANE provide both support and educational material to patients and their families.

Cyclothymia

Previously regarded as a disorder of personality ('cyclothymic temperament'—see opposite) mainly because of its early age of onset and relative stability throughout adult life, cyclothymia is now considered to be a mood disorder.

Clinical features

- Persistent instability of mood, with numerous periods of mild depression and mild elation, not sufficiently severe or prolonged to fulfil the criteria for bipolar affective disorder or recurrent depressive disorder.
- The mood swings are usually perceived by the individual as being unrelated to life events.

The diagnosis is difficult to establish without a prolonged period of observation or an unusually good account of the individual's past behaviour.

In DSM-IV the symptoms must have been present for at least 2 years, with no period lasting longer than 2 months in which they have been at a normal state, and no mixed episodes may have occurred.

Epidemiology Prevalence 3–6% of general population. Age of onset: usually early adulthood (i.e. teens or 20s), but sometimes may present later in life. More common in the relatives of patients with bipolar affective disorder.

Differential diagnosis Bipolar affective disorder, recurrent depressive disorder, drug or alcohol misuse, ADHD, conduct disorder, personality disorder (emotionally unstable), medical conditions (as for bipolar affective disorder, see p. 305).

Course Onset is often gradual, making it difficult to pinpoint exactly when symptoms began. The alternating ups and downs may fluctuate in hours, weeks, or months. Because the mood swings are relatively mild and the periods of mood elevation may be enjoyable (with increased activity and productivity, self-confidence, and sociability), cyclothymia frequently fails to come to medical attention. Often the person may present either because of the impact of the depressive episodes on their social and work situations, or because of problems related to comorbid drug or alcohol misuse. Usually runs a chronic course, persisting throughout adult life. In some cases symptoms may cease temporarily or permanently, or develop into more severe mood swings meeting the criteria for bipolar affective disorder or recurrent depressive disorder.

Management

- If pharmacological treatment is contemplated this usually consists of a trial of a mood stabiliser (e.g. lithium).
- Recently there has been a tendency to use anticonvulsants such as valproate, carbamazepine, gabapentin, or lamotrigine, as these may be better tolerated. As yet there is no clear evidence to suggest any of these approaches is superior.

- Psychoeducation and insight-orientated psychotherapy may help the person to understand the condition, and allow them to develop better ways of coping.
- There is often a reluctance to continue to take medication as this not only treats the depressive episodes, but also may be perceived as 'blunting' creativity, productivity, or intellectual capacity.

Kraepelin's 'cyclothymic temperament'

These are the people who constantly oscillate hither and thither between the two opposite poles of mood, sometimes 'rejoicing to the skies', sometimes 'sad as death'. Today lively, sparkling, beaming, full of the joy of life, the pleasure of enterprise, and the pressure of activity, after some time they meet us depressed, enervated, ill-humored, in need of rest, and again a few months later they display the old freshness and elasticity.

Emil Kraepelin (1896) *Manic-Depressive Insanity and Paranoia*. (Extract from translation of the 8th edition of Kraepelin's textbook *Psychiatrie*)

Lithium

Despite problems with tolerability, lithium[1] still remains the 'gold standard' in the treatment of bipolar affective disorder against which other treatments are measured. The effectiveness of long-term treatment with lithium is supported by at least 9 controlled, double-blind studies[2,3]. This evidence far exceeds the available support for other possible alternatives to lithium treatment, although the last decade has seen an emerging body of research supporting the use of anticonvulsant, antipsychotic, or sedative agents.

Mode of action Uncertain—numerous effects on biological systems (particularly at high concentrations). Lithium can substitute for Na^{2+}, K^+, Ca^{2+}, Mg^{2+} and may have effects on cell membrane electrophysiology. Within cells, lithium interacts with systems involving other cations, including the release of neurotransmitters and 2nd messenger systems, (e.g. adenylate cyclase, inositol 1,4,5,-triphosphate, arachidonate, protein kinase C, G proteins and calcium), effectively blocking the actions of transmitters and hormones. There is also a reduction in receptor up-regulation, perhaps explaining lithium's value as an adjunctive treatment.

Interactions

Increased plasma concentration (risk of toxicity even at therapeutic serum levels) ACE inhibitors/angiotensin II antagonists, analgesics (esp. NSAIDs), antidepressants (esp. SSRIs), antiepileptics, antihypertensives (e.g. methyldopa), antipsychotics (esp. haloperidol), calcium-channel blockers, diuretics, metronidazole

Decreased plasma concentration (risk of decreased efficacy) Antacids, theophylline

Other interactions Anti-arrhythmics (e.g. amiodarone: increased risk of hypothyroidism), antidiabetics (may sometimes impair glucose tolerance), antipsychotics (increased risk of EPSEs), muscle relaxants (enhanced effect), parasympathomimetics (antagonises neostigmine and pyridostigmine)

Initiating and monitoring lithium therapy

Prior to commencing lithium therapy
Physical examination, FBC, U&Es, TFTs, creatinine clearance (CC), ECG.

Starting dose
Usually 400–600 mg given at night, increased weekly depending on serum monitoring to max. 2 g (usual dose 800 mg-1.2 g)—actual dose depends upon preparation used (as molar availability varies even when milligram amounts are the same)—see opposite.

Monitoring
Check lithium level 5 days after starting and 5 days after each change of dose. Blood samples should be taken 12hrs post-dose.

Once a therapeutic serum level (0.6–1.2mmol/L) has been established
Continue to check lithium level/U&Es every 3 mths, TFTs every 6–12 mths, CC every 12 mths.

Information for the patient

Starting lithium should be fully discussed with the patient, highlighting the relevant issues discussed in the pages following on adverse effects. Emphasis should be on a number of issues:
- How and when to take their lithium dose.
- What to do if a dose is missed.
- What the common side-effects are.
- What the longer-term problems may be.
- The need for regular monitoring of blood levels, kidney, and thyroid functioning.
- What medicines/illnesses may change the levels of lithium in the blood.
- A reminder of these issues is usually given in the form of a 'lithium card'.

Lithium preparations

Preparation	Active component	Available dosages
Camcolit (tablets)	Lithium carbonate	250/400 mg (scored)
Li-liquid(oral solution)	Lithium citrate	509 mg/5 ml
Liskonum (tablets)	Lithium carbonate	450 mg (scored)
Litarex (tablets)	Lithium citrate	564 mg
Priadel (tablets)	Lithium carbonate	200/400 mg
Priadel (liquid)	Lithium citrate	520 mg/5 ml

1 The use of lithium salts in the treatment of 'psychotic excitement' is usually credited to John Cade in 1949 (*Medical Journal of Australia* **2**, 349–352). However, this was a 'rediscovery' of the application of lithium to the treatment of 'insanity' first described by W.A. Hammond in 1871 ('The treatment of insanity' in *A Treatise on Diseases of the Nervous System*, New York: Appleton, 325–84). The use of a *specific* agent for a *specific* disorder heralded the start of the modern era of psychopharmacology.

2 Price LH and Heninger GR (1994) Lithium in the treatment of mood disorders *NEJM* **331**, 591–8.

3 Burgess S, Geddes J, Hawton K, *et al.* (2002) Lithium for maintenance treatment of mood disorders. *The Cochrane Library*, 1 Oxford: Update Software.

Lithium—adverse effects

As lithium is a highly toxic ion, safe and effective therapy requires monitoring of serum levels. Up to 75% of patients treated with lithium will experience some side-effects[1].

Dose-related side-effects

Polyuria/polydipsia (reduced ability to concentrate urine due to antidiuretic hormone [ADH] antagonism), weight gain (effects on carbohydrate metabolism and/or oedema), cognitive problems (e.g., dulling, impaired memory, poor concentration, confusion, mental slowness), tremor, sedation or lethargy, impaired coordination, gastrointestinal distress (e.g., nausea, vomiting, dyspepsia, diarrhoea), hair loss, benign leucocytosis, acne, and oedema.

Management Usually dealt with by lowering the dose lithium, or altering the dose schedule or formulation. If side-effects persist, additional medications may be necessary: e.g. β-blockers (tremor), thiazide or loop diuretics (polyuria, polydipsia or oedema), topical antibiotics or retinoic acid (acne). Gastrointestinal problems can be managed by administering lithium with meals or switching lithium preparations, such as lithium citrate.

Cardiac conduction problems

Usually benign ECG changes: (e.g. T wave changes, widening of QRS). Rarely, exacerbation of existing arrhythmias or new arrhythmias due to conduction deficits at the SA or AV nodes (contraindicated in heart failure, sick sinus syndrome).

Long-term effects

Renal function ~10–20% of patients on long-term therapy demonstrate morphological kidney changes (interstitial fibrosis, tubular atrophy, and sometimes glomerular sclerosis.) >1% may develop irreversible renal failure (rising serum creatinine) after 10 years or more of treatment.

Subclinical/clinical hypothyroidism 5–35%, more frequent in women, tends to appear after 6 to 18 months of treatment, and may be associated with 'rapid cycling' bipolar disorder. N.B. Although lithium-induced hypothyroidism is generally reversible on discontinuation, it does not constitute an absolute contraindication for continuing lithium treatment as the associated hypothyroidism is readily treated with thyroxine[2].

It is worth noting that, in addition to the classic signs and symptoms of hypothyroidism, patients with bipolar disorder are also at risk of developing depression and/or rapid cycling as a consequence of suboptimal thyroid functioning. Should these symptoms occur and suboptimal thyroid functioning is confirmed, thyroid supplementation with or without lithium discontinuation is the treatment of choice[3].

Teratogenicity (see p. 876)

The much-quoted 400-fold increased risk of Ebstein's anomaly (a congenital malformation of the tricuspid valve) due to first trimester lithium exposure[4], now appears to be substantially less than first reported—at most an 8-fold relative risk[5]. Other reported second and third trimester problems include polyhydramnios, premature delivery, thyroid abnormalities, nephrogenic diabetes insipidus, and floppy baby syndrome. The estimated risk of major congenital anomalies for lithium-exposed babies is 4–12% compared with 2–4% in untreated control groups.

Management A balance needs to be struck between the risks of teratogenicity and the risks of relapse following discontinuation. Cohen *et al.* (1994)[5] have suggested guidelines, dependent on the severity of the bipolar disorder and the risk of relapse:

• Mild, stable forms of bipolar disorder—lithium may be tapered down and stopped pre-pregnancy.
• Moderate risk of relapse—lithium should be tapered and discontinued during the first trimester (4–12 weeks after last menstrual period).
• Severe forms of bipolar disorder, who are at high risk of relapse—lithium should be maintained during pregnancy (with informed consent, appropriate counselling, prenatal diagnosis and detailed ultrasound and echocardiography at 16–18 weeks gestation).

Toxicity

The usual upper therapeutic limit for 12-hour post-dose serum lithium level is 1.2 mmol/l. With levels >1.5 mmol/l most patients will experience some symptoms of toxicity; >2.0 mmol/l definite, often life-threatening, toxic effects occur. There is often a narrow therapeutic window where the beneficial effects outweigh the toxic effects (esp. in older patients).

Early signs and symptoms Marked tremor, anorexia, nausea/vomiting, diarrhoea (sometimes bloody), with associated dehydration and lethargy.

As lithium levels rise Severe neurological complications—restlessness, muscle fasciculation/myoclonic jerks, choreoathetoid movements, marked hypertonicity. This may progress to ataxia, dysarthria, increased lethargy, drowsiness, and confusion/delirium. Hypotension and cardiac arrhythmias precede circulatory collapse, with emerging seizures, stupor, and eventual coma (high risk of permanent neurological impairment or death).

Management

• Education of patients (methods of avoiding toxicity—e.g. maintaining hydration and salt intake, and being alert to early signs and symptoms).
• Careful adjustment of dosage may be all that is required.
• In severe toxicity (e.g. following OD), rapid steps to reduce serum lithium level are urgently necessary. This may involve forced diuresis with intravenous isotonic saline, or in cases where toxicity is severe or accompanied by significant renal failure, hemodialysis.

1 Goodwin FK and Jamison KR (1990) *Manic-Depressive Illness.* Oxford University Press.

2 Jefferson JW (ed.) (1987) *Lithium Encyclopedia for Clinical Practice*, 2nd ed. Washington, American Psychiatric Press.

3 Bocchetta A, Bernardi F, Pedditzi M, *et al.* (1991) Thyroid abnormalities during lithium treatment. *Acta Psychiatr Scand.* 1991 **83**, 193–8.

4 Weinstein MR (1980) In: Johnson FN (ed.) *Handbook of Lithium Therapy.* MTP Press, 421–29.

5 Cohen LS, Friedman JM, Jefferson JW, *et al.* (1994) A reevaluation of risk of in utero exposure to lithium. *JAMA* **271**, 146–50.

Valproate/valproic acid

In the UK, despite the widespread use of sodium valproate as a mood stabiliser, the only *licensed* preparation for bipolar affective disorder is Depakote® (see below). There are no published placebo-control trials of the efficacy of sodium valproate in bipolar affective disorder—despite data being published on tolerability (suggesting GI side-effects are less with Depakote®).

Psychiatric indications

- Acute mania (up to 56% effective).
- Acute depressive episode (in bipolar affective disorder) in combination with an antidepressant—data limited.
- Prophylaxis of bipolar affective disorder—possibly more effective in rapid cycling.

Pharmacokinetics

Sodium valproate is available in tablet, liquid, suspension, syrup, enteric-coated, and slow-release (Epilim Chrono®) forms. Semisodium valproate (divalproex sodium or Depakote®) comes as enteric-coated tablets containing valproic acid and sodium valproate. They are both rapidly absorbed when taken orally (peak serum level for sodium valproate ~2hrs; semi-sodium valproate 3–8hrs) with a plasma half-life of 6–16hrs.

Interactions

- Raised serum levels with phenobarbitone, phenytoin, and antidepressants (TCAs, fluoxetine).
- Decreased serum levels with carbamazepine.
- Toxicity may be precipitated by other highly protein-bound drugs (e.g. aspirin), which can displace valproate from its protein-binding sites.

Side-effects and toxicity

Dose-related side-effects GI upset (anorexia, nausea, dyspepsia, vomiting, diarrhoea), raised LFTs, tremor, and sedation—if persistent, may require dose reduction, change in preparation, or treatment of specific symptoms (e.g. β-blocker for tremor; H2-blocker for dyspepsia).

Unpredictable side-effects Mild, asymptomatic leukopenia and thrombocytopenia (reversible upon drug reduction/discontinuation), hair loss (usually transient), increased appetite, and weight gain.

Rare, idiosyncratic side-effects Irreversible hepatic failure, pancreatitis, agranulocytoses, polycystic ovaries/hyperandrogenism.

Toxicity/overdose Wide therapeutic window, hence unintentional overdose is uncommon. Signs of overdose include somnolence, heart block, eventually coma, and even death (haemodialysis may be needed).

Treatment guidelines for sodium valproate

- Full medical history (particularly liver disease, haematological problems, and bleeding disorders)/full physical examination; check FBC, LFTs, baseline ECG.
- **Sodium valproate**: Start with a low, divided dose (e.g. 200 mg bd or tds), increase every few days or every week by 200–400 mg/day according to response and side-effects, up to a maximum of 2500 mg/day, or until serum levels are 50–125 mmol/l (see below). Usual maintenance dose 1000–1500 mg/day.
- **Depakote®**: Start with 250 mg tds (or up to 20 mg/kg for acute manic episode) and increase every few days or every week by 250–500 mg/day to a maximum of 2000 mg/day, or until serum levels are 50–125 mmol/l (see below). Usual maintenance dose 1000–2000 mg/day.
- Once the patient is stable, simplify regime.
- If GI upset is a problem with sodium valproate, consider changing to enteric-coated, slow-release (Epilim Chrono®), or Depakote®.
- If poor compliance is an issue, consider use of slow-release tablets.
- Once established, check FBC, LFTs, and serum valproate level every 6 mths.

Points to note

- There is no well-established correlation between serum concentrations and mood-stabilising effects. Best advice is to use similar doses and serum levels that are considered therapeutic for epilepsy.
- Closer clinical monitoring for side-effects may be necessary for patients who cannot reliably report early signs.

Carbamazepine

Psychiatric indications

- Acute mania (less effective than lithium/equivalent efficacy to antipsychotics)—alone or in combination with lithium.
- Acute depressive episode (in bipolar affective disorder)—alone or in combination with lithium.
- Prophylaxis of bipolar affective disorder—data limited.

Pharmacokinetics

Carbamazepine is available in a variety of forms (solutions, suspensions, syrups, and chewable or slow-release formulations), all with similar bioavailability. Peak plasma concentrations between 4–8 hrs (usually), may be as late as 26 hrs. Plasma half-life 18–55 hrs. With long-term use, carbamazepine induces its own metabolism, decreasing the half-life 5–26 hrs.

Interactions

- Carbamazepine decreases the plasma levels of many drugs metabolised by the liver e.g. antipsychotics, BDZs (except clonazepam), TCAs, other anticonvulsants, hormonal contraceptives, thyroid hormones.
- Carbamazepine serum concentrations can be increased by certain drugs e.g. erythromycin, calcium channel blockers (diltiazem and verapamil, but not nifedipine or nimodipine), SSRIs.

Side-effects and toxicity

Unpredictable side-effects Antidiuretic effects leading to hyponatremia (6–31%), probably more common in the elderly, sometimes developing many months after starting treatment; decrease in total and free thyroxine levels/increase in free cortisol levels (rarely clinically significant).

Idiosyncratic side-effects Agranulocytosis, aplastic anaemia, hepatic failure, exfoliative dermatitis (e.g. Stevens-Johnson syndrome), and pancreatitis (these side effects usually occur within the first 3–6 mths of treatment, rarely after longer periods). N.B. Routine blood monitoring does not reliably predict blood dyscrasias, hepatic failure, or exfoliative dermatitis—patient education about early symptoms and signs essential.

Other rare side-effects Systemic hypersensitivity reactions, cardiac conduction problems, psychiatric symptoms (including occasional cases of mania and psychosis), and, extremely rarely, renal problems (failure, oliguria, hematuria, and proteinuria).

Toxicity/overdose *Early signs:* dizziness, ataxia, sedation, and diplopia. Acute intoxication may present as marked irritability, stupor, or even coma. May be fatal in overdose (if >6 g ingested). *Symptoms of overdose:* nystagmus, ophthalmoplegia, cerebellar/extrapyramidal signs, impairment of consciousness, convulsions, respiratory depression, cardiac problems (tachycardia, hypotension, arrhythmias/conduction disturbances), GI upset, and other anticholinergic symptoms. Significant overdose requires emergency medical management (i.e. close monitoring, symptomatic treatment, gastric lavage, and possible haemodialysis.)

Treatment guidelines for carbamazepine

- Full medical history (particularly liver disease, haematological problems, and bleeding disorders); physical examination; check FBC, LFTs, U&Es, baseline ECG.
- Start with a low, divided dose (e.g. 200–600 mg/d in 2–4 divided doses), increase every few days or every week by 200 mg/day according to response and side-effects, up to 800–1200 mg/day, with slower increases thereafter as indicated, to a maximum of 2000 mg/day, or until serum levels are 4–15 g/ml (trough level—taken immediately prior to morning dose, and 5 days after dose change).
- Maintenance doses are usually around 1000 mg/day (range 200–1600 mg/day). *Doses higher than 1600 mg/day are not recommended.*
- Check FBC, LFTs, and serum carbamazepine level every 2 wks during first 2 mths of treatment, then reduce monitoring to every 3 mths.
- Once the patient is stable, simplify regimen and consider use of slow-released preparation, to enhance compliance.

Points to note

- Closer clinical monitoring for side-effects may be necessary for patients who cannot reliably report early signs.
- If carbamazepine is combined with lithium, there may be an increased risk of developing an acute confusional state. Closer monitoring is advisable and minimisation of the use or dose of other medications (e.g. antipsychotics, anticholinergics, BDZs) that may contribute to confusion.

Anxiety and stress-related disorders

Introduction

If schizophrenia is 'the heartland of psychiatry', then neurotic disorders are surely the rest of the continent, in view of their prevalence in the general population (see opposite) and, the morbidity they cause.

As unpopular as the term 'neurosis' has become (for a historical, perspective see p. 340), it is still retained in the ICD-10 in the rubric 'neurotic, stress-related, and somatoform disorders'. DSM-IV has effectively carved up the neuroses into 'anxiety disorders', 'somatoform disorders', 'dissociative disorders', and 'adjustment disorders'. Here, we retain the use of 'neuroses' as shorthand for all these disorders, but will use the subdivisions when talking about the particular disorders.

We have all experienced anxiety symptoms, perhaps suffer from a particular 'phobia', or are a little bit obsessive about certain things—but to be 'clinically' significant, these problems must be severe enough to cause marked distress and/or substantially interfere with our day-to-day lives. Because of the 'recognisable' quality of some of the symptoms of neurotic disorders, it may be helpful to divide them into three categories:

1. The common neuroses
- Anxiety/phobic disorders—e.g. panic, agoraphobia, generalised anxiety disorder (GAD), specific (understandable) phobias (e.g. snakes, spiders), hypochondriasis, social phobia.
- Stress-related disorders—e.g. acute stress reactions, adjustment disorder, post-traumatic stress disorder (PTSD).
- Obsessive-compulsive disorder (OCD).

2. The unusual neuroses (i.e. outwith 'normal' experience)
- Anxiety/phobic disorders—e.g. 'non-understandable' phobias (e.g. dirt, feathers), dysmorphophobia.
- 'Hysterical' conversion disorders.
- Dissociative/depersonalisation-derealisation disorder.
- Somatoform disorders.

3. 'Culture-specific' disorders (seen only in certain populations)
- Chronic fatigue syndrome (CFS)/ eating disorders (see p. 840)
- Other 'culture-bound' disorders

In this section, we deal only with the anxiety and stress-related disorders. The other disorders may be found in the **Liaison psychiatry** section (conversion, somatisation, CFS, hypochondriasis, dysmorphophobia), the **Behavioural disorders** section (eating disorders), and a specific section on **Transcultural psychiatry** (culture-bound disorders).

Points to note
- 'Symptoms' are common in the general population.
- Comorbidity frequent (other neuroses, depression, substance misuse, personality disorder).
- May often present with physical symptoms.
- Must be recognised if they are to be treated appropriately.
- Management will usually involve a combined approach (pharmacological and psychological).

Prevalence of psychiatric disorders in the general population

Disorder	Rate%	
	Previous 6 mths	Lifetime
Schizophrenia	0.9	1.5
Affective disorders	5.8	8.3
Substance abuse disorders	6.0	16.4
Anxiety disorders	8.9	14.6

(Data derived from multiple community surveys.)

Historical perspective

The term 'neurosis' was coined by William Cullen in 1777, replacing 'illness of the nerves' (coined by Robert Whytt in 1764 to replace the old 'vapours'), and meaning any disease of the nervous system without a known organic basis (which at the time also included epilepsy). Clinical descriptions of neurotic symptoms can be found in the works of Hippocrates. However, the 'illness' vanished under the cloak of both pagan and Christian beliefs, with typical symptoms attributed to the work of 'spirits', possession, or divine punishment. It did not resurface properly until the Renaissance (the 1500s) thanks (in part) to the witchcraft trials, when doctors were called in to present diagnoses of known illnesses which could be mistaken for demonic possession (the first recorded 'medical defence'!). Although there was much debate, the brain became the final resting place as the organ most likely to be involved in the aetiology of the condition.

The history of the neuroses is tightly bound to the (re)discovery of hypnosis (formerly the remit of 'faith healing'). The work of Franz-Anton Mesmer [1734–1815] ('mesmerism') and James Braid [1795–1860] ('braidism') was brought to France by Azam in 1859, coming to the attention of Charcot, whose experiments with 'hysterics' would have a profound influence on one particular 'assistant'—Sigmund Freud. Freud's first paper, published in 1886, shortly after his return to Vienna, was of a case of 'traumatic hysteria' in a male patient. It was his *Studies on Hysteria*, written with Josef Breuer and published in 1895, which provided the starting point of all his subsequent major concepts of psychoanalytical theory—including repression, psychic reality, and the subconscious.

The idea of repression of trauma (out of consciousness) and the appearance of 'defences' was highly influential, with the neuroses regarded as illnesses of the mind, needing psychotherapeutic treatment. Old arguments of 'emotional' versus 'physical' factors resurfaced in the aftermath of the First World War, as some authorities found it difficult to attribute the illnesses seen in fit, healthy, young men (who had indisputably experienced 'traumatic events') to 'conversion hysteria' or 'phobic neurosis'. The 'encephalitis lethargicans' epidemic in 1919, and the presence of numerous 'hysterical' symptoms (e.g. convulsions, mutism, feelings of passion, obsessions/compulsions, spasms) argued in favour of at least some of the 'neuroses' having an organic basis.

In the 1920s, Walter Cannon proposed the concept of the 'emergency reaction', believing this 'fight-or-flight' response was mediated by the autonomic nervous system (sympathetic response). He also noted that the physiological responses were too slow to account for feelings, and that some other 'neural mechanism' must be at work.

The dominance of the behaviourists in psychology relegated 'emotion' to just another 'way of acting' in a particular situation (albeit internally perceived). Although an oversimplification, this led to the development of the 'conditioning theory' of anxiety. John Watson, the father of behaviourism, claimed to have produced an animal phobia in an eleven-month-old boy, 'little Albert', by making a loud clanging noise whilst the boy was happily playing with a rat. Watson proposed that neuroses arose out of traumatic learning situations and then persist to influence behaviour throughout life.

This was adapted by the 1930s to include the concept of 'instrumental conditioning' (the association of an emotionally arousing stimulus and a neutral response), and, in the 1940s, Mowrer attempted to translate Freud's theory of anxiety neurosis into the language of learning theory: responses that reduce anxiety are learned (in a behavioural way)—sometimes these reinforced behaviours may be aberrant, unhelpful, or simply bizarre, and present as 'neuroses'. 'Avoidance' was postulated as the behaviour that was reinforced due to successfully removing a 'negative reinforcer' (e.g. fear). These ideas led to the rational treatment of phobias with 'desensitisation' techniques.

In the search for Cannon's 'neural mechanism' neurophysiologists used lesioning experiments to identify the thalamus as a critical gateway for stimuli, and the hypothalamus as mediating the physiological response (via the HPA axis) the Cannon-Bard Theory. Other theories emerged over the years (e.g. the Papez Circuit, 1937) and understanding the 'emotional life' of the brain remains at the forefront of research (see *The Emotional Brain* by Joseph LeDoux, 1998).

Inviting as psychological explanations appeared, the late 1950s also heralded the arrival of the benzodiazepines. 'Tranquilisers' (e.g. Miltown, Librium, Valium) became the 'housewives' choice', effectively treating a multitude of 'neurotic' symptoms. Unfortunately, the indiscriminate use of these drugs led to them being 'demonised' as causing dependence problems (despite evidence for their effectiveness when properly used). The advent of the 'antidepressants' artificially separated 'neurotic depression' from the other neuroses, but nonetheless some utility was also seen in treating the anxiety disorders. A key study was the use of clomipramine in the treatment of OCD (see *The Boy Who Couldn't Stop Washing* by Judith Rapoport, 1989). The fact that clomipramine was the most serotonergic of the TCAs, paved the way for the 2nd generation antidepressants (the SSRIs) to be used in 'neuroses' (previously thought only to be amenable to psychological approaches).

Brain imaging demonstrated underlying functional changes in OCD patients (in the frontal cortex [left orbital gyrus] and bilateral caudate nuclei), which 'normalised' after successful treatment with medication (and interestingly with CBT techniques—although this took longer). For many patients with panic attacks, structural and functional changes were found in the temporal lobes. These findings resonated with the long-held observation that neurotic symptoms (e.g. anxiety, panic, somatic symptoms, depersonalisation/derealisation) were often reported in other 'organic' conditions (e.g. temporal lobe epilepsy).

Modern views are eclectic in their approach—e.g. the biopsychosocial model (see p. 255). For the neuroses, early environmental influences (including 'social' factors like maternal deprivation) can alter the sensitivity of physiological stress responses in adulthood. Hence, the experience of stressors (psychological or physical) may lead (e.g. through the effects of 'stress hormones' such as cortisol, and other neurophysiological mechanisms) to alterations in the structure and/or function of the brain, which in turn manifest as clinical symptoms (i.e. behavioural and/or emotional change).

Hyperventilation syndrome (HVS)*

Essence HVS is a relatively common presentation which may be mistaken for panic disorder and there is considerable overlap (hence its inclusion in this section):

- 50–60% of patients with panic disorder or agoraphobia have symptoms of HVS.
- 25% of HVS patients have symptoms of panic disorder.

It may also be confused for other organic diseases, particularly of the cardio-respiratory system, due to the physical symptoms manifest.

Minute ventilation exceeds metabolic demands, leading to haemodynamic and chemical changes that produce characteristic symptoms (dyspnoea, agitation, dizziness, atypical chest pain, tachypnoea and hyperpnoea, paraesthesias, and carpopedal spasm) usually in a young, otherwise healthy patient.

Aetiology Unknown—however, certain stressors do provoke an exaggerated respiratory response in some individuals (e.g. emotional distress, sodium lactate, caffeine, isoproterenol, cholecystokinin, and CO_2.) HVS patients tend to use accessory muscles to breathe, rather than the diaphragm, resulting in hyperinflated lungs and perceived effort or dyspnoea when stressors induce the need to take a deep breath. This leads to anxiety, and triggers further deep breathing, setting up a vicious cycle.

Epidemiology ♀:♂ = 7:1, usually presents between 15–55 yrs, but can occur at any age.

Symptoms and signs

- **Cardiac**—chest pain/angina ('atypical':may last hours, not minutes; often relieved by exercise; GTN ineffective), ECG changes (prolonged QT, ST depression or elevation, and T-wave inversion).
- **Respiratory**—hyperpnoea, tachypnoea, dyspnoea, wheeze (bronchospasm secondary to low P_aCO_2)
- N.B. *In chronic forms hyperventilation may not be clinically apparent.*
- **CNS** (due to reduced CBF secondary to hypocapnia)—dizziness, weakness, confusion, agitation, depersonalisation, visual hallucinations, syncope or seizure (rare), paraesthesias (usually upper limbs and bilateral), perioral numbness.
- **GI**—bloating, belching, flatus, epigastric pressure (due to aerophagia), dry mouth (due to mouth breathing and anxiety).
- **Metabolic** (due to electrolyte disturbance secondary to respiratory alkalosis)—acute hypocalcaemia (signs carpopedal spasm, muscle twitching, positive Chvostek and Trousseau signs, and prolonged QT interval), hypokalaemia (with generalised weakness), acute hypophosphataemia (may contribute to paraesthesias and generalized weakness).

Differential diagnosis Extensive: diagnosis of exclusion—ARDS, asthma, AF, atrial flutter, cardiomyopathy, COPD, costochondritis, DKA, hyperthyroidism, metabolic acidosis, methaemoglobinaemia, MI, panic (and other anxiety) disorder, pleural effusion, pneumonia, pneumothorax, PE, withdrawal syndromes.

Investigations
- Unless there is a clear history of HVS, any first presentations of hyperventilation should be referred for exclusion of serious underlying medical problems (see 'Differential diagnosis' opposite).
- These investigations may include full physical, FBC, U&Es, TFTs, glucose, Ca^{2+}, PO_4, pulse oximetry, ABG (in HVS: pH normal, P_aCO_2 and HCO_3 low), toxicology, ELISA d-dimer (PE), ECG, CXR, and possibly V/Q scan.
- Repeating these investigations at later presentations should only be done if there are new clinical findings.

Management
- **Acute management** If serious underlying pathology has been excluded, management includes:
  - Reassurance of the patient.
  - Alleviation of severe anxiety (e.g. use of BDZs).
  - Establishment of normal breathing pattern (instructing the patient to breath more abdominally using the diaphragm; physically compressing the upper chest and instructing the patient to exhale maximally to reduce hyperinflation).

N.B. Use of rebreathing techniques (e.g. into a paper bag) may be unsuccessful because patients have difficulty complying with the technique and because CO_2 itself may be a chemical trigger for anxiety in these patients.

- **Further management**
  - Education about hyperventilation, relaxation, and breathing techniques may be helpful ('provocation' should not be performed except in this setting).
  - Use of beta-blockers and BDZs may have some utility, and some success is reported for the use of antidepressants in prevention of further episodes.
  - If there is clear psychiatric morbidity (e.g. anxiety or depression) this should also be specifically addressed.

*Formerly known as Da Costa syndrome. Other archaic terms include: cardiac neurasthenia, cardiac neurosis, circulatory neurasthenia, disordered action of the heart (DAH), effort syndrome, hyperdynamic-adrenergic circulatory state, hyperkinetic heart syndrome, irritable heart, neurocirculatory asthenia, soldier's heart, vasoregulatory asthenia.

Panic[1] disorder (1)—clinical features

Essence

Panic attack A period of intense fear characterised by a constellation of symptoms (see opposite) that develop rapidly, reach a peak of intensity in about 10 mins, and generally do not last longer than 20–30 mins (rarely over 1 hr). Attacks may be either *spontaneous* ('out of the blue') or *situational* (usually where attacks have occurred previously). Sometimes attacks may occur during sleep (*nocturnal panic attacks*), and rarely, physiological symptoms of anxiety may occur without the psychological component (*non-fearful panic attacks*).

Panic disorder[2] Recurrent panic attacks, which are not secondary to substance misuse, medical conditions, or another psychiatric disorder. Frequency of occurrence may vary from many attacks a day, to only a few attacks a year. There is usually the persistent worry about having another attack or the consequences of the attack (which may lead to phobic avoidance of places or situations—see *Agoraphobia*), and significant behavioural changes related to the attack.

Symptoms/signs (see opposite)

- Physical symptoms/signs are related to autonomic arousal (e.g. tremor, tachycardia, tachypnoea, hypertension, sweating, GI upset) which are often compounded by HVS (in 50–60% of cases see pp. 342–3).
- Concerns of death from cardiac or respiratory problems may be a major focus, leading to patients presenting (often repeatedly) to emergency medical services.
- Panic disorder may be undiagnosed in patients with 'unexplained' medical symptoms[3] (chest pain, back pain, GI symptomsincluding IBS, fatigue, headache, dizziness, or multiple symptoms[4]).
- Thoughts of suicide (or homicide) should be elicited as acute anxiety (particularly when recurrent) can lead to impulsive acts (usually directed towards self). **N.B. Risk of attempted suicide is substantially raised where there is comorbid depression, alcohol misuse, or substance misuse**.

Epidemiology Lifetime prevalence: 4.2% for panic disorder, 8% for panic attacks (mean value derived from American ECAS[4] and NCS[5]); 1.5–5% for panic disorder, 3–5.6% for panic attacks (ECA). Women are 2–3 times more likely to be affected than men. Age of onset has a bimodal distribution with highest peak incidence at 15–24 yrs and a second peak at 45–54 yrs. Rare after age 65.

Comorbidity Agoraphobia (community surveys: 30–50%; psychiatric clinics: 75%), depressive disorder (up to 68%), other anxiety and related disorders (up to 50%—e.g. social phobia, OCD), alcohol (up to 30%) and substance misuse, bipolar affective disorder (20%), medical conditions (e.g. mitral valve prolapse, hypertension, cardiomyopathy, COPD, IBS, migraine).

Differential diagnosis Other anxiety or related disorder (panic attacks may be part of the disorder), substance or alcohol misuse/withdrawal (e.g. amphetamines, caffeine, cocaine, theophylline, sedative-hypnotics, steroids), mood disorders, psychiatric disorders secondary to medical conditions, medical conditions presenting with similar symptoms (e.g. *endocrine*: carcinoid syndrome, Cushing's disease/syndrome, hyperthyroidism, hypoglycemia, hypoparathyroidism, phaeochromocytoma; *haematological*: anaemia, *cardiac*: arrhythmias, mitral valve prolapse, MI; *respiratory*: COPD/asthma, HVS; *neurological*: epilepsy—esp. TLE, vestibular dysfunction).

Investigations There are no specific tests for panic disorder, however basic investigations should be performed to exclude physical causes (e.g. FBC, U&Es, glucose, TFTs, ECG, and if supported by history/physical examination: toxicology, Ca^{2+}, urinary VMA/pHVA, ECHO, and EEG).

Symptoms associated with panic attacks (in order of frequency of occurrence)

- Palpitations, pounding heart, or accelerated heart rate.
- Sweating.
- Trembling or shaking.
- Sense of shortness of breath or smothering.
- Feeling of choking or difficulties swallowing ('*globus hystericus*').
- Chest pain or discomfort.
- Nausea or abdominal distress.
- Feeling dizzy, unsteady, light-headed, or faint.
- Derealisation or depersonalisation (feeling detached from oneself or one's surroundings).
- Fear of losing control or going crazy.
- Fear of dying ('*angor animus*').
- Numbness or tingling sensations (paraesthesia).
- Chills or hot flashes.

---

1 'Panic' derives from the Greek god 'Pan' who was in the habit of frightening humans and animals 'out of the blue'.

2 ICD-10 and DSM-IV disagree on the nature of panic disorder. ICD-10 regards true panic attacks as not being *situational*, and DSM-IV allows for both *spontaneous* and *situational*. Hence DSM-IV includes agoraphobia within panic disorder, seeing it as a special case of *situational panic disorder* (panic disorder with agoraphobia), whereas ICD-10 separates agoraphobia (under the rubric 'phobic anxiety disorders') from panic disorder (under the rubric 'other anxiety disorders'). 'Agoraphobia with panic disorder' is allowed in ICD-10 when there is avoidance of places or situations where to have a spontaneous panic attack would be difficult or embarrassing.

3 Katon W (1984) Panic disorder and somatization. Review of 55 cases. *American Journal of Medicine* **77**, 101–8.

4 Simon GE and Van Korff M (1991) Somatization and psychiatric disorder in the NIMH Epidemiologic Catchment Area study. *AJP* **148**, 1494–500.

5 Eaton WW, Kessler RC, Wittchen HU, Magee WJ(1994) Panic and panic disorder in the United States. *AJP* **151**, 413–20.

Panic disorder (2)—aetiological models

There are a number of theories, based primarily on successful pharmacological treatment, to explain the biological basis of panic disorder:

The serotonergic model

Exaggerated post-synaptic receptor response to synaptic serotonin, possibly secondary to subsensitivity of $5HT_{1A}$ receptors.

The noradrenergic model

Increased adrenergic activity, with hypersensitivity of presynaptic alpha₂ receptors. (Locus coeruleus activity affects the hypothalamic-pituitary-adrenal axis and the firing rate is increased in panic.)

The GABA model

Decreased inhibitory receptor sensitivity, with resultant excitatory effect.

Cholecystokinin-pentagastrin model

Pentagastrin induces panic in a dose-dependent fashion in patients with panic disorder.

The lactate model

Postulated aberrant metabolic activity induced by lactate, from studies involving exercise-induced panic attacks (replicated by IV lactate infusion).

The false suffocation carbon dioxide hypothesis

Explains panic phenomena by hypersensitive brainstem receptors.

The neuroanatomical model

Suggests that panic attacks are mediated by a 'fear network' in the brain that involves the amygdala, the hypothalamus, and the brainstem centres.

The genetic hypothesis

Panic disorder has moderate heritability of around 30–40% (from family and twin studies). Most studies to date suggest that *vulnerability* is genetically determined, but critical stressors are required to develop clinical symptoms. The recently discovered genomic duplication (DUP25) on chromosome 15 (found in 7% of the population, but ~95% of patients with panic disorder) is perhaps the best evidence yet for genetic susceptibility[1].

---

1 Gratacos M, Nadal M, Martin-Santos R, et al. (2001) A polymorphic genomic duplication on human chromosome 15 is a susceptibility factor for panic and phobic disorders. *Cell* **106**, 367–79.

Panic disorder (3)—management guidelines

Combination of pharmacological and psychological treatments may be superior to single approach.

Pharmacological

- **SSRIs** (e.g. paroxetine [at least 40 mg], fluoxetine, fluvoxamine, citalopram, sertraline) are recommended as the drug of choice (unless contraindicated—see p. 280). In view of the possibility of initially increasing panic symptoms, start with low dose and gradually increase. Beneficial effect may take 3–8 weeks.
- **Alternative antidepressant** TCAs (e.g. imipramine or clomipramine) although not specifically licensed in the UK have been shown to be 70–80% effective (possible alternatives include: desipramine, doxepin, nortryptiline, or amitriptyline.) MAOIs (e.g. phenelzine) again not licensed, but may be superior to TCAs (for severe, chronic symptoms). There is also some favourable evidence for RIMAs (e.g. moclobemide).
- **BDZs** (e.g. alprazolam or clonazepam) should be used with caution (due to potential for abuse/dependence/cognitive impairment) but may be effective for severe, frequent, incapacitating symptoms. Use for 1–2 weeks in combination with an antidepressant may 'cover' symptomatic relief until the antidepressant becomes effective. N.B. 'Anti-panic' effects do not show tolerance, although sedative effects do.
- **If initial management is ineffective** Consider change to a different class agent (i.e. TCA, SSRI, MAOI) or combination (e.g. TCA+Lithium, SSRI+TCA). If 'treatment-resistant' consider alternative agent (e.g. carbamazepine, valproate, gabapentin, low-potency BDZ [diazepam—may need high dose], venlafaxine, inositol, verapamil).
- **If successful** Continue treatment for ~1yr before trial discontinuation (gradual tapering of dose). Do not confuse 'withdrawal' effects (10–20% of patients) with re-emergence of symptoms (50–70% of patients). If symptoms recur, continue for ~1yr before considering second trial discontinuation. (N.B. Patient may wish to continue treatment, rather than risk return of symptoms).

Psychological

- **Behavioural methods**: to treat phobic avoidance by exposure, use of relaxation, and control of hyperventilation (have been shown to be 58–83% effective[1]).
- **Cognitive methods**: teaching about bodily responses associated with anxiety/education about panic attacks, modification of thinking errors[2].
- **Psychodynamic methods**: there is some evidence for brief dynamic psychotherapy, particularly 'emotion-focused' treatment (e.g. 'panic-focused psychodynamic psychotherapy'), where typical fears of being abandoned or trapped are explored.

Issues of comorbidity

- In view of high levels of comorbidity, treatment of these conditions should not be neglected.

- For the other anxiety disorders and depression, this issue is somewhat simplified by the fact that SSRIs and other antidepressants have been shown to be effective for these conditions too. However, behavioural interventions (e.g. for OCD, social phobia) should also be considered.
- Alcohol/substance abuse may need to be addressed first, but specific treatment for persistent symptoms of panic ought not to be overlooked.

Emergency treatment of an acute panic attack

- Maintain a reassuring and calm attitude (most panic attacks spontaneously resolve within 30 mins).
- If symptoms are severe and distressing consider prompt use of BDZs (immediate relief of anxiety may help reassure the patient, provide confidence that treatment is possible, and reduce subsequent 'emergency' presentations).
- If 'first presentation', exclude medical causes (may require admission to hospital for specific tests).
- If panic attacks are recurrent, consider differential diagnosis for panic disorder and address underlying disorder (may require psychiatric referral).

1 Ballenger JC et al. (1997) Panic disorder and agoraphobia. In *Treatments of psychiatric disorders* (2nd ed.) Vol.2. American Psychiatric Press, Washington DC, pp 1421–52.

2 Barlow DH and Craske MG (1988) *Mastery of your anxiety and panic.* Center for Stress and Anxiety Disorders, State University for New York at Albany.

Agoraphobia[1]

Essence Symptoms of anxiety (psychological and/or autonomic) are not secondary delusional or obsessive thoughts and are restricted to places or situations where escape may be difficult or embarrassing, leading to avoidance (e.g. of crowds, public places, travelling away from home or alone).

Epidemiology Prevalence (6 month) 2.8–5.8 % (ECA); $\male:\female = 1:3$; as for panic disorder, there is a bimodal distribution with the first being somewhat broader (15–35 yrs). In later life agoraphobic symptoms may develop secondary to physical frailty, with the associated fear of exacerbating medical problems or having an accident.

Aetiology *Genetic* Both genetic and environmental factors appear to play a role. The predisposition towards overly interpreting situations as dangerous may be genetic, and some commentators suggest an ethological factor involving an evolutionarily determined vulnerability to unfamiliar territory[2]. First-degree relatives also have an increased prevalence of other anxiety and related disorders (e.g. social phobia), alcohol misuse, and depressive disorders. *Psychoanalytical* Unconscious conflicts are repressed and may be transformed by displacement into phobic symptoms. *Learning theory* Conditioned fear responses lead to learned avoidance.

Comorbidity Panic disorder, depressive disorder, other anxiety and related disorders (e.g. 55% also have social phobia), alcohol and substance misuse

Differential diagnosis Other anxiety and related disorders (esp. generalised anxiety disorder, social phobia, OCD), depressive disorders, secondary avoidance due to delusional ideas in psychotic disorders.

Management

- **Pharmacological** *Antidepressants* As for panic disorder. *BDZs* short-term use only (may reinforce avoidance)—most evidence for alprazolam/clonazepam.
- **Psychological** *Behavioural methods* Exposure techniques (focused on particular situations or places), relaxation training, and anxiety management. *Cognitive methods* Teaching about bodily responses associated with anxiety/education about panic attacks, modification of thinking errors.

1 Literally 'fear of the market place' (Greek.)

2 Lelliott P, Marks I, McNamee G, Tobena A (1989) Onset of panic disorder with agoraphobia. Toward an integrated model. *Archives of General Psychiatry* **46**, 1000–4.

Simple or specific phobias

Essence Recurring excessive and unreasonable psychological or autonomic symptoms of anxiety, in the (anticipated) presence of a specific feared object or situation leading, whenever possible, to avoidance. DSM-IV distinguishes 5 subtypes: animals, aspects of the natural environment, blood/injection/injury, situational, and 'other'.

Epidemiology Prevalence: lifetime 11.3%, 12-mth (NCS) 8.8%, 6-mth (ECA) 4.5–11.9%; ♀:♂variable 1:3–1:20; animal/situational phobias may be more common in ♀; occurrence mainly in childhood/adolescence (mean 15yrs): animal phobias ~7yrs, claustrophobia ~20yrs.

Aetiology Genetic Both genetic and environmental factors play a role. MZ:DZ = 25.9%:11.0%[1] for animal phobia, situational phobia roughly equal suggesting stronger role for the environment. **Psychoanalytical** ↑The manifest fear is the symbolic representation of an unconscious conflict, which has been repressed and displaced into phobic symptoms. **Learning theory** Regarded as a conditioned fear response related to a traumatic situation, with learned avoidance (the trigger to the conditioned fear response may be a reminder of the original situation). Observational learning also appears to be important, and the 'preparedness' theory (Marks[2]) suggests that fear of certain objects may be evolutionarily adaptive (related to survival of the individual or species), selectively acquired, and difficult to extinguish as this is a 'non-cognitive' process.

Comorbidity The lifetime risk for patients with specific phobias experiencing at least one other lifetime psychiatric disorder is reportedly over 80% (NCS), particularly other anxiety disorders (panic, social phobia) and mood disorders (mania, depression, dysthymia). However, rates of substance misuse are considerably less than in other anxiety disorders.

Differential diagnosis Panic disorder (fear of having further panic attack), agoraphobia, social phobia, hypochondriasis (fear of having a specific serious illness), OCD (avoidance/fear of an object or situation due to obsessional thoughts, ideas, or ruminations), psychosis (avoidance due to delusional idea of threat—fears tend to be overly excessive).

Management **Psychological** Behavioural therapy—treatment of choice: methods aim to reduce the fear response e.g. Wolpe's systematic desensitisation[3] with relaxation and graded exposure (either imaginary or in vivo). Other techniques: reciprocal inhibition, flooding (not better than graded exposure), and modelling. Cognitive methods: education/anxiety management, coping skills/strategies—may enhance long-term outcomes. **Pharmacological** Generally not used, except in severe cases to reduce fearavoidance (with BDZs e.g. diazepam) and allow the patient to engage in exposure techniques (2°-blockers may be helpful, but benefit is not sustained). Clear 2° depression may require an antidepressant.

Course Without treatment, tend to run a chronic course. However, individuals may not present unless life changes force them to confront the feared object or situation.

Specific phobias—selected glossary

Accidents	Dystychiphobia
Animals	Zoophobia
Ants	Myrmecophobia
Automobiles	Amaxophobia, motorphobia
Bees	Apiphobia, melissophobia
Birds	Ornithophobia
Blood	Haemophobia
Bridges	Gephyrophobia
Cats	Felinophobia
Choking/being smothered	Anginaphobia, pnigophobia, pnigerophobia
Contamination, dirt, or infection	Molysomophobia, mysophobia
Creepy, crawly things	Herpetophobia
Crossing streets	Agyrophobia
Darkness	Nyctophobia, scotophobia
Dentists	Dentophobia, Odontophobia
Depth	Bathophobia
Doctors	Iatrophobia
Dogs or rabies	Cynophobia
Everything	Panophobia, panphobia, pamphobia
Feathers	Pteronophobia
Flying	Aviophobia
Forests, at night	Nyctohylophobia
Frogs	Batrachophobia
Hair, fur, or animal skins	Chaetophobia, Trichophobia, doraphobia
Horses	Equinophobia, hippophobia
Hospitals	Nosocomephobia
Injections	Trypanophobia
Jumping	Catapedaphobia
Lightning and thunder	Brontophobia, karaunophobia
Moths	Mottephobia
Needles	Aichmophobia, belonephobia
Open high places	Aeroacrophobia
Operations: surgical	Tomophobia
Place: enclosed	Claustrophobia
Railways/trains	Siderodromophobia
Rain	Ombrophobia, Pluviophobia
Rats	Zemmiphobia
Reptiles	Herpetophobia
Snakes	Ophidiophobia
Spiders	Arachnophobia.
Vomiting	Emetophobia
X-rays	Radiophobia

1 Kendler KS, Neale MC, Kessler RC,et al. (1992) The genetic epidemiology of phobias in women. The interrelationship of agoraphobia, social phobia, situational phobia, and simple phobia. *Archives of General Psychiatry* **49**, 273–81.

2 Marks IM (1969) *Fears and Phobias* Academic Press: New York.

3 Wolpe J (1973) *The practice of behaviour therapy (2nd* ed.) Pergamon: New York.

Social phobia

Essence Symptoms of incapacitating anxiety (psychological and/or autonomic) are not secondary delusional or obsessive thoughts and are restricted to particular social situations, leading to a desire for escape or avoidance (which may reinforce the strongly held belief of social inadequacy).

Epidemiology Lifetime rates vary from 2.4% (ECA) to 13.3% (NCS), 12mth prevalence 7.9% (NCS); ♂=♀ for those seeking treatment (however community surveys suggest ♂>♀); bimodal distribution with peaks at 5 yrs and between 11–15 yrs (ECA)—often patients do not present until they are in their 30s.

Aetiology Both genetic and environmental factors play a role. MZ:DZ = 24.4%:15.3%[1]. The predisposition towards overly interpreting situations as dangerous may be genetic, whereas individual interpretations of social cues may be environmentally determined[2] (i.e. the particular trigger for the conditioned fear response depends on the social situation in which first episode of anxiety experienced).

Symptoms/signs Somatic symptoms include blushing, trembling, dry mouth, perspiration when exposed to the feared situation, with excessive fear (which is recognised as such by the patient) of humiliation, embarrassment, or others noticing how anxious they are. Individuals are often characteristically self-critical and perfectionistic. Avoidance of situations may lead to difficulty in maintaining social/sexual relationships, educational problems (difficulties in interactions with other students/oral presentations), or vocational problems (work in less demanding jobs, well below their abilities). Thoughts of suicide are relatively common.

Comorbidity[3] There is a high level of psychiatric comorbidity with the most common disorders including simple phobia, agoraphobia, panic disorder, generalised anxiety disorder, PTSD, depression/dysthymia, and substance misuse.

Differential diagnosis Other anxiety and related disorders (esp. generalised anxiety disorder, agoraphobia, OCD), poor social skills, anxious/avoidant personality traits, depressive disorders, secondary avoidance due to delusional ideas in psychotic disorders, and substance misuse.

Management
- **Psychological** CBT, in either an individual or group setting, should be considered as a first-line therapy (along with SSRIs/MAOIs) and may be better at preventing relapse. Components of this approach include relaxation training/anxiety management (for autonomic arousal), social skills training, and integrated exposure methods (modelling and graded exposure).
- **Pharmacological** β-blockers (e.g. atenolol) may reduce autonomic arousal, particularly for 'specific social phobia' (e.g. performance anxiety). For more generalised social anxiety, both SSRIs (e.g. fluoxetine, paroxetine, sertraline) and MAOIs (e.g. phenelzine) are significantly more effective. Other treatment possibilities include RIMAs (e.g. moclobemide) or the addition of a BDZ (e.g. clonazepam, alprazolam) or buspirone.

Course
- Without treatment, social phobia may be a chronic lifelong condition.
- With treatment, response rates may be up to 90%, especially with combined approaches.
- Medication best regarded as long-term, as relapse rates are high on discontinuation.

1 Kendler KS, Neale MC, Kessler RC, et al. (1992) The genetic epidemiology of phobias in women. The interrelationship of agoraphobia, social phobia, situational phobia, and simple phobia. *Archives of General Psychiatry* **49**, 273–81.

2 Rapee RM and Heimberg RG (1997) A cognitive-behavioral model of anxiety in social phobia. *Behaviour Research and Therapy* **35**, 741–56.

3 Schneier FR, Johnson J, Hornig CD, et al. (1992) Social phobia. Comorbidity and morbidity in an epidemiologic sample. *Archives of General Psychiatry* **49**, 282–8.

Generalised anxiety disorder (GAD)

Essence 'Excessive worry' (generalised free-floating persistent anxiety) and feelings of apprehension about everyday events/problems, with symptoms of muscle and psychic tension, causing significant distress/functional impairment.

Signs/symptoms See opposite.

Epidemiology Prevalence: 6mth (ECA) 2.5–6.4%, lifetime (NCS) 3–4%; early gradual onset (mean 21, range 2–60yrs); ♀ > ♂ esp. early onset (associated with childhood fears and marital/sexual disturbance); later onset often after a stressful event; single (~30% never marry), unemployed.

Aetiology *Genetic* Heritability ~30% (environmental factors important). *Neurobiological* ANS responsiveness (? downregulation of α_2 receptors); loss of regulatory control of cortisol (HPA axis) in ~1/3 of GAD patients (DMST—reduced cortisol suppression). Possible sustained activation of stria terminalis (increased startle) following prolonged CRF stimulation (chronic stress). Abnormalities in the 'behavioural inhibition system' (septohippocampal-Papez circuit-amygdala). Neurotransmitter abnormalities (e.g. ↓GABA activity, dysregulation of 5-HT systems, CCK). *Psychological* Experience of unexpected negative events (e.g. early death of parent, rape, war) or chronic stressors (dysfunctional family/marriage). Overprotective or parenting lacking warmth and responsiveness (theoretically leading to low perceived control over events).

Comorbidity Other anxiety disorders (simple phobias, social phobia, panic disorder), depression/dysthymia, alcohol and drug problems, other 'physical' conditions: (e.g. IBS, HVS, atypical chest pain).

Differential diagnosis 'Normal worries', depression, mixed anxiety/depression, other anxiety disorders (the anxiety is more focused), drug and alcohol problems, medical conditions (see opposite), side-effects of prescribed medications (see opposite).

Management *Psychological* Generally less effective than in the other anxiety disorders (lack of situational triggers); some evidence for CBT. *Behavioural methods:* may help treat avoidance by exposure, use of relaxation and control of hyperventilation. *Cognitive methods*: teaching about bodily responses related to anxiety/education about panic attacks, modification of thinking errors. **Pharmacological** Directed towards predominant anxiety symptoms: *psychic symptoms*—buspirone[1] (beneficial effects may take 2–4 wks); *somatic symptoms*—BDZs (e.g. lorazepam, diazepam); *depressive symptoms*—TCAs (imipramine, clomipramine), trazodone, venlafaxine, SSRIs; *cardiovascular symptoms* or *autonomic symptoms*—β-blockers (e.g. atenolol). If initial approach ineffective/partially effective, use combined approaches (e.g. buspirone + antidepressant). **Physical** Psychosurgery (rare)—for severe/intractable anxiety.

Symptoms of GAD (present most days for at least 6mths)

DSM-IV At least 3 (or 1 in children) out of: restlessness or feeling keyed up or on edge; easy fatiguability; concentration difficulties or 'mind going blank'; irritability; muscle tension; sleep disturbance.

ICD-10 At least 4 (with at least 1 from 'autonomic arousal') out of:
- Symptoms of autonomic arousal: palpitations/tachycardia; sweating; trembling/shaking; dry mouth.
- 'Physical' symptoms: breathing difficulties; choking sensation; chest pain/discomfort; nausea/abdominal distress.
- Mental state symptoms: feeling dizzy, unsteady, faint or lightheaded; derealisation/depersonalisation; fear of losing control, 'going crazy', passing out, dying.
- General symptoms: hot flushes/cold chills; numbness or tingling sensations.
- Symptoms of tension: muscle tension/aches and pains; restlessness/ inability to relax; feeling keyed up, on edge, or mentally tense; a sensation of a lump in the throat or difficulty swallowing.
- Other: exaggerated responses to minor surprises/being startled; concentration difficulties/'mind going blank' due to worry or anxiety; persistent irritability; difficulty getting to sleep due to worrying.

Course Chronic and disabling, prognosis generally poor, remission rates low (~30% after 3yrs, with treatment), 6yr outcome—68% mild residual symptoms, 9% severe persistent impairment. Often comorbidity becomes more significant (esp. alcohol misuse) and this worsens the prognosis.

Medical conditions that may be associated with anxiety-like symptoms

Cardiovascular Arrhythmias, IHD, mitral valve disease, cardiac failure

Respiratory Asthma, COPD, HVS, PE, hypoxia

Neurological TLE, vestibular nerve disease

Endocrine Hyperthyroidism, hypoparathyroidism, hypoglycaemia, phaeochromocytoma

Miscellaneous Anaemia, porphyria, SLE, carcinoid tumour, pellagra

Prescribed medications causing anxiety-like symptoms

Cardiovascular Antihypertensives, antiarrhythmics

Respiratory Bronchodilators, α-adrenergic agonists

Neurological Anticholinergics, anticonvulsants, antiparkinsonian agents

Psychiatric Antidepressants, antipsychotics, antabuse (disulfiram) reactions, withdrawal from BDZs and other sedatives

Miscellaneous Thyroxine, NSAIDs, antibiotics, chemotherapy

1 Buspirone should be considered as an alternative to BDZs when sedative effects are unwanted (e.g. drivers of vehicles, pilots, machine operators), in patients with a personal/family history of drug misuse, or for those already taking other CNS depressants.

Obsessive–compulsive disorder (OCD)

Essence A common, chronic condition, often associated with marked anxiety and depression, characterised by 'obsessions' (see p. 96) and 'compulsions' (see p. 85). Obsessions/compulsions must cause distress or interfere with the person's social or individual functioning (usually by wasting time), and should not be the result of another psychiatric disorder. At some point in the disorder, the person recognises the symptoms to be excessive or unreasonable.

Clinical features Checking (63%), washing (50%), contamination (45%), doubting (42%), bodily fears (36%), counting (36%), insistence on symmetry (31%), aggressive thoughts (28%).

Epidemiology Mean age: 20 yrs, 70% onset before age 25 yrs, 15% after age 35 yrs. Sex distribution equal. Prevalence: 0.5–2% of general population.

Associations Avoidant, dependent, histrionic traits (~40% of cases), anankastic/obsessive-compulsive traits (5–15%) prior to disorder. In schizophrenia, 5–45% of patients may present with symptoms of OCD ('schizo-obsessive's' poorer prognosis). Sydenham chorea (up to 70% of cases) and other basal ganglia disorders (e.g. TS, post-encephalitic parkinsonism).

Comorbidity Depressive disorder (50–70%), alcohol- and drug-related disorders, social phobia, specific phobia, panic disorder, eating disorder, tic disorder (up to 40% in juvenile OCD) or TS.

Differential diagnosis 'Normal' (but recurrent) thoughts, worries, or habits; anankastic PD/OCPD; schizophrenia; phobias; depressive disorder; hypochondriasis; body dysmorphic disorder; trichotillomania.

Management

- **Psychological** *Psychotherapy* Supportive: valuable (including family members, use of 'groups'); psychoanalytical: no unequivocal evidence of effectiveness (insight-orientated psychotherapy may be useful in some patients). *Behavioural therapy* Response prevention useful in ritualistic behaviour; thought stopping may help in ruminations; exposure techniques for obsessions. *Cognitive therapy* so far not proven effective.
- **Pharmacological** *Antidepressants* SSRIs: fluoxetine, fluvoxamine, sertraline, or paroxetine should be considered first-line (no clear superiority of any one agent, high doses usually needed—e.g. 40–60 mg fluoxetine allow at least 4–12 wks for treatment response, regard as 'long-term'). Clomipramine (e.g. 200–300 mg) has specific anti-obsessional action (first-or second-line choice). MAOIs: phenelzine should be considered as third-line if patient resistant to 2 different SSRIs/or clomipramine and SSRI and there are associated panic attacks. *Augmentative strategies*: buspirone—if marked anxiety; antipsychotic (risperidone, haloperidol, pimozide)—if psychotic features, tics, or schizotypal traits; lithium—if marked depression. Other possibilities include enhancing 5HT function with L-tryptophan or fenfluramine (controversialmay—have serious cardiac adverse effects).
- **Physical** *ECT* consider if patient suicidal or severely incapacitated. *Psychosurgery* may be considered for severe, incapacitating, intractable

cases (i.e. 'treatment-resistant':2 antidepressants, 3 combination treatments, ECT, and behavioural therapy), where the patient can given informed consent—e.g. stereotactic cingulotomy (reported up to 65% success). In theory, disrupts the neuronal loop between the orbitofrontal cortex and the basal ganglia.

Course Often sudden onset (e.g. after stressful 'loss' event), symptom intensity may fluctuate (contact-related/phasic) or be chronic.

Outcome 20–30% significantly improve, 40–50% show moderate improvement, but 20–40% have chronic or worsening symptoms. Relapse rates are high for stopping medication.

Prognostic factors
- **Poor prognosis**: Giving in to compulsions, longer duration, early onset, bizarre compulsions, symmetry, comorbid depression, delusional beliefs or overvalued ideas, personality disorder (esp. schizotypal PD).
- **Better prognosis**: Good premorbid social and occupational adjustment, a precipitating event, episodic symptoms.

Aetiology of OCD
- **Neurochemical** Dysregulation of the 5HT system, or 5HT/DA interaction.
- **Immunological** Cell-mediated autoimmune factors may be associated (e.g. against basal ganglia peptides).
- **Imaging** CT and MRI: bilateral reduction in caudate size. PET/SPECT: hypermetabolism in orbitofrontal gyrus and basal ganglia (caudate nuclei) that 'normalises' following successful treatment (either pharmacological or psychological).
- **Genetic** Suggested by family and twin studies (3–7% of first-degree relatives affected, MZ: 50–80% DZ: 25%.), no candidate genes as yet identified.
- **Psychological** Defective arousal system and/or inability to control unpleasant internal states. Obsessions are conditioned (neutral) stimuli, associated with an anxiety-provoking event. Compulsions are learned (and reinforced) as they are a form of anxiety-reducing avoidance.
- **Psychoanalytical** 'Regression' from Oedipal stage to pre-genital anal-erotic stage of development as a defence against aggressive or sexual (unconscious) impulses. Associated defences:isolation, undoing, and reaction formation.

'Exceptional stressors' and 'traumatic events'

ICD-10 definition

'Commonsense' approach: 'a stressful event or situation...of an exception-ally threatening or catastrophic nature, which is likely to cause pervasive distress in almost anyone.' Includes 'traumatic' events (e.g. rape, criminal assault, natural catastrophe) and 'unusually sudden changes' in the social position and/or network of the individual (e.g. domestic fire, multiple bereavement).

DSM-IV definition

Narrower criteria. The traumatic event must have involved actual or threatened death or serious injury, or a threat to the physical integrity of self or others. The person's response to the traumatic event must have involved intense fear, helplessness, or horror (disorganised/agitated behaviour in children).

Type I and Type II trauma

The above definitions describe what has been termed:

'*Type I trauma*'—single, dangerous and overwhelming events com-prising isolated (often rare) traumatic experiences of sudden, surprising, devastating nature, with limited duration.

'*Type II trauma*'—that due to sustained and repeated ordeal stressors (a series of traumatic events or exposure to prolonged trauma) that may be variable, multiple, chronic, repeated, and anticipated, and are usually of intentional human design (e.g. ongoing physical or sexual abuse, combat). This may lead to 'complex PTSD', with somatisation, dissociation, detach-ment from others, restricted range/dysregulation of affect, and emotional lability (poor impulse control, self-destructive behaviour, and pathological patterns of relationships).

ICD-10 acknowledges this type of reaction with the diagnosis **'enduring personality changes after catastrophic experience'**, whereas DSM-IV does not currently include the much debated diagnosis 'DESNOS' (disorders of extreme stress not otherwise specified).

How common are these events?

Using DSM-IV criteria, up to 80% of men and 75% of women[1] may experi-ence at least one traumatic event in their lifetime. Common events include sudden death of a loved one, accidents, fire, flood, natural disasters, or being a witness to severe injury (or murder).

Continued debate

• Controversy surrounds both of the above definitions, as they exclude 'low-magnitude stressors' (e.g. divorce, job loss, failing exams) although ~0.4% of the population may develop 'PTSD-like' symptoms.

- Equally, 'common' events (e.g. RTAs, sexual assault) quite often lead to PTSD-like symptoms.
- Even perpetrators (albeit 'unwilling') of traumatic events (e.g. war-related crimes, torture) may experience PTSD-like symptoms (associated with feelings of shame or guilt).
- Emphasis on 'life-threatening' events/threats to 'physical integrity' may also be too restrictive. The perception of threat to, or loss of, autonomy may actually be more significant than physical assault—seen in studies of victims of sexual/physical assault and political prisoners.
- Whether 'diagnosis' should be made on the basis of symptom clusters, rather that any definition of what constitutes a 'valid' traumatic event becomes 'academic' when a patient presents with clinically significant problems, (although it may generate much heat when issues of 'compensation' are involved).

1 Stein MB, Walker JR, Hazen AL, Forde DR (1997) Full and partial posttraumatic stress disorder: findings from a community survey. *AJP* **154**, 1114–19.

Acute stress reaction

(ICD-10)

Essence A transient disorder (lasting hours or days) that may occur in an individual as an immediate (within 1hr) response to exceptional stress (e.g. natural catastrophe, major accident, serious assault, warfare, rape, multiple bereavement, fire). The stressor usually involves severe threat to the security or physical integrity of the individual or of a loved person(s).

Symptoms/signs Symptoms tend to be mixed/changeable with an initial state of daze, followed by depression, anxiety (as for GAD, see p. 356), anger, or despair. Presence of social withdrawal, narrowed attention, disorientation, aggression, hopelessness, overactivity, or excessive grief defines mild (none), moderate (2 of these symptoms present), or severe (4 present, or dissociative stupor) forms.

Epidemiology Incidence variable across studies, but estimated around 15–20% of individuals following exceptional stress.

Aetiology No specific theories, as it is a transient disorder.

Risk factors Physical exhaustion, presence of other organic factors, elderly.

Differential diagnosis PTSD ('exceptional trauma', delayed or persistent symptoms, re-experiencing of the traumatic event), adjustment disorder (not necessarily 'exceptional' stressor, wider range of symptoms), concussion/mild brain injury, brief psychotic disorder, dissociative disorders (no clear stressor), substance misuse.

Management By definition—no specific treatment needed.

Outcome

- Once the stressor is removed, symptoms resolve (usually) within a few hours.
- If the stress continues, the symptoms tend to diminish after 24–48 hrs and are minimal within about 3 days.

Acute stress disorder

(DSM-IV)
Essence Clear overlap with 'acute stress reaction' (symptoms of dissociation, anxiety, hyperarousal), but greater emphasis on dissociative symptoms, onset within 4wks, lasting 2d to 4wks (after which diagnosis changes to PTSD).

Symptoms/signs As for PTSD (except for duration).

Epidemiology Incidence quoted as 13–14% of RTA survivors, 19% of victims of assault.

Aetiology Similar to PTSD.

- **Psychological** 'Re-experiencing symptoms'. Fear response to harmless situations associated with original trauma, perhaps due to 'emotional' memories, rather than verbally accessible (declarative) memory. Part of the process of remodelling underlying 'schemas' (about self and the world) which requires the holding of trauma experiences in 'active' memory until the process is complete ('working through'). *Dissociation* A cognitive mechanism to protect the individual from being overwhelmed by the experience (i.e. to allow 'thinking without feeling'), which, if persistent, delays the process of integration.
- **Biological** Neurophysiological changes leading to permanent neuronal changes as a result of the effects of chronic stress or persistent re-experiencing of the stressful event. Neurotransmitters implicated include catecholamines, serotonin, GABA, endogenous opioids, and glucocorticoids.

Risk factors Previous history of psychiatric disorder, previous traumatic event(s), premorbid depression, or dissociative symptoms.

Comorbidity Similar to PTSD (i.e. depression, substance misuse).

Differential diagnosis PTSD (time-frame. >1mth duration), adjustment disorder (doesn't meet criteria for 'traumatic' event—see p. 360; wider range of symptoms), concussion/mild brain injury, brief psychotic disorder, dissociative disorders (no clear stressor), substance misuse.

Management

- **Simple practical measures** e.g. support, advice regarding police procedures, insurance claims, dealing with the media, course and prognosis, may be all that is required.
- **Psychological** *Debriefing* May be useful for certain individuals (needing 'supportive' therapy), but reviews suggest there is little positive benefit and may worsen outcome! *CBT* Brief interventions (education, relaxation, graded *in vivo* exposure, and cognitive restructuring) may reduce development of chronic problems/PTSD (not immediate, but ~2wks after the event appears best).
- **Pharmacological** TCAs, SSRIs, and BDZs may be useful for clinically significant symptoms (evidence lacking).

Outcome By definition this is either a self-limiting condition or continues into PTSD.

Adjustment disorders

Adjustment disorders sit uneasily between what are regarded as normal or just 'problematic' difficulties and the major psychiatric diagnoses. They must occur with 1mth (ICD-10) or 3mths (DSM-IV) of a particular psychosocial stressor, and should not persist for longer than 6mths after the stressor (or its consequences) is removed (except in the case of 'prolonged depressive reaction' in ICD-10). Symptoms are 'clinically significant' due to marked distress, or impairment of normal functioning, and may be 'sub-threshold' (due to symptom or duration criteria) manifestations of mood disorders, anxiety disorders, stress-related disorders, somatoform disorders, or conduct disorders.

Sub-classification

ICD-10 Brief depressive reaction (>1mth), prolonged depressive reaction (<6mths but >2yrs), mixed anxiety and depressive reaction, predominant disturbance of other emotions, predominant disturbance of conduct, mixed disturbance of emotion and conduct, and other specified predominant symptoms. Allows inclusion of bereavement/grief reactions.

DSM-IV Depressed mood, anxious mood, mixed anxious and depressed mood, disturbance of conduct, mixed disturbance of emotions and conduct, and unspecified. Specifically excludes bereavement reactions (see p. 366). 'Acute' disorders >6mths; 'chronic' disorders <6mths.

Epidemiology Prevalence in inpatient/outpatient psychiatric populations is conservatively estimated at around 5%. In general hospital settings it may be as high as 20% (physical illness being the primary stressor for up to 70% of these cases). For child and adolescent psychiatric cohorts: ~70%.

Aetiology By definition the problems are caused by an identifiable stressor. Individual predisposition plays a greater role than other conditions, but symptoms would not have arisen without the stressor.

Comorbidity Possibly higher incidence of alcohol-related problems than the general population, but no different from other psychiatric disorders.

Differential diagnosis Diagnostic uncertainty may arise if debate surrounds whether the stressor is sufficiently severe to be labelled 'exceptional' or 'traumatic' (acute stress reaction/disorder or PTSD may be considered). Equally, it may be difficult to determine whether symptoms (e.g. low mood, anxiety, sleep disturbance, anorexia, lack of energy) are attributable to a medical disorder or are primarily psychiatric in nature. Use of alcohol and drugs (illicit and prescribed) may complicate the picture.

Management

* **Psychological** The mainstay of management is essentially supportive psychotherapy to enhance the capacity to cope with a stressor that cannot be reduced or removed, and to establish sufficient support (esp. practical help—e.g. provision of carers/child-care, financial support and benefits, OT assessment, contact with specific support groups.) to maximise adaption. Ventilation/verbalisation of feelings may be useful in preventing maladaptive behaviours (e.g. social isolation, destructive behaviours, suicidal acts) and understanding the 'meaning' of the stressor to the individual may help correct 'cognitive' distortions.
* **Pharmacological** The use of antidepressants or anxiolytics/hypnotics may be appropriate where symptoms are persistent and distressing (e.g. prolonged depression/dysphoria), or where psychological interventions have proved unsuccessful.

Outcome

* 5yr follow-up suggests recovery in ~70% (adolescents:~40%), intervening problems in ~10% (adolescents: ~15%), and development of major psychiatric problems in ~20% (adolescents: ~45%).
* In adults, psychiatric problems are usually depression/anxiety or alcohol-related problems.

Normal and 'abnormal' grief reactions

Controversy surrounds how we ought to regard normal/abnormal grief, and whether they are distinct from depression or other stress-related disorders[1]. It is very common for those suffering bereavement to have depressive symptoms. However, it is less common for people to experience a clear depressive episode that requires treatment[2]. Normal grief is variable in its intensity and duration. Some commentators regard bereavement as just another 'stressor' and argue that, depending on the phenomenology, grief may be regarded as an acute stress reaction/disorder, an adjustment disorder, or even a form of PTSD ('traumatic grief'). Just as the former reactive/endogenous debate surrounding depression has led to recommendations that 'clinical' symptoms should be treated, a bereaved person should not be denied effective treatment on the basis of 'understandibility', nor should arbitrary time-frames (e.g. less than 4 wks [ICD-10], less than 2 mths [DSM-IV]) dictate against clinical need.

Definitions

Bereavement Any loss event, usually referring to the death of someone.

Grief The feelings, thoughts, and behaviour associated with bereavement.

'Normal' grief The typical symptoms experienced after bereavement. These include: disbelief, shock, numbness, and feelings of unreality; anger; feelings of guilt; sadness and tearfulness; preoccupation with the deceased; disturbed sleep and appetite and, occasionally, weight loss; seeing or hearing the voice of the deceased. Usually these symptoms gradually reduce in intensity, with acceptance of the loss and readjustment. A typical 'grief reaction' lasts up to 12 mths (mean 6 mths), but cultural differences exist.

'Abnormal (pathological/morbid/complicated) grief' A grief reaction that is very intense, prolonged, delayed (or absent), or where symptoms outside the normal range are seen: e.g. preoccupation with feelings of worthlessness (or thoughts of death), excessive guilt, marked slowing of thoughts and movements, a prolonged period of not being able to function normally, hallucinatory experiences (other than the image or voice of the deceased)[3].

Risk factors for depression following a bereavement Previous history of depression, intense grief or depressive symptoms early in the grief reaction, few social supports, little experience of death, 'traumatic' or unexpected death.

Management Generally 'normal' grief does not require specific treatment, although BDZs may be used to reduce severe autonomic arousal or treat problematic sleep disturbance in the short-term. Where there are features of 'abnormal' grief, or where there are clinical symptoms of depression/anxiety, treatment with antidepressants ought to be considered, along with supportive counselling (e.g. through organisations such as CRUSE).

Near the end of his life Sigmund Freud was consulted by a woman who had become depressed following the death of her husband. After listening to her, Freud quietly stated, 'Madam, you do not have a neurosis, you have a misfortune'.

Wahl CW (1970) Archives of the Foundations of Thanatology 1, p. 137

'I know of only one functional psychiatric disorder, whose cause is known, whose features are distinctive, and whose course is usually predictable, and this is grief, the reaction to loss. Yet this condition has been so neglected by psychiatrists that until recently it was not even mentioned in the indexes of most of the best-known general textbooks of psychiatry'.

Parkes CM (1986)

1 Stroebe M, van Son M, Stroebe W, et al. (2000) On the classification and diagnosis of pathological grief.Clinical Psychology Review 20, 57–75.

2 The results from studies vary. A study by Zisook et al looked at the rate of depression in late-life widows. The results showed that 16% of them had depression 13 mths after bereavement. (Zisook S, Paulus M, Shuchter SR, Judd LL (1997) The many faces of depression following spousal bereavement. J Affect Disord 45, 85–95.)

3 Parkes CM (1986) Bereavement: studies of grief in adult life (2rd ed.) International Universities Press.

Post-traumatic stress disorder (1)— diagnosis

Essence Severe psychological disturbance following a traumatic event (see p. 360) characterised by involuntary re-experiencing of elements of the event, with symptoms of hyperarousal, avoidance, and emotional numbing.

Symptoms/signs Symptoms arise within 6mths (ICD-10) of the traumatic event (delayed onset in ~10% of cases) or are present for at least 1mth, with clinically significant distress or impairment in social, occupational, or other important areas of functioning (DSM-IV).

Both ICD-10 and DSM-IV include:

- 2 or more 'persistent symptoms of increased psychological sensitivity and arousal' (not present before exposure to the stressor):
  - Difficulty falling or staying asleep
  - Irritability or outbursts of anger
  - Difficulty in concentrating
  - Hypervigilance
  - Exaggerated startle response

Other ICD-10 Criteria:

- Persistent remembering or 'reliving' of the stressor in intrusive 'flashbacks', vivid memories, or recurring dreams; and in experiencing distress when exposed to circumstances resembling or associated with the stressor.
- Actual or preferred avoidance of circumstances resembling or associated with the stressor which was not present before exposure to the stressor.
- Inability to recall, either partially or completely, some important aspects or the period of exposure to the stressor.

Other DSM-IV criteria: (more specific—see opposite)

Epidemiology Risk of developing PTSD after a traumatic event 8–13% for men, 20–30% for women. Lifetime prevalence estimated as 7.8% ($\male : \female = 1:2$)[1]. Cultural differences exist.

Aetiology

- **Psychological/biological** see *Acute Stress Disorder* (p. 363)
- **Neuroimaging** Reduced (right) hippocampal volume (may relate to enhanced reactivity to stimulation and memory deficits). Dysfunction of the amygdala and associated projections (hippocampus, septum, PFC) may lead to enhanced fear response.
- **Genetic** Higher concordance rates seen in MZ than DZ twins.

Risk factors

- **Vulnerability factors** Low education, lower social class, Afro-Carribbean/Hispanic, female gender, low self-esteem/neurotic traits, previous (or family) history of psychiatric problems (esp. mood/anxiety disorders), previous traumatic events (including childhood experiences).

- **Protective factors** High IQ, higher social class, Caucasian, male gender, psychopathic traits, chance to view body of dead relative/friend.

Comorbidity (may be primary or secondary) Depressive/mood disorders, other anxiety disorders, alcohol and drug misuse disorders, somatisation disorders.

Differential diagnosis Acute stress reaction/disorder, enduring personality change after a catastrophic event (duration at least 2 yrs, see p. 363), adjustment disorder (less severe stressor/different symptom pattern), other anxiety disorder, depressive /mood disorder, OCD, schizophrenia (or associated psychosis), substance-induced disorders.

Other DSM-IV criteria

The traumatic event is persistently re-experienced in 1 (or more) of the following ways:
- Recurrent and intrusive distressing recollections of the event, including images, thoughts, or perceptions (or repetitive play in which themes or aspects of the trauma are expressed in children).
- Recurrent distressing dreams of the event (or frightening dreams without recognisable content in children).
- Acting or feeling as if the traumatic event were recurring (or trauma-specific re-enactment in children).
- Intense psychological distress at exposure to internal or external cues that symbolise or resemble an aspect of the traumatic event.
- Physiological reactivity at exposure to internal or external cues that symbolise or resemble an aspect of the traumatic event.

Persistent avoidance of stimuli associated with the trauma and numbing of general responsiveness (not present before the trauma), as indicated by 3 (or more) of:
- Efforts to avoid thoughts, feelings, or conversations associated with the trauma.
- Efforts to avoid activities, places, or people that arouse recollections of the trauma.
- Inability to recall an important aspect of the trauma.
- Markedly diminished interest or participation in significant activities.
- Feeling of detachment or estrangement from others.
- Restricted range of affect.
- Sense of foreshortened future.

1 Kessler RC, Sonnega A, Bromet E, et al (1995) Posttraumatic stress disorder in the National Comorbidity Survey. *Archives of General Psychiatry* **52**, 1048–60.

Post-traumatic stress disorder (2)—management

Psychological

- **CBT** Treatment of choice—should include elements of: education about the nature of PTSD, self-monitoring of symptoms, anxiety management (stress inoculation), exposure to anxiety-producing stimuli in a supportive environment, cognitive restructuring (esp. for complicated trauma), anger management.
- **Eye movement desensitisation and reprocessing (EMDR)** A novel (controversial) treatment using voluntary multi-saccadic eye movements to reduce anxiety associated with disturbing thoughts.
- **Psychodynamic therapy** Aims to understand the meaning of the traumatic event for the individual and to work through and resolve the provoked unconscious conflict.

Pharmacological

- There is limited evidence for the efficacy of any particular medication in PTSD (although comorbid conditions should be addressed with specific interventions).
- Treatments should be directed towards predominant symptoms:
  - **Depressive symptoms**—SSRIs (reasonable evidence for fluoxetine, fluvoxamine, sertraline); TCAs (some evidence for amitriptyline, desipramine, imipramine); MAOIs (e.g. phenelzine) may also reduce anxiety (overarousal) and intrusiveness.
  - **Anxiety symptoms**—consider use of BDZs (clonazepam, alprazolam), buspirone, antidepressants.
  - **Sleep disturbance**—may be improved by use of sedative antidepressants (e.g. trazodone), cyproheptadine, or specific hypnotics.
  - **Intrusive thoughts**—possibilities include carbamazepine, lithium, fluvoxamine.
  - **Hyperarousal**—some evidence for SSRIs, propranolol/clonidine, lithium, valproate.
  - **Hostility/impulsivity**—carbamazepine, valproate.
  - **Psychotic symptoms/severe aggression or agitation**—may warrant use of an antipsychotic.

Outcome

- ~50% will recover within 1st year, ~30% will run a chronic course.
- Outcome depends on initial symptom severity.
- Recovery will be helped by:
  - Good social support
  - Lack of negative responses from others
  - Absence of 'maladaptive' coping mechanisms (e.g. avoidance, denial of problems, 'safety behaviours', not talking about the experience, thought suppression or rumination)
  - No further traumatic life events (including secondary problems such as physical health, acquired disability, disfigurement, disrupted relationships, financial worries, ongoing litigation.)

Depersonalisation (derealisation) syndrome

Essence A rare disorder, characterised by persistent or recurrent episodes of a distressing feeling of unreality or detachment. This may be in relation to the outside world (derealisation) or the person's own body, thoughts, feelings, or behaviour (depersonalisation). It is viewed as a dissociative disorder (DSM-IV) or an anxiety/stress-related disorder (ICD-10)

Clinical features
- Patients may find it difficult to describe their experiences, often reporting feeling 'as if' they are a passive observer of what is going on around them or their own actions. This may be accompanied by an emotional numbness (inability to experience feelings) and the impression of being in a dream- or trance-like state.
- There may also be the experience of alterations in the perception of objects or people, appearing unfamiliar or different in respect to usual colour, shape, distance, or size. Insight tends to be preserved (unlike 'passivity phenomena' in psychoses), the patient recognises the experiences as abnormal, and often finds them unpleasant, distressing, and anxiety-provoking

Epidemiology Up to 50% of 'normal' individuals may experience depersonalisation in their lifetime (usually in the context of psychological distress). In psychiatric populations it is a very common experience (lifetime prevalence ~80%), with persistent symptoms (and associated functional impairment) in ~12%. Clinical populations show ♂:♀ = 1:2. Age of onset usually adolescence or early adulthood (may go undetected in children).

Aetiology Psychoanalytical An ego defence against painful and conflicting memories, impulses, or affects, which usually have their roots in childhood trauma[1]. **Psychological** An adaptive response to overwhelming stress, allowing continued function by protecting against potentially overwhelming anxiety. **Biological** Altered function in systems central to the integrated processing of information in the brain (with functional localisation in the parietotemporal and limbic areas), where serotonergic mechanisms play a key role[2].

Comorbidity Anxiety disorders (particularly phobias, panic disorder, OCD), depressive disorders, personality disorders (anankastic/obsessional, BPD)

Differential diagnosis Depersonalisation may be experienced by persons in the context of sleep or sensory deprivation, being in unfamiliar surroundings, or an acutely stressful/traumatic situation. It may also be a symptom in schizophrenia/psychosis, mood or anxiety disorders, acute intoxication/withdrawal from alcohol, illicit substances (particularly hallucinogens), or medication, and in organic disorders such as hyperventilation, hypoglycaemia, migraine, epilepsy, or other neurological conditions.

Management

- Organic causes should be excluded with appropriate investigations, which may sometimes include brain imaging (CT/MRI) and EEG.
- Comorbid psychiatric conditions should also be identified and treated, although despite successful alleviation of these conditions, depersonalisation may persist.
- Evidence for successful management of depersonalisation syndrome is poor, with perhaps the exception of a role for SSRIs.
- Recurrent episodes, which are associated with particular stressors, may respond to behavioural methods (exposure, flooding, paradoxical intention [to gain control], negative reinforcement).
- Other psychotherapeutic approaches involve acceptance and understanding of symptoms, identification of 'putative' defence functions, identifying underlying psychopathology, and integration of traumatic experiences and memories.

Course

- Onset is usually sudden, with symptoms persisting only for a brief period.
- Occasionally symptoms may persist for hours, days, weeks, months, or even years (rare).
- Resolution tends to be gradual. Recurrent episodes generally occur in the context of recurring (perceived) stressful situations.
- Chronic symptoms run a fluctuating course, and may be treatment-resistant.

---

1 The dangers of attributing present psychopathology to childhood events cannot be overstated—recently illustrated by high-profile cases of alleged 'recovered memories'. Unsubstantiated claims of childhood (or other) abuse should be regarded with extreme caution. The psychodynamic notion of 'repression' is at best intellectually dubious, and the significance of childhood trauma even in empirical studies finds little consistent support. (See Pope HG (1997) *Psychology astray: fallacies in studies of 'repressed memory' and childhood trauma* Upton, Boca Raton, FL.)

2 Even as early as 1935, Mayer Gross thought psychological explanations to be of 'limited value', seeing depersonalisation as 'an unspecific preformed functional response of the brain'. (Mayer-Gross W (1935) On depersonalisation. *British Journal of Medicine and Psychology*, **XV(2)**, 103–26.)

Disorders of behaviour

Anorexia nervosa (1)—overview

Essence Condition, usually in young women, with marked distortion of body image, pathologically low weight, and weight-loss behaviours. Significant mortality: 10–15% (2/3 physical complications, 1/3 suicide).

Epidemiology ♂:♀ = 1:10; mean age of onset: ♀ 16–17yrs (rarely > 30yrs); ♂ ~12yrs. Incidence ~0.5% of adolescent and young women. Community samples suggest equal distribution across the social classes, but clinic samples show excess of upper/middle classes.

Diagnostic criteria

- Low body weight-15% + below expected, BMI 17.5 or less (see opposite for calculation).
- Self-induced weight loss—avoidance of 'fattening' foods, vomiting, purging, excessive exercise, use of appetite suppressants.
- Body image distortion—'dread of fatness': overvalued idea, imposed low weight threshold.
- Endocrine disorders—HPA axis: e.g. amenorrhoea, reduced sexual interest/impotence, raised GH levels, raised cortisol, altered TFTs, abnormal insulin secretion.
- Delayed/arrested puberty—if onset pre-pubertal.

N.B. In 'atypical' cases one or more of these key features may be absent, or all are present but to a lesser degree.

Aetiology

- **Genetic** concordance rates MZ:DZ = 65%:32%, female siblings: 6–10%.
- **Adverse life events** no excess of childhood physical or sexual abuse (compared to psychiatric controls).
- **Psychodynamic models**
  - Family pathology—enmeshment, rigidity, overprotectiveness, lack of conflict resolution, weak generational boundaries.
  - Individual pathology—disturbed body image (due to dietary problems in early life, parents' preoccupation with food, lack of a sense of identity).
  - Analytical model—regression to childhood, fixation on the oral stage, escape from the emotional problems of adolescence.
- **Biological**
  - Hypothalamic dysfunction—? cause or consequence.
  - Neuropsychological deficits—reduced vigilance, attention, visuospatial abilities, and associative memory (correct with weight gain).
  - Brain imaging *CT*: 'pseudoatrophy'/sulcal widening and ventricular enlargement (correct with weight gain). *Functional imaging*: unilateral temporal lobe hypoperfusion perhaps related to visuospatial problems/body image distortion.

Differential diagnosis

- Chronic debilitating physical disease
- Brain tumours
- GI disorders (e.g. Crohn's disease, malabsorption syndromes)
- Loss of appetite (may be secondary to drugs e.g. SSRIs, amphetamines)
- Depression/OCD (features of which may be associated)

BMI (body mass index)[*]

BMI is a ratio between weight and height, which correlates with body fat, and is used to evaluate if a person is at an unhealthy weight (given a certain height). BMI value is more useful for predicting health risks than the weight alone (for adults aged 18 + yrs).

To calculate BMI the following formulae are used:

$$BMI = \frac{Weight\ (in\ kilogram)}{Height\ (in\ meter)^2}$$

or

$$BMI = \frac{Weight\ (in\ pounds) \times 704.5}{Height\ (in\ inches)^2}$$

Range		Interpretation	Risk to health
Women	Men		
<19.1	<20.7	Underweight	The lower the BMI, the greater the risk
19.1–25.8	20.7–26.4	Ideal weight	Normal, very low risk
25.8–27.3	26.4–27.8	Marginally overweight	Some risk
27.3–32.2	27.8–31.1	Overweight	Moderate risk
32.3–44.8	31.1–45.4	Very overweight or obese	High risk
>44.8	>45.4	Morbid obesity	Very high risk

N.B. BMI is less reliable for: children and teenagers (ranges are based on adult heights), competitive athletes and bodybuilders (muscle weight may skew the results), pregnant or nursing women, and people over 65.

[*]The formula for BMI was developed by the Belgian statistician Adolphe Quetelet in the 19th Century and is sometimes referred to as 'Quetelet's formula'.

Anorexia nervosa (2)—physical consequences

Common problems
Mainly due to the effects of starvation or vomiting:
- **Oral** Dental caries.
- **Cardiovascular** Hypotension; prolonged QT; arrhythmias; cardiomyopathy.
- **Gastrointestinal** Prolonged GI transit (delayed gastric emptying, altered antral motility, gastric atrophy, decreased intestinal mobility); constipation. N.B. Prokinetic agents may accelerate gastric emptying and relieve gastric bloating, which can accelerate resumption of normal eating habits.
- **Endocrine and metabolic** Hypokalemia; hyponatremia; hypoglycemia; hypothermia; altered thyroid function; hypercortisolaemia; amenorrhea; delay in puberty; arrested growth; osteoporosis.
- **Renal** Renal calculi.
- **Reproductive** Infertility; low birth-weight infant.
- **Dermatological** Dry scaly skin and brittle hair (hair loss); lanugo (fine downy) body hair.
- **Neurological** Peripheral neuropathy; loss of brain volume: ventricular enlargement, sulcal widening, cerebral atrophy, ('pseudoatrophy'—corrects with weight gain).
- **Hematologic** Anaemia; leucopaenia; thrombocytopaenia.

Cardiac complications
- The most common cause of death (mortality rate ~10%).
- Findings may include
  - Significant bradycardia (30–40bpm)
  - Hypotension (systolic <70 mmHg)
  - ECG changes (sinus bradycardia, ST-segment elevation, T wave flattening, low voltage, and right axis deviation) may not be clinically significant unless there are frequent arrhythmias (QT prolongation may indicate increased risk for arrhythmias and sudden death).
  - ECHO may reveal decreased heart size, decreased left ventricular mass (with associated abnormal systolic function), and mitral valve prolapse (without significant mitral regurgitation). These changes reflect physiological response to malnutrition and will recover on refeeding.

Amenorrhoea
- Included in the diagnostic criteria, due to hypothalamic dysfunction (hypothalamic-pituitary-ovarian axis) with low levels of FSH and LH, despite low levels of oestrogen (reversion to the prepubertal state occurs with LH response to GnRH blunted leading to amenorrhea).
- Consequences include reduced fertility, multiple small follicles in the ovaries, decreased uterine volume, and atrophy.

N.B. Weight loss, excessive exercise, and stress are also important. However, amenorrhea can persist (in 5–44% of cases) even after recovery and return to normal weight.

Osteopenia

Both cortical and trabecular bone are affected, and osteopenia persists despite oestrogen therapy. Contributing to bone loss are low levels of progesterone and decreased IGF-1 levels.

Treatment

- No specific treatment exists; however, 1000–1500 mg/d of dietary calcium and 400 IU of vitamin D is recommended to prevent further bone loss and maximise peak bone mass.
- Exercise and HRT, although of benefit in adult women, may be harmful for adolescents with anorexia nervosa (causing premature closure of bone epiphysis).

Physical signs

- loss of muscle mass
- dry skin
- brittle hair and nails
- callused skin over interphalangeal joints (Russell sign)
- anaemia
- hypercarotinemia (yellow skin and sclera)
- fine, downy, lanugo body hair
- eroded tooth enamel
- peripheral cyanosis
- hypotension
- bradycardia
- hypothermia
- atrophy of the breasts
- swelling of the parotid and submandibular glands
- swollen tender abdomen (intestinal dilatation due to reduced motility and constipation)
- peripheral neuropathy

Anorexia nervosa (3)—assessment

Full psychiatric history

- Establish the context in which the problems have arisen (to inform development of a treatment plan).
- Confirm the diagnosis of an eating disorder.
- Assess risk of self-harm/suicide.

Commonly reported psychiatric symptoms

- Concentration/memory/decision-making problems
- Irritability
- Depression
- Low self-esteem
- Loss of appetite
- Reduced energy
- Insomnia
- Loss of libido
- Social withdrawal
- Obsessiveness regarding food

Full medical history

- Focus on the medical complications of altered nutrition (p. 378).
- Detail weight changes, dietary patterns, and excessive exercise.

Symptoms commonly elicited on systemic enquiry

- General physical health concerns
- Amenorrhoea
- Cold hands and feet
- Weight loss
- Constipation
- Dry skin
- Hair loss
- Headaches
- Fainting or dizziness
- Lethargy

Physical examination

- Determine weight and height (calculate BMI—see p. 377).
- Assess physical signs of starvation and vomiting (p. 379).
- Routine and focused blood tests (see opposite).
- ECG (and ECHO if indicated).

Blood tests

FBC Hb usually normal or elevated (dehydration); if anaemic, investigate further. Leucopaenia and thrombocytopaenia seen.

ESR Usually normal or reduced; if elevated, look for other organic cause of weight loss.

U&Es Raised urea and creatinine (dehydration), hyponatraemia (excessive water intake or SIADH—neurogenic diabetes insipidus, affecting 40%, may be treated with vasopressin, but is reversible following weight gain), hypokalaemic hypochloraemic metabolic alkalosis (from vomiting), metabolic acidosis (laxative abuse). Other abnormalities may include hypocalcaemia, hypophosphataemia, hypomagnesaemia.

Glucose Hypoglycaemia (prolonged starvation and low glycogen stores).

LFTs Minimal elevation.

TFTs Low T3/T4, increased rT3 (euthyroid sick syndrome—an adaptive mechanism; hormonal replacement not necessary; reverts to normal on re-feeding).

Albumin/total protein Usually normal.

Cholesterol May be dramatically elevated (starvation)—secondary to decreased T3 levels, low cholesterol binding globulin, and leakage of intrahepatic cholesterol.

Endocrine Hypercortisolaemia, ↑GH levels, ↓LHRH, ↓LH, ↓FSH, ↓oestrogens, and ↓progestogens.

Anorexia nervosa (4)—management

General principles
- Most patients will be treated as outpatients.
- A combined approach is better:
  - **Pharmacological** Fluoxetine (especially if there are clear obsessional ideas regarding food); previously TCAs or chlorpromazine used for weight gain.
  - **Psychological** Family therapy (more effective in early onset), individual therapy (behavioural therapy = CBT; may improve long-term outcome).
  - **Education** Nutritional education (to challenge overvalued ideas), self-help manuals ('bibliotherapy').
- Hospital admission should only be considered if there are serious medical problems (see below).
  - Compulsory admission may be required: feeding is regarded as 'treatment' (N.B. Ethical issue regarding patient's 'right to die' vs. their 'right to treatment').

Criteria for admission to hospital
Inpatient management may be necessary for patients with significant medical or psychiatric problems:
- Extremely rapid or excessive weight loss that has not responded to outpatient treatment.
- Severe electrolyte imbalance (life-threatening risks due to hypokalaemia or hyponatraemia).
- Serious physiological complications, e.g. temperature $< 36\,^{\circ}$C; fainting due to bradycardia (PR < 45 bpm) and/or marked postural drop in BP.
- Cardiac complications or other acute medical disorders.
- Marked change in mental status due to severe malnutrition.
- Psychosis or significant risk of suicide.
- Failure of outpatient treatment (e.g. inability to break the cycle of disordered eating or engage in effective outpatient psychotherapy).

Admission should not be viewed as punishment by the patient and the goals of inpatient therapy should be fully discussed with the patient (and their family):
- Addressing physical and/or psychiatric complications.
- Development of a healthy meal plan.
- Addressing underlying conflicts (e.g. low self-esteem, planning new coping strategies).
- Enhancing communication skills.

Risks of re-feeding
With re-feeding, cardiac decompensation may occur, especially during the first 2 wks (when the myocardium cannot withstand the stress of an increased metabolic demand). Symptoms include excessive bloating, oedema, and, rarely, congestive cardiac failure (CCF).

To limit these problems:
- Measure U&Es and correct abnormalities before re-feeding.
- Recheck U&Es every 3 days for the first 7 days and then weekly during re-feeding period.
- Attempt to increase daily caloric intake slowly by 200–300 kcal every 3–5 days until sustained weight gain of 1–2 pounds per week is achieved.
- Monitor patient regularly for development of tachycardia or oedema.

Prognosis
- If untreated, this condition carries one of the highest mortality figures for any psychiatric disorder (10–15%).
- If treated, 'rule of thirds' (1/3 full recovery, 1/3 partial recovery, 1/3 chronic problems).
- Poor prognostic factors include:
  - chronic illness
  - late age of onset
  - bulimic features (vomiting/purging)
  - anxiety when eating with others
  - excessive weight loss
  - poor childhood social adjustment
  - poor parental relationships
  - male sex

Bulimia nervosa

Essence Characterised by recurrent episodes of binge eating, with compensatory behaviours and overvalued ideas about 'ideal' body shape and weight. Often there is a past history of anorexia nervosa (30–50%) and body weight may be normal.

Epidemiology Incidence 1–1.5% of women, with mid-adolescent onset, and presentation in early 20s.

Aetiology Similar to anorexia nervosa, but also evidence for associated personal/family history of obesity, and family history of affective disorder and/or substance misuse. Possible 'dysregulation of eating', related to serotonergic mechanisms (?supersensitivity of $5HT_{2C}$ secondary to $\downarrow5HT$).

Diagnostic criteria

- Persistent preoccupation with eating
- Irresistible craving for food
- 'Binges'—episodes of overeating
- Attempts to counter the 'fattening' effects of food (self-induced vomiting, abuse of purgatives, periods of starvation, use of drugs e.g. appetite suppressants, thyroxine, diuretics)
- Morbid dread of fatness, with imposed 'low weight threshold'

N.B. In 'atypical' cases, one or more of these features may be absent.

Physical signs

- May be similar to anorexia nervosa (p. 378); tend to be less severe.
- Specific problems related to 'purging' include:
  - Arrhythmias
  - Cardiac failure (sudden death)
  - Electrolyte disturbances ($\downarrow K^+$, $\downarrow Na^+$, $\downarrow Cl^-$, metabolic acidosis [laxatives] or alkalosis [vomiting])
  - Oesophageal erosions
  - Oesophageal/gastric perforation
  - Gastric/duodenal ulcers
  - Pancreatitis
  - Constipation/steatorrhea
  - Dental erosion
  - Leucopaenia/lymphocytosis.

Investigations As for **Anorexia nervosa** (p. 381).

Differential diagnosis

- Upper GI disorders (with associated vomiting)
- Brain tumours
- Personality disorder
- Depressive disorder
- OCD
- Drug-related increased appetite (see pp. 852–3)
- Other causes of recurrent overeating (e.g. menstrual-related syndromes—p. 434, Kleine-Levin syndrome—p. 404)

Comorbidity
- Anxiety/mood disorder
- 'Multiple dyscontrol behaviours' e.g.:
  - Cutting/burning
  - Overdose
  - Alcohol/drug misuse
  - Promiscuity
  - Other impulse disorders (pp. 386–7)

Treatment
- **General principles**
  - Full assessment (as for **anorexia nervosa**, p. 380).
  - Usually managed as an outpatient.
  - Admission only for suicidality, physical problems, extreme refractory cases, or if pregnant (due to increased risk of spontaneous abortion).
  - Combined approaches improve outcome.
- **Pharmacological**
  - Most evidence for 'high-dose' SSRIs (fluoxetine 60mg)—long-term treatment necessary (>1yr).
- **Psychotherapy**
  - Best evidence for CBT.
  - IPT may be as effective long-term, but acts less quickly.
  - 'Guided self-help' is a useful first step (e.g. bibliotherapy), with education and support often in a group setting.

Prognosis
Generally good, unless there are significant issues of **low self-esteem** or evidence of **severe personality disorder**.

The SCOFF[1] questions
These questions are useful as a *screening* tool for eating disorders (both anorexia and bulimia nervosa) in primary care. They have low sensitivity, and a score of 2+ 'yes' answers indicates that further more detailed history is indicated, before considering treatment or referral.
- Do you make yourself **Sick** because you feel uncomfortably full?
- Do you worry you have lost **Control** over how much you eat?
- Have you recently lost more than **One** stone in a 3-month period?
- Do you believe yourself to be **Fat** when others say you are too thin?
- Would you say that **Food** dominates your life?

---

1 Morgan JF, Reid F, Lacey JH (1999) The SCOFF questionnaire: assessment of a new screening tool for eating disorders. BMJ **319**, 1467–8.

Other impulse-control disorders

Impulse-control disorders are disorders in which a person acts on a certain impulse, that is potentially harmful, but they cannot resist.

Pathological gambling disorder[1]

Persistent and recurrent maladaptive patterns of gambling behaviour. Relatively common and may lead to significant personal, family, and occupational difficulties.

Clinical features

* Preoccupation with gambling (thinking of past gambling experiences, planning the next experience, or thinking of ways to get money to gamble).
* Needing to gamble with larger amounts of money to get the same feeling of excitement.
* Unsuccessful attempts to stop gambling or to cut down.
* Restlessness or irritability when trying to cut down or stop gambling.
* Gambling to escape from problems or to get away from feeling anxious, depressed, or guilty.
* Chasing losses (return after losing to get even).
* Lying to family or friends about gambling.
* Committing illegal acts to finance gambling.
* Losing or jeopardising relationships, jobs, or career opportunities because of gambling.
* Relying on family or friends for money because of financial problems caused by gambling.

Treatment Exclusion and treatment of any comorbid psychiatric disorder (e.g. depression); proposed specific treatments to control addictive behaviour include: SSRIs (fluoxetine, fluvoxamine, paroxetine, citalopram) and naltrexone, CBT may also help reduce the preoccupation with gambling.

Kleptomania[2]

Failure to resist impulses to steal items that are not needed or sought for personal use or monetary value. Usually women, mean age 36, mean duration of illness 16 years (often childhood onset).

Differential diagnosis Shoplifting (actions are usually well-planned and motivated by need or monetary gain); OCD; depression.

Comorbidity Eating disorders and substance abuse disorders; may be precipitated by major stressors (e.g. loss events).

Treatment SSRIs (e.g. fluoxetine); psychotherapy (CBT, family therapy).

Pyromania[3]

The presence of multiple episodes of deliberate and purposeful fire-setting, leading to property damage, legal consequences, and injury or loss of life. It is rare in children; more common in male adolescents, particularly those with poor social skills and learning difficulties.

Clinical features
- Tension or affective arousal before the act.
- Fascination with, interest in, or attraction to fire and its situational contexts.
- Pleasure, gratification, or relief when setting fires, or when witnessing or participating in the aftermath.
- Evidence of advance preparation.
- Indifference to consequences on property or life.
- Not for financial gain, to express socio-political ideology, to conceal criminal activity, as an expression of anger or vengeance, to improve one's living circumstances, due to delusions or hallucinations, or as a result of impaired judgement.

Differential diagnosis Conduct disorder, ADHD, adjustment disorder, other major affective or psychotic disorder.

Comorbidity Substance misuse, past history of sexual or physical abuse, antisocial personality disorder.

Treatment Should address any underlying or comorbid psychiatric disorder. Psychotherapeutic intervention may be helpful (e.g. CBT).

Trichotillomania[4]

Stereotyped recurrent pulling of hair, exacerbated by stress or even relaxation (e.g. reading, watching TV). Feelings of tension are relieved by pulling hair. Usually involves the scalp, but may include eyelashes, eyebrows, axillae, body, or pubic regions. *In children*, $♀ = ♂$, limited course. *In adults*, $♀ > ♂$, chronic or episodic course. Lifetime prevalence: 1–2%.

Associated features Examining hair root, pulling strands between teeth, trichophagia (eating hairs), nail biting, scratching, gnawing, excoriation.

Differential diagnosis OCD, Tourette's syndrome, pervasive developmental disorder (e.g. autism), stereotyped behaviour, factitious disorder.

Comorbidity Depressive disorder, generalised anxiety disorder, OCD, personality disorder.

Treatment Address any comorbid disorder; behavioural modification (substitution, positive/negative reinforcement); evidence for specific use of: SSRIs, clomipramine, pimozide, risperidone, and lithium.

1 Raylu N and Oei TP (2002) Pathological gambling. A comprehensive review. *Clin Psychol Rev* **22**, 1009–61.

2 McElroy SL, Pope HG Jr, Hudson JI, *et al.* (1991) Kleptomania: a report of 20 cases. *AJP* **148**, 652–7.

3 Puri BK, Baxter R, Cordess CC (1995) Characteristics of fire-setters. A study and proposed multiaxial psychiatric classification. *BJP* **166**, 393–6.

4 Walsh KH and McDougle CJ (2001) Trichotillomania. Presentation, etiology, diagnosis and therapy. *Am J Clin Dermatol* **2**, 327–33.

Normal sleep—stages and cycles[1]

Sleep stages

Sleep normally follows a typical pattern of stages and cycles as revealed by electroencephalography (EEG).

Stage 1 (light sleep)

As wakefulness declines, posterior alpha activity disappears, with slow theta (4–7 Hz) and delta (2–3 Hz) activity emerging, plus occasional vertex waves. This stage lasts only a few minutes, but may recur briefly during the night during sleep stage transitions or following body movements.

Stage 2

Typical features include: *K complexes* (symmetrical high-voltage vertex waves) that arise both spontaneously and in response to sudden stimuli; *sleep spindles* (0.5s phases of 12–14Hz fast activity, maximal at the vertex). This lasts 15–30 mins, followed by the gradual appearance of high voltage waves (>75mV) in the delta range in a semi-symmetrical distribution over both hemispheres occupying less than 20% of the EEG recording.

Stage 3 and 4 (delta sleep, slow wave sleep, [SWS])

Greater than 20% (but less than 50%) delta wave activity indicates stage 3 sleep, and greater than 50% defines stage 4 sleep. Sleep spindles can occasionally be seen in stage 3. Together, these stages are called SWS and last 30–45 mins, before reversion to stage 2.

REM sleep

The end of the first sleep cycle is marked by a brief period of arousal before the onset of REM sleep. This has characteristic low-voltage, desynchronised EEG activity with associated muscle atonia and episodic *rapid eye movements (REM)*. Occasional bursts of EMG activity (myoclonia) may be seen in association with the phasic eye movements. There are no sleep spindles or K complexes and alpha activity is rarely seen.

Sleep cycles

A typical night's sleep has 4 or 5 cycles of these sequential stages, each lasting 90–110 mins. As the night progresses, the amount of time spent in delta sleep decreases, with consequent increase in REM sleep. Hence, the 1st REM period may last only 5–10 mins, whereas the last REM period, just before waking, may last up to 40 mins. Although the total amount of sleep needed will vary between individuals and with age, total sleep time in adults is usually between 5 and 9hrs. Remarkably, REM sleep occupies 20–25% of total sleep time in all ages.

1 Rechtschaffen A and Kales A (1968) *A Manual of Standardized Terminology, Techniques and Scoring System for Sleep Stages of Human Subjects.* Washington D.C, U.S Government Printing Office, Public Health Service.

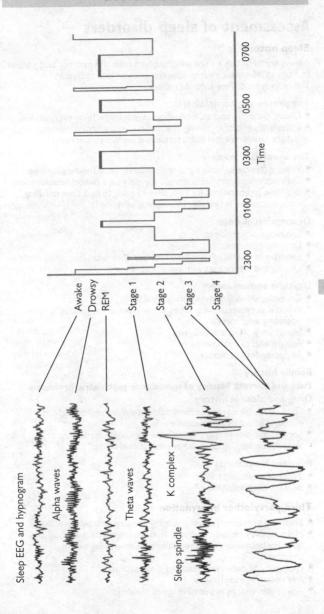

Assessment of sleep disorders

Sleep history

Always try to obtain a third-party account from the patient's bed partner, or from an informant such as a parent or carer (see opposite).
The main areas covered should include:

The presenting complaint(s)
- Onset, duration, course, frequency, severity, effects on everyday life
- Pattern of symptoms, timing, fluctuations, exacerbating/relieving factors, environmental factors, relevant current stressors

The usual daily routine
- Waking (time, methode e.g. alarm, natural), usual morning routine
- Daily activities (start/finish times), any daily naps (when, how long for)
- Bed time (preparations for bed, time of going to bed, time of falling asleep, activities in bed e.g. TV, reading, sex)

Description of sleep
- Behaviour whilst asleep
- Dreams/nightmares
- Episodes of wakening (and how they are dealt with)
- Quality and satisfaction with sleep

Daytime somnolence
- General level of alertness during the day
- When/if sleep occurs (e.g. when active meal times, walking, driving, operating machinery)
- Effects on work/social activities
- Any periods of confusion
- Any episodes of collapse

Family history
Past and current history of medical or psychiatric problems
Drug and alcohol history
- General review of regular medications (alerting/sedating effects), including timing of administration
- Specific questions regarding: caffeine-containing drinks (tea, coffee, soft drinks), smoking, alcohol, other recreational drugs

Previous treatments
- Types of treatment tried
- Benefits/problems/side-effects

Third-party/other information
- Breathing problems (snoring, gasping, choking, stopping breathing)
- Motor activity (muscle twitches, limb movements, other unusual or complex behaviours e.g. sleep-talking/sleep-walking/dream enactment)
- Frequency of occurrence and any clear pattern
- Any recent mood changes
- Any recent change in use of drugs or alcohol

Methods of further assessment

Sleep diary To create a record of the sleep-wake pattern over a two-week period in order to clarify any pattern or particular factors that may be present. Important information includes: daily activities, pattern of sleeping, mealtimes, consumption of alcohol/caffeine/other drugs, exercise, and daytime sleepiness/napping.

Video recording A useful component of assessment, particularly for the parasomnias. Routinely used in sleep laboratory studies; however, home videos of sleep-related behaviour may be just as informative.

Actigraphy A method of both quantifying circadian sleep-wake patterns and identifying movement disorders occurring during sleep. Actigraphs incorporate a piezoelectric motion sensor, often in a wristwatch-like unit, that collects data on movement over several days, for later computer analysis. *Indications* Circadian rhythm sleep disorders, jet lag, paediatric sleep disorders, monitoring leg movements (e.g. in 'restless leg syndrome' or periodic movements of sleep) or other movement disorders (e.g. parkinsonian tremor).

Polysomnography Detailed recording of a variety of physiological measures including EEG, electro-oculogram (EOG), and electromyogram (EMG). Other parameters may be added as required: ECG, respiratory monitoring (nasal/oral airflow, diaphragm EMG), pulse oximetry, actigraphy, penile tumescence, and oesophageal pH (for oesophageal reflux). Audio and video recording help to assess nocturnal behaviours, vocalisations, and snoring. Time coding of all these measures allows temporal correlations to be made of the various parameters. In general, one night of testing, followed by a daytime multiple sleep latency test (MSLT—see below) is sufficient to diagnose most conditions.

Indications Hypersomnia (where common extrinsic causes e.g. medication, shift work, have been excluded; to diagnose suspected periodic limb movements of sleep, sleep apnoea, or narcolepsy), insomnia (where periodic limb movements of sleep or sleep apnoea are suspected and initial treatment has been ineffective), parasomnias (where the clinical history is unclear, initial treatment has been unsuccessful, and polysomnography is likely to aid the diagnosis e.g. REM sleep behaviour disorder or multiple parasomnias), to validate the accuracy of a sleep complaint (where a more objective measure is needed), to assess the benefits of treatment (e.g. continuous positive airway pressure—CPAP), suspected nocturnal epilepsy, serious cases of sleep-related violence.

Multiple sleep latency test (MSLT) Devised to assess daytime somnolence, but also helps in identifying daytime REM sleep, for example in narcolepsy. The patient is put to bed at 2-hour intervals starting at 8 a.m. with the objective of measuring time to sleep onset (*sleep latency*). In adults a mean sleep latency of 5 mins or less indicates a pathological level of daytime somnolence; 5–10 mins is 'indeterminate' but may reflect a primary psychiatric disorder; over 10 mins is regarded as normal. The ICSD-R suggests specific MSLT criteria for a diagnosis of narcolepsy (see p. 402).

Insomnia (1)—overview

Essence Persistent problems (at least 3 days/wk for 1 mth) falling asleep, maintaining sleep, or poor quality of sleep. Individuals are preoccupied and excessively concerned with their sleep problems, distressed by them, and social or occupational functioning is affected.

Prevalence A common complaint (~30% general population), F > M, greater in the elderly. 'Clinically significant insomnia' (causing marked personal distress or interference with social and occupational functioning) ~6%.

Differential diagnosis

Intrinsic causes Psychophysiological insomnia (difficulty initiating and maintaining sleep, with associated somatised tension anxiety: learned sleep prevention), sleep state misperception (no objective evidence of sleep disturbance), idiopathic insomnia (lifelong inability to obtain adequate sleep—rare), sleep apnoea syndromes, periodic limb movement disorder, restless legs syndrome.

Extrinsic causes Inadequate sleep hygiene, environmental sleep disorder, adjustment sleep disorder, limit-setting sleep disorder, sleep-onset association disorder, nocturnal eating (drinking) disorder, food allergy insomnia, altitude insomnia, dependency-related sleep disorder (hypnotics, alcohol, stimulants).

Circadian rhythm disorders Delayed/advanced sleep-phase syndromes (p. 408).

Medical disorders Pain (arthritis, peptic ulcer, headache), respiratory disorders (COPD, cystic fibrosis, asthma), diabetes, Parkinson's disease, endocrine disorders (Addison's disease, Cushing's syndrome).

Psychiatric disorders Depression, bipolar affective disorder, anxiety disorder, panic disorder, PTSD, anorexia nervosa, schizophrenia.

Drugs and alcohol (see opposite page.)

Management (see p. 398–9)
- Identify and address any underlying problems (drug dependency, medication issues, primary medical or psychiatric conditions)
- Education
- Sleep hygiene measures
- Relaxation training
- Sleep restriction
- Use of hypnotics (if unresponsive to other measures.)

Common drug-related causes of insomnia

- Antidepressants (e.g. MAOIs, SSRIs, venlafaxine, reboxetine)
- Antiparkinsonian medication
- Bronchodilators (e.g. aminophylline, theophylline, pseudoephedrine)
- Cardiovascular medication (e.g. beta-blockers, clonidine, high-dose digoxin, verapamil)
- Chemotherapy agents
- Corticosteroids/anabolic steroids
- NSAIDs (high-dose)
- Stimulants (e.g. dexamphetamine, methylphenidate, amphetamine, cocaine, caffeine, nicotine)
- Thyroxine
- Withdrawal (e.g. hypnotics, opiates, alcohol, or cannabis)

Insomnia (2)—intrinsic causes

Sleep apnoea syndromes

- *Obstructive sleep apnoea syndrome (Pickwickian syndrome)* Repetitive episodes of upper airway obstruction during sleep, usually associated with reduced blood oxygen saturation, daytime somnolence, loud snoring, and dry mouth. Usually middle-aged, overweight males. Prevalence 1–2%.

- *Central sleep apnoea syndrome* Cessation or decrease of ventilatory effort during sleep, more common in the elderly, but also seen in degenerative neurological disorders. Snoring is intermittent and not as loud as in obstructive sleep apnoea. Considered pathological when the events are sufficient to disturb sleep, result in hypoxia, or cause cardiac changes.

- *'Ondine's curse'* The total inability to breath while asleep, extremely rare, usually due to central alveolar hypoventilation syndrome.

Investigation Polysomnography (diagnosis, assessment of severity, and measurement of the impact on sleep architecture and oxygen saturation).

Management *General* weight loss, avoidance of sedative drugs, reduction of alcohol consumption. *Specific* Oral appliances (for mild cases)—e.g. the 'sleep and nocturnal obstructive apnoea redactor' [SNOAR]), 'continuous positive airway pressure' (CPAP), or 'bi-level positive airways pressure' (Bi-PAP). *Surgical* (for severe cases): nasal reconstruction, tonsillectomy, uvulopalatopharyngoplasty, bimalleolar advancement, and rarely tracheostomy.

Periodic limb movement (in sleep) disorder (PLMS)

Periodic episodes of repetitive, stereotyped limb movements. Rare in children, common in over 60s (~34%). May be a feature in up to 15% of patients with insomnia. Movements usually reported by bed partner. Associated daytime somnolence. Polysomnography may aid diagnosis.

Differential diagnosis Sleep starts (p. 416), drug-related exacerbation (e.g. TCAs, lithium).

Management Reassurance, removal of exacerbating factors, clonazepam.

Restless legs syndrome (Ekbom's syndrome)

Unpleasant, often painful sensations in the legs, particularly on sleep onset, which significantly interfere with the ability to get to sleep. Usually idiopathic or familial. Exacerbated by caffeine, fatigue, or stress.

Prevalence ~10% general population, ♂ = ♀, greater in the elderly.

Associations PLMS, pregnancy, uraemia, rheumatoid arthritis, iron deficiency anaemia, folate deficiency, hypothyroidism, poliomyelitis, peripheral neuropathy (e.g. diabetes), chronic myelopathy, Parkinson's disease, drug-related (e.g. antidepressants; phenothiazines; lithium; calcium channel blockers; withdrawal from barbiturates, other sedatives and opiates).

Differential diagnosis Antipsychotic-induced akathisia, ADHD.

Investigations Full history, examination, routine blood tests (polysomnography rarely needed).

Management *General* Movement (walking, stamping) or stimulation of the legs (rubbing, squeezing, hot showers, hot packs, ointments). *Medication* Clonazepam (alone or in combination with sinemet, bromocriptine, or opiates).

Insomnia (3)—extrinsic causes

Inadequate sleep hygiene Clinically significant disruption of the normal sleep-wake schedule due to a wide range of daily living activities (e.g. level of coffee consumption, frequent late nights) is inconsistent with the maintenance of good quality sleep and full daytime alertness.

Management Understand the contribution of each factor and take steps to eliminate or minimise their effects.

Environmental sleep disorder Common transient sleep disturbance due to disturbing environmental factor(s), (e.g. heat, cold, noise, light, excessive movement of bed partner, danger, allergens, hospitalisation, unfamiliar surroundings.) leading to insomnia or excessive sleepiness.

Altitude insomnia Unusual form of acute insomnia, accompanied by headaches, loss of appetite, and fatigue, occuring at high altitudes in the absence of administered oxygen. Seen in 25% of individuals who ascend above 2000m above sea level and in most individuals above 4000m.

Adjustment sleep disorder Sleep disturbance temporally related to stress, conflict, or environmental change, causing emotional arousal.

Limit-setting sleep disorder Primarily a child disorder, estimated prevalence 5–10% in children, characterised by inadequate enforcement of bedtimes by a caregiver, with resultant stalling or refusal to go to bed at an appropriate time.

Sleep-onset association disorder Occuring mainly in children aged 6 months to 3 years, sleep onset is impaired by the absence of a certain object (e.g. favourite toy) or set of circumstances.

Food allergy insomnia A rare disorder of initiating and maintaining sleep due to an allergic response to food allergens.

Nocturnal eating (drinking) syndrome Primarily a childhood problem (prevalence 5% in children aged 6 months to 3 years), with marked decrease after weaning. Characterised by recurrent awakenings and inability to return to sleep without eating or drinking.

Insomnia (4)—general management strategies

Education about sleep
There are many myths surrounding sleep and the clinician should be able to educate the patient about the stages of sleep, sleep cycles, changes in sleep patterns with age, and the nature of the particular sleep problem or disorder the patient presents with.

Sleep hygiene
Establishing good sleep habits
Control of environmental factors (noise, light, temperature); 'wind down' time (~1hr) before going to bed with the use of distractions from the days' stresses (reading, watching television, listening to music, having a warm bath); avoidance of caffeine-containing drinks after about 4pm; not smoking at least for an hour before bed; regular exercise (not late at night); a late 'tryptophan' snack (warm milk or other milky drink); avoidance of naps during the day (or confining naps to the early afternoon, not longer than ~40mins); learning to set aside a time during the day to reflect on problems and stresses.

Stimulus control
Go to bed only when sleepy; avoid other activities (with the exception of sex) whilst in bed; if sleep does not occur, do not remain in bed for more than 10–20 mins, get up and go to another room (without turning on all the lights), returning to bed only when sleepy; establish a regular time to get up, with no more than 1 hour's variation (even at weekends and during holidays).

Relaxation training
The regular practice of relaxation techniques during the day (particularly progressive relaxation) may help to provide patients with the means to reduce general arousal, which can be used if necessary whilst in bed.

Sleep restriction
When sleep is fragmented, a sleep restriction strategy may help to reduce the total time spent in bed and improve the quality of sleep by 'consolidation'. There are a number of steps to sleep restriction, and to complete the programme does require motivation and encouragement (see opposite.)

Medication
Despite the prevailing public perception that insomnia is best treated by the use of a 'sleeping tablet', prescribing should be the last option, rather than the first. Before an hypnotic is prescribed the cause of insomnia should be established, possible underlying factors adequately addressed, and any primary medical or psychiatric disorder effectively treated. They should only be used to treat insomnia when it is severe, disabling, or subjecting the individual to extreme distress. Ideally hypnotics should be used as short-term adjuncts to other forms of therapy and prolonged administration should be avoided. Interrupted courses (i.e. 5 nights with

medication, 2 without) for no more than 4 weeks may help avoid tolerance and reduce the 'rebound insomnia' that often accompanies cessation. Choices include: benzodiazepines (see below), zopiclone/zolpidem, chloral hydrate, and sedating antidepressants (e.g. trazodone).

Sleep restriction
- Keep a sleep diary for 5–14 days to allow the calculation of total sleep time (TST) and sleep efficiency (SE).
- TST = (total time spent in bed)-(hrs spent awake during the night).
- $SE = \dfrac{TST \times 100}{\text{total time spent in bed}}$
- For the first few nights of a sleep restriction programme only spend the same number of hours in bed as the average TST for the past week. No naps during the day are allowed (despite initial tiredness).
- Continue to keep a sleep diary and when the calculated mean SE for 5 nights reaches 85% or better, go to bed 15 mins earlier.
- Repeat the procedure with increases of 15 mins if the mean SE remains 85% or better, or decreases of 15 mins if the mean SE falls below 85%, until a satisfactory amount of night-time sleep is acheived.

Benzodiazepines

Length of action	Examples	Comments
Ultra short	Midazolam Triazolam	Facilitate the onset of sleep and do not cause daytime sedation. Not suitable if a more potent effect is required as higher doses increase the risk of rebound insomnia in the second half of the night.
Intermediate	Temazepam	Effective in initiating, maintaining, and consolidating fragmented sleep.
Long	Diazepam Nitrazepam Flurazepam Flunitrazepam	Lead to 'hang-over' effects the following day, but do help to consolidate fragmented sleep.

N.B. Benzodiazepines may worsen sleep apnoea and should not be given to patients unless the respiratory syndrome is controlled by other means (e.g. CPAP).

Hypersomnia (1)—overview

Essence The term 'hypersomnia' covers a number of different forms of excessive daytime sleepiness. Individuals may complain of 'sleep attacks'—recurrent daytime sleep episodes that may be refreshing or unrefreshing, 'sleep drunkenness' (prolonged transition to a fully aroused state on waking), lengthening of night-time sleep, almost constant excessive daytime sleepiness, or even recurrent periods of more or less permanent sleep lasting several days over several months. Diagnosis and treatment are particularly relevant when the individual works in an industry or profession where vigilance and concentration are essential (e.g. hospital workers, pilots, train drivers, the military) N.B. Excessive sleepiness is a leading cause of road traffic accidents.

Prevalence Common—up to 15% in the general population.

Differential diagnosis

Intrinsic causes Narcolepsy (p. 402), recurrent hypersomnia (Kleine-Levin syndrome, menstrual-related hypersomnia—p. 404), idiopathic hypersomnia, post-traumatic hypersomnia, sleep apnoea syndromes (p. 394), PLMS (p. 394).

Extrinsic causes Insufficient sleep syndrome, dependency-related sleep disorders (alcohol, hypnotics, opiates), toxins (arsenic, bismuth, mercury, copper, other heavy metals, carbon monoxide, vitamin A).

Circadian rhythm disorders (p. 408) Time zone change (jet lag) syndrome, shift work sleep disorder, delayed/advanced sleep-phase syndromes, non-24-hour sleep-wake syndrome.

Medical disorders Neurological, infectious, metabolic, and endocrine disorders.

Psychiatric disorders Mood disorders.

Medication-related Anticonvulsants, antidepressants, antiemetics, antihistamines, antiparkinsonian drugs, antipsychotics, anxiolytics/hypnotics, other (clonidine, methyldopa, prazosin, reserpine, scopolamine, progestogens).

Hypersomnia (2)—narcolepsy*

The most common neurological cause of hypersomnia, estimated prevalence 0.047%[1]. Sex ratio is equal. Age range: 10–50+yrs (70–80% before 25 yrs).

Aetiology May be due to hypocretin deficiency.

Clinical features The classical 'tetrad' of symptoms[2]—**excessive sleepiness, cataplexy, sleep paralysis**, and **hypnagogic hallucinations**—are suffered by only a minority of patients with narcolepsy. Excessive daytime sleepiness and associated cataplexy (sudden bilateral loss of muscle tone triggered by a strong emotional reaction such as laughter or anger) are by far the most common complaints. Other REM sleep phenomena also occur, but are not necessary for the diagnosis to be made. These include sleep paralysis and hallucinations on falling asleep (hypnagogic) or, less commonly, waking up (hypnopompic). Sleep may also be disturbed due to frequent awakenings, sleep talking, and REM-related sleep behaviours.

Course Usually chronic, although some of the symptoms may improve or remit. Hallucinations and sleep paralysis present variably, and sometimes cataplexy may disappear over time. Poor sleep quality tends to persist. Treatments are directed at the most troublesome symptoms.

Differential diagnosis
- Sleep attacks in narcolepsy are usually irresistible and refreshing, whereas in other forms of hypersomnia they tend to be more frequent, of longer duration, easier to resist, and unrefreshing.
- The attacks also tend to occur in unusual and often dangerous situations in narcolepsy, (e.g. talking, eating, standing, walking, or driving).
- Disturbances and shortening of nocturnal sleep are more common in narcolepsy, compared to other causes of hypersomnia where nocturnal sleep is usually prolonged and there is difficulty in waking in the morning.

Investigation
- **HLA (human leucocyte antigen) typing**—there is a strong association between HLA-DR2 haplotypes coded on chromosome 6 and narcolepsy: HLA DQB1*0602 and DQA1*0102 are found in up to 85–95% of individuals, compared with 12–38% in the general population.
- **Polysomnography**—sleep EEG and multiple sleep latency test (MSLT). *ICSD-R criteria*: sleep latency of 10 mins or less, REM sleep latency of 20 mins or less, MSLT demonstrating a mean sleep latency of 5 mins or less, and two or more sleep-onset REM periods.

Management
- **Daytime somnolence**—regular naps, stimulants (methylphenidate, methamphetamine, mazinol, pemoline, modafinil).
- **Cataplexy**—TCAs or SSRIs (and possibly 'newer' antidepressants and venlafaxine, nefazodone, and mirtazepine). These drugs may also improve REM-related symptoms, hypnagogic/hypnopompic hallucinations, and sleep paralysis. N.B. Abrupt withdrawal of antidepressants may potentially cause cataplectic episodes or even 'status cataplecticus'.

- Other treatments for poor sleep and REM-related symptoms include benzodiazepines (e.g. clonazepam) and possibly gamma-hydroxybutyrate (GHB).

* First described by Gélineau (1880) De la narcolepsie. *Gaz Hôp (Paris)* **53**, 626.

1 Ohayon MM, Priest RG, Zulley J, et al. (2002) Prevalence of narcolepsy symptomatology and diagnosis in the European general population. *Neurology* **58**, 1826–33.

2 Yoss RE and Daly DD (1957) Criteria for the diagnosis of the narcoleptic syndrome. *Mayo Clin Proc.* **32**, 320–8.

Hypersomnia (3)—recurrent hypersomnia

Kleine-Levin syndrome[*]

A rare syndrome of 'periodic somnolence and morbid hunger', occurring almost exclusively in male adolescents, usually following a course of decreasing frequency of attacks, which may persist for many years before complete cessation.

Clinical features Periods lasting from days to weeks of attacks of hypersomnia accompanied by excessive food intake (megaphagia). Other behavioural symptoms may occur including sexual disinhibition (which may appear compulsive in nature), along with a variety of other psychiatric symptoms such as confusion, irritability, restlessness, euphoria, hallucinations, delusions, and schizophreniform states. Attacks may occur every 1 to 6 months and last from 1 day to a few weeks. Between attacks the patients recover completely, and the syndrome may easily be confused for other neurological, metabolic, or psychiatric disease.

Management
- Hypersomnia—stimulants (only effective for short periods of time).
- Preventative measures—for sufficiently frequent episodes causing major disruption of social or occupational functioning—lithium, carbamazepine, or valproate.

Menstrual-related hypersomnia

Characterised by excessive daytime sleepiness preceding menstruation, with detectable alterations in polysomnography when symptomatic.

Aetiology Unknown; no clear hormonal differences have been found.

Management Stimulants—reserved only for symptomatic periods.

[*] Originally described by Willi Kleine in 1925 and subsequently by Max Levin in 1936, the eponym 'Kleine-Levin syndrome' was coined by Critchley and Hoffman in 1942.

Hypersomnia (4)—other intrinsic/ extrinsic causes

Idiopathic hypersomnia[1]

Clinical features
* *Polysymptomatic form* Nocturnal sleep is prolonged (10 hrs or more), with sleep drunkenness on waking, and constant or recurrent excessive daytime sleepiness associated with frequent, unrefreshing naps.
* *Monosymptomatic form* Excessive daytime sleepiness alone.

Course A chronic condition with marked impact on social and occupational functioning.

Diagnosis Detailed history (to exclude other causes of hypersomnia), polysomnography.

Differential diagnosis Sleep apnoea syndromes, periodic limb movement disorder, or upper airways resistance syndrome.

Management As for narcolepsy (avoid naps as they are unrefreshing).

Post-traumatic hypersomnia

Excessive sleepiness occuring after traumatic injury of the CNS. Prevalence unknown.

Aetiology Lesions generally involve the brain stem (the tegmentum of the pons or thalamic projections) or the posterior hypothalamus.
N.B. It is more usual following head injury or concussion that patients complain of insomnia rather than hypersomnia.

Insufficient sleep syndrome

Persistently failing to obtain sufficient nocturnal sleep required to support normally alert wakefulness.

Prevalence Unknown, but thought to be common in the general population, particularly amongst parents of young children, doctors, students, long-distance lorry drivers, and other occupations where 'unsociable' long hours of work are commonplace.

Clinical features Periods of excessive sleepiness concentrated in the afternoon and early evening. Rest days usually characterised by late rising from bed and frequent naps. Associated reduced productivity, difficulty in concentration and attention, low mood or irritability, and somatic symptoms (usually gastrointestinal or musculoskeletal).

Diagnosis Made on history alone.

Management Directed towards scheduling increased time asleep, either at night or with regular short naps during the day.

1 Roth B (1976) Narcolepsy and hypersomnia: review and classification of 642 personally observed cases. *Schweiz Arch Neurol Neurochir Psychiatr.* **119**, 31–41.

Circadian rhythm sleep disorders (1)—overview

When an individual's sleep-wake schedule is not in synchrony with the sleep-wake schedule of their cultural environment or society, this may lead to complaints of insomnia or excessive daytime sleepiness, causing marked distress or interference with social or occupational functioning.

Extrinsic causes

Time zone change (jet lag) syndrome Symptoms include varying degrees of difficulty in initiating or maintaining sleep, daytime fatigue, decrements in subjective daytime alertness and performance, feelings of apathy, malaise or depression, and somatic symptoms (gastrointestinal upset, muscle aches, or headaches).

Shift work sleep disorder Symptoms of insomnia or excessive sleepiness occur as transient phenomena in most people working shifts. Adaptation to a change in shift-work schedule usually takes 1–2 weeks; however, rotating day/night shifts may present particular difficulties. Often sufferers consult with somatic complaints (general malaise, gastrointestinal upset) rather than the underlying disorder of sleep.

Intrinsic causes

Irregular sleep-wake pattern Sleep occurrence and waking behaviour are very variable, leading to considerable disturbance of the normal sleep-wake cycle and complaints of insomnia (inadequate nocturnal sleep and daytime somnolence/frequent napping). The idiopathic form is rare, and it is associated with Alzheimer's disease, head injury, developmental disorders, and hypothalamic tumours.

Delayed sleep phase syndrome (DSPS) The late appearance of sleep (typically around 2am), but normal total sleep time and architecture, which may lead to complaints of sleep-onset insomnia and difficulty awakening at the desired time in the morning. Cause is unknown, although some cases are related to head injury. Usually presents in adolescence, running a continuing course until old age. Individuals may adapt to the condition by taking evening or night jobs.

Advanced sleep phase syndrome (ASPS) The opposite of DSPS, this syndrome leads to complaints of evening sleepiness, early sleep onset (e.g. 6–8 pm), and early morning wakening. May be confused with depression (due to early morning wakening), particularly in elderly patients in whom the syndrome occurs more frequently.

Non-24-hour sleep-wake disorder Rare occurrence of a greater than 24-hour sleep-wake period, leading to a chronic pattern of 1–2 hour daily delays in sleep onset and wake times, with an 'in-phase' period every few weeks (free of symptoms). Associated with schizoid personality traits and may occur more frequently in blind individuals.

Investigations
- Comprehensive history
- Use of a 14-day sleep-wake chart
- Actigraphy—objective measurement of the rest-activity cycle
- Polysomnography is rarely needed

Differential diagnosis
- Poor sleep hygiene
- Depressive disorder
- Misuse of drugs (particularly stimulants or sedatives) and alcohol
- Physical conditions such as: dementia, head injury, other causes of brain damage or injury, and recovery from coma.

Circadian rhythm sleep disorders (2)—management

General measures

These include education about the nature of sleep and establishing good sleep habits. This is particularly important for shift work sleep disorder in which alcohol, nicotine, and caffeine may be used to self-medicate symptoms. Other advice for shift-workers should emphasize: maintenance of regular sleep and mealtimes whenever possible, use of naps to limit sleep loss, and minimisation of environmental factors (noise, light, other interruptions) when sleeping during the day.

Chronotherapy

DSPS

- Establishing a regular waking time, with only 1 hour's variability at weekends and holidays, may help initially.
- If unsuccessful, '**phase-delay**'[1] methods may be employed to achieve a phase shift of the sleep-wake cycle. This involves:
  - Establishing a 27-hour day to allow progressive delay of the usual onset of sleep by about 3 hours in each sleep cycle.
  - Sleep should only be permitted for 7–8 hours, with no napping.
  - The disruption to the person's normal routine caused by undergoing this regime (which may take 5–7 days to complete) requires appropriate measures to be taken to ensure other family and work commitments are attended to.
- An alternative strategy is to advise the individual to remain awake at the weekend for one full night, and to go to bed the next evening 90 minutes earlier than usual.
  - Sleep periods should again be limited to 7–8 hours, with no napping.
  - The procedure can then be repeated each weekend until a normal bedtime is achieved.

ASPS

- Slowly delaying sleep onset by gradual increments of 15 minutes may be effective.
- Alternatively '**phase-advance**'[2] methods may be used:
  - The patient goes to bed 3 hours earlier each night until the sleep cycle is advanced back to a normal bedtime.
  - This may be difficult to implement, particularly with elderly patients.

Light therapy[3] This includes both the use of bright light (2500–10000 lux) with ultraviolet rays filtered out, and light restriction. Bright light is assumed to suppress melatonin (which is sleep-promoting).

DSPS Exposure to bright light is scheduled on waking to prevent morning lethargy, usually for 2 hours daily for 1 week, often with adjunctive light restriction after 4pm.

ASPS Exposure to bright light is recommended 2 hours before scheduled bedtime, to delay this to a more sociable time. N.B. Evidence for the effectiveness of light therapy in other intrinsic circadian rhythm disorders of sleep (e.g. shift work sleep disorders, jetlag) is lacking.

Medication

- The entrainment of circadian rhythms through the use of appropriately timed **short-acting benzodiazepines**[4] (e.g. triazolam) has been advocated, particularly for the treatment of jet lag.
- **Melatonin**[5] (0.5–5mg) also appears capable of advancing the sleep phase and resetting the circadian rhythm in Travellers with jet lag syndrome flying across five or more time zones, particularly in an easterly direction, and especially if they have experienced jet lag on previous journeys.

1 Czeisler CA, Richardson GS, Coleman RM, et al. (1981) Chronotherapy: resetting the circadian clocks of patients with delayed sleep phase insomnia. *Sleep* **4**, 1–21.

2 Moldofsky H, Musisi S, Phillipson EA (1986) Treatment of a case of advanced sleep phase syndrome by phase advance chronotherapy. *Sleep* **9**, 61–5.

3 Terman M, Lewy AJ, Dijk DJ, et al. (1995) Light treatment for sleep disorders: consensus report. IV. Sleep phase and duration disturbances. *J Biol Rhythms* **10**, 135–47.

4 Buxton OM, Copinschi G, Van Onderbergen A, et al. (2000) A benzodiazepine hypnotic facilitates adaptation of circadian rhythms and sleep-wake homeostasis to an eight hour delay shift simulating westward jet lag. *Sleep* **23**, 915–27.

5 Herxheimer A and Petrie KJ (2002) Melatonin for the prevention and treatment of jet lag. *Cochrane Database Syst. Rev.* CD001520.

Parasomnias (1)—overview

Parasomnias include unusual behaviours and motor acts with or without autonomic changes that accompany sleep. Sometimes the events occur when arousal is incomplete, or they are associated with REM sleep. Other episodes may arise during the transition form sleep to wakefulness, from wakefulness to sleep, or in transitions between sleep stages.

Points to note

- The often 'bizarre' nature of the parasomnias frequently leads them to being misdiagnosed as psychiatric disorders, particularly if they appear temporally related to stressful situations.
- This may in turn lead to inappropriate treatment, with associated problems, including exacerbation of the parasomnia.
- Often there will be associated psychological distress or psychiatric problems secondary to the parasomnia.
- Rarely there may also be forensic implications, where there is a history of sleep-related violence.

The International Classification of Sleep Disorders (Revised)[1]

The ICSD-R subdivides parasomnias according to the sleep stages they occupy:

Arousal disorders (disorders of non-REM sleep)

Confusional arousals, sleep walking, sleep terrors.

Sleep-wake transition disorders

Rhythmic movement disorder, sleep starts, sleep talking, nocturnal leg cramps.

Parasomnias usually associated with REM sleep

Nightmares, sleep paralysis, impaired sleep-related penile erections, sleep-related painful erections, REM sleep-related sinus arrest, REM sleep behaviour disorder.

Other parasomnias

Sleep bruxism, sleep enuresis, sleep-related abnormal swallowing syndrome, nocturnal paroxysmal dystonia, sudden unexplained nocturnal death syndrome, primary snoring, infant sleep apnoea, congenital central hypoventilation syndrome, sudden infant death syndrome, benign neonatal sleep myoclonus, other parasomnia not otherwise stated.

Parasomnia overlap disorder[2]

Sometimes disorders of non-REM sleep (e.g. sleep walking and sleep terrors) may occur along with REM sleep behaviour disorder. 70% of cases are in young men (mean age 34 yrs). Idiopathic cases, occurring at a younger

1 American Sleep Disorders Association (1997).

2 Schenck CH, Boyd JL, Mahowald MW (1997) A parasomnia overlap disorder involving sleepwalking, sleep terrors, and REM sleep behavior disorder in 33 polysomnographically confirmed cases. *Sleep* **20**, 972–81.

age are associated with other medical (brain injury, nocturnal paroxysmal atrial fibrillation), psychiatric (PTSD, depression, schizophrenia), or substance abuse (alcohol, amphetamine) disorders. There is no increased risk of psychiatric disorder.

Management Clonazepam (0.5–2 mg nocte).

Parasomnias (2)—arousal disorders (of non-REM sleep)

Confusional arousals ('sleep drunkenness')

Clinical features Confusion during and following arousals from sleep, most typically from deep sleep in the first part of the night. Individuals appear disorientated, incoherent, hesitant and slow, but may walk about, get dressed, and even perform complex motor behaviours. Violence, assault, and even homicide may occur (rare)—planning or premeditation is not possible.

Polysomnography Arousal out of SWS, usually in the 1st third of the night.

Prevalence Almost universal in young children (before aged 5 yrs), become less common in older childhood. Fairly rare in adulthood, usually occurring in the context of sleep deprivation, exacerbated by alcohol or other depressant drugs.

Associated disorders Sleep apnoea syndromes, narcolepsy, idiopathic hypersomnia, encephalopathy.

Differential diagnosis Acute confusional states, sleep terrors (evident autonomic arousal), somnambulism (usually docile, not aggressive when challenged), and REM sleep behaviour disorder (evident dream enactment.)

Management
- Prevent the patient from falling into deep, prolonged SWS: avoidance of sleep deprivation
- The restricted use of alcohol and other sedative drugs (illicit and prescribed)
- Sleep hygiene measures (p. 398)

Sleepwalking (somnambulism)

Clinical features Complex, automatic behaviours (automatisms) (e.g. aimless wandering, attempting to dress or undress, carrying objects, eating, urinating in unusual places, and, rarely, driving a car). Episodes of variable duration usually occur 15–120 mins following sleep onset, but may occur at other times. Eyes usually wide open, glassy, and talk is incoherent with communication usually impossible. Injury may occur (e.g. falling down the stairs, exiting through a window). Activity never appears intentional or planned, and only rarely aggressive behaviour occurs. The person is usually easily returned to bed, falls back into normal sleep, and has no recollection of the episode the following morning. If awakened during the episode—confused and disorientated. Dream content (if present) is fragmented, without specific themes.

Polysomnography Light, non-REM sleep, with episodes sometimes preceded by hypersynchrony of generalised (non-epileptic) high-voltage delta waves.

Prevalence Up to 17% in childhood (peak age 4–8 yrs); 4–10% in adults. Familial forms do occur. Precipitants similar to confusional arousals.

Associated disorders Sleep apnoea syndromes, PLMS, nocturnal seizures, medical/neurological disorders, febrile illness, alcohol use/abuse, pregnancy, menstruation, psychiatric medication (lithium, anticholinergics), stress (no clear association with psychiatric illness).

Differential diagnosis Confusional arousals, episodic wandering (Stage 2 sleep, 2nd half of the night), epileptic fugue states, and REM sleep behaviour disorder in the elderly.

Management
- Reassurance
- Protect the patient from coming to harm (e.g. closing windows, locking doors, sleeping downstairs)
- Relaxation techniques and minimisation of stressors
- Sleep hygiene measures (p. 398)
- Avoidance of sleep deprivation
- Medication (for patients with frequent episodes/high-risk behaviours)— small doses of a benzodiazepine (e.g. diazepam 2–10 mg, clonazepam 1–4 mg), or antidepressant (imipramine, paroxetine) at night.

N.B. Treatment of any concurrent psychiatric disorder does not control the parasomnia.

Sleep terrors (parvor nocturnes, incubus)

Clinical features Sudden awakening with loud terrified screaming (the person may sit up rapidly) with marked autonomic arousal (tachycardia, tachypnoea, diaphoresis, mydriasis). Sometimes frenzied activity occurs, which may lead to injury. Episodes usually last for 10–15 mins, with evident increase in muscle tone and resistance to physical contact. If wakened, the individual appears confused and incoherent, but soon falls asleep, wakening the next morning with no memory of the event. In children, usually occurs in the first 3rd of the night. In adults, can occur at any time of night.

Polysomnography Abrupt wakening out of Stage 3 or 4 sleep is seen on EEG, with generation of alpha activity, usually in the 1st third of the night. Partial arousals out of SWS, occurring up to 10–15 times in one night, are also seen even when a full episode is not recorded.

Prevalence Children ~3%, adults ~1% (may be more common in males), evidence for heritability. Deep and prolonged SWS is a predisposing factor, precipitated by fever, sleep deprivation, and depressant medication. *Associated disorders* As for sleepwalking.

Differential diagnosis Nightmares, nocturnal epilepsy, nocturnal panic attacks.

Management
- Reassurance of the individual (and partner/parents) of the benign character of the disorder.
- If the episodes are frequent (more than once a week)—use similar methods as for sleepwalking.

Parasomnias (3)—sleep-wake transition disorders

Rhythmic movement disorder

Clinical features Stereotyped, repetitive movements involving large muscles, usually of the head and neck, typically immediately prior to sleep, sustained into light sleep. Common forms include headbanging ('jactatio capitis nocturna'), head rolling, and body rocking. Sometimes movements become so violent that head injury results.

Polysomnography Rhythmic movement artifacts during light non-REM sleep, without evidence of epileptiform activity.

Prevalence Common in young children (60% at 9 mths), decline with age (25% at 18 mths, 8% at 4 yrs). More frequent in boys.

Associated problems Developmental problems/psychopathology (older children).

Management
- Unnecessary in most cases, and parents can be reassured that in the majority of infants the disorder will resolve by around the age of 18 months.
- If injury or socially disruption occurs, medication may be used (e.g. low-dose benzodiazepine or antidepressant), with variable reported success.

Sleep starts ('hypnic jerks')

Clinical features Occur at sleep onset and present as sudden abrupt contractions of muscle groups, usually the legs, but sometimes also involving the arms, neck, or even the entire body. When wakened by jerks, an individual may have the feeling of falling in space ('siderealism'). Sometimes this feeling is so intense and frightening that it can lead to fear of going to sleep with subsequent sleep-onset difficulties.

Polysomnography Occasional vertex waves, associated with muscular contraction.

Prevalence 60–70% (essentially a universal component of the sleep-onset process).

Differential diagnosis Nocturnal myoclonic jerks (with evident epileptiform activity on EEG), fragmentary myoclonus (during non-REM sleep), nocturnal leg myoclonus/PLMS (often associated with restless legs syndrome), and the rare 'startle disease' or hyperkplexia syndrome (myoclonus occurs following minor stimuli both during wakefulness and sleep).

Management
- Treatment usually unnecessary.
- If there is significant interference with sleep—general measures (e.g. avoidance of stimulants such as caffeine, nicotine) or low-dose clonazepam at night.

Sleep talking (somniloquy)

Clinical features The common uttering of words or sounds during sleep, without subjective awareness, and speech generally devoid of meaning. Rarely, emotionally charged long 'tirades' occur with content related to the person's occupation or preoccupation.

Polysomnography Brief partial arousal during non-REM sleep is usually seen on EEG in about 60% of cases. Less commonly, somniloquy may occur during REM sleep, if related to dream content or in association with another disorder of REM sleep.

Associated disorders Confusional arousals, sleep terrors, REM sleep behaviour disorder.

Management
● Unless the problem is leading to disruption of sleep in a bed partner, or is a secondary symptom of other sleep pathology, treatment is rarely necessary.

Nocturnal leg cramps

Clinical features Sensations of painful muscular tightness or tension, in the calf (or the foot), occurring during sleep, which awaken the sufferer.

Prevalence Up to 16% of healthy individuals, more common in the elderly.

Associated problems Excessive muscular activity, dehydration, diabetes, arthritis, pregnancy, and Parkinson's disease.

Differential diagnosis Periodic leg movements of sleep (painless), muscle spasm due to spasticity following stroke, other neurological causes of muscle spasticity.

Management
● Treatment only for severe, recurrent symptoms
● Palliative measures (heat, massage, muscle stretching)
● Quinine sulphate (325mg nocte)

Parasomnias (4)—disorders associated with REM sleep

Nightmares

Clinical features Frightening dreams that usually awaken the sleeper from REM sleep, without associated confusion. May be preceded by a frightening or intense real-life traumatic event.

Polysomnography Increased REM density, lasting about 10 mins, terminated by an awakening, usually in the 2nd half of the night.

Prevalence Common (occasional occurrence in ~50 % of adults). Frequent nightmares (one or more a week) occur in about 1% of adults.

Differential diagnosis Sleep terrors, REM sleep behaviour disorder, nocturnal panic attacks.

Management
Treatment usually unnecessary. If episodes are frequent, distressing, or causing a major disturbance to the individual's carers or bed partner:
- *General measures* Avoidance of stress, discontinuation of drugs that may potentially promote nightmares (see opposite page), principles of sleep hygiene (p. 398),
- *Medication* REM-suppressing drugs (e.g. antidepressants). N.B. sudden discontinuation may lead to exacerbation of the problem with REM-rebound.

Sleep paralysis

Clinical features The frightening experience of being unable to perform voluntary movements either at sleep onset (hypnagogic or predormital form) or awakening (hypnopompic or postdormital form), either during the night or in the morning.

Polysomnography Atonia in peripheral muscles (as in REM sleep) despite desynchronised EEG with eye movements and blinking (i.e. awake). H-reflex activity is also abolished during an episode (as in REM sleep).

Prevalence As an isolated phenomenon, reported to occur at least once in the lifetime of 40–50% of normal individuals (usually due to sleep-deprivation). As a chronic complaint, however, it is much less common. Familial sleep paralysis (without sleep attacks or cataplexy) is exceptionally rare.

Differential diagnosis Narcolepsy (occurs in up to 40% of cases), periodic hypokalaemia (in adolescents, following a high carbohydrate meal, and with low-serum potassium during the attack).

Management
- Sleep hygiene (p. 398) esp. avoidance of sleep deprivation, may help to prevent episodes.
- Persistent problems may respond to REM-suppressant medication (e.g. clomipramine 25mg or an SSRI).

REM sleep behaviour disorder (RSBD)[1]

Clinical features Vivid, intense, action-packed, violent dreams (reported as 'nightmares'), dream-enacting behaviours (verbal and motor), sleep injury (ecchymoses, lacerations, fractures—of self and bed partner), general sleep disruption.

Polysomnography Elevated submental EMG tone and/or excessive phasic submental/limb EMG twitching during REM sleep, in the absence of EEG epileptiform activity.

Prevalence A rare sleep disorder, more common in older males.

Associated disorders 50% of cases associated with neurological disorders, usually degenerative (e.g. Parkinson's disease), and narcolepsy (may be an early sign of neurological disease that manifests fully several years later—full neurological examination should be performed.) Rarely associated with other psychiatric disorders, but may be induced or aggravated by psychiatric drugs (e.g. TCAs, MAOIs, high-dose SSRIs, SNRIs), cessation/misuse of REM-suppressing agents (e.g. alcohol, amphetamine, cocaine), or severe stress related to traumatic experiences.

Differential diagnosis Sleepwalking, sleep terrors, nocturnal dissociative disorders, nocturnal epilepsy, obstructive sleep apnoea (where arousals from REM sleep associated with aggressive behaviour and vivid REM-related dreams), states of intoxication, malingering.

Management
- Ensure a safe sleeping environment (for patient and sleeping partner).
- Eliminate any factors that might be inducing or aggravating the condition (including treatment of any primary neurological, medical, or psychiatric disorder).
- If symptoms persist and are problematic, clonazepam (0.5–1.0mg nocte) is the treatment of choice, effectively controlling both behaviours and dreams, with good evidence of long-term safety and sustained benefit. Alternatives include carbamazepine, melatonin, l-dopa, and imipramine.

Drugs associated with vivid dreams or nightmares
- Baclofen
- Beta-blockers
- Clonidine
- Digoxin toxicity
- Famotidine
- Indomethacin
- Methyldopa (alcohol, BDZs, opiates)
- Nalbumetone
- Nicotine patches (atenolol, propranolol)
- Pergolide
- Reserpine
- Stanozolol
- Verapamil
- Withdrawal

---

1 Schenck CH, Mahowald MW (2002) REM sleep behavior disorder: clinical, developmental, and neuroscience perspectives 16 years after its formal identification in SLEEP. *Sleep* **25**, 120–38.

Sleep disorders related to psychiatric disorders

Although it is unusual for psychiatric patients to present with a primary sleep disorder, it is not uncommon for psychiatrists to have to deal with secondary problems of **insomnia** (not getting enough sleep or feeling 'unrefreshed') or **hypersomnia** (feeling excessively sleepy during the day or sleeping too much), in the context of a primary psychiatric disorder, or as a consequence of medication. Equally, **sleep deprivation** may have its own psychological consequences, or may precipitate the onset of a psychiatric illness, particularly a manic episode.

Major affective disorders

Alterations in sleep are central symptoms in the mood disorders. Initial insomnia, frequent waking (for often prolonged periods), early morning waking, vivid or disturbing dreams, daytime fatigue are frequently seen in major depressive disorder. Occasionally, hypersomnia may be a feature in 'atypical' cases, bipolar affective disorder, and 'seasonal affective disorder'. Episodes of mania may be characterised by marked insomnia and a decreased need for sleep.

Management
- Treat the primary disorder.
  - *Initial insomnia*—more sedating antidepressants (tricyclics, trazodone, nefazodone, mirtazepine).
  - *Hypersomnia*—more 'activating' antidepressants (SSRIs, reboxetine, bupropion, MAOIs, RIMAs).
N.B. Most antidepressants are REM-suppressant and may exacerbate underlying primary sleep disorders (e.g. parasomnias and sleep-related movement disorders) either on commencement or cessation.

Anxiety disorders

Anxiety disorders commonly disrupt the normal sleep pattern leading to insomnia—which may be triggered by an acute stressful event. Symptoms include: initial insomnia, frequent waking, reduced total sleep time, and early morning waking.
- *Panic disorder* 'Sleep-related' (nocturnal) attacks may occur with associated intense fear, feelings of impending doom, autonomic arousal, somatic symptoms, and fear of going to sleep (leading to avoidance behaviour that may present as 'insomnia').
- *PTSD* Recurrent distressing dreams related to a traumatic event are a core feature of this disorder.

Differential diagnosis 'Night terrors' (patient not awake, usual onset in childhood, and not accompanied by daytime anxiety); 'Nightmares' (intense dream content and usually occur in early hours of the morning).

Treatment
- Treatment of the primary anxiety disorder will generally improve the patient's ability to initiate and sustain sleep.
- Most anxiolytics tend to be sedating, and it is usual to prescribe a higher dose at night.

- When less sedating drugs, such as the SSRIs are used, additional treatment may be necessary to target persistent sleep problems (e.g. cognitive behavioural techniques, short-term use of hypnotics, or a small dose of a more sedating antidepressant at bedtime).

Schizophrenia

Patients with schizophrenia demonstrate increased nocturnal wakefulness and daytime somnolence. It is often difficult to disentangle the effects of medication, active positive symptoms, persistent negative symptoms, and disorganised behaviour.

Management

- Daytime somnolence—monitor the effects of antipsychotic medication and adjust timing and dosage.
- Insomnia—general sleep hygiene measures, with an emphasis on a behavioural approach when 'disorganisation' is a central feature; judicious use of hypnotics or higher dose of sedating antipsychotic at night-time.

Dementia

Normal aging is associated with increased sleep latency, reduced total sleep time, loss of SWS, frequent arousals leading to fragmentation of nocturnal sleep, and an increase in daytime napping.

- Some sleep disorders (e.g. sleep apnoea syndromes, PLMS) occur more frequently in the elderly population.
- Dementia generally causes further increases in sleep latency, further reductions in total sleep time, and increased fragmentation of nocturnal sleep, in proportion to the severity of the illness.
- Disorders of normal circadian rhythm are also commonly seen, with a characteristic 'sundown syndrome' of confusion and agitation at bedtime.

Management

- General sleep hygiene measures (with an emphasis on establishing and reinforcing a normal 24-hour circadian cycle through the use of environmental cues, daily routine, avoidance of daytime napping, and regular activities).
- 'Sundown syndrome' may respond to low-dose antipsychotic medication (e.g. haloperidol, risperidone) or sedating antidepressants (e.g. trazodone).

The effects of psychiatric medication on sleep

Antidepressants

Sedating

- TCAs are usually sedative due to their anticholinergic effects:
  - Most sedating—amitriptyline, trimipramine, doxepin, imipramine, clomipramine
  - Least sedating—nortriptyline, protriptyline, desipramine; (paroxetine)
- Tetracyclic antidepressants (maprotiline, mianserin) and trazodone also have marked sedating properties, although these are less related to their anticholinergic properties and may be due to their 5HT2 and histamine antagonism—properties shared by some of the newer antidepressants, (e.g. nefazodone, mirtazepine).

Alerting MAOIs, SSRIs, NARIs (reboxetine), DARIs (bupropion), SNRIs (venlafaxine) all tend to have alerting effects which may, be useful in the treatment of hypersomnolence associated with 'atypical' depression, and should be taken in the morning or early afternoon.

Mood-stabilising drugs

Lithium tends to be mildly sedating.

Carbamazepine may cause drowsiness at the start of treatment or when the dose is being increased, but this is usually a transient effect.

Sodium valproate is less sedative than carbamazepine, with only mild effects on sleep.

Antipsychotic drugs

Most antipsychotics cause drowsiness and impaired performance. There is a great degree of variability even within groups of antipsychotics (see opposite page).

Benzodiazepines and associated hypnotics

By definition, benzodiazepines and barbiturates are sedating. Problems arise due to 'REM rebound' on discontinuation, tolerance to the beneficial hypnotic effects after long-term use, and problems of dependence Newer hypnotics, such as zopiclone and zolpidem, share the sleep-enhancing properties of the benzodiazepines, but may be less likely to cause 'rebound' or dependence.

Psychostimulant drugs

Although very useful in the treatment of hypersomnia (particularly in narcolepsy), ADHD, and to suppress appetite, this group of drugs all tend to cause insomnia with fragmented sleep due to frequent awakenings (e.g. dexamphetamine, methylphenidate, methamphetamine, mazinol, pemoline, and modafinil) and should not be taken in the evening. Cessation, with the notable exception of modafinil, leads to increases in total sleep time and REM 'rebound'.

Sedative effects of antipsychotics

Marked sedation	Moderate sedation	Minimal Sedation
Chlorpromazine	Benperidol	Amisulpiride
Clozapine	Droperidol	Flupenthixol
Methotrimeprazine	Fluphenazine	Haloperidol
Pericyazine	Loxapine	Pimozide
	Olanzapine	Quetiapine
	Perphenazine	Risperidone
	Promazine	Sulpiride
	Thioridazine	Trifluoperazine
	Zuclopenthixol	Zotepine

The effects of drugs and alcohol on sleep

Alcohol

Alcohol most probably exerts its sedative effects through a combination of GABA facilitation and glutamate inhibition. The acute effects of alcohol lead to reduced sleep latency, increased total sleep time, increased SWS, mild suppression of REM sleep in 1st half of the night, and subsequent increased REM sleep in 2nd half of the night, associated with sleep disruption, intense dreaming, and even nightmares. Chronic effects of alcohol abuse include the loss of SWS, sleep disruption, and significant insomnia. Withdrawal from alcohol is also associated with insomnia. Sleep architecture is disrupted, with increased sleep latency, reduced total sleep time, loss of SWS, increased REM density and/or amount. 'Delirium tremens', with marked agitation, confusion, and hallucinations, is characterised by intense REM rebound.

Nicotine

This tends to cause initial insomnia, and may be associated with sleep disruption and increased REM sleep. Use of nicotine patches has been associated with vivid dreams and nightmares.

Cannabis

The hypnotic effects of cannabis are modulated by the cannabinoid-1 receptors in the brain and appear to be similar to the effects of benzodiazepines and alcohol, increasing SWS and suppressing REM sleep. Cessation may lead to problems of initial insomnia, sleep disruption and REM rebound.

Opiates

Although sleep is improved when opiates are used therapeutically for pain relief or in the treatment of restless legs, misuse is associated with generalised sleep disruption. Particular changes in sleep architecture include decreased sleep efficiency, decreased total sleep time, decreased SWS, and decreased REM sleep. Withdrawal symptoms include insomnia, with fragmentation of sleep and disruption of normal sleep architecture, related to increased arousal and REM rebound.

Stimulants

This group encompasses a range of different types of compounds. The effects of amphetamine and cocaine include reduced REM sleep, and increased sleep and REM latency. Xanthines (caffeine, theophylline) also have similar effects, exerting their influence on sleep mechanisms through adenosine receptors, directly interfering with the generation of sleep. The amphetamine derivatives fenfluramine and MDMA (3,4-methylene-dioxy-methamphetamine, 'Ecstasy') have a pharmacological action that is primarily serotonergic. This may lead to both daytime sedation and disturbed sleep (due to periods of drowsiness and wakefulness), as well as a reduced duration of REM sleep. SWS may be increased during the 'withdrawal' phase as a 'rebound' phenomenon.

Sexual dysfunction (1)—general principles

A brief note on 'talking about sex'

Discussing sexual issues, particularly sexual dysfunction, may be embarrassing for the individual, and this is compounded if the clinician is also uncomfortable. Aside from experience of asking about these issues, a few general principles should be borne in mind.

- An empathic, non-judgemental, understanding approach is essential.
- Acknowledge the difficulty in talking about sexual problems.
- Reassure that such problems are common and are treatable.
- Avoid 'medical' terminology (or adequately explain any terms used).
- Start with general enquiries before moving on to more specific issues.
- Do not make *any* assumptions (esp. orientation, practices, experience, number of partners).
- Be aware of common sexual myths (see *opposite*.)

Defining sexual dysfunction

Despite disagreement about what constitutes 'normal', there is general consensus that sexual dysfunction is present when there are persistent impairments of normal patterns of sexual interest or response. Usually these manifest as lack or loss of interest/enjoyment of sexual activities, the inability to experience or control orgasm, or a physiological barrier to successful sexual intercourse. Criteria for a diagnosis of sexual dysfunction include:

- Inability to participate in a preferred sexual relationship
- Presence of the sexual dysfunction on (almost) all occasions
- Duration of at least 6 months
- Significant stress or interpersonal difficulties
- Not accounted for by a physical disorder, drug treatment (or use), or other mental or behavioural disorder

Sub-clinical problems

Certain individuals will not meet strict criteria for a specific diagnosis, but nevertheless experience significant distress. Usually these problems are adjustment difficulties related to timing, frequency, and method of initiating sexual activity. Any treatment tends to be supportive (for the patient and their partner) and educative (sex education).

Common triggers for sexual problems

Psychological Relationship problems; life stressors; anxiety/depression; low self-esteem; sexual performance anxiety; excessive self-monitoring of arousal; feelings of guilt about sex; fear of pregnancy or STDs; lack of knowledge about sexuality/'normal' sexual responses; previous significant negative sexual experience (esp. rape or childhood sexual abuse issues).

Environmental (Fear of) interruptions (e.g. from children, parents); physical discomfort.

Physical Use of drugs or alcohol; medication side-effects; pain or discomfort due to illness; feeling tired or 'run down'; recent childbirth.

Factors related to the partner Sexual attractiveness (gender, physical characteristics); evidence of disinterest, constant criticism, inconsideration, and inability to cope with difficulties (esp. sexual); sexual inexperience/ poor technique; preference for sexual activities that are unappealing to the partner.

Common sexual myths[1]
- Men should not express their emotions.
- All physical contact must lead to sex.
- Good sex leads to a wild orgasm.
- Sex = intercourse.
- The man should be the sexual leader.
- Women should not initiate sex.
- Men feel like sex all the time.
- Women should always have sex when her partner makes sexual approaches.
- Sex is something we instinctively know about.
- 'Respectable' people should not enjoy sex too much and certainly never masturbate.
- All other couples have 'great' sex, several times a week, have an orgasm every time, and always orgasm simultaneously.
- If sex is not good, there is something wrong with the relationship.

1 Adapted from Andrews G and Jenkins R (eds) (1999) *Management of Mental Disorders* (U.K. edition, vol.2). Sydney: World Health Organisation Collaborating Centre for Mental Health and Substance Abuse, pp 612–3.

Sexual dysfunction (2)—problems common to men and women

Sexual dysfunction is common in the general population with lifetime prevalence in young adults estimated as[1]:

Problem	Male	Female
Reduced libido	30%	40%
Arousal difficulties	50%	60%
Reaching orgasm too soon	15%	10%
Failure to have orgasm	2%	35%
Dyspareunia	5%	15%

Lack or loss of sexual desire

Lack of pleasure in anticipating, or reduced urge to engage in, sexual activity. May be **primary** (always has been absent) or **secondary** (has declined recently), **situational** (specific settings or partners), or **total** For a diagnosis, loss of desire ought not to be secondary to other sexual problems (e.g. dyspareunia or erectile failure).

Differential diagnosis Sexual aversion, lack of sexual enjoyment, depression, physical causes (chronic pain, endocrine disturbance, effects of drugs or alcohol).

Management
• Treat any primary cause found (physical, psychological, or psychiatric).
• Establish the reasons for seeking help, provide information (e.g. 'common triggers' [p. 427])
• Address general relationship issues.
• Consider specialist referral (behavioural work, graded individual and couple exercises require experienced therapist (e.g. 'sensate focus' techniques, see opposite page).

Sexual aversion and lack of sexual enjoyment

Sexual aversion Strong negative feelings, fear, or anxiety due to the prospect of sexual interaction; of sufficient intensity to lead to active avoidance of sexual activity.

Lack of sexual enjoyment Lack of appropriate pleasure, despite normal sexual responses and achievement of orgasm.

Management Both of these conditions tend to be related to difficult and complex psychosocial factors, often stemming from a previous traumatic sexual experience (e.g. rape or molestation). For this reason, only a skilled, experienced therapist should attempt treatment. Where possible, refer to a specialist service. Establishing the reasons for seeking help may clarify sensible outcome goals.

Excessive sexual desire

Occasionally increased sexual drive may occur, presenting as a problem for individuals, partners (on whom 'unreasonable' demands are made), or carers (when sexual disinhibition occurs). Referred to as **nymphomania** (women) or **satyriasis** (men). Usually occurs in late teenage/early adulthood, secondary to a mood disorder (e.g. mania), in the early stages of dementia, associated with learning disability, secondary to brain injury, or as a side-effect of some drugs.

Management Treatment should address any primary problem, general relationship issues. When the problem is persistent, specialist referral may be appropriate (for cognitive, behavioural, or, rarely, pharmacological therapy).

'Sensate focus' (Masters and Johnston, 1966[2])

A series of specific exercises for couples (essentially a form of *in vivo* 'desensitisation' to reduce sexual anxiety), initially encouraging each partner to take turns in paying increased attention to their own senses. There are a number of stages to a course of therapy:

Stage one The couple take turns to touch each other's body (with the breasts and genitals off limits), to establish an awareness of sensations (touching and being touched) and usually in silence (to avoid distractions). If sexual arousal does occur, they are not to proceed to intercourse. If any touch is uncomfortable, the partner being touched must let his or her partner know, either verbally or non-verbally.

Stage two Touching is expanded to include the breasts and genitals, still with an emphasis on awareness of sensations and not the expectation of a sexual response (intercourse and orgasm are still prohibited). A 'hand riding' technique is used (placing one hand on top of the partner's hand while being touched) to indicate more or less pressure, faster or slower pace, or change to a different spot.

Stage three The couple try mutual touching (not taking turns), to practice a more natural form of physical interaction. Intercourse is still off limits.

Stage four Mutual touching continues, moving to the female-on-top position without attempting penetration. The woman can rub the penis against her clitoral region, vulva, and vaginal opening regardless of whether or not there is an erection, still focusing on the physical sensations, and stopping or returning to non-genital touching if either partner becomes orgasm orientated or anxious. In later sessions, she may progress to putting the tip of the penis into the vagina if there is an erection, and after completing a few sessions in this way, couples are usually comfortable enough to proceed to full intercourse.

1 Haas K and Haas A (1993) *Understanding Human Sexuality.* Mosby.

2 Masters WH and Johnson VE (1966) *Human Sexual Response.* New York: Bantam Books.

Sexual dysfunction (3)—problems specific to women

Failure of genital response

This is usually due to vaginal dryness or lack of lubrication, due to psychological factors (e.g. anxiety), physical problems (e.g. infection), oestrogen deficiency (esp. post-menopausally), or secondary to lack or loss of sexual desire.

Management

- General aims: increasing arousal levels during periods of sexual activity (see below), alleviating vaginal dryness (with use of lubricating gel, oestrogen replacement), and reducing factors that may inhibit arousal (see *Common triggers* p. 427).
- If problems persist, referral to a specialist should be considered.

Orgasmic dysfunction

The most common sexual complaint in women. Experience of orgasm is delayed or does not occur at all, despite normal sexual arousal and excitement. Individuals may consider this to be normal and not complain of dysfunction. Problems may be **primary** (never had an orgasm in any situation), **secondary** (previously able, but not currently), **situational** (problems only occur in certain situations), or **total** (in all situations). Complicating factors may include secondary lack or loss of sexual desire, other sexual dysfunctions, and relationship problems.

Management

- Complex cases should be referred to a specialist sex therapist.
- Less complex cases may respond to a directed self-help programme[1]. This usually includes directed masturbation, 'sensate focus' for couples, Kegel's pelvic floor exercises, and use of sexual fantasy.

Non-organic vaginismus

Penetration is impossible or painful due to blockage of the vaginal opening caused by spasms of the pelvic floor muscles. Usually related to anxieties or fearful thoughts—e.g. fear of pain on penetration, previous sexual assault, belief in premarital sex being wrong or sinful, childhood punishment for masturbation, general fear of sex (esp. the first experience of intercourse is likely to be painful or bloody), fear of pregnancy and painful labour. Vaginismus leads to pain during intercourse, thus reinforcing these beliefs.

Management

- Physical examination (to exclude vaginal obstruction due to a growth, a tumour, or the hymen).
- Vaginismus is best treated by an expert and management will include:education (to dispel myths and tackle misunderstandings or negative attitudes), relaxation techniques, and strategies to achieve penetration (e.g. self-exploration, Kegel's exercises, use of graded trainers, sensate focus exercises, involvement of partner, graded attempts at intercourse, reassurance for the partner).

Non-organic dyspareunia

Pain during intercourse that may be felt superficially (at the entrance of) or deep within the vagina.

Management

- Exclude physical causes of pain (e.g. infection, tender episiotomy scar, endometriosis, ovarian cyst).
- Provide information about ensuring adequate arousal, variation of intercourse positions to avoid 'deep' penetration.
- Relaxation techniques (including Kegel's exercises) and 'positive self-talk' may help reduce anxiety and ensure the woman feels 'in control'.
- Where deep pain is experienced *after* intercourse, this may be due to *pelvic congestion syndrome* (with symptoms similar to pre-menstrual syndrome) caused by accumulation of blood during arousal without occurrence of orgasm. Achieving orgasm (by intercourse, masturbation, or use of a vibrator) may help to alleviate this congestion.
- For complex cases, with vague or intermittent problems, associated secondary sexual or psychiatric problems, or when initial treatment is unsuccessful, referral to a specialist is indicated.

Kegel's exercises

These are pelvic floor muscle exercises. The muscle can be identified by attempting to stop urine flow, and contraction of this muscle may need to be practised before voluntary control is mastered. The exercises should be practised for a few minutes every day. Repeat a) and b) ten times initially (building up to 30 times over 4–6 weeks) and c) and d) five times (building up to 20 times over 4–6 weeks).

a) Breathing normally, quickly contract and relax the muscle.
b) Breathing normally, contract the muscle for a count of three, and then relax.
c) Inhale slowly, contracting the muscle for a count of three, hold for a count of three, then, exhaling slowly, relax to a count of three.
d) With the muscle relaxed, bear down (as if trying to push something out of the vagina) for a count of three

---

1 Heiman JR and LoPiccolo J (1988) *Becoming Orgasmic*. Piatkus Books.

Sexual dysfunction (4)—problems specific to men

Erectile failure (failure of genital response) Inability to develop or maintain an erection, leading to failure of coitus or sexual intercourse. **Subtypes** *Primary* Never been able to sustain an erection; *Secondary* Able to do so in the past; *Situational* Only successful under certain circumstances; *Total* Not under any circumstances. **Contributing factors** Moral/religious views on sex and masturbation; previous negative sexual experiences (may undermine sexual confidence and increase 'performance anxiety'); secondary to other sexual dysfunction (e.g. premature ejaculation); use of alcohol and drugs; stress and fatigue.

Management Physical assessment to exclude organic causes (disease or surgery affecting the blood supply of the penis, side-effects of drugs or medication) especially in older men; refer to expert on sexual problems if *primary, total, long-standing* (years), or not associated with obvious triggers. **General** Education (about physical and psychological factors that may contribute to erectile failure) and self-help exercises[1,2] (better if partner involved). **Physical** Sildenafil (Viagra); training in self-administration of papaverine or prostaglandin E_1 into the penis prior to intercourse; use of a vacuum constriction device; surgical implantation of semi-rigid or inflatable penile prostheses. N.B. Relapse common (~75%), usually related to clear triggers, and will improve naturally or through use of previously successful techniques. (Seeing this as a 'normal' situation may help relieve anxiety and reduce the sense of failure which might otherwise prolong problems further.)

Orgasmic dysfunction (or 'inhibited ejaculation') Relatively rare in men. Orgasm delayed/does not occur at all, despite normal sexual excitement and arousal. **Situational dysfunction** usually has a psychological cause (see *Common triggers* p. 427); **total dysfunction** may have a variety of causes.

Management Main aims: reducing 'performance anxiety', increasing arousal and physical stimulation i.e. addressing any common triggers, relationship problems, associated feelings of anxiety or guilt, or memories of past traumatic/unpleasant sexual experiences. Education (dispelling myths, understanding 'normal' physiology, the effects of alcohol); use of sensate focus techniques. Persistent problems should be referred to an expert.

Premature ejaculation The inability to control ejaculation adequately for both partners to enjoy the sexual interaction. Ejaculation may occur immediately after penetration, or in the absence of an erection.

Differential diagnosis Delayed erection (prolonged stimulation needed to achieve adequate erection; short time to ejaculation); organic impairment (esp pain); 'normal' rapid ejaculation in young or sexually inexperienced men (control is learned with practice); secondary to psychological stressors; transient problem following a period of reduced sexual activity.

Management Expert advice should be sought for complex cases or where there is associated orgasmic dysfunction/lack or loss of sexual desire. Sympathetic partner is crucial to successful management. General education (specific issues of 'normal' time before ejaculation occurs). Reduction of 'performance anxiety' (as for *Orgasmic dysfunction*). Use of self-help guides[2]. Specific exercises may include: the 'stop-start' technique (see below), the 'squeeze technique' (see below), and sensate focus (see p 000).

Non-organic dyspareunia Pain during intercourse in men; usually has a physical cause (e.g. urethral infection, scarring secondary to STD, tight foreskin) that can be directly treated. If psychological factors are the root cause, reassurance, education, and use of relaxation and cognitive techniques may be helpful. Complex cases require expert management.

The 'stop-start' technique (Semans' technique)

Developed by Masters and Johnson[3,4]; effective in up to 90% of cases of premature ejaculation.

Aims: To increase the frequency of sexual contact and increase the sensory threshold of the penis.

Setting: Best performed in the context of *sensate focus* exercises—to ensure non-genital areas are focused on first (less threatening for anxious individuals, allowing the recognition of sensations leading up to ejaculation, and may make the 'quality' of the sexual experience better), to limit the number of 'accidental' ejaculations (that may discourage couples early on), and increase good communication and cooperation.

Technique:
• Stimulation of the penis until high arousal (but not the ejaculation threshold) is achieved.
• Cessation of stimulation for a few minutes to allow arousal to subside.
• Repetition 4–5 times until ejaculation is permitted.

'Squeeze technique'

If control does not develop using the 'stop-start' technique, this method may be used to inhibit the ejaculatory reflex:
• Stimulation of the penis until high arousal (but not the ejaculation threshold) is achieved.
• The man (or his partner) applies a firm squeeze to the head of the penis for 15–20 seconds. (Forefinger and middle finger are placed over the base of the glans and shaft of the penis, and the thumb applies pressure on the opposite side at the base of the undersurface of the glans.)

N.B. This technique should be practised before high arousal occurs to establish how firmly the penis may be squeezed without causing pain.

1 Williams W (1985) *It's Up To You.* Sydney: Maclennan and Petty.

2 Zilbergeld B (1980) *Men and Sex.* London: Fontana.

3 Masters WH and Johnson VE (1966) *Human Sexual Response.* New York: Bantam Books.

4 Masters WH and Johnson VE (1980) *Human Sexual Inadequacy.* New York: Bantam Books.

Menstrual-related disorders

Premenstrual syndrome (PMS) or tension (PMT)

Refers to a constellation of menstrually related, chronic, cyclical, physical and emotional symptoms occurring in the luteal phase (the second half) of the menstrual cycle.

Symptoms Breast tenderness, fatigue, cramping, bloating, irritability, aggressiveness, depression, inability to concentrate, food cravings, lethargy, and libido change.

Aetiology Unknown (thought to reflect hormonal/neurotransmitter abnormalities).

Prevalence May affect up to 40% of women of reproductive age with severe impairment in about 5% including associated premenstrual dysphoric disorder (PMDD) (*see below*).

Psychiatric consultation is not usual unless emotional symptoms are marked.

Differential diagnosis Fewer than 50% of women complaining of PMS have the diagnosis confirmed by rigorous criteria. Many self-referrals with PMS meet the criteria for a depressive or anxiety disorder[1]. Hypothyroidism and gynaecological disorders (dysmenorrhoea, postpartum status, polycystic ovary disease, and endometriosis) should be excluded. Possible nutrient deficiencies (e.g. manganese, magnesium, B vitamins, vitamin E, and linoleic acid).

Investigations
- No specific tests diagnose PMS, including measurements of specific nutrient deficiencies and reproductive hormones.
- TFTs and gynaecological consultation are appropriate.
- Charting of daily symptoms for at least two menstrual cycles may aid in confirming cyclical pattern.

Management (PMS and PMDD)
- Conservatively managed (unless there is significant psychiatric comorbidity)—e.g. a diet low in salt, fat, caffeine, and sugar; restriction of alcohol and tobacco; aerobic exercise; and measures to reduce stress.
- Consider medication if there is failure to adequately respond after 2–3 months (SSRIs—e.g. fluoxetine, paroxetine, sertraline; diuretics for severe oedema—e.g. frusemide, spironolactone; danazol for mastalgia.)
- RCTs have failed to demonstrate the effectiveness of OCP in treating PMS, but some women report improvement of PMDD[2].
- Bilateral oophorectomy is a last resort for patients with severe symptoms when medical therapy has either failed or has produced unacceptable side-effects.
- No evidence for other treatment options—e.g. progesterone, dietary supplements (evening primrose oil, magnesium, vitamin B6 or E), bromocriptine, benzodiazepines, buspirone, GnRH agonists, hysterectomy, and endometrial ablation.

Premenstrual dysphoric disorder (PMDD)

A more severe form of PMS, characterised by markedly depressed mood, anxiety, affective lability, and reduced interest in activities. Symptoms may be indistinguishable from a mixed affective disorder, although classically they have occurred regularly during the last week of the luteal phase in most menstrual cycles over the preceding 12 months, begin to disappear within several days of the onset of menses, and are always absent in the week after menses.

Menopausal disorders

There is an increased incidence of anxiety and depression in peri- or post-menopausal women. This is not related directly to hormonal changes. Rather, patients presenting with mood-related problems around the menopause experience coincident psychosocial stressors[3], and the changes in gonadal hormones may exacerbate pre-existing mood disorders[4].

Assessment

- Exclude other causes of mood disturbance.
- Particular attention should be paid to past psychiatric history and current social history.

Management

- Evidence for HRT is inconclusive, although if mood symptoms are secondary to physical symptoms this may have a role (HRT may also augment effects of antidepressants)[5].
- Treatment is with standard approaches for depression/anxiety.

1 Keenan PA, Stern RA, Janowsky DS, Pedersen CA (1992) Psychological aspects of premenstrual syndrome. I: Cognition and memory. *Psychoneuroendocrinology* **17**, 179–87.

2 Rubinow DR, Schmidt PJ, Roca CA (1998) Hormone measures in reproductive endocrine-related mood disorders: diagnostic issues. *Psychopharmacology Bulletin* **34**, 289–90.

3 Cooke DJ (1985) Psychosocial vulnerability to life events during the climacteric. *BJP* **147**, 71–5.

4 Sagsoz N, Oguzturk O, Bayram M, Kamaci M (2001) Anxiety and depression before and after the menopause. *Arch Gynecol Obstet.* **264**, 199–202.

5 Birkhauser M (2002) Depression, menopause and estrogens: is there a correlation? *Maturitas* **41** (Suppl 1), S3–8.

Disorders associated with pregnancy

Normal pregnancy

Although there is usually an increase in symptoms of anxiety and depression during pregnancy, these are quite normal and usually related to 'adjustment' in the 1st trimester and 'fears' in the 3rd trimester. Unless there is a past history of psychiatric illness, there is no reported increase in the incidence of psychiatric disorders[1].

Risk factors Family or personal history of depression; ambivalence about the pregnancy; high levels of neuroticism; lack of marital, family, or social supports.

Treatment Usually will focus on psychosocial interventions; specific psychiatric disorders should be identified and treated appropriately (see *Prescribing in Pregnancy* p. 876).

Miscarriage and abortion[2]

There is an increase in psychiatric morbidity, with over 50% of women experiencing an adjustment disorder (grief reaction) with significant depressive symptoms. Chronic symptoms are rare, but risk is increased when there is a history of previous miscarriage or abortion, or where conflict is experienced related to religious or cultural beliefs.

Hyperemesis gravidarum[3]

Vomiting in pregnancy that is sufficiently pernicious to produce weight loss, dehydration, acidosis from starvation, alkalosis from loss of HCl in vomitus, and hypokalaemia. Occurs in 1–20/1000 pregnant women. Although psychological factors may be important in benign forms, these are now regarded as secondary rather than primary (i.e. *not* a somatoform disorder).

Complications Muscle weakness, ECG abnormalities, tetany, psychological disturbance, and more seriously (but rarely): oesophageal rupture, Wernicke encephalopathy, central pontine myelinosis, retinal hemorrhage, renal damage, spontaneous pneumomediastinum, intrauterine growth retardation, and foetal death.

Associations Transient hypothyroidism (60% of cases), *H. pylori* infection.

Management Admission to hospital (~24%), parenteral fluid, electrolyte replacement, vitamin supplementation, antiemetics or short-term steroids, diazepam (for nausea and associated distress).

Psuedocyesis[4]

A condition in which a woman firmly believes herself to be pregnant and develops objective pregnancy signs (abdominal enlargement, menstrual disturbance, apparent foetal movements, nausea, breast changes, labour pains, uterine enlargement, cervical softening, urinary frequency, positive pregnancy test) in the absence of pregnancy.

Differential diagnosis Possible medical disorders should be excluded (ectopic pregnancy, corpus luteal cyst, placenta praevia, pituitary tumour, pelvic tumour).

Aetiology Regarded as a somatoform disorder or variant of depression, it may present as a complication of postpartum depression or psychosis with amenorrhoea. It may be related to Couvade's syndrome in expectant fathers (see p. 85).

Treatment Tends to include supportive or insight-orientated psychotherapy and a trial of an antidepressant.

1 Klein MH and Essex MJ (1995) Pregnant or depressed? The effect of overlap between symptoms of depression and somatic complaints of pregnancy on rates of depression in the second trimester. *Depression* **2**, 308–14.

2 Clare AW and Tyrrell J (1994) Psychiatric aspects of abortion. *Ir J Psychol Med* **11**, 92–8.

3 Kuscu NK and Koyuncu F (2002) Hyperemesis gravidarum: current concepts and management. *Postgrad Med J* **78**, 76–9.

4 Small GW (1986) Pseudocyesis: an overview. *Can J Psych* **31**, 452–7.

Personality disorders

Introduction

Personality disorder is one of the most contentious diagnoses in psychiatry. Although there are clear diagnostic criteria, the term is often used as a pejorative label for patients whom we dislike, following an inadequate assessment. Diagnostic reliability is poor and current categorical classifications lack validity. The concept has been attacked for being nothing more than medicalisation of socially unacceptable behaviour.

Although the vast majority of people with personality disorders are not violent, much discussion has focused on personality disordered offenders and 'psychopaths'. There have been numerous attempts in various countries to devise legislative measures to protect society from 'dangerous psychopaths', and the role of psychiatry in this endeavour has been a point of argument within the profession and between the profession and others (particularly politicians and lawyers) for over a century.

There are many psychiatrists who believe that psychiatry has no role in the treatment of people with personality disorders. They argue that:
- Personality is by definition unchangeable
- There is no evidence that psychiatry can do anything
- These people are disruptive and impinge negatively on the treatment of other patients
- These people are not ill and are responsible for their behaviour
- Psychiatry is being asked to deal with something that is essentially a social problem.

On the other hand there are those who believe that people with personality disorder clearly fall within the remit of psychiatry, arguing:
- People with personality disorder suffer from the symptoms of their disorder
- They have high rates of suicide, other forms of premature death, and of other mental illness
- There are treatment approaches which are effective
- Their opponents are rejecting patients because they dislike them
- The problem is not that these people cannot be helped but that traditional psychiatric services do not provide the type of approach and services that are necessary

The focus of this chapter is on the clinical assessment and management of people with personality disorders. The place of personality disorder in mental health legislation is covered in Chapter 19 and personality disorder and offending is mentioned in Chapter 15. Disorders of sexual preference are also covered in this chapter, as they are grouped with personality disorders in ICD-10.

The concept of personality disorder

Essence

'Personality' can be seen as the enduring characteristics and attitudes of an individual. We all recognise, amongst people we know well, some who manifest certain characteristics more than others: shyness, confidence, anger, generosity, tendency to display emotions, sensitivity, and being per-nickety to name but a few. When these enduring characteristics of an individual are such as to cause distress or difficulties for themselves or in their relationships with others then they can be said to be suffering from personality disorder. Personality is separate from illness, although the two interact.

Definition

The following definition is based on ICD-10 and DSM-IV (both are very similar). Personality disorders are enduring (starting in childhood or adolescence and continuing into adulthood), persistent and pervasive disorders of inner experience and behaviour that cause distress or significant impairment in social functioning. Personality disorder manifests as problems in **cognition** (ways of perceiving and thinking about self and others), **affect** (range, intensity, and appropriateness of emotional response), and **behaviour** (interpersonal functioning, occupational and social functioning, and impulse control). To diagnose personality disorder, the manifest abnormalities should not be due to other conditions (such as psychosis, affective disorder, substance misuse, or organic disorder) and should be out of keeping with social and cultural norms.

Development of the concept[1]

The development of clinical concepts of conditions which would today be recognised as personality disorder started in the early 19th Century, at a time when the main two groups of mental conditions acknowledged by psychiatrists were insanity and idiocy. It became clear that there were individuals who were neither insane (not suffering from delusions or hallucinations) nor clearly idiots, imbeciles, or morons (to use the then contemporary terminology for learning disability), but who nevertheless manifested abnormalities in their behaviour.

The term 'moral insanity' was introduced by Prichard in 1835. 'Moral' meant 'psychological' (rather than the modern meaning concerning ethics), and amongst the patients described were people who had affective disorders as well as people who were personality disordered.

As the concept has developed various labels have been used, but the term 'psychopathy' dominated the 20th Century. The term was used in various ways:

- Broadly and literally, covering any psychopathology at all.
- More narrowly, covering all personality disorders.
- More narrowly still, covering personality disorders manifesting antisocial behaviour.
- At its narrowest, referring to cold, callous, self-centred, predatory individuals.

Until relatively recently personality disorder manifesting antisocial behaviour has dominated the literature. Clinical developments have been complicated by legal definitions (such as 'moral imbecile' in 1913 and 'psychopathic disorder' in 1959).

Kraeplin (1896) and Schneider (1923) introduced classification systems which can be seen as forerunners of the current categorical approaches in DSM-IV and ICD-10.

Key contributions to the development of concepts related to personality disorder

1809	Pinel describes 'manie sans délire'.
1812	Rush describes 'perversion of the moral faculties'.
1835	Prichard describes 'moral insanity'.
1838	Ray describes 'moral mania'.
1891	Koch describes 'psychopathic inferiority'.
1896	Kraepelin describes and categorises 'psychopathic personalities'.
1913	Category 'moral imbecile' introduced in Mental Deficiency Act.
1919	Kretschmer suggests relationship between body types and personality.
1923	Schneider describes and categorises 'psychopathic personalities'.
1930	Partridge describes 'sociopathy'.
1939	Henderson describes 'psychopathic states'.
1941	Cleckley publishes *Mask of Sanity* describing psychopaths.
1959	Category 'psychopathic disorder' introduced in Mental Health Act.

1 Saß H and Herpertz S (1995) Personality disorders. Clinical section. In *A History of Clinical Psychiatry* (eds. Berrios G and Porter R). London: Athlone.

'Normal' personality

The term 'normal' personality can be used to refer to an ideal state or that which is statistically normal, but here it describes aspects of personality psychology which offer a descriptive and explanatory framework for the understanding of personality. There are two main approaches: **nomothetic** and **ideographic**[1].

Nomothetic approaches

Personality seen in terms of attributes shared by individuals. Two subdivisions: **type (or categorical) approaches** (discrete categories of personality); and **trait (or dimensional) approaches** (a limited number of qualities, or traits, account for personality variation). Type approaches dominate the description and classification of personality disorder, but trait approaches are pre-eminent in modern personality psychology.

Type approaches These describe individual personality by similarity to a variable number of predefined archetypes. These may attempt to include all aspects of personality and behaviour—the 'broad' models—or they may describe one aspect of personality—the 'narrow' models. An example of the former is the humoral model of Hippocrates which described four fundamental personality types, (choleric, sanguine, melancholic and phlegmatic); an example of the later is the type A vs. type B model which describes groups of behaviours exhibited by people at higher and lower risk of cardiac disease.

Trait approaches These view a variable number of traits as continuous scales along which each person will have a particular position; the positions on all the traits represent a number of dimensions which describe personality. Examples include: *Eysenck's three factor theory* (neuroticism, extraversion, psychoticism); *Costa and McCrae's five factor model* (neuroticism, extraversion, openness, agreeableness, conscientiousness); *Cloninger's seven factor model* (novelty seeking, harm avoidance, reward dependence, persistence, self-directedness, cooperativeness, self-transcendence; originally only first 3 factors); *Cattell's 16 factor theory*. A consensus has emerged from personality questionnaire research and from lexical approaches that there are five fundamental traits (the 'big five') similar to those of Costa and McCrae. The heritability of personality traits in twin and adoptive studies has been found to be moderately large (about 30%).

Ideographic approaches

Unlike nomothetic approaches, emphasise individuality and seek to understand an individual's personality by understanding that individual and their development rather than by reference to common factors. Examples are psychoanalytic, humanistic, and cognitive-behavioural approaches. The first two have little scientific validity and the last has compromised with trait theorists.

Is personality stable?

Are there traits which are persistent and predict a person's behaviour over time in a number of situations? Situationists have argued that the situation was a stronger determinant of behaviour than personality traits.

However, more recent research has demonstrated the long-term stability of a number of personality traits and, perhaps unsurprisingly, most now agree that both the situation and personality traits are important in determining behaviour.

1 Deary I and Power M (1998) Normal and abnormal personality. In *Companion to Psychiatric Studies* (eds. Johnstone EC, Freeman CPL and Zeally AK). Edinburgh: Churchill Livingstone.

Classification of personality disorder

It is largely accepted that normal personality is best described and classified in terms of dimensions or traits. Although this also applies to personality disorder, our current psychiatric classifications are categorical. The various categories of personality disorder described in ICD-10 and DSM-IV have a number of origins: psychodynamic theory, apparent similarities between certain personality disorders and certain mental illnesses, and descriptions of stereotypical personality types. The various categories used come together in a piecemeal and arbitrary fashion and do not represent any systematic understanding or study of personality disorder. The categorical classification of personality disorder is psychiatric classification at its worst.

There are a number of important points to bear in mind when using standard categorical approaches in the diagnosis of personality disorders:

- Due to their heterogeneous origins, there is overlap between the criteria for some categories.
- It is more common for individuals to meet the criteria for more than one category of personality disorder than to meet only the criteria for a single category.
- When making a diagnosis one should use all the categories for which a person meets the criteria.
- If a person meets criteria for more than one category, then they do not suffer from more than one actual disorder. A person has a personality and this may or may not be disordered. If it is disordered it may have various features which are rarely described adequately by a particular category.
- Clinically it is more important to understand and describe the specific features of a person's personality than it is to assign them to a particular category.
- The diagnosis of personality disorder is a particular area where one may believe, wrongly, that one has a better understanding of a person by assigning them to a specific category (an example of 'tautology'*).

ICD-10 and DSM-IV

The personality disorder categories in ICD-10 and DSM-IV are set out opposite. The two schemes are similar, but there are categories that appear in one but not the other, and for some categories different terms are used. Each category has a list of features, a number of which should be present for the person to be diagnosed as manifesting that particular aspect of personality disorder. DSM III (and subsequent editions) placed personality disorder on a separate axis (along with other developmental disorders in axis II) from mental illness (axis I). See p. 9.

---

* Tautology (the restatement of the same information using different words) is a particular danger in psychiatry generally, and the diagnosis of personality disorder in particular. For example, saying that someone has 'borderline' traits gives a gloss of understanding to the simple fact that a person repeatedly self-harms, without actually communicating any new information (except perhaps the 'therapeutic despair' of the psychiatrist).

ICD-10 and DSM-IV classifications of personality disorder

ICD-10	DSM-IV*	Description
Paranoid	Paranoid	Sensitive, suspicious, preoccupied with conspiratorial explanations, self-referential, distrust of others.
Schizoid	Schizoid	Emotionally cold, detachment, lack of interest in others, excessive introspection and fantasy.
(Schizotypal disorder classified with schizophrenia and related disorders)	Schizotypal	Interpersonal discomfort with peculiar ideas, perceptions, appearance, and behaviour.
Dissocial	Antisocial	Callous lack of concern for others, irresponsibility, irritability, aggression, inability to maintain enduring relationships, disregard and violation of others' rights, evidence of childhood conduct disorder.
Emotionally unstable—impulsive type	—	Inability to control anger or plan, with unpredictable affect and behaviour.
Emotionally unstable—borderline type	Borderline	Unclear identity, intense and unstable relationships, unpredictable affect, threats or acts of self-harm, impulsivity.
Histrionic	Histrionic	Self-dramatisation, shallow affect, egocentricity, craving attention and excitement, manipulative behaviour.
—	Narcissistic	Grandiosity, lack of empathy, need for admiration.
Anxious (avoidant)	Avoidant	Tension, self-consciousness, fear of negative evaluation by others, timid, insecure.
Anankastic	Obsessive-compulsive	Doubt, indecisiveness, caution, pedantry, rigidity, perfectionism, preoccupation with orderliness and control.
Dependent	Dependent	Clinging, submissive, excess need for care, feels helpless when not in relationship.

*DSM-IV uses 3 broader clusters to organise the categories of personality disorder—cluster A (odd/eccentric)—paranoid, schizoid, schizotypal cluster B (flamboyant/dramatic)—antisocial, histrionic, narcissistic, borderline; and cluster C (fearful/anxious)—avoidant, dependent, obsessive-compulsive. Although this may seem sensible, there is no particular validity to this clustering.

Psychopathy and 'severe' personality disorder

Psychopathy

The terms 'psychopathy', 'psychopathic personality disorder', 'psychopathic disorder' and 'psychopath' have dominated much of the personality disorder literature until relatively recently. As mentioned on p. 442, the term has been used in various ways, but there are probably only two legitimate ways in which these terms should be used:

- The legal category of 'psychopathic disorder' under the MHA1983.
- 'Psychopathy' as defined by the Psychopathy Checklist—Revised (PCL-R) as an extreme form of antisocial or dissocial personality disorder.

Psychopathic disorder under the MHA1983

Psychopathic disorder is one of four categories of mental disorder under the MHA1983, defined as *'a persistent disorder or disability of mind (whether or not including significant impairment of intelligence) which results in abnormally aggressive or seriously irresponsible conduct on the part of the person concerned'*. Patients detained under this category display a range of personality and other pathology. Only a minority are 'psychopaths' as defined below.

Psychopathy Checklist—revised (PCL-R)[1]

In *The Mask of Sanity* Cleckley[2] described various features of psychopathy referring to cold, callous, self-centred, predatory, parasitic individuals. This concept has led to the development of the PCL-R, which measures the extent to which a person manifests the features of this prototypical psychopath. The items of the PCL-R are listed opposite. Psychopathy as defined by the PCL-R is strongly correlated with risk of future violence. It defines a narrower group of individuals than antisocial or dissocial personality disorder, and individuals scoring highly commonly fulfil the criteria for antisocial, narcissistic, histrionic, paranoid, and perhaps borderline categories in DSM-IV.

Severe personality disorder[3]

The term 'severe personality disorder' is often used but has no clear meaning or definition. Severity of personality disorder has been defined in various ways:

- In terms of severe impact on social functioning.
- By using the PCL-R cut-off and being synonymous with psychopathy.
- By defining severity as the presence of features fulfilling the criteria for multiple categories of DSM-IV or ICD-10 personality disorders (sometimes this is further defined by stating that the categories should be from at least 2 DSM-IV clusters, and perhaps that one must be from cluster B).

None of these approaches are entirely satisfactory, and each defines different but overlapping groups of individuals.

Notes on the PCL-R
The items of the PCL-R cover the affective, interpersonal, and behavioural features of psychopathy. Assessment is based on a comprehensive records' review and in-depth interview(s). Each item is rated 0 (absent), 1 (some evidence but not enough to be clearly present), or 2 (definitely present). There are detailed descriptions of each item in the coding manual. The summed score (out of 40) gives an indication of the extent to which a person is psychopathic and may be converted into a percentile using reference tables for different populations. In the USA a score of 30 or above is used as a cut-off to diagnose 'psychopathy'; in the UK this cut-off is 25 or above.

PCL-R items
1. Glibness/superficial charm
2. Grandiose sense of self-worth
3. Need for stimulation/proneness to boredom
4. Pathological lying
5. Conning/manipulative
6. Lack of remorse or guilt
7. Shallow affect
8. Callous/lack of empathy
9. Parasitic lifestyle
10. Poor behavioural control
11. Promiscuous sexual behaviour
12. Early behaviour problems
13. Lack of realistic, long-term goals
14. Impulsivity
15. Irresponsibility
16. Failure to accept responsibility for own actions
17. Many short-term marital relationships
18. Juvenile delinquency
19. Revocation of conditional release
20. Criminal versatility

---

1 Hare RD (1991) *The Hare Psychopathy Checklist-Revised.* Toronto: Multi-Health Systems.

2 Cleckley H (1941) *The Mask of Sanity.* London: Henry Klimpton.

3 Tyrer P (2004) Getting to grips with severe personality disorder. *Criminal Behaviour and Mental Health* **14,**1–4.

Aetiology of personality disorder

While there is no single, convincing theory explaining the genesis of personality disorder, the following observations are suggestive of possible contributing factors.

Genetic

Evidence of heritability of 'normal' personality traits; some evidence of heritability of cluster B personality disorders; familial relationship between schizotypal personality disorder and schizophrenia, between paranoid personality disorder and delusional disorder, and between borderline personality disorder and affective disorder. No good evidence for relationship between XYY genotype and psychopathy.

Neurophysiology

'Immature' EEG (posterior temporal slow waves) in psychopathy; functional imaging abnormalities in psychopathy (e.g. decreased activity in amygdala during affective processing task); low 5-HT levels in impulsive violent individuals; autonomic abnormalities in psychopathy (slowed galvanic skin response).

Childhood development

Difficult infant temperament may proceed to conduct disorder in childhood and personality disorder; ADHD may be a risk factor for later antisocial personality disorder; insecure attachment may predict later personality disorder (particularly disorganised attachment); harsh and inconsistent parenting and family pathology are related to conduct disorder, and may therefore be related to later antisocial personality disorder; severe trauma in childhood (such as sexual abuse) may be a risk factor for borderline personality disorder and other cluster B disorders.

Psychodynamic theories

Freudian explanations of arrested development at oral, anal, and genital stages leading to dependent, obsessional, and histrionic personalities; 'borderline personality organisation' described by Kernberg (diffuse unfiltered reaction to experience prevents individuals from putting adversity into perspective leading to repeated crises); narcissistic and borderline personalities seen as displaying primitive defence mechanisms such as splitting and projective identification; some see antisocial personalities as lacking aspects of superego, but more sophisticated explanation is in terms of a reaction to an overly harsh superego (representing internalisation of parental abuse).

Cognitive-behavioural theories

There are maladaptive schemata (stable cognitive, affective, and behavioural structures representing specific rules that affect information processing). These schemata represent core beliefs which are derived from an interaction between childhood experience and pre-programmed patterns of behaviour and environmental responses. Schemata are unconditional compared with those found in affective disorders (e.g. 'I am unlovable' rather than 'If someone important criticises me, then I am unlovable') and are formed early, often pre-verbally.

Theories synthesising cognitive-behavioural and psychodynamic aspects

The following are two quite similar models that underlie relatively recently introduced therapies for borderline personality disorder.

Cognitive-analytical model (p. 792) Borderline patients experience a range of partially dissociated 'self-states', which arise initially as a response to unmanageable external threats and are maintained by repeated threats or internal cues (such as memories). Abusive experiences in childhood lead to internalisation of the harsh parental object leading to intrapsychic conflict which is repressed or produces symptomatic behaviours. Deficits in self-reflection, poor emotional vocabulary, and narrow focus of attention lead to incoherent sense of self and others.

Dialectical behavioural model (p. 794) Innate temperamental vulnerability interacts with certain dysfunctional ('invalidating') environments leading to problems with emotional regulation. Abnormal behaviours which are manifested represent products of this emotional dysregulation or attempts to regulate intense emotional states by maladaptive problem solving.

Epidemiology of personality disorder[1]

The measurement of the prevalence of personality disorder of any type and of specific categories of personality disorder in any population has a number of problems: in earlier studies personality disorder and other mental disorders were mutually exclusive, not allowing for the recording of comorbidity; studies differ in the method used to make a diagnosis (interviews/case-notes/informants; clinical diagnosis versus research instruments; emphasis on current presentation or on life history); and in some studies subjects were only allowed to belong to one category of personality disorder.

Findings regarding personality disorder of any type will be considered separately from findings related to specific personality disorder categories.

Personality disorder of any type

Community Rates of personality disorder in the community have been found to be 2–18% (the generally accepted approximate is 10%). It is more prevalent in younger adults, and may be more prevalent in males.

Primary care Of patients presenting with conspicous psychiatric morbididty, 5–8% will have a primary diagnosis of personality disorder. The rate of comorbid personality disorder in patients with other primary diagnoses is 20–30%.

Psychiatric patients 30–40% of outpatients and 40–50% of inpatients have a personality disorder, not usually as a primary diagnosis. A primary diagnosis of personality disorder occurs in about 5–15% of inpatients.

Other populations 25–75% of prisoners have a personality disorder. Antisocial personality disorder is most prevalent, but many prisoners fulfil the criteria for more than one diagnostic category, and many personality disordered prisoners do not meet the criteria for the antisocial category.

Specific categories of personality disorder

The prevalence rates of the categories of personality disorder (most studies have used DSM categories, so these are used here) in the general population are approximately:

DSM-IV	Prevalence
Paranoid	0.5–3%
Schizoid	0.5–7%
Schizotypal	0.5–5%
Antisocial	2–3.5%
Borderline	1.5–2%
Histrionic	2–3%
Narcissistic	0.5–1%
Avoidant	0.5–1%
Dependent	0.5–5%
Obsessive-compulsive	1–2%

1 Casey P (2000) The epidemiology of personality disorder. In *Personality disorders: diagnosis, management and cause* (ed. Tyrer P). Oxford: Butterworth Heinemann.

Relationship between personality disorder and other mental disorders

The current state of classification and understanding of the aetiology and pathogenesis of mental disorders is such that most psychiatric diagnoses are based on descriptive criteria. It is common to find that an individual meets the criteria for an axis I disorder along with a personality disorder. At one extreme, both may be a manifestation of the same underlying condition; at the other, they may represent two completely separate aetio-pathogenic entities.

The relationship between personality disorder and other mental disorders may be:

- *Mutually exclusive* Personality disorder cannot be diagnosed in an individual with another mental disorder. The personality pathology displayed is a manifestation of the other mental disorder, and giving a separate personality diagnosis has no purpose. This was the only approach possible prior to DSM-III's introduction of multi-axial diagnosis. This approach is not favoured by current classification systems, even where the two appear to be manifestations of the same condition.
- *Coincidental* In an individual, personality disorder and another disorder may come together by chance. However, epidemiologically there is support for an association between personality disorder and other mental disorders.
- *Associative* Both in individual cases and epidemiologically there are a number of reasons why the coexistence of personality disorder and other mental disorders may be more than just coincidental:
  - Sharing common aetiology (but separate disorder)
  - Prodromal (part of the development of the axis I disorder)
  - Part of a spectrum (a 'partial' manifestation of the axis I disorder)
  - Vulnerability (a separate disorder, manifestations of which make an individual more likely to suffer from an axis I disorder)

Problems in assessing personality in patients with other mental disorders

A number of problems may arise in the diagnosis of personality disorder in people who appear to have axis I disorders:

- Underlying personality disorder may be missed as assessment may focus on the current mental state disorder.
- Personality disorder may be misdiagnosed as axis I disorder and vice versa.
- In an individual with personality disorder, an axis I disorder may be missed or misconstrued as being part of the personality disorder.

In such cases it is important to remember that axis I pathology is common in people with personality disorders and any change in the presentation of a patient with personality disorder may be due to this. Equally, it is important to base assessment of personality on information (preferably from a number of sources) on the pre-morbid functioning of an individual, rather than on their current functioning or just their own account of their previous functioning (their memory or interpretation of which may be coloured by their current mental state).

Comorbidity between personality disorders and other specific mental disorders[1]

Strong associations

- Avoidant personality disorder and social phobia (possibly because they both describe a group of people with the same condition).
- Substance misuse and cluster B personality disorders.
- Eating disorders and cluster B and C personality disorders (particularly bulimia nervosa and cluster B).
- Neurotic disorders and cluster C personality disorders (it has been suggested that these individuals have a 'general neurotic syndrome').
- Somatoform disorders and cluster B and C personality disorders.
- Habit and impulse disorders and cluster B personality disorders (unsurprisingly).
- PTSD and borderline personality disorder (this is not borderline personality disorder redefined as chronic PTSD, but is probably due to the increased rate of life events and vulnerability of such individuals).

Moderate associations

- Schizotypal personality disorder and schizophrenia (also a weaker association between schizophrenia and antisocial personality disorder).
- Depression and cluster B and C personality disorders.
- Delusional disorder and paranoid personality disorder.

Impact of personality disorders on manifestation, treatment, and outcome of other mental disorders

Although the concept of 'comorbid personality disorder' may seem spurious from an aetio-pathological perspective, its presence has an impact on the presentation, treatment, and outcome of axis I disorders, and it is therefore useful to recognise such comorbidity from a clinical perspective.

- **Presentation** The presentation of axis I disorders may be distorted, exaggerated, or masked by the presence of an underlying personality disorder.
- **Treatment and outcome** The presence of comorbid personality disorder will usually make treatment more difficult and worsens the outcome of axis I disorders. This may be due to problems in the following areas:help-seeking behaviours, compliance with treatment, coping styles, risk-taking, lifestyle, social support networks, therapeutic alliance, alcohol and substance misuse.

Some contend that it is the presence of this comorbidity which makes it more likely for a person to fail to respond to standard primary care treatment approaches, therefore necessitating referral to psychiatric services.

1 Tyrer P (2000) Comorbidity of personality disorder and mental state disorders. In *Personality disorders: diagnosis, management and cause* (ed. Tyrer P). Oxford: Butterworth Heinemann.

Assessment of personality disorder[1]

Potential pitfalls

There are a number of potential pitfalls in the assessment and diagnosis of personality disordered patients:

- Relying on diagnoses made by others (psychiatrists are notoriously poor at diagnosing personality disorder).
- Failing to recognise comorbidity.
- Misdiagnosing personality disorder as mental illness and vice versa.
- Inadequate information.
- Negative counter-transference (basing diagnosis on your negative reaction to a patient rather than on an objective assessment; transference and countertransference may be a part of this but negative feelings towards an individual should not be the primary basis for a diagnosis of personality disorder).
- Applying ICD-10 or DSM-IV categories without a broader assessment of personality.

Making the diagnosis of personality disorder

- A clinical diagnosis of personality disorder should be based on an accurate assessment of a person's enduring and pervasive patterns of emotional expression, interpersonal relationships, social functioning, and views of self and others *when they are not suffering from another mental disorder.*
- In many cases information from *sources* other than the patient will be essential. Potential sources of information include:clinical interviews (perhaps repeated); observation (usually repeated); previous records (medical, prison, school, social work); independent accounts (perhaps from several sources such as relatives and other professionals).
- Information from various areas of the *psychiatric history* (childhood and adolescence; work record; forensic history/other aggression or violence; relationship history; psychiatric contact/self-harm) will give an indication of a person's personality and whether it may be disordered.
- In addition, specific enquiry can be made regarding the following aspects of *personality*:interests and activities; relationships; mood/emotions; attitudes (religious, moral, health); self-concept; coping with difficulties; specific characteristics or traits (perhaps based on personality disorder categories); include both positive and negative aspects.
- In describing personality and personality disorder, first the features of a person's personality should be described, then a decision should be made as to whether the degree of distress and disruption due to personality traits is such as to indicate the presence of personality disorder, then the features that are pathological should be described. If one wants to make categorical diagnoses then the category or categories for which the criteria are met may be stated.

Instruments to assess personality disorder

There are a number of instruments available for assessing personality disorder. Such instruments are mainly used in research and are rarely seen in clinical practice. Most require training and some take a considerable amount of time to complete.

Self-report questionnaires Millon Clinical Multiaxial Inventory (MCMI), Personality Disorder Questionnaire (PDQ-IV), Wisconsin Personality Inventory (WISPI)

Structured clinical interviews with patient only Structured Clinical Interview for DSM-IV Personality Disorder (SCID-II), Diagnostic Interview for DSM-IV Personality Disorders (DIPD-IV)

Structured clinical interviews with informant only Standardized Assessment of Personality (SAP)

Structured clinical interviews with patient and/or informant Personality Assessment Schedule (PAS), Structured Interview for DSM-IV Personality Disorders (SIDP-IV), International Personality Disorder Examination (IPDE)

Instruments assessing specific personality disorders Schedule for Interviewing Borderlines (SIB), Diagnostic Interview for Borderline Patients (DIB), Borderline Personality Disorder Scale (BPD-Scale), Psychopathy Checklist-Revised (PCL-R), Psychopathy Checklist-Screening Version (PCL-SV), Schedule for Schizotypal Personalities (SSP).

Diagnostic instruments including an assessment of antisocial personality disorder Diagnostic Interview Schedule (DIS), Feigner Diagnostic Criteria.

Functional assessment

The functional assessment of personality and associated problems has been proposed as a useful clinical approach which can produce a formulation identifying issues to be addressed in management.
• **List abnormal personality traits**—thoughts about self and others (e.g. identity problems, paranoia, grandiosity, magical thinking, exaggerating, suggestibility, preoccupation with death, obsessionality, self-esteem), feelings and emotions (e.g. depression, elation, mood instability, callousness, loneliness, anger, irritability), behaviour (e.g. stubbornness, quarrelsomeness, sadism, self-destructiveness, compliance, impulsivity, theatricality, attention seeking), social functioning (e.g. social isolation, controlling others, dependence on others, mistrust of others, inviting rejection, forming unstable intense relationships, manipulating and using others), insight (including the ability to understand and integrate one's thoughts, feelings and actions).
• **Describe associated distress and comorbid axis I disorders.**
• **Describe interference with functioning**—occupational, family and relationships, offending/violence.

---

1 Gunn J (2000) Personality disorder: a clinical suggestion. In *Personality disorders: diagnosis, management and cause* (ed. Tyrer P). Oxford: Butterworth Heinemann.

Management of personality disorder (1)—general aspects

It is generally felt that personality disorder is resistant to specific psychiatric treatment. However, there is no good evidence to either refute or support this statement. Patients often present at a time of crisis and/or when they develop a comorbid axis I disorder. Although some may wish to, psychiatrists cannot avoid having to manage patients with personality disorder.

Principles of successful management plans

A successful management plan in personality disorder is tailored to the individual's needs and explicitly states jointly agreed and realistic goals. The approach to these patients should be consistent and agreed across the services having contact with the patient. Plans should take a long-term view, recognising that change, if it comes, will only be observable over a long period.

Possible management goals

Potential management goals include: psychological and practical support; monitoring and supervision; intervening in crises; increasing motivation and compliance; increasing understanding of difficulties; building a therapeutic relationship; limiting harm; reducing distress; treating comorbid axis I disorders; treating specific areas (e.g. anger, self-harm, social skills); and giving practical support (e.g. housing, finance, child care).

Managing comorbid axis I disorders

It is important to recognise and treat comorbid axis I pathology in patients with personality disorder. Standard treatment approaches should be used, taking into account aspects of the patient's personality (e.g. impulsivity and an anti-authoritarian attitude may lead to non-compliance with medication).

Understanding and managing the relationship between the patient and staff[2]

Rejection for treatment of patients with personality disorder (even when they present with mental illness) is often due to the intense negative feelings these patients may engender, and the disruptive and uneasy relationships they form with those that try to help them. Just as they do in many of their interpersonal relationships, patients with personality disorders display disordered attachment in their relationships with staff (whether with individuals or with a service). When dealing with such patients this needs to be recognised, acknowledged, and managed. An acceptance of, and tolerance for these difficulties needs to be combined with continuing commitment to the patient. However, patients, staff, and other agencies need to realise there are no instant solutions and that psychiatric services cannot take responsibility for all adverse behaviours.

Admission to hospital

Patients with personality disorder benefit little from prolonged admissions to conventional psychiatric units. Admission to such units may be necessary when there is a specific crisis (usually in the short term) or the patient presents with an axis I disorder. Longer-term admission for the treatment of personality disorder could be undertaken in a therapeutic community. Involuntary long-term hospitalisation of patients with personality disorder primarily to prevent harm to others where there is little prospect of clinical benefit to the patient is ethically dubious.

Managing crises

Individuals with personality disorder often present in crisis. This may follow life events, relationship problems, or occur in the context of the development of comorbid mental illness. In some cases the crisis may follow what appears to the outside observer to be a relatively minor or non-existent stressor. Where patients repeatedly present in crisis it can be helpful for the various professionals involved to plan what the response should be in such situations. A consistent response is important, but there should be sufficient flexibility to deal with changes in circumstances. For example, where a patient repeatedly presents with self-harm it may be appropriate for outpatient treatment to continue following any necessary medical treatment; however, if this patient presents threatening suicide following the death of a partner, then it may be appropriate to arrange admission to hospital. Other approaches to individuals presenting with threats of self-harm or of violence and to manipulative patients are covered on pp. 902–5.

1 Davison SE (2002) Principles of managing patients with personality disorder. *Advances in Psychiatric Treatment* **8:** 1–9.

2 Adshead G (1998) Psychiatric staff as attachment figures. Understanding management problems in psychiatric services in the light of attachment theory. *BJP* **172,** 64–9.

Management of personality disorder (2)—specific treatments[1,2]

Medication[3]

The main indication for medication in patients with personality disorder is the development of comorbid mental illness. There is no good evidence that medication has any effect on personality disorder itself. The positive findings from studies have been short-term, and probably due to the effects of medication on comorbid disorders rather than on the personality disorder itself. Bearing this in mind, the following have been suggested:

- **Antipsychotics** may be of some benefit in cluster B (particularly borderline) and cluster A (particularly schizotypal and perhaps paranoid) disorders.
- **Antidepressants** may be of benefit in impulsive, depressed, or self-harming patients (particularly borderline), and in cluster C (particularly avoidant and obsessive-compulsive) disorders.
- **Anticonvulsants and lithium** have been suggested where there is affective instability or impulsivity.

Therapeutic community

A therapeutic community is a consciously designed social environment and programme within a residential or day unit, in which the social and group process is harnessed with therapeutic intent. It is an intense form of psychosocial treatment in which every aspect of the environment is part of the treatment setting, in which interpersonal behaviour can be challenged and modified. The main principles are democratisation, permissiveness, communalism, and reality confrontation. There are various interactions between patients and staff both individually and in groups, particularly in the daily community groups, which contribute towards achieving these principles. There is some evidence that such treatment is effective with some patients with personality disorders.

Dialectical behavioural therapy (DBT) (p. 794)

Combination of individual and group therapy lasting at least 12 months. In stage 1, individual therapy focuses on a detailed cognitive-behavioural approach to self-harm and other 'therapy interfering' behaviours. Internal and external antecedents are explored, and alternative problem-solving strategies are developed. Group therapy focuses on tolerance of distress, emotional regulation and interpersonal skills. 'Mindfulness training' based on Eastern meditation techniques is a key part of this. In stage 2, patients are helped to process previous trauma, but only when stage 1 skills are developed. In stage 3, the focus is on developing self-esteem and realistic future goals. Another aspect of DBT is that patients may contact therapists by telephone between sessions to help them apply skills when difficulties arise. There is evidence that DBT may be an effective therapy for outpatients with borderline personality disorder.

Cognitive-analytic therapy (pp. 792–3)

May be appropriate for some patients with borderline personality disorder. Aims to identify different 'self states' and associated 'reciprocal role procedures' (patterns of relationships learned in early childhood). Patients are helped to observe and change thinking and behaviour related to these 'self states'. Countertransference helps provide useful information about 'reciprocal role relationships' either through identification with the patient or reacting to their projections. The aim is for patients to be able to recognise their various 'self states' and to be aware of them without dissociating.

Psychodynamic therapy (pp. 776–81)

Classic Freudian or Jungian psychoanalysis is of no proven benefit for patients with personality disorder, and is probably contraindicated in patients with severe personality disorders. However, psychodynamic concepts are extremely useful in understanding personality disordered patients and the reactions they provoke in others, including ourselves. Modified psychodynamic approaches for patients with borderline and narcissistic personality disorders have been developed.

Cognitive-behavioural therapy (pp. 786–7)

Schema-focused therapy concentrates on identifying and modifying early maladaptive schemas and related behaviours. Patients are educated about schemas and led to expect that they will be difficult to change (for example, patients will distort new information to fit in with their existing schemas). 'Empathic confrontation' is used to help patients to repeatedly and persistently challenge their core beliefs about themselves and others. Issues related to interpersonal schemas may arise in the therapeutic relationship and be used as 'data' for dealing with these schemas.

There are other models used in cognitive-behavioural therapy to treat personality disorder, but all have in common: the goal-directed problem-solving approach; the teaching of specific skills; a longer time-scale than the relatively brief length of therapy for most other disorders; emphasis on developing, maintaining, and utilising the therapeutic relationship; a focus on underlying core beliefs (schemas) regarding self and others; and, a longer-term historical perspective in therapy as opposed to the here-and-now focus with many other disorders.

1 Davidson K and Tyrer P (2000) Psychosocial treatment in personality disorder. In *Personality disorders: diagnosis, management and cause* (ed. Tyrer P). Oxford: Butterworth Heinemann.

2 Deary I and Power M (1998) Normal and abnormal personality. In *Companion to Psychiatric Studies* (eds. Johnstone EC, Freeman CPL, Zeally AK). Edinburgh: Churchill Livingstone.

3 Tyrer P (2000) Drug treatment of personality disorder. In *Personality disorders: diagnosis, management and cause* (ed. Tyrer P). Oxford: Butterworth Heinemann.

Outcome of personality disorder[1]

Morbidity and mortality

High rates of accidents, suicide, and violent death, particularly where cluster B features are prominent. As mentioned already, there are high rates of other mental disorders (see p. 454).

Outcome of other disorders in patients with personality disorder

The outcome of mental illness and physical illness is worse in patients with personality disorders. The potential reasons for this are covered on p. 455.

Persistence of personality disorder

Some contend that personality disorder is by definition life-long and there-fore has a poor prognosis, but the evidence for this is far from conclusive.

Comparison between different age groups

Personality disorder is less prevalent in older adults than younger adults, particularly for cluster B disorders. In terms of 'normal' personality, compared with young adults the elderly are more likely to be cautious and rigid, and less likely to be impulsive and aggressive. However, cross-sectional studies looking at different age groups at one point in time tell us little about the development of personality in individuals over time.

Follow-up of individuals over time

Antisocial/dissocial Children presenting to child services with antisocial behaviour are 5–7 times as likely to develop antisocial personality disorder as those presenting with other problems. May show some improvement in antisocial behaviour by fifth decade. However, may just change with time from 'overt' criminal behaviour to more 'covert' antisocial behaviour such as domestic violence and child abuse. There is contra-dictory evidence as to whether 'burn-out' or 'maturation' in later life really does occur.

Borderline A third to a half of patients fulfilling the criteria for borderline personality disorder do not have personality disorder at all when followed up after 10–20 years. About a third continue to have borderline personality disorder and others have other predominating personality disorders. Poor prognostic indicators are severe repeated self-harm and 'comorbid' antisocial personality; a good prognostic indicator may be an initial presentation with comorbid affective disorder.

Schizotypal Generally have poorer prognosis than borderline patients. About 50% may develop schizophrenia.

Obsessional May worsen with age. More likely to develop depression than OCD.

Clusters There is some evidence that cluster A traits worsen with age, cluster B traits improve, and cluster C traits remain unchanged.

---

1 Tyrer P and Seivewright H (2000) Outcome of personality disorder. In *Personality disorders: diagnosis, management and cause* (ed. Tyrer P). Oxford: Butterworth Heinemann.

Disorders of sexual preference (1)—general aspects[1]

Essence

Disorders of sexual preference (the term used in ICD-10) or paraphilias (the term used in DSM-IV) are disorders in which an individual is sexually aroused by inappropriate stimuli. Other terms used include sexual deviation and perversion. There is some overlap between these disorders, sex offending, and inappropriate sexual behaviour, but the three are separate concepts (see p. 636). Homosexuality was previously included, but this is no longer the case.

Disorders of sexual preference are one of three broad types of sexual disorders. The others are gender identity disorders and sexual dysfunctions (see opposite). In some cases two or more of these are present.

Definition

DSM-IV defines each paraphilia as at least 6 months of recurrent, intense, sexually arousing fantasies, sexual urges, or behaviours involving a particular inappropriate act or object. These fantasies, urges, or behaviours must cause clinically significant distress or impairment in social functioning. ICD-10 has less strict and less detailed criteria, referring to the particular object or act as being the most important source of sexual arousal or essential for satisfactory sexual response.

Classification

There are many different objects and acts that may be the focus of disorders of sexual preference. Most of the defined categories are extreme forms of behaviours that are common parts of 'normal' sexual activity. The classification systems in DSM-IV and ICD-10 are very similar (see opposite). A disorder of sexual preference may be present in addition to other mental disorders.

Aetiology

Physiological factors These may include genetic factors, prenatal influence of hormones in utero, hormonal abnormalities in adults, and perhaps brain abnormalities.

Psychological theories These include absence of effective father with over-protective/close binding/intimate mother; failure of successful resolution of oedipal conflict; modelling and conditioning; masculine insecurity.

The various factors may lead to sexual deviation by (a) preventing normal sexual development and relationships, and/or (b) promoting deviant sexual interest.

Epidemiology

It is difficult to estimate the prevalence of these disorders as many individuals do not present for help and are unlikely to admit to sexually deviant

1 Abel GG and Osborn CA (2000) The paraphilias. In *New Oxford Textbook of Psychiatry* (eds. Gelder MG, López-Ibor, Andreasen N). Oxford: Oxford University Press.

arousal in surveys. Rates of sexual offending do not give a good approximation of rates of disorders of sexual preference, as these disorders represent one of many factors that may lead to such offending (see p. 636). There is probably a wide range of sexual practices in the 'normal' population. Disorders of sexual preference are more common in males than females (perhaps 30 times more common). From clinical samples, age of onset is usually between 16 and 20, and many individuals have multiple paraphilias, in series and/or in parallel.

Classification of disorders of sexual preference

ICD-10	DSM-IV	Sexually arousing object or act
Fetishism	Fetishism	Non-living object (e.g. clothing, shoes, rubber).
Fetishistic transvestism	Transvestic fetishism	Cross-dressing (not few articles but complete outfit, perhaps with wig and make-up). Clear association with sexual arousal distinguishes from transsexual tranvestism. However, may be an early phase in some transsexuals.
Exhibitionism	Exhibitionism	Exposure of genitals to strangers.
Voyeurism	Voyeurism	Watching others who are naked, disrobing, or engaging in sexual acts.
Paedophilia	Paedophilia	Children (usually prebubertal or early pubertal). May be specified as attracted to males, females, or both, or as limited to incest.
Sadomasochism	Sexual masochism	Being humiliated, beaten, bound, or made to suffer.
	Sexual sadism	Psychological or physical suffering of others.
—	Frotteurism	Touching and rubbing against non-consenting person.
Other disorders of sexual preference	Paraphilia not otherwise specified	Includes telephone scatalogia (obscene phone calls), necrophilia (corpses), partialism (exclusive focus on part of body), zoophilia (animals), coprophilia (faeces), urophilia (urine), klismaphilia (enemas), autoerotic asphyxia (self asphyxiation).
Multiple disorders of sexual preference	—	Many individuals manifest multiple disorders. Term 'polymorphous perversity' has been used. Most common combination is fetishism, transvestism, and sadomasochism.

Disorders of sexual preference (2)—assessment and management[1]

Assessment

Why is the person presenting now?

• May present directly or at request of spouse when behaviour is discovered or starts to cause problems in relationships. Occasionally present as sexual dysfunction, with disorder of preference coming to light on further assessment.

• May present at own request, or more likely at request of court, prosecutor, or solicitor, after committing offence.

Is there another mental disorder?

Various psychiatric disorders may lead to release of sexually deviant behaviour, perhaps in individuals who have experienced fantasies but not acted on them previously. Particularly important to exclude in someone presenting for first time in middle age or later. So full psychiatric history, MSE, and perhaps neurological examination/investigation important.

Psycho-sexual assessment

Full psycho-sexual assessment essential in anyone presenting with sexual problems. Interviewer should put person at ease and be able to facilitate by being open, sensitive, and able to discuss sexual matters. Involvement of sexual partner in assessment (either at the same time or through another interview) is usually helpful. Following areas should be covered: • *Sexual knowledge* and sources of information • *Sexual attitudes* to self and others • Age of onset and development of *sexual interest, masturbation,* dating, *sexual intercourse* • *Relationship history*, including: age of self and partner, gender of partners, duration, quality, problems, abuse • *Fantasy* (content/use/development) • *Orientation* • *Drive* (frequency of masturbation/intercourse) and *dysfunction* (specific inquiry about arousal, impotence, premature ejaculation) • *Experience* (range of sexual behaviours with specific enquiry about paraphilias) • *Current sexual practices*: mood, thoughts, visual images, material used, and conditions for arousal during both intercourse and masturbation (many men with paraphilias report 'normal' intercourse although at the time they are imagining deviant scenarios); where various forms of arousal are reported estimate proportion of sexual practice devoted to each.

What does the person want from treatment?

• Do they want help at all or have they just come as they have been forced to (by spouse, courts, etc.)?

• Do they want to change the focus of their sexual arousal and/or desist from the overt behaviour?

• Do they want to adapt better to the behaviour without changing it?

• Are they motivated to engage in treatment?

Further investigations

Physical examination and investigations may be indicated, particularly if sexual dysfunction coexists. Penile plethysmography, polygraphy, and visual reaction times may be useful in assessing paraphilias.

Management
General issues
Treatment should not be imposed on people who do not want it. Patients should realise that treatment will take considerable effort on their part. The aims of treatment should be clear from the beginning. Broadly, there are three possible aims:
• Better adjustment without changing the behaviour.
• Desisting from overtly problematic behaviour but retaining 'deviant' arousal.
• Changing the focus of the arousal.

Where treatment is aimed at change, the following may need to be addressed:
• Encouraging development of 'normal' relationships.
• Addressing sexual inadequacy (perhaps using approaches similar to those for sexual dysfunction).
• Develop interests, activities, and relationships that will fill the time previously taken up by fantasising about, preparing for, and taking part in the deviant activity.
• Decreasing masturbation to deviant fantasies and encouraging masturbation to more appropriate fantasies.

Specific treatment approaches
Physical treatments Neurosurgery and bilateral orchidectomy ('castration') of historical interest only. Various medications have been used: antipsychotics, oestrogens, progestogens, luteinising-hormone releasing analogue, antiandrogens, and SSRIs. There is evidence for the efficacy of cyproterone acetate (an antiandrogen) and medroxyprogesterone acetate (a progestogen) in the treatment of hypersexuality and paraphilias. Recently, SSRIs have been used increasingly, and some use them first-line due to their relative lack of side-effects.

Psychodynamic psychotherapy Individual and group approaches have been used, ranging from sophisticated psychoanalysis to primarily supportive therapy.

Cognitive-behavioural therapy Specific techniques may be used to decrease deviant (covert sensitisation, aversive therapy, masturbatory satiation, biofeedback) and increase 'normal' arousal (orgasmic reconditioning, shaping, fading, exposure to explicit stimuli, biofeedback, systematic desensitisation). Controversially used to treat homosexuality until the 1970s. Social skills training, assertiveness training, sexual education, and relapse prevention can also be helpful. Addressing cognitive distortions regarding sex, women, or children may also be important.

1 Brockman B and Bluglass R (1996) A general psychiatric approach to sexual deviation. In *Sexual Deviation* (ed. Rosen I). Oxford: Oxford University Press.

Old age psychiatry

Psychiatric illness in older people and psychogeriatrics

Psychogeriatrics, or old age psychiatry, is a new specialty which has arisen over the last 40 years in response to demographic changes and the growth of geriatric medicine. It was inspired by the 'social psychiatry' movement and growing emphasis on the care and welfare of vulnerable sectors of the population.

Psychiatric illnesses in older people include:

- Pre-existing psychiatric disorders in the ageing patient
- New disorders related to the specific stresses and circumstances of old age (e.g. bereavement, infirmity, dependence, sensory deficits, isolation)
- Disorders due to the changing physiology of the ageing brain, as well as psychiatric complications of neurological and systemic illnesses

Psychiatric problems often coexist with physical problems, and treatment strategies need to take account of this (as well as the different pharmacokinetics of the older patient). Furthermore, the elderly are more likely to manifest physical symptoms of psychiatric disorder than younger adults. Cognitive assessment and physical examination are always essential parts of psychiatric management of the older person. Dementia is generally the main focus of interest in psychogeriatrics, but the discipline also concerns itself with depressive illness, paranoid states, and other late-onset problems.

Since older people are often dependent on others, consideration of the role and the needs of carers are important aspects of holistic care. Psychiatric care of the elderly interfaces with multiple services, both state and independent (e.g. social services, housing and welfare services, the legal system, charity organisations, and religious institutions).

The demographics of old age

In developed countries such as the UK, the elderly population has been increasing steadily over the last century. For example, in the UK the percentage of the population older than 65 yrs was 5% in 1900, is 15% in 2003, and is projected to be 24% in 2034[1]. This trend is largely attributed to the decline in infant mortality, control of infectious diseases, and improvement in sanitation, living standards, and nutrition as well as a declining birth rate. The implications of increasing elderly people in society are many, including a drop in the proportion of the working population, an increase in overall disability and health needs, and a corresponding increase in the need for both health and social services.

In terms of psychiatric disorders, it is well known that certain disorders increase in frequency with advancing age. For example, 5% of people older than 65 yrs suffer from moderate to severe dementia and the prevalence increases to over 30% of those over 85 yrs[2]. The prevalence of other disorders in people >65 yrs is approximately: 1.1% for schizophrenia; 1.4% for bipolar disorder; and 12.5% for neurosis and personality disorder[3]. Other research has shown a particularly high prevalence of mental disorder among numbers of elderly people in sheltered accommodation (~30% in old age homes have cognitive impairment) and in hospital (30–50% patients >65 yrs in general hospital wards have psychiatric disorder)[4]. Finally, it is regrettably the case that psychiatric disorders are commonly either undiagnosed or misdiagnosed at primary care level. Having said this, research has demonstrated a marked improvement over the last decade in both diagnosis and management at this level.

The role of the old age psychiatrist[5]

- **Advocate** Together with various pressure groups, the old age psychiatrist (OAP) is an active proponent of the interests of the elderly, whether it comes to sourcing funding or providing education to the public in an effort to dispel the stigma attached to ageing.
- **Teacher** The OAP is well placed to provide education in both medical and non-medical contexts. Medical and nursing students, across-discipline specialists and trainees, school pupils, community forum and service organisers may all benefit from the expertise of the OAP.
- **Health educationalist/promoter** Holistic care of the elderly includes both health education and preventative intervention.
- **Student** Psychogeriatrics is a major arena of new research, while the changing demography of ageing requires the OAP to make academic forays into other disciplines such as sociology, history, and human geography.
- **Innovator** The relative infancy of the discipline means that individuals working in this area have had the opportunity to be creative and innovative in developing appropriate services.
- **Team player** The multidisciplinary nature of old age psychiatry means that the OAP engages with professionals and lay people both in the community and in institutions.
- **'Missionary'** The concept and practice of psychogeriatrics originated in the UK and was spread to North America, Australia, and the rest of Europe by a core of zealots. A number of international organisations have formed and the global challenges for the 21st Century include expanding the discipline within developing countries as well as finding new strategies for caring for the growing numbers of elderly people within the first world.

1 Butler R and Brayne C (1998) Epidemiology In: *Seminars in Old Age Psychiatry* Eds: Butler R and Pitt B. Gaskell, London.

2 Jorm AF, Korten AE, Henderson AS (1987) The prevalence of dementia: a quantitative integration of the literature. *Acta Psychiatrica Scandinavia* **76**, 465–79.

3 Kay DW, Beamish P, Roth M (1964) Old age mental disorders in Newcastle upon Tyne. I. A study of prevalence. *British Journal of Psychiatry* **110**, 146–58.

4 Mayou RA and Hawton KE (1986) Psychiatric disorder in the general hospital. *British Journal of Psychiatry* **149**, 172–90.

5 Jolley D (1999) The importance of being an old age psychiatrist. In: *Everything you need to know about old age psychiatry…* Ed. R Howard. Wrightson Biomedical Publishing Ltd.

Normal ageing[1]

Neurobiology of ageing

- The **weight** and **volume** of the brain decreases by 5% between ages 30 and 70 yrs, by 10% by the age of 80, and by 20% by the age of 90. There is a proportionate increase in **ventricular size** and size of the **subarachnoid space**.
- **MRI** shows ↓cortical grey matter with little change to white matter.
- **CBF** in frontal and temporal lobes and thalamus decreases with age.
- There is some **nerve cell loss** in the cortex, hippocampus, substantia nigra, and purkinje cells of the cerebellum. There may also be reduction in **dendritic processes**. The cytoplasm of nerve cells accumulates a pigment, (**lipofuscin**), while there are also changes in the components of the cytoskeleton.
- **Tau protein** (links neurofilaments and microtubules) can accumulate to form **neuro-fibrillary tangles (NFTs)** in some nerve cells. In normal ageing NFTs are usually confined to cells of the hippocampus and entorhinal cortex.
- **Senile plaques** (extra-cellular amyloid and neuritic processes) are found in the normal ageing brain in the neocortex, amygdala, hippocampus, and entorhinal cortex.
- **Lewy bodies** (intra-cellular inclusions) occur normally and are confined to the substantia nigra and the locus coeruleus.
- **Hirano bodies** (rod-shaped actin) occur in new hippocampal pyramidal cells.
- **Amyloid deposits** (β-amyloid and A4 amyloid) may be widespread in superficial cortical and leptomeningeal vessels as well as patchy within the cortex.

Psychology of ageing

- **Cognitive assessment** is often complicated by physical illness or sensory deficits.
- **IQ** peaks at 25 yrs, plateaus until 60–70, and then declines.
- **Performance IQ** drops faster than *verbal IQ*, which may be due to reduced processing speed or to the fact that verbal IQ depends largely on familiar 'crystallised' information while performance IQ involves novel, fluid information.
- **Problem solving** deteriorates due to declining abstract ability and increasing difficulty applying information to another situation.
- **Short-term memory (STM)** does not alter with age. However, **working memory (WM)** shows a gradual decrease in capacity and this is worse with ↑complexity of task and ↑memory load.
- **Long-term memory (LTM)** declines, except for remote events of personal significance which may be recalled with great clarity.
- There is a characteristic pattern of **psychomotor slowing** and impairment in the manipulation of new information.
- Tests of well-rehearsed skills such as **verbal comprehension** show little or no decline.

Social problems of old age

With the breakdown of traditions and family structures in many societies, increasing numbers of elderly live alone or in homes for the aged. Losses include: loss of status, loss of independence, and loss of spouse/partner. Most elderly have limited income and are unemployed. Increase in medical problems compounds the dependency and care needs. The elderly face variable degrees of isolation, marginalisation, and stigmatisation.

1 Gelder M, Gath D, Mayou R, Cowen P (1996) *Oxford Textbook of Psychiatry*, 3rd Edition, Oxford University Press, Oxford.

Multidisciplinary assessment

Elderly people suffering from mental health problems often have a range of psychological, physical, and social needs. This implies that individual assessment, management, and follow-up requires collaboration between health, social, and voluntary organisations and family carers. Assessment of the older patient with mental illness includes the following:

- Full history from the patient, family, and carers
- Full physical and neurological examination
- MSE, including full cognitive assessment
- Functional assessment (evaluation of ability to perform functions of everyday living)
- Social assessment (accommodation; need for care; financial and legal issues; social activities)
- Assessment of carers' needs

The best place for performing an assessment is in the patient's home. A domiciliary visit has the advantage of being more convenient and relaxing for the patient and it provides the health carer with an opportunity to assess living conditions, social activities, and medications kept in the house. In addition, family members, neighbours, and carers may be available for interviewing. A follow-up visit to the day hospital may be required in order to perform physical examination and medical investigations. Sometimes brief admission is indicated, especially if the elderly person has pressing physical or psychiatric needs or if support is unavailable (or desperately needs respite). Obviously a full assessment may involve doctors, nurses, occupational therapists, psychologists, social workers, voluntary workers, legal professionals, and others involved with the elderly.

In obtaining a thorough history it is important to allow the patient to tell their own story. One needs to enquire about the presenting problem and how it has evolved, whether it is a new or longstanding problem, and whether the individual has a personal or family history of mental problems. In addition, enquire about losses, social history, and social circumstances (housing, income, social activities, etc), medical problems and medications, alcohol history, and presence or absence of family support and carers. It is particularly important to assess activities of daily living such as level of independence, ability to cook, shop, pay accounts, maintain the home, and cope with bathing, toilet, laundry, etc.

MSE needs to include an assessment of sight and hearing as well as determining the presence or absence of anxiety or mood symptoms, suicidality, abnormal beliefs or perceptions, and cognitive impairment. Cognitive assessment must include: orientation; memory; concentration and attention; language, praxis, and simple calculation; intelligence; insight; and judgement. An MMSE will incorporate these elements (see p. 66). There is a wide range of rating scales for assessing mental state, cognitive performance, activities of daily living, and carer burden—see Burns et al [1] (2002) for an overview.

Key questions for carers include:[2]

- Relationship to the patient
- Amount of care provided
- Degree of stress they are under
- What help they would accept
- Understanding and knowledge of the patient's illness
- What expectations they have from services
- Their awareness of support or voluntary organisations

1 Burns A, Lawlor B, Craig S (2002) Rating scales in old age psychiatry. *BJP* **180**, 161–7.

2 Butler R and Pitt B (1998) Assessment. In: *Seminars in Old Age Psychiatry* Ed. R Butler and B Pitt. Gaskell.

Specific aspects of psychiatric illnesses in the elderly (1)—overview and neuroses

Overview

The range of psychiatric illnesses in the elderly is very similar to that in younger people. However, the individual factors that contribute to aetiology, clinical presentation, and management strategy differ due to the specific biopsychosocial conditions of old age. In order to grasp a full understanding of elderly psychopathology it is necessary to appreciate the physiological, psychological, and socio-cultural factors unique to this age group. Disorders in the elderly may present with some 'classic' symptoms (common to adult psychopathology), but very often their clinical manifestation varies significantly due to the unique conditions of old age. The following pages focus on the 'unique' features of psychiatric illnesses in the elderly.

Neuroses

Prevalence Depression and anxiety are more prevalent than dementia in old age. There is no decline in their prevalence with advancing age, but of concern is the fact that there is a reduction in referrals to psychiatry. This may be due to increased acceptance of symptoms by the elderly or due to deficiencies in detection by health professionals. The estimated prevalence of neurotic disorders is 1–10% with a female predominance and roughly equal frequency of 'old' and 'new' cases.

Clinical features Non-specific anxiety and depressive symptoms predominate and hypochondriacal symptoms are often prominent. Obsessional, phobic, dissociative, and conversion disorders are less common. Factors such as physical ill health, immobility, and lack of social support may give rise to fear and a lack of confidence about going out of the home—this has been termed 'space phobia'.

Aetiology Multiple factors may contribute to new neurotic symptoms in the elderly. Among these, major life events, physical illness, feelings of loneliness, impaired self-care, and 'insecure' personality style are most common.

Differential diagnosis Physical illness; acute or chronic organic brain disease; affective disorders.

Management

- The mainstay of treatment is to identify and manage aetiological factors. This obviously very often calls for social interventions and thus a multidisciplinary approach is essential.
- Counselling may be difficult especially where older people have had limited exposure to psychological methods.
- Antidepressants may be indicated for severe and disabling symptoms and are certainly preferable to benzodiazepines.

Specific aspects of psychiatric illnesses in the elderly (2)—mood disorders

Epidemiology

Aetiology

Clinical features

Depression

Specific aspects of psychiatric illnesses in the elderly (2)—mood disorders[1]

Epidemiology Less than 10% of new cases of mood disorder occur in old age and very few are bipolar. Episodes occur more frequently and last longer. Studies suggest that mood disorders in the elderly have a worse prognosis and there may be a tendency towards chronicity. Gender differences in prevalence also diminish with advancing age. Prevalence of clinically significant **depression** is 10% for those >65 yrs, with 2–3% being severe. Rates of depression differ depending on setting: 0.5–1.5% in the community; 5–10% of clinical outpatients; 10–15% of clinical inpatients; 15–30% of those in residential and nursing homes. **Mania** accounts for 5–10% of mood disorders in the elderly.

Aetiology Positive family history becomes less relevant in older-onset mood disorder. Physical illnesses are associated in 60–75% of cases. Major life events are common, as is the lack of a confiding and supportive relationship. Older patients are less likely to complain as losses are 'expected'. Neuroimaging yields conflicting results and brain changes noted may relate to the normal ageing process. The strongest imaging evidence for brain changes is for mania in men.

Clinical features
Depression
There are no clear distinctions between the clinical presentation of depression in the elderly and that in younger people. However, some symptoms are often more striking:

- Severe psychomotor retardation or agitation occurs in up to 30% of depressed elderly patients.
- A degree of cognitive impairment has been detected in 70% (esp. with effortful tasks).
- Depressive delusions regarding poverty, physical illness, or nihilistic in nature, are common (e.g. Cotard's syndrome, p. 85).
- Paranoia is also common, while derogatory and obscene auditory hallucinations may occur.
- Classic symptoms may not even be evident and the patient may instead present with somatic, anxiety, or hypochondriacal complaints. A high index of suspicion is required when older patients present with these symptoms, especially abnormal illness behaviour.

'Pseudodementia' A minority of retarded depressed elderly present with 'pseudodementia' (i.e. marked difficulties with concentration and memory), but careful testing excludes dementia.

Features suggestive of pseudodementia: previous history of depression; depressed mood; biological symptoms; 'islands of normality'; exaggerated symptoms; response to antidepressant medication.

Mania presents a similar clinical picture as in younger patients; however, it is more often followed immediately by a depressive episode in older patients.

Hypomania may occur but there is usually a history of BAD. First episode of mania or hypomania in an elderly person requires careful screening for cerebral (or systemic) pathology (e.g. stroke or hyperthyroidism).

Differential diagnosis **Dementia**—difficult to distinguish and can occur together, if in doubt best to treat; **Paranoid disorder**—depressive paranoia and delusions may be difficult to distinguish from psychoses; **Stroke**—especially after left frontal CVA or 2° to the lability, reactive stress, organic apathy, ↓motivation, or drug side-effects associated with stroke; **Parkinson's disease**—drug side-effects in treating PD may suggest depressive illness; **other physical disorders** e.g. infection, hypothyroidism, tumours, alcohol, drug side-effects. NB Full physical investigation is vital.

Management

- **Antidepressants** TCAs are not absolutely contraindicated in the elderly, but care must be exercised in prescribing. ECG and BP monitoring is important due to postural drops as well as other cardiac problems. Also suicide risk may exclude TCAs. First-line is probably SSRIs due to ↓side-effects and relative safety in OD. Others include: trazodone; SNRIs such as venlafaxine; and, occasionally, moclobemide (delayed hypotension a problem). General rules include: low starting dose; gradual increases; prolonged trial periods (2–3 months); long maintenance periods (up to 2 years); beware of suicide risk; consider lithium augmentation.
- **ECT** First-line treatment for severe illness and specifically where there is marked agitation, life-threatening stupor, suicidality, or contra-indications, failure, or excessive side-effects of drugs. ECT is generally safe and effective. Dementia is not a contraindication. Post-ECT confusion may be a problem, in which case treatments should be given at longer intervals. Following ECT, antidepressant medication should be given for a longer maintenance period than in younger patients. ECT may also be used for maintenance therapy.
- **Psychological treatments** Therapies include: CBT for depression; supportive psychotherapy; bereavement counselling.
- **Treatment of mania** Age-appropriate doses of neuroleptics may be used, in particular haloperidol or atypicals such as risperidone. Lithium is first-line in prophylaxis but lower dosages are indicated (levels: 0.4–0.7 mmol/L) and regular thyroid and renal checks are essential. Also note that levels may easily change in the presence of infection, dehydration, and use of other medications (e.g. diuretics).

Prognosis Generally prognosis is good, especially: onset <70 yrs short illness; good previous adjustment; absent physical illness; good previous recovery. Poor outcome is associated with: severity of initial illness; psychotic symptoms; physical illness; poor medication compliance; severe life events during follow-up period.

---

1 Gelder M, Gath D, Mayou R, Cowen P (1996) *Oxford Textbook of Psychiatry*, 3rd Edition, Oxford University Press, Oxford.

Specific aspects of psychiatric illnesses in the elderly (3)—psychoses

Psychotic illness in the elderly may be classified as follows:
1 'Old psychosis'—the 'graduate' population
2 'New psychosis'—late-life schizophrenia or late paraphrenia
3 Other conditions with paranoid and/or hallucinatory symptoms

'Old psychosis'

With the advent of antipsychotic drugs in the 1950s, there followed a progressive decrease in the numbers of long-stay patients with schizophrenia in institutions. Thus more and more ageing patients with chronic schizophrenia moved into the community, and in countries such as the UK and USA, many of these patients are increasingly referred to psychogeriatric services.

'New psychosis'

Paraphrenia—a term coined by Emil Kraepelin in 1909; described a psychotic illness characterised by delusions and hallucinations, without changes in affect, form of thought, or personality.

Late paraphrenia—described by Roth and Morrisey in 1952; they noted that this type of illness was the most common form of psychosis in old age (defined as >60 yrs).

NB Some controversy remains as to whether late paraphrenia represents schizophrenia of late onset or whether it is a distinct entity (most evidence supports the former).

Epidemiology Relatively rare condition; population studies estimate <1% prevalence. Approximately 10% of admissions to psychiatric wards for the elderly will have the condition. One study showed that when ICD-10 criteria were used, 60% cases were classified as paranoid schizophrenia, 30% as delusional disorder, and 10% as schizo-affective disorder[1]. Gender distribution is estimated at 4–9:1 female: male predominance. (NB Schizophrenia has a later onset in women.)

Aetiology

- **Genetics** The risk of schizophrenia in 1st degree relatives is 3.4% in late paraphrenics, compared with 5.8% in young schizophrenics, and less than 1% in the general population[2].
- **Premorbid personality** of people with late paraphrenia is characterised by poor adjustment and it is estimated that nearly 45% show lifelong paranoid and/or schizoid traits.
- **Sensory impairments** such as deafness, of onset in middle life, increases risk of late paraphrenia.
- **Social isolation** and major **life events** may also be contributory factors.
- **Organic factors** Structural imaging demonstrates mild ventricular enlargement; cerebrovascular pathology is a common comorbid finding.

Clinical features Persecutory delusions are the most common symptom of late paraphrenia (roughly 90% of patients) and tend to relate to commonplace themes (such as neighbours spying). Other common delusions include: referential, misidentification, hypochondriacal, and religious. Auditory hallucinations occur in approximately 75%, while visual (13%), somatic/tactile (12%), and olfactory (4%) hallucinations are not uncommon[3]. Schneiderian 1st rank symptoms are common (46%), while negative symptoms, thought disorder, and catatonia are extremely uncommon. 10–20% may present with delusions only.

Treatment
- Relieve isolation and sensory deficits
- Establish rapport and develop a therapeutic alliance (often difficult!)
- Exclude cognitive or medical disorders
- Hospital admission is often required
- Low-dose atypical antipsychotics preferred as elderly are very sensitive to side-effects.

Other conditions with paranoid or hallucinatory symptoms
These include the following conditions:
- **Secondary paranoid states**—due to organic disorders or substances (see p. 130)
- **Delirium** (see pp. 734–5)
- **Dementia** (see pp. 132–45)
- **Affective disorders** (see pp. 478–9)
- **Schizoaffective disorder** (see p. 228)

Hallucinations of sensory deprivation In the elderly, complex visual hallucinations can occur as a non-specific phenomenon, secondary to visual impairment—this is sometimes referred to as Charles Bonnet syndrome. These hallucinations may be well-formed and contain animals, people, or scenes. There may be partial or complete insight. Differential diagnosis includes: DLB (pp. 140–1), acute confusional state (pp. 734–5). Reassurance may be adequate, but in some cases a small dose of antipsychotic medication may reduce distressing symptoms.

1 Howard R, Castle D, Wessely S, Murray R (1993) A comparative study of 470 cases of early-onset and late-onset schizophrenia. *BJP* **163**, 352–7.

2 Kay DWK and Roth M (1961) Environmental and hereditary factors in the schizophrenias of old age (late paraphrenia) and their bearing on the general problem of causation in schizophrenia. *Journal of Mental Science* **107**, 649–686.

3 Almeida O (1998) Late paraphrenia. In: *Seminars in Old Age Psychiatry*, eds. Butler R and Pitt B, Gaskell.

Other mental health problems in the elderly

Alcohol problems

With decreasing tolerance for alcohol in advancing age, there is a corresponding increase in risk of intoxication and adverse effects. Males predominate, although there is an increase in prevalence of alcohol problems in women in their 8th and 9th decades.

Risk factors for late onset of alcohol problems include: women; higher socioeconomic class; physical ill-health; precipitating life events; neurotic personality; psychiatric illness.

Korsakoff psychosis is an important sequel in 'old cases'—see p. 530

Principles of management

- Prognosis is good if alcohol problems commence secondary to practical problems.
- Encourage and facilitate involvement in non-drinking social activities.
- In extreme cases consider need for supervision of finances.
- Orientate towards reducing physical problems.
- Moving to residential care may reduce social isolation.

Drug abuse

Generally, illicit substance abuse is not a significant problem in the elderly. However, misuse of prescription drugs such as benzodiazepines, opiates, and analgesics frequently becomes a problem in this age group. Dependence on these medications may result from careless prescription of long-term treatments for common problems of ageing such as insomnia and arthritis. With the best of intentions, doctors sometimes believe that it is 'cruel' to withdraw patients from these medications, especially if the patient has been using the drug for years and is advanced in age. However, it is important to consider whether withdrawal may actually enhance quality of life by diminishing chronic side-effects such as depression.

Sexual problems

Factors influencing the sexual life of younger adults are relevant to older people too (e.g. social stresses, illness, and side-effects of medications). In addition, the elderly may experience added problems related to the specific physiological changes that accompany ageing. Dementia sufferers may become sexually demanding as part of the disinhibition that frequently characterises this disorder. Health carers may fail to detect sexual problems experienced by older people as a sexual history is commonly overlooked. This may result from incorrect assumptions that carers often make regarding sexuality in this age group. The client too may assume that his or her sexual dysfunction is a 'normal' aspect of ageing. Some practical remedies are: hormone replacement therapy; vaginal lubricants and topical oestrogen; and, of course, Viagra.

Personality problems

Personality traits often become more prominent and rigid in old age; in particular traits such as cautiousness, introversion, and obsessionality.

Paranoid traits may intensify, especially in situations where there is increasing social isolation. In some cases increasing paranoia may be mistaken for a paranoid psychotic state such as delusional disorder. Psychopathy is said to 'burn-out' with advancing age and criminal behaviour is rare in the elderly (approximately 1% of male offenders are >60 yrs). Roughly 5–10% of older people exhibit features of personality disorder and these individuals often come to the attention of health services when they are residents in homes for the elderly. Since personality disorder is by definition lifelong, any significant change in personality needs explanation. Both organic and functional brain disorders may manifest as 'a change in personality'. Personality problems are often the cause of **Diogenes syndrome**—also called senile squalor syndrome—in which eccentric and reclusive individuals become increasingly isolated and neglect themselves, living in filthy, poor conditions. They are often oblivious to their condition and resistant to help, necessitating intervention.

Suicide

Old age is a risk factor for suicide and it is estimated that approximately 20% of all suicides are of the elderly. There is a male predominance of 2:1 in this age group, as suicide rates tend to increase with age in men and decrease with age in women. The rate of elderly suicides declined markedly during the 1960s due to the detoxification of the mains gas supply.

Predictive factors for suicide in the elderly:
- Increasing age
- Male
- Physical illness (35–85% cases)
- Social isolation
- Widowed or separated
- Alcohol abuse
- Depressive illness, current or past (80% cases)
- Recent contact with psychiatric services

Parasuicide

Parasuicide is relatively uncommon with older people, accounting for only 5% of cases. Gender distribution is roughly equal. An apparent parasuicide in this age group is much more likely to be a failed suicide and thus all para-suicides should be taken very seriously. It is important to exclude depression and also personality disorder as 90% have a depressive illness. Also 60% are physically ill; 50% have been previously admitted to a psychiatric hospital; and 8% go on to complete a suicide within 3 years of a parasuicide.

Issues of elder abuse[1,2]

In recent decades the unfortunate problem of elder abuse has become increasingly recognised. It is often overlooked and requires an integrated response from multiple disciplines and agencies, including health and social services, the criminal justice system, and government. The need for a unified multidisciplinary approach cannot be emphasised enough as a fragmented response is fraught with problems, as some countries have learned from bad experience.

Types of elder abuse Elder abuse is an all-inclusive term representing all types of mistreatment or abusive behaviour towards older adults. This mistreatment can be an act of commission (abuse) or omission (neglect), intentional or unintentional, and of one or more types:
- Physical, sexual verbal, or psychological abuse
- Physical or psychological neglect
- Financial exploitation

The abuse or neglect results in unnecessary suffering, injury, pain, or loss and leads to a violation of human rights and a decrease in the quality of life.

Epidemiology of elder abuse Occurs in both domestic and institutional settings:
- **Domestic setting** Approximately 4–6% of elderly people report incidents of abuse or neglect in domestic settings. The most common forms of abuse are verbal abuse and financial exploitation by family members and physical abuse by spouses. Gender distribution (of victims) is equal and economic status and age are unrelated to risk of abuse. Importantly, elder abuse is underreported—450 000 older adults in domestic settings were abused, neglected, or exploited in the USA during 1996, of which only 70 000 were self-reported.
- **Institutional settings** No data exists for the extent of abuse within institutional settings. However, one survey of nursing home staff in a US state disclosed that 36% of staff had witnessed at least one incident of physical abuse in the preceding year, while 10% admitted having committed at least one act of physical abuse themselves.

Explaining elder abuse The main risk factors for elder abuse are: dependency and social isolation of the victim; carer has mental or substance misuse problems; absence of a suitable guardian. Factors vary according to the type of abuse; for example, dependency is a risk factor for financial or emotional abuse, but not necessarily for physical abuse. Also the causes of spouse abuse may differ from the causes of abuse by adult offspring.

An integrative response to elder abuse Prevention is the best approach and a number of measures have proved effective: training and support of carers; reducing isolation of elders; respite care; CPN visits; etc. Responding to abuse effectively requires a multidisciplinary approach and a proactive system of assessment of suspicious cases (a number of assessment instruments have been developed[3,4]).

1 Payne BK (2002) An integrated understanding of elder abuse and neglect. *Journal of Criminal Justice* **30**, 535–47.

2 Wolf RS (1999) Suspected abuse in an elderly patient. *Am Fam Physician.* **59**, 1319–20.

3 Fulmer T (2003) Elder abuse and neglect assessment. *Journal of Gerontological Nursing* **29**, 8–9.

4 Reis M (1998) Validation of the indicators of abuse (IOA) screen. *Gerontologist.* **38**, 471–80.

Psychopharmacology in the elderly[1,2]

Pharmacokinetics The physiological changes associated with ageing mean that the older patient's system 'handles' drugs quite differently from that of a younger individual.

* *Absorption* generally remains the same, although there are reductions in gastric pH and mesenteric blood flow.
* *Distribution* of drugs is altered however: reduced body mass, body water, and plasma proteins, together with increased body fat causes increased levels of free drug and longer half-lives (especially of psychotropics).
* *Drug metabolism* is reduced due to decreased blood flow to the liver and loss of efficiency of liver microsomes.
* *Excretion* is reduced with the drop in renal clearance that accompanies old age. Thus drug effects are generally prolonged and cumulative and the risk of toxicity is high.

Pharmacodynamics Technology such as PET is enlightening our understanding of the direct effects of drugs in the CNS. Specific differences in these effects in the elderly include:

* **Dopaminergic system**—there are less DA cells in the basal ganglia; thus there is increased sensitivity to the EPSEs of neuroleptics (not dystonias).
* **Cholinergic system**—there is a normal reduction in cholinergic receptors with advancing age (and a gross reduction in DAT).
* **Noradrenergic system**—NA levels decrease with age, which may cause this age group to become increasingly vulnerable to mood disorders.
* **Narcotics and sedative hypnotics**—there is increased sensitivity to sedatives in the elderly due to a reduction in the number of available receptors.

The implications of these changes are that elderly patients are more sensitive to almost all drugs used in psychiatry.

1 Baldwin R and Burns A (1998) Pharmacological treatments. *Seminars in Old Age Psychiatry* Eds. Butler R and Pitt B, Gaskell.

2 Gareri P, Falconi U, De Fazio P, De Sarro G (2000) Conventional and new antidepressant drugs in the elderly. *Progress in Neurobiology* **61**, 353–96.

General principles of prescribing include:

1 Start with a very low dose.
2 Increases should be made slowly.
3 Maximum efficacy is often achieved at significantly lower doses than in younger adults.
4 Beware of dangerous side-effects such as postural hypotension and arrhythmias.
5 The elderly are particularly sensitive to EPSEs and anti-cholinergic side-effects.
6 Beware of drug interactions due to common problem of polypharmacy in the elderly.
7 Atypical neuroleptics are generally better tolerated than conventionals.
8 SSRIs, SNRIs, and NARIs are generally safer than TCAs; while MAOIs and lithium may be useful in resistant depression.
9 Monitor lithium therapy closely as levels can fluctuate easily and long-term effects on thyroid and renal function are not infrequent.
10 Always consider suicide risk as old age is a risk factor for suicide.

Services for the elderly[1,2]

Services for the elderly are organised differently according to government policies and availability of resources. In principle though, the ideal service should plan to:

- Maintain the elderly person at home for as long as possible
- Respond quickly to medical and social problems as they arise
- Ensure coordination of the work of those providing continuing care
- Support relatives and others who care for the elderly at home
- Promote liaison between medical and social and voluntary services

Primary care services At the primary care level GPs, health visitors, community nurses, and health workers will deal with most of the problems of elderly people.

Acute and long-term hospital services Elderly patients often require admission for acute assessment and treatment, respite care, or long-term care. Services may be situated within general medical wards for the elderly or within specialised old age psychiatry units. The advantage of acute services being located in general hospitals rather than in psychiatric hospitals is that a range of associated specialist services (such as old age medicine, neurology, and radiology) is often more readily available.

Day and outpatient care Ideally a service should have outpatient facilities for the assessment, treatment, and follow-up of mobile elderly patients with mental health problems. Sometimes these clinics offer a specialist service such as the 'memory clinic'. Day-care services may take the form of a general or psychiatric day hospital, and local authorities often provide day centres and social clubs for functional and social support.

Community psychiatric nurses (CPNs) CPNs provide a vital link between primary care and specialist services. They often perform assessments on patients after receiving a referral from a GP. They also monitor treatment in collaboration with GPs and the psychiatric services. In addition, they take part in the organisation of home support for the demented elderly.

Informal carers These are the unpaid relatives, neighbours, or friends who care for the elderly person at home. Demographic changes and the move to community care have increased the burden on carers. Informal carers are twice as likely to be women. Carers often suffer considerable stress, especially where the patient is suffering from advanced dementia. Relieving carer burden is a challenge for any service. Active involvement of medical and social personnel, as well as provision of education and respite, are important aspects of carer support.

Domiciliary services These include; home helps; meals at home; laundry and shopping services; emergency call systems. In some countries such as the UK, local authorities provide these services; however, in many others these services are either privately engaged, obtained from voluntary organizations, or are unavailable.

Residential and nursing care In most countries the local authorities take responsibility for providing old people's homes and other sheltered accommodation. These range in standard from large crowded institutions to small independent units and, ideally, they need to balance individual privacy with involvement in outside activities. In many communities private homes are available, but financial constraints put these out of the reach of the majority of older people. In planning residential care for the elderly, authorities need to provide for a wider range of accommodation: a small supported unit with 2 or 3 people may be ideal for the still independent and mobile individual; while larger homes with nursing support are required for those who are more dependent, with a number of physical and/or psychiatric needs.

1 Wertheimer J (1997) Psychiatry of the elderly: a consensus statement. *International Journal of Geriatric Psychiatry* **12**, 432–5.

2 Gelder M, Gath D, Mayou R, Cowen P (1996) *Oxford Textbook of Psychiatry*, 3rd Edition, Oxford University Press, Oxford.

Capacity, powers of attorney, and guardianship[1]

Civil law governs the management of individuals and their affairs in cases where he/she becomes incapable of managing for themselves. These issues are most relevant to the psychotically ill, the learning disabled, and the elderly. Decisions regarding treatment of the individual as well as his/her capacity to enter into contracts are dealt with under civil law. (See general discussion on p. 822). Different countries vary in respect of specific details and provisions within their legal systems, but there are a number of general principles which are discussed below.

Capacity refers to the individual's ability to make a clear and informed decision regarding a specific contract (e.g. a financial transaction; marriage and divorce; making a will; decision about treatment). It is important to recognise that an individual may have capacity to make a specific decision (e.g. get married) regardless of his/her general competence (e.g. may be learning disabled). **Testamentary capacity** is the ability to make a valid will, and the test for this capacity is whether the individual was of 'sound disposing mind' at the time of making the will. Psychiatrists may be asked to report on testamentary capacity and are sometimes required to report on whether the testator was subjected to undue influence. It is important to see the testator alone, although factual accuracy should be checked with others (e.g. family members, carers, etc.).

There are 4 legal criteria for determining testamentary capacity:

1 Testator must understand what a will is and what its consequences are.
2 Testator must understand the nature and extent of his/her property (though not in detail).
3 Testator must know the names of close relatives and beneficiaries and be able to assess their claims to his/her property.
4 Testator must not be acting on delusional ideas or be in such an emotional state that might distort feelings or judgements relevant to making the will.

Powers of attorney (POA) In a case where an individual suffers from a fluctuating (e.g. schizophrenia) or deteriorating (e.g. dementia) mental disorder, it is advisable for him/her to appoint a power of attorney during a 'lucid interval'. This involves the patient and the attorney signing a document with a witness present (a doctor may be an appropriate witness where the patient's mental state and capacity may be in question). When the patient becomes ill and no longer has capacity, the attorney applies to register the POA with the court (Court of Protection in the UK) and is then able to act on behalf of the patient. This form of POA is sometimes called a 'durable' or 'enduring' POA.

Guardianship Where no provision has been made in advance of the patient losing capacity, a more formal procedure is required involving the courts. This is known as guardianship, receivership (UK), or curatorship. This is most commonly invoked with the elderly. In most cases a relative, close friend, business advisor, or officer of the local authority applies to the court for guardianship. Where the patient is in hospital, the doctor may become involved in either notifying relatives of the patient's change in capacity, or making the application him/herself (if relatives are absent or unwilling). A doctor (usually specialist) is required to examine the patient and complete a certificate affirming that the patient is incapable, by reason of mental disorder, of managing and administering his/her affairs. In cases where the patient's estate is very small, the court may direct one of its officers to take a specific action. However, in most cases, a guardian is appointed by the court to administer the patient's affairs. The guardian is usually a relative but is sometimes a professional person if there is a conflict of interest. The guardian is required to visit the patient regularly, investigate and manage his/her affairs, and report back to the court regarding decisions made. Guardianship is usually a costly business for the patient and/or his/her family.

1 Jeffreys P (1998) Law. In: *Seminars in Old Age Psychiatry* Eds. Butler R and Pitt B, Gaskell.

The end of life, living wills, and withdrawal of active treatment

The end of life Managing a patient's final weeks or days and ensuring that their death is a 'good death' is a challenge that has only recently been addressed in our health services and training programmes[1]. Many health professionals have never received any guidance regarding their involvement in this common and extremely important phase of people's lives. Contemporary palliative services stress the following components in providing a 'good death':

• A multidisciplinary approach
• Ability to 'diagnose dying'
• Communication with patient and family
• Provision of adequate physical support (e.g. analgesia, hydration)
• Minimise unnecessary interventions
• Establish a non-resuscitation plan
• Psychological, social, cultural, and spiritual support

Living wills[2] A living will is an advance directive (usually written and witnessed) made by an individual regarding their preferences for future treatment during their final illness. Usually the person specifies the degree of irreversible deterioration after which they want no further life-sustaining treatment. They may also give clear instructions refusing certain medical interventions. If a health professional is asked to assist someone in drawing up a living will, the following issues should be considered; the patient should be fully informed about the illness and treatment options; the patient should be mentally competent; the patient should be reflecting his/her own views, free from influence. The health carer is required to abide by the living will, although basic care (i.e. analgesia, catheter, fluids) should be provided in all cases. (The BMA has a code of practice entitled **Advance Statements about Medical Treatment**).

Withdrawal of treatment[3,4] The active or passive involvement of a carer in hastening an individual's death is highly controversial and morally complex. There are differing degrees of involvement that should be distinguished:

• Withdrawal of active interventions such as medications, blood transfusion, etc. This is an accepted aspect of palliative care and draws little debate.
• Withdrawal of life-sustaining treatment such fluids, food, etc. This is equivalent to 'allowing a patent to die'. Since the current emphasis is on preserving human dignity rather than preserving life, this is morally acceptable for many and should not be considered euthanasia.
• Active intervention which hastens or precipitates the patient's death-euthanasia. This is distinguishable from homicide in that the patient has either consented to the assisted death or is unable to (e.g. comatose) and the intervention is regarded as a 'mercy killing'.

That time of year thou mayst in me behold
When yellow leaves, or none, or few, do hang
Upon those boughs which shake against the cold,
Bare ruin'd choirs, where late the sweet birds sang.
In me thou see'st the twilight of such day
As after sunset fadeth in the west;
Which by and by black night doth take away,
Death's second self, that seals up all in rest.
In me thou see'st the glowing of such fire,
That on the ashes of his youth doth lie,
As the death-bed whereon it must expire
Consum'd with that which it was nourish'd by.
This thou perceiv'st, which makes thy love more strong,
To love that well which thou must leave ere long.

Shakespeare: *Sonnet 72*

1 Ellershaw J and Ward C (2003) Care of the dying patient: the last hours or days of life. *BMJ* **326**, 30–34.

2 Ramsay S (1995) UK doctors get advance-directive guidance. *Lancet* **345**, 913–14.

3 Hermsen MA and ten Have HA (2002) Euthanasia in palliative care journals. *Journal of Pain and Symptom Management* **23**, 517–25.

4 Sharma BR (2003) To legalize physician-assisted suicide or not?—a dilemma. *Journal of Clinical Forensic Medicine* **10**, 185–90.

Substance misuse

The psychiatry of substance misuse

The sub-specialty of substance misuse is concerned with the assessment and treatment of patients with problems arising from the misuse of harmful or addictive substances. These include: 1) alcohol, 2) illegal or 'street' drugs, 3) prescription and over-the-counter medicines, and 4) volatile chemicals. The resultant problems include both mental and physical illnesses and family, housing, employment, and legal difficulties. In treatments, both psychological and pharmacological interventions are used; these may include detoxification and substitute prescribing.

The majority of interventions in patients with substance use problems are undertaken by GPs. In areas where there are no substance misuse specialists the majority of more complex cases are seen by general psychiatrists, with management of the acute medical problems, including overdose and withdrawals, treated in the general hospital. All psychiatrists will have ample opportunity to see patients whose problems derive from substance use.

Around the UK there is variable provision of services for drug and alcohol abusers. Drug and alcohol problems may be dealt with within a combined 'addiction service', or may be managed separately. Some services will restrict themselves to the primary substance misuse and its problems, while others will address all mental health needs. In the field of treatment services for those with substance use problems, specialists will work alongside voluntary and non-medical treatment agencies, many of which provide a good and very vital service. Strong links between psychiatry/ substance use services and the non-medical agencies should be fostered.

Drug treatment services within the health care system make up only one part of the wider range of centrally and locally funded and volunteer services for problem drug users. Within the health service sector most of drug user contact and service provision is with GPs who will have a variable degree of experience of, and enthusiasm for, such work. The availability of specialist services will vary by area and setting (e.g. rural/urban) and may range from the special interest of an individual psychiatrist or GP, to a specialist service with support staff and dedicated facilities. Local pharmacists can also be a useful resource in supervising consumption of substitute drugs.

Non-health care provision will also vary by setting but may include: advice shops offering leaflets and education about drugs and harm reduction strategies; self-help groups, some adhering to an AA style 'twelve-step approach', usually involving peer support from ex-users; residential facilities offering detoxification and abstinence programs. The practitioner working in the field of drug misuse should develop an awareness of these services and their referral criteria and encourage a collaborative approach to client management.

The skills required for those working in the field of substance misuse are:

- **Knowledge of the psychiatric syndromes associated with misused substances** Both knowledge of the patterns of physical and mental disorders associated with substance misuse and the presentations of mental disorder when there is comorbid substance use.

- **Experience of interviewing and counselling methods** Skills at interviewing and motivating patients who may have very ambivalent feelings about changing behaviour.
- **Experience of the pharmacological and psychological treatment methods** An area undergoing constant development where there is a need to keep abreast of changes in guidelines over time.
- **Awareness of the pattern of drug use within a community** Patterns of drug use change over time, and the types and strengths of drugs available in a community will also change. Information from police and the voluntary sector can be helpful here.
- **Willingness to be involved with other agencies** Valuable work in the field of substance misuse is done by agencies outside the health-care system. Practitioners should attempt to understand the work of these agencies and refer to them where appropriate.
- **Ability to take a long-term view** Substance misuse disorders can be chronic, some would say lifelong, conditions and patients may relapse many times before showing improvement.
- **Ability to consider health in its wider context** Substance misuse gives rise to health risks beyond the effect of the drug, (e.g. drink driving deaths, HIV infection). In addition, substance misuse is a community problem leading to lost productivity, crime, road accidents, violence, and family break-up.
- **Consider change beyond change in an individual patient** Patterns of substance misuse in a society are susceptible to political manipulation (e.g. licensing hours, decriminalisation, legalisation, availability of treatment services). One role of substance misuse specialists is to understand these factors and to present the case for political change.

Sometimes there is a perception that drug or alcohol users are difficult or unrewarding patients to treat. It should be noted that GMC guidelines direct that it is 'unethical for a doctor to withhold treatment from any patient on the basis of a moral judgement that the patient's activities or lifestyle may have contributed to the conditions for which treatment was being sought'.

N.B. For the purposes of this chapter, we refer to alcohol misuse and drug misuse separately and refer to them collectively as substance misuse. Alcohol is of course a drug and should be thought of as such, but we believe this terminology to be clearer and more understandable to patients.

Substance use and misuse

'Mankind cannot bear very much reality' - T.S. Eliot
'The urge to escape, the longing to transcend themselves, if only for a few minutes, is and always has been one of the principal appetites of the soul' - Aldous Huxley

People in all cultures, at all times through history, have sought out mood- or perception-altering substances. 25% of adults smoke; 90% drink alcohol; 33% have lifetime experience of one illegal drug (mostly cannabis). Society's attitude to substance use and to those with substance use problems has varied from prohibition and condemnation to tolerance and treatment. Within British society at the moment caffeine use is legal and accepted; alcohol and tobacco use are accepted with legal limitations; and other substances have severe legal limitations—some available only on prescription, others not at all. Despite this, the harmful effects of alcohol dwarf those of other drugs.

Many of the abused substances subsequently described have been used in their naturally occurring form throughout history (e.g. the chewing of coca leaves by Peruvian Indians). There has been a tendency for the development of more potent drug preparations which contain a higher concentration of the active ingredient (e.g. freebase cocaine), and the development of routes of administration which produce more rapid and intense effects (e.g. IV use). This has generally been associated with an increase in the attendant problems.

Patients presenting with drug misuse problems represent only a small percentage of those who take drugs. Little is known about the non-presenting drug users. Their numbers may be revealed by community surveys but they are otherwise poorly studied. It is clear, however, that the normal route from use of to abstinence from a substance is the individual deciding to discontinue use and then doing so, without medical consultation or help.

The reasons for substance use are varied, may be mixed, and may change over the course of a patient's life. They include: a search for a 'high'; a search for a repeat of initial pleasurable effects; cultural norm in some sub-cultures; self-medication for anxiety, social phobia, insomnia etc; self-medication for negative symptoms of psychotic illness; and to prevent development of withdrawal symptoms.

The pattern of risks associated with substance use varies with the substance taken, the dose and route of administration, and the setting. They include: acute toxicity; behavioural toxicity (e.g. jumping from height due to believing one can fly); toxic effects of drug contaminants; secondary medical problems; secondary psychiatric problems; risk of development of dependency; and negative social, occupational, marital, and forensic consequences.

Substance misuse disorders

Acute intoxication The pattern of reversible physical and mental abnormalities produced by the direct effects of intoxicating substances. Some physical and psychological signs and symptoms (e.g. disinhibition) are highly specific and also transitory depending on [...]. Most syndromes have both chronic effects and impairment of the ability to learn. The full effect of a particular substance is dependent on dose and comorbidity.

Acute use A relatively short-term use with no pain [...] or physical or mental consequences may occur in parts to physical harm to health. It is not a disorder. Can enter acute states into both nominal continuous and if excessive use persists or in the presence of other [...] absolute minimum intake of the substance.

Harmful use This is a pattern of psychoactive substance use that is actually causing harm to the user's physical or mental health or to others. The pattern of use is often criticized by others, and is associated with being [...]. The damage may be linked to medical or psychological consequences.

Dependence The syndrome of dependence is a cluster of behavioural, cognitive, and physiological phenomena that develop after repeated substance use [...] and as a syndrome generalized with a range of substances. The stimulus given priority to the user over other behaviours that once had value. The central characteristic is an intense desire and persistent tendency to take [...] the substance, there is a strong sense of the presence of other features may occur.

Withdrawal When there are other considerations a diagnosis of withdrawal is a group of symptoms of variable clustering and severity occurring on withdrawal [...] These are time-limited and related to the type of substance. Symptoms [...] can be associated with any number of [...], some with physical symptoms [...].

Complicated withdrawal Where [...] the acute withdrawal [...] features.

Substance-induced psychotic disorder A cluster of psychotic phenomena that occur during or following psychoactive substance use [...].

Cognitive impairment syndromes [...] a syndrome in which a presumed aetiology is a direct consequence of psychoactive substance use is classified for [...].

Substance misuse disorders

Acute intoxication The pattern of reversible physical and mental abnormalities caused by the direct effects of the substance. These are specific and characteristic for each substance, (e.g. disinhibition and ataxia for alcohol, euphoria and visual sensory distortions for LSD). Most substances have both pleasurable and unpleasant acute effects; for some, the balance of positive and negative effects is situation-, dose- and route-dependent.

At-risk use A pattern of substance use where the person is at increased risk of harming their physical or mental health. This is not a discrete point but shades into both normal consumption and harmful use. At-risk use depends not only on absolute amounts taken but the situations and associated behaviours, (e.g. any alcohol use is risky if associated with driving).

Harmful use The continuation of substance use despite evidence of damage to the user's physical or mental health or to their social, occupational, and familial well-being. This damage may be denied or minimised by the individual concerned.

Dependence The layman's 'addiction'. Encompasses a range of features initially described in connection with alcohol abuse (p. 502), now recognised as a syndrome associated with a range of substances. Dependence includes both physical dependence (the physical adaptations to chronic, regular use) and psychological dependence (the behavioural adaptations). In some drugs (e.g. hallucinogens), no physical dependence features are seen.

Withdrawal Where there is physical dependence on a drug, abstinence will generally lead to features of withdrawal. These are characteristic for each drug. Some drugs are not associated with any withdrawals; some with mild symptoms only; and some with significant withdrawal syndromes. Clinically significant withdrawals are recognised in dependence on alcohol, opiates, nicotine, benzodiazepines, amphetamines, and cocaine. Symptoms of withdrawal are often the 'opposite' of the acute effects of the drug, (e.g. agitation and insomnia on benzodiazepine withdrawal).

Complicated withdrawal Withdrawals can be simple, as above or complicated by the development of seizures, delirium, or psychotic features.

Substance-induced psychotic disorder Illness characterised by hallucinations and/or delusions occurring as a direct result of substance-induced neurotoxicity. Psychotic features may occur during intoxication and withdrawal states, or develop on a background of harmful or dependent use. There may be diagnostic confusion between these patients and those with primary psychotic illness and comorbid substance misuse. Substance-induced illnesses will be associated in time with episodes of substance misuse and may have atypical clinical features, (e.g. late first presentation with psychosis, prominence of non-auditory hallucinations).

Cognitive impairment syndromes Reversible cognitive deficits occur during intoxication. Persisting impairment (in some cases amounting to dementia) caused by chronic substance use is recognised for alcohol, volatile chemicals, benzodiazepines, and, debatably, cannabis. Cognitive impairment is associated with heavy chronic harmful use/dependence and shows gradual deterioration with continued use and either a halt in the rate of decline or gradual improvement on abstinence.

Residual disorders Several conditions exist (e.g. alcoholic hallucinosis, p. 526; persisting drug-induced psychosis, p. 560; LSD flashbacks, p. 92) where there are continuing symptoms despite continuing abstinence from the drug.

Exacerbation of pre-existing disorder All other psychiatric illnesses, especially anxiety and panic disorders, mood disorders, and psychotic illnesses may be associated with comorbid substance use. Although this may result in exacerbation of the patient's symptoms and a decline in treatment effectiveness, it can be understood as a desire to self-medicate (e.g. alcohol taken as a hypnotic in depressive illness) or escape unpleasant symptoms (e.g. opiates taken to 'blot out' derogatory auditory hallucinations). Sometimes there is debate about whether there is, for example, a primary mood disorder with secondary alcohol use or vice versa. Careful examination of the time course of the illness may reveal the answer. In any case, it is advisable to address substance misuse problems first as this may produce secondary mood improvements and continuing substance misuse will limit antidepressant treatment effectiveness.

The dependence syndrome

This is a clinical syndrome describing the features of substance dependence. It was described initially by Edwards & Gross[1] as a provisional description of alcohol dependence but may be applied to the description of drug dependence. These features form the core of both ICD-10 and DSM-IV descriptions of substance dependence.

- **Primacy of drug-seeking behaviour** Also called 'salience' of drug use. The drug and the need to obtain it become the most important things in the person's life, taking priority over all other activities and interests. Thus drug use becomes more important than retaining job or relationships, remaining financially solvent, and in good physical health and may diminish moral sense leading to criminal activity and fraud. This diminishes the 'holds' on a person's continued use. If he rates drug use above health, then stern warnings about impending illness are likely to mean little.

- **Narrowing of the drug-taking repertoire** The user moves from a range of drugs to a single drug taken in preference to all others. The setting of drug use, the route of use, and the individuals with whom the drug is taken may also become stereotyped.

- **Increased tolerance to the effects of the drug** The user finds that more of the drug must be taken to achieve the same effects. They may also attempt to combat increasing tolerance by choosing a more rapidly acting route of administration, (e.g. IV rather than smoked), or by choosing a more rapidly acting form, (e.g. freebase cocaine rather than cocaine hydrochloride). In advanced dependence there may be a sudden loss of previous tolerance; the mechanism for this is unknown. Clinically, tolerance is exhibited by individuals who are able to display no or few signs of intoxication while at a blood level in which intoxication would be evident in a non-dependent individual.

- **Loss of control of consumption** A subjective sense of inability to restrict further consumption once the drug is taken.

- **Signs of withdrawal on attempted abstinence** A withdrawal syndrome, characteristic for each drug, may develop. This may be only regularly experienced in the mornings because at all other times the blood level is kept above the required level.

- **Drug taking to avoid development of withdrawal symptoms** The user learns to anticipate and avoid withdrawals, (e.g. having the drug available on waking).

- **Continued drug use despite negative consequences** The user persists in drug use even when threatened with significant losses as a direct consequence of continued use, (e.g. marital break-up, prison term, loss of job).

- **Rapid reinstatement of previous pattern of drug use after abstinence** Characteristically, when the user relapses to drug use after a period of abstinence, they are at risk of a return to the dependent pattern in a much shorter period than the time initially taken to reach dependent use.

---

1 Edwards G and Gross MM (1976) Alcohol dependence: provisional description of a clinical syndrome. *BMJ* **1**, 1058–61.

Stages of change and harm reduction

Stages of change

A model for understanding motivation and action towards change in harmful patterns of drug use proposed by Prochaska and DiClemente[1]. Motivation is regarded as a prerequisite for and a precursor to action towards abstinence or more controlled drug use.

- **Pre-contemplation** The user does not recognise that problem use exists, although this may be increasingly obvious to those around them.
- **Contemplation** The user may accept that there is a problem and begins to look at both the positive and negative aspects of continued drug use.
- **Decision** The point at which the user decides on whether to continue drug use or attempt change.
- **Action** The point of motivation, where the user attempts change. A variety of routes exist by which change may be attempted, which may or may not include medical services.
- **Maintenance** A stage of maintaining gains made and attempting to improve those areas of life harmed by drug use.
- **Relapse** A return to previous behaviour but with the possibility of gaining useful strategies to extend the maintenance period on the user's next attempt.

Harm reduction

Harm reduction is a method of managing drug users in which it is accepted that steps can be taken to reduce the mortality and morbidity for the user without necessarily insisting on abstinence from drugs. This approach gained currency during the 80s in an attempt to halt the projected AIDS epidemic. Perhaps the majority of patients will present before abstinence is a realistic or achievable goal for them. Optimum care for this group of patients will involve engaging them with the service, exploring and encouraging motivation to change, and suggesting harm reduction strategies. Examples of such strategies include:

- Advice directed at use of safer drugs or safer routes of administration.
- Advice regarding safer injecting practice (p. 539).
- Advice regarding safe sex.
- Prescription of maintenance opiates or benzodiazepines.
- Assessment and treatment of comorbid physical or mental illness.
- Engagement with other sources of help, (e.g. social work, housing).

Drug misuse is a community problem and some aspects of harm reduction include consideration of reduction of morbidity to the community more generally. Prescription of methadone may reduce criminality in a dependent individual, with consequent community benefit. Equally, there is a responsibility with the prescriber to consider the potential for community harm via leakage and accidental overdose when monitoring the prescription of any drug.

1 Prochaska JO and DiClemente CC (1986) Towards a comprehensive model of change. In Miller WR and Heather N pp3–27 (eds) *Treating addictive behaviours: processes of change*, Plenun Press, New York.

Alcohol misuse

In the UK, roughly 93% of men and 87% of women drink alcohol. Minimal alcohol consumption can of course be pleasurable, socially enjoyable, and associated with health benefits (reduction in deaths from coronary artery disease). There is a tendency to view most people as normal drinkers and a subset as vulnerable to the development of alcohol problems. In fact on a population level, increasing the overall alcohol consumption (e.g. by reducing the real price of alcohol) tends to increase the total number of problem drinkers.

Alcohol consumption in the community is roughly normally distributed with a long 'tail' to the right. The distinction between normal and heavy drinking is arbitrary. On both a population and individual level, increased consumption is associated with increased risk of harm of all kinds. However, the fact that normal drinkers heavily outnumber heavy drinkers means that, despite their lower rates of problems, greater numbers of alcohol-related problems occur in normal rather than heavy drinkers. This gives rise to the so-called 'prevention paradox'—that to significantly reduce overall alcohol related morbidity we must look to reduce problems in normal rather than heavy drinkers. This applies more to problems such as drink driving and drink-related trauma rather than to medical complications of heavy use such as cirrhosis.

The term 'alcoholic' is often used by patients themselves and is the preferred term of Alcoholics Anonymous. It has unfortunately acquired a pejorative meaning to the general public, and images of the 'down and out' or 'skid row' alcoholic, drinking strong drink from brown paper bags, have damaged this word's use in clinical contexts. It is not used in DSM-IV or ICD-10 where the preference is to make the diagnosis of alcohol dependence or harmful use (abuse in DSM-IV).

A history of alcohol use

Alcohol has been used in all societies throughout recorded history, with documentary evidence of brewing and wine making as early as 3000 B.C. The intoxicating effects of alcohol were most probably discovered independently in many cultures around the time of the evolution of agriculture, possibly on noting fermentation in fruit. Ancient peoples produced alcoholic beverages from a wide variety of materials including fruits, berries, honey, corn, barley, wheat, sugar cane, and potatoes. The use of alcohol by individuals has been variously regarded, from complete tolerance through to outright prohibition.

Alcohol has always had a place in the lifestyles and formal rituals of many peoples around the world. It was used as an intoxicant in religious rituals, as a celebration, as a gift, as a greeting, and to mark births and deaths. For almost as long as alcohol use is recorded there are recorded attempts at control on its use by the authorities. In AD 92 The Roman emperor, Domitian, attempted to restrict wine production and its distribution and sale. Similar restrictions were attempted at various times by other leaders, sometimes accompanied by moral disapproval of drinking or drunkenness in particular. In Medieval Britain, ale was a staple part of the diet and was consumed in huge quantities, while drunkenness, particularly among the clergy was frowned upon by the Christian churches. Consumption of wine is of course the centrepiece of Christian worship. After initially preaching moderation, Mohammed later forbade the use of alcohol to followers of his religion, possibly as a way of differentiating his converts from the Christians around them.

The process of natural fermentation of alcohol by yeasts can produce beverages of up to 13% proof: above this concentration the yeast dies. Stronger concentrations of alcohol are produced by the process of distillation which was discovered in the Middle East in 1000 AD. Public consumption of distilled liquor became prevalent in the 18th Century and the accompanying social problems together with the conservative attitudes of the emerging Protestant clergy led to a developing moral disapproval of alcohol consumption.

In the mid 18th Century, as part of a continuing military and trade dispute with France, the British government imposed heavy taxes on French wine imports and encouraged the distillation of cheap domestic spirits—in particular, gin. This change in the drinking practice in the general population from low- to high-strength alcohol produced significant alcohol-related problems in the general public, immortalised in the lithographs of the 'gin palaces' by George Cruikshank. In an effort to control the problem the government passed laws to restrict the time and place at which alcohol could be sold and began to levy increasing taxes on distilled spirits. This had the positive effect of reducing consumption but the negative effect of introducing a government interest in continuing consumption. The late 18th Century writings of Benjamin Rush describe habitual drunkenness as a 'disease of the mind'.

18th-century America saw the development of an increasingly widespread temperance movement (those signing a pledge 'TA' for total abstinence becoming known as teetotalers). The temperance movement lobbied for a complete ban on alcohol consumption, and succeeded in 1921 following the passing of the 18th amendment to the US Constitution which provided for prohibition. The period of 11 years until the repeal of prohibition in the 21st amendment did indeed see a reduction in social problems and mortality; however, its unpopularity, widespread flouting of the law, and the flourishing of illegal activity in gangsterism led to its repeal.

Today, in most western countries, alcohol use is widely tolerated and socially accepted. Interestingly though, moral disapproval of drinking during pregnancy and drinking while driving a motor vehicle has resulted in substantial decreases in these activities. Despite improvement in these limited areas, most western countries have seen an increase in absolute consumption and alcohol-related medical harm compounded by an increasing passion for drug misuse.

Alcohol as a drug

Preparations The active ingredient in alcoholic drinks is ethyl alcohol which makes up a variable percentage of the volume. The flavour of drinks comes from 'congeners'—the additional organic substances derived from the brewing materials.

Pattern of use Of all drugs, alcohol has the widest range of patterns of use, ranging from yearly light consumption to continuous consumption throughout the waking hours.

Drug actions The effects of alcohol on the CNS were traditionally described as being due to non-specific effects on neuronal cell wall fluidity and permeability. It is now believed that in addition to these general effects there are neurotransmitter-specific effects, including: enhancement of GABA-A transmission (anxiolytic effects), release of dopamine in the mesolimbic system (euphoriant effects), and inhibition of NMDA-mediated glutaminergic transmission (amnesic effects). Ethyl alcohol is oxidised by alcohol dehydrogenase (ADH) to acetaldehyde, which in turn is oxidised by acetaldehyde dehydrogenase (ALDH) to carbon dioxide and water. 98% of alcohol metabolism takes place in the liver. Approximately one unit, (or 8 g), of alcohol can be metabolised per hour. Illicitly brewed alcohol may contain methanol, which is broken down to formaldehyde, which has marked toxic effects in the retina.

Acute effects Alcohol is absorbed rapidly from mouth, stomach, and small intestine, and from a single consumption maximum blood levels are obtained in ~60 minutes. Absorption is slowed by the presence of food in the stomach and is speeded-up by taking effervescent drinks. Alcohol is hydrophilic and is widely distributed throughout the body organs including the brain, placenta, lungs, and kidneys. Blood alcohol concentration (BAC) is consistent throughout the body with the exception of fat and can be estimated from breath samples. In normal drinkers BAC correlates with the subjective and the observable CNS effects of alcohol. Heavy drinkers may have high BAC with limited outward signs of intoxication due to the development of tolerance. Because of their different body fat distribution, women will have a higher BAC than men following the same oral intake. Initial symptoms of alcohol intoxication are subjective elevation of mood, increased socialisation, and disinhibition. Continuing consumption, intended to prolong these effects, can lead to lability of mood, impaired judgement, aggressiveness, slurred speech, unsteady gait, and ataxia.

Societal factors The prevalence of alcohol-related harm increases with the mean population consumption. This mean consumption is increased by increased availability of alcohol, increased societal tolerance of drinking, decreased restrictions on the sale of alcohol, and a decreased 'real price' of alcohol. Price is the most influential factor in demand, the real price of a pint of beer or bottle of whiskey having dropped considerably since the war. Where societies forbid all alcohol consumption (e.g. prohibition America, Islamic counties), there is a decrease in alcohol related problems but an increase in the level of personality abnormality in those who continue to drink.

Risk factors Heavy drinking is more common in men, in lower socio-economic groups, in those with lower educational levels, and in the young. Some professions are also associated with heavy drinking and drink-related harm. These include drinks industry workers (easy availability and effect of heavy drinkers seeking out jobs here); travelling salesmen (boredom, periods away from home, acceptance of drinking on the job); doctors (stress, freedom from direct supervision, reluctance to seek help with incipient problems).

Genetics First-degree relatives of alcoholics have double the risk of alcohol problems themselves. Significantly higher rates in identical compared with fraternal twins (although not 100% concordance). Children of alcoholics have increased risk of development of alcohol problems themselves even when adopted into families without alcohol problems. A metabolically relatively inactive form of ALDH is common in oriental people, leading to accumulation of acetaldehyde and an unpleasant 'flushing' reaction in affected individuals who take alcohol. This may account for the significantly lower rate of alcohol problems found in affected individuals. No causative genes for alcoholism have been identified and it is expected that it will show polygenic inheritance. Problem drinkers contain a significant sub-group of individuals with dissocial personality traits which predisposes to alcoholism and is itself heritable.

Medical complications Acute toxicity occurs at levels over 300 mg% (see p. 524), with clouding of consciousness and coma, risk of aspiration, hypoglycaemia, and acute renal failure. Associated with a wide range of chronic medical problems (pp. 532–3).

Psychiatric complications Harmful use and dependent use (p. 524) distinguished by the presence of withdrawals on abstinence; withdrawals may be complicated by seizures and development of acute confusional state—delirium tremens (p. 516); acute alcohol induced amnesia; alcoholic hallucinosis, (p. 526); alcohol-induced delusional disorder, (p. 526); Wernicke-Korsakoff syndrome (pp. 530–1); pathological jealousy, (p. 526); alcohol-related cognitive impairment and alcoholic dementia, (p. 526); alcohol misuse also associated with development of or exacerbation of anxiety/depressive symptoms and with deliberate self-harm and suicidal behaviour.

Interventions Advice regarding safer drinking patterns in those with 'at risk' or harmful use, (p. 512); strategies towards encouraging and maintaining abstinence in those with dependency and those with established medical or psychiatric damage; medically managed detox, (p. 518); Psychological and pharmacological support of abstinence or changed drinking pattern, (pp. 520–3.)

Screening for alcohol problems

Diseases related to alcohol abuse are common, significant, and amenable to improvement by early intervention. They are therefore suitable for screening. There are low rates of detection in primary care and hospital settings which may be improved by increased vigilance, increased awareness of alcohol problems, awareness of routes of referral, asking routine alcohol-screening questions (e.g. **CAGE**—see opposite), and paying special attention to at-risk groups. Many patients give reasonably accurate drinking histories if asked, although some may underestimate consumption.

Disorders suggesting occult alcohol problem Hepatitis; cryptogenic (i.e. medically unexplained) cirrhosis; seizures—particularly late onset; gastritis; anaemia; unexplained raised MCV or deranged LFTs; cardiomyopathy; accidents, particularly repeated and poorly explained; TB; head injury; hypertension persisting despite apparently adequate treatment; treatment resistance in other psychiatric conditions; impotence in men.

Breath testing Blood alcohol concentration (BAC) is a measure of recent alcohol consumption. Measured in mg alcohol per 100ml blood (mg%). Correlates well with breath alcohol measured by breathalyser (see opposite). Useful in assessing recent drinking, (e.g. in supervised detox regimes) and as objective measure of intoxication, (e.g. in A&E). Discrepancy between high BAC and lack of apparent intoxication suggests the development of tolerance.

Blood tests Elevated red cell mean corpuscular volume (MCV), gamma glutamyl transferase (γGT), and carbohydrate deficient transferrin (CDT) act as markers for excess alcohol consumption. They are best used to monitor consumption in patients in follow-up. Not sensitive/specific enough for routine screening purposes.

- **MCV** Sensitivity 20–50%, specificity 55–100%. Remains raised for 3–6 months due to 120-day lifespan of RBC. False positive in B12 and folate deficiency
- **γGT** Sensitivity 20–90%, specificity 55–100%. Raised for 2–4 weeks Other LFTs are less specific for alcoholic-related. liver damage. False positive in liver diseases of other cause and may remain raised in chronic alcoholic liver disease despite abstinence.
- **CDT** Sensitivity 70%, specificity 95%. Increased levels in response to heavy drinking. More expensive than γGT and not available in all areas.

Cage questionnaire

A brief screening questionnaire for identification of at-risk drinking:

C: Have you ever felt you should **C**ut back on your drinking?

A: Has anyone ever **A**nnoyed you by criticising your drinking?

G: Have you ever felt **G**uilty about your drinking?

E: Have you ever had a drink early in the morning as an **E**ye-opener?

More than two positive responses suggests possible at-risk drinking and should prompt further assessment.

NB The **'Cage + 2'** adds two additional questions:

1. What is the most alcohol you have drunk in a single day?
2. What is the most alcohol you have drunk in a single week?

Breath and blood alcohol levels

Breath alcohol reading (mcg%)	BAC (mg%)
0.35	80
0.52	120
0.70	160
0.87	200
1.05	240
1.40	320
1.75	400

A breathalyser allows an objective measurement of the breath alcohol and hence an approximation of the BAC. Breath alcohol reading should form part of the routine assessment of a patient presenting with alcohol problems and of patients in follow-up (e.g. supervised detox), rather than being prompted by suspicion of inaccuracy of oral report.

Assessment of the patient with alcohol problems

Patients with a primary alcohol problem, or where it is thought that alcohol consumption is a contributory factor in their presentation, should have a more detailed assessment of their alcohol use, in addition to standard psychiatric history and MSE.

Lifetime pattern of alcohol consumption Age at first alcoholic drink. Age when first drinking regularly. Age when first drinking most weekends. Age when first drinking most days. When did they first begin to drink more than their peers? When (if ever) did they first feel they had an alcohol problem? Pattern of drinking throughout life until present—describe periods of abstinence and more heavy drinking and the reasons for these.

Current alcohol consumption Describe a current day's drinking. When is the first drink taken? What types of drink are taken and in what setting? What is the total number and volume of drinks taken in a day? Some patients find it hard to describe a typical day or easy to over-rationalise recent heavy consumption. Ask them to describe the previous day's drinking, then the day before that etc., until a pattern emerges. Describe a typical and a 'heavy' day's drinking.

Signs of dependence Do they experience withdrawals in the morning or when unable to get alcohol? Have they ever drunk more alcohol as way of relieving withdrawals? Are they having to drink more to get the same intoxicating effect? Do they no longer get 'drunk' at all? Do they find it difficult to stop drinking once started? Have they tried and failed to give up, and if so why? Do they have episodes of 'lost' memory?

Physical/mental health Have they been told of any physical health problems due to drinking? Have they previously been told to stop drinking by a doctor? Any previous or current psychiatric diagnoses.

Problems related to alcohol Have they missed days at work, or had warnings about poor performance, or lost a job as a result of alcohol? Are there relationship difficulties or a relationship breakdown due to drinking? Are there financial problems? Have they been in trouble with the police or have outstanding charges against them?

Previous treatment attempts Describe the nature and type of previous treatments. Describe the subsequent return to drinking. Describe any periods of abstinence since the development of the drinking problem. How were they maintained and what ended them?

Family history Drinking problems in parents and extended family. Quality of relationships in past and present. Childhood environment.

Attitude to referral Why have they attended the appointment today? Do they feel they have an alcohol problem and if so will they accept help for it? What sort of help do they want and are there types of treatment they will not accept?

Patient goals What (if anything) do they want to change about their drinking? What pattern of drinking do they aspire to?

Physical examination Note general condition; evidence of withdrawals including tremor in hands or protruded tongue; degree of facial capilliarisation; stigmata of liver disease (palpable liver edge, jaundice, spider naevi, ascites, palmar erythema); evidence of peripheral neuropathy; ataxia of gait; breath alcohol reading.

Blood testing FBC, LFTs, other blood tests as indicated on history/ examination.

Giving drinking advice

There are a variety of situations where the doctor will be called on to give 'safe drinking' advice: individuals whose histories reveal evolving risky drinking patterns; patients with comorbid psychiatric illness; and individuals with alcohol problems who are attempting controlled drinking rather than abstinence.

There are a wide variety of types of alcoholic drink, each of a different 'strength', (i.e. percentage alcohol by volume). It is the amount of alcohol taken rather than the type of drink which contributes to physical/mental health effects—avoiding spirits or other drinks perceived as 'strong' will not protect from health risks if the absolute amount of alcohol is above safe limits.

Sensible drinking Men should drink no more than 21 and women no more than 14 units of alcohol per week. There should be at least two non-drinking days per week. The amounts should be spread over several days, not drunk all at once. Amounts should not be 'saved up' from a light week and drunk on top of the following week's allowance. The amounts quoted are not 'safe' amounts but represent levels of drinking not associated with significant risks to health. In some situations (e.g. driving, operating machinery) the 'safe amount' is zero. Some individuals (e.g. previously alcohol-dependent, chronic medical conditions, pregnant) should not drink at all.

Techniques of controlled drinking Patients who are seeking advice about avoiding potential alcohol problems and those individuals who are seeking to change from 'at risk' or harmful drinking patterns to controlled drinking patterns may find a selection of the following strategies helpful:
- Set a weekly and daily alcohol limit and keep to it.
- Do not drink alone.
- Do not drink with individuals who drink heavily themselves.
- Pace drinking, matching the consumption of a light or slow drinker.
- Don't buy rounds.
- Alternate soft and alcoholic drinks. Drink with a meal.
- Rehearse what to say if offered a drink that you don't want.
- Plan alternative, enjoyable non-drinking activities to replace drinking periods, (e.g. cinema, sports).

Amounts of alcohol in common drinks

The amount of alcohol in drinks is measured in units. One unit contains ~8 grams of alcohol. In alcoholic drinks where the percentage of alcohol by volume is given, the number of units = volume in litres x % alcohol. Numbers of units in common drinks are given below. In calculating numbers of units in an alcohol history, remember that home measures of drinks are usually more generous than those in pubs.

Drink	Alcohol % by volume	Measure	Alcohol units
Beer and stout	4.0	Pint	2.0
Continental lager	5.0	440 ml can	2.2
Strong lager	9.0	440 ml can	4.0
Normal cider	4.5	Pint	2.5
		1 litre	4.5
Strong cider	8.4	1 litre	8.4
Wine	9–14	125 ml glass	1.5
		750 ml bottle	6.8–10.5
Gin/vodka/rum	37.5	25 ml measure	1
		700 ml bottle	26.3

Planning treatment in alcohol misuse

Patients presenting with alcohol problems often display marked ambivalence about whether there is even a problem, let alone about the need for change. This reflects both the perceived positive as well as negative roles alcohol plays in their lives and the memory of previous failure or difficulties in attempting change. The aim in counselling such patients is to guide them in making their own decision towards change, or if change is not likely or possible now, to guide them towards harm reduction and considering the possibility of future change.

Motivational interviewing This is a technique aimed at enabling a patient to move through the stages of change (p. 503) to the point where action can be contemplated. It is based on the principle that: 'people believe what they hear themselves say'. The interviewer aims to aid the patient in explaining why they should change their behaviour and how this will be achieved.

- Therapist does not take a directive or prescriptive role but expresses interest and concern for the patient's problems and explores the consequences of their behaviour.
- Uses open-ended questions, reflective listening and summarising with identification of discrepancy between individual statements.
- Aids the assessment of the pros and cons of current behaviour, avoiding confrontation or direct challenge.
- Emphasises patient's own perceptions of degree of risk rather than telling them about risks which they may not believe.
- Encourages personal responsibility and patient's choice of treatment options.

Planning interventions The initial assessment interview forms the beginning of intervention. Its aims are to gather and impart information, promote the possibility of positive action, and to plan treatment. The ongoing therapeutic relationship aims to maintain purpose, monitor progress, aid self-monitoring and self-awareness. The process of planning treatment should proceed along the following lines:

- Make diagnosis (alcohol dependence, harmful, or 'at-risk' use).
- Assess stage of change, (p. 503).
- Decide with patient the goal of intervention:
  - **Continue current drinking pattern** In some patients there will be no need for change at all. In others there will be a clear history of alcohol problems but the patient presents as 'pre-contemplative' regarding change. In these cases give harm-reduction advice and 'leave the door open' to further assessment and help rather than alienating the patient.
  - **Change to safer drinking pattern** Many individuals will be able to modify risky or harmful drinking patterns given appropriate advice and help (perhaps monitored by a 'drinking diary', which is later reviewed).
  - **Attempt abstinence from alcohol** In some individuals the only safe course is to aim to abstain from alcohol completely.
- For abstinence in a dependent drinker, consider the need for and setting of detox (p. 518).

- Plan support methods and follow-up (pp. 520–1).
- At follow-up contact, review progress, emphasise changes made, review mental health.
- Anticipate and deal with relapse if it occurs.

Abstinence vs. controlled drinking The decision to try for controlled drinking rather than abstinence is one for individual patient choice. The doctor should offer suitable advice.

- **Factors suggesting possibility of success of controlled drinking:** previous prolonged periods of controlled drinking, alcohol misuse primarily in context of other mental disorder which has responded to treatment, otherwise stable lifestyle, absence of drinking problem in family and friends.
- **Factors against controlled drinking:** previously alcohol-dependent, previous failure at controlled drinking, comorbid mental illness, comorbid drug use, established organ damage, risk of job loss/ marriage loss.

Relapse Alcohol misuse is a chronic illness and many patients will 'fall off the wagon' several times before achieving long-standing change. The possibility of relapse should be anticipated with the patient and appropriate strategies should be in place to deal with it (e.g. early OP review). *Causes of relapse:* ambivalent motivation, insufficient support, novel events, overconfidence, new mental illness.

Counselling families The family of a patient with alcohol problems may contact you directly to ask for advice regarding their relative.

- Patient's relatives sometimes request that their relative be detained in hospital 'to stop them drinking'. The MHA in the UK specifically does not allow detention of patients solely for reason of drug or alcohol dependency.
- Aim to encourage and reward moves by the drinker to achieve change in their drinking pattern, while avoiding rewarding and hence reinforcing drinking, but avoiding confrontation or ultimatums.
- Sometimes continued family involvement, despite their best intentions, serves only to support the drinker in their chosen lifestyle. In this case the family may have to be aided to step back, (AA call this 'disengaging with love').

Prognostic factors There is ~3.6-fold excess mortality cf. age-matched controls. Of 100 45-year-old patients at 20 years follow-up: 40% dead, 30% abstinent, 30% problem drinking. **Positive factors** Motivated to change; supportive family or relationship; in employment; treatable comorbid illness (e.g. anxiety disorder, social phobia); accepting of appropriate treatment goal; AA involvement. **Negative factors** Ambivalent to change; unstable accommodation or homeless; drinking embedded into lifestyle (e.g. limited pursuits outside alcohol, all friends are drinkers); repeated treatment failures; cognitive impairment.

Alcohol withdrawal syndromes

In a patient with alcohol dependence, stopping alcohol completely or substantially reducing the usual amount taken causes the development of characteristic withdrawal syndromes. These syndromes should be anticipated and prophylaxis considered in any patient:

- With a history of dependence.
- Who has previously experienced withdrawal syndromes.
- Who has consumed more than 10 units of alcohol on a daily basis for the previous 10 days.
- Currently experiencing withdrawals.

Uncomplicated alcohol withdrawal syndrome

- Occurs 4–12 hours after the last alcoholic drink.
- Features—coarse tremor, sweating, insomnia, tachycardia (pulse > 100), nausea and vomiting, psychomotor agitation, and generalised anxiety.
- Occasionally, transitory visual, tactile, or auditory hallucinations or illusions.
- There may be increasing craving for alcohol both in itself and as a relief from the withdrawal symptoms.
- Symptoms increase in severity in rough proportion to the habitual alcohol consumption, peaking at 48 hours and lasting 2–5 days, with more severe symptoms being more prolonged.

Alcohol withdrawal syndrome with seizures

- In 5–15% of cases withdrawals are complicated by grand mal seizures occurring 6–48 hours after the last drink.
- If seizures occur only during withdrawal they do not signify the development of idiopathic epilepsy.
- Predisposing factors: previous history of withdrawal seizures, idiopathic epilepsy, history of head injury, hypokalaemia.

Delirium tremens

Acute confusional state (p. 534) secondary to alcohol withdrawal. A medical emergency requiring inpatient medical care.

- Occurs in 5% of episodes of withdrawal. Onset 1–7 days after the last drink with a peak incidence at 48 hours.
- Risk is increased by severe dependence, comorbid infection, and pre-existing liver damage.
- In addition to the features of uncomplicated withdrawal there is:
  - Clouding of consciousness
  - Disorientation
  - Amnesia for recent events
  - Marked psychomotor agitation
  - Visual, auditory, and tactile hallucinations (characteristically of diminutive people or animals—'Lilliputian' hallucinations).
  - Marked fluctuations in severity hour by hour, usually worse at night.
  - In severe cases: heavy sweating, fear, paranoid delusions, agitation, suggestibility, raised temperature, sudden cardiovascular collapse.

- Reported mortality of 5–10%. It is most risky when it develops unexpectedly and its initial manifestations are misinterpreted (e.g. in a patient not known to be alcohol-dependent developing symptoms post-operatively).
- Differential diagnosis—hepatic encephalopathy, head injury, pneumonia, acute psychotic illness, acute confusional state with other primary cause.

Management of alcohol withdrawal

Detoxification (detox) is the medical management of withdrawal symptoms in a patient with substance dependence. Alcohol detox involves: psychological support; medication to relieve withdrawal symptoms (usually via a reducing benzodiazepine regime); observation for development of features of complicated withdrawal; nutritional supplementation; and integration with follow-up. Detox may be carried out as inpatient or, with support, in the community. The need to medically manage the complications of alcohol withdrawal can also arise in an unplanned fashion, (e.g. in an alcohol-dependant patient in police custody or following emergency surgery). Most of the problems of alcohol use are related to inability to maintain abstinence rather than to the initial problems of withdrawal.

Detox procedure
- Decide on setting.
- Assess need for benzodiazepine-reducing regime.
- Consider need for other medications.
- Provide verbal and written advice.
- Inform GP of the plans.
- Give the patient a contact in case of emergency.
- Decide on explicit follow-up after detox.

Setting
Outpatient detox
- Treatment of choice for most uncomplicated alcohol-dependent patients, with comparable completion rates to inpatient detoxification and comparable percentage remaining abstinent at 6 months.
- Where there are doubts about compliance or concerns about drinking 'on top of' the prescribed drug, the patient should be seen daily in the morning and breathalysed before dispensing that day's and the following morning's supply of the drug.

Indications for inpatient detox
- Past history of complicated withdrawals (seizures or delirium).
- Current symptoms of confusion or delirium.
- Comorbid mental/physical illness, polydrug misuse, or risk of suicide.
- Symptoms of Wernicke-Korsakoff syndrome (pp. 530–1).
- Severe nausea/vomiting; severe malnutrition.
- Lack of stable home environment.

Reducing regime
Benzodiazepines are prescribed in alcohol withdrawal to ameliorate unpleasant withdrawal symptoms (e.g. tremor, anxiety) and to reduce the risk of withdrawal seizures. They are prescribed in a rapidly reducing regime in order to avoid the development of secondary, iatrogenic dependence, while covering the period of maximum risk.
- Many units prefer chlordiazepoxide to diazepam for outpatient use as it has a lower abuse potential.
- Diazepam is often preferred for inpatient use as it is faster acting, allowing dose titration against effect, and can be given parenterally.

Indications for prescribing a reducing regime
• Clinical symptoms of withdrawal.
• History of alcohol dependence syndrome.
• Consumption is greater than 10 units/day over the previous 10 days.

Not required if
• <10 units daily.
• No history of withdrawals/drinking to avoid anticipated withdrawals.
• BAC =0 and no withdrawal features.

Symptom monitoring
Review patients regularly to assess withdrawals. Continuing symptoms should be managed by increasing the next day's planned dosages, rather than increasing the length of the course or relying on 'prn' dosage.

Benzodiazepine withdrawal regime
Suggested outpatient reducing regime using chlordiazepoxide.

	On waking	Midday	Early evening	At bedtime
Day 1	—	30 mg	30 mg	30 mg
Day 2	20 mg	20 mg	20 mg	20 mg
Day 3	20 mg	10 mg	10 mg	10 mg
Day 4	10 mg	10 mg	—	20 mg
Day 5	10 mg	—	—	10 mg

Other medications
• **Anticonvulsants** Benzodiazepines in sufficient dosage are the most effective anticonvulsants in alcohol withdrawal. Other oral drugs (e.g. phenytoin, carbamazepine) do not reach therapeutic level until after the time of maximal risk.
• **Antipsychotics** Where hallucinations or delusions develop they can usually be managed by temporarily increasing the benzodiazepine dose. The addition of an antipsychotic (e.g. haloperidol 5–10mg orally up to tds) should be considered if this fails. Antipsychotics do reduce the seizure threshold, but given sufficient benzodiazepine cover this should not be a concern.
• **Supplementary vitamins** Where there are symptoms suggestive of Wernicke-Korsakoff syndrome or evidence of malnourishment give parenteral B vitamins (p. 530). In other patients give a 4-week course of 100mg thiamine, tds.
• **Other psychotropics** While many patients withdrawing from alcohol complain of anxiety and/or depressive symptoms, many will be directly secondary to alcohol use/withdrawal. They should not be treated with psychotropics until they have been assessed when abstinent from alcohol. Generally speaking, do not start new psychotropics at this time.

Maintenance interventions in alcohol misuse (1)—psychological methods

In planning treatment in alcohol problems, attention should be focused not only on achieving, but on maintaining change. Many patients find the initial change (e.g. moving to abstinence or controlled drinking) surprisingly easy, but find it difficult to maintain change in the longer term. Alcohol misuse is a chronic illness characterised by relapse and in dependent drinkers there is the tendency for dependent drinking patterns to recur rapidly on abstinence. For this reason, maintenance interventions should support change, and in every patient, relapse should be anticipated and strategies to deal with it should be in place.

Individual counselling In addition to monitoring agreed change, individual counselling can address the following:
- Social skills training (e.g. 'saying no').
- Problem-solving skills.
- Relaxation training.
- Anger management.
- Cognitive restructuring.
- Relapse prevention.

In selected patients there may be a role for more formal psychotherapies.

Group support Variety of group methods both within the health service and in the voluntary sector. Variable local provision. Most widespread and best known is AA (see opposite).

Pharmacological support (pp. 522–3).

Residential abstinence In selected patients, time in a residential facility may offer a period of abstinence which is unachievable 'outside', allowing interventions in physical and mental health and a chance to plan social change to permit continued abstinence on discharge. A variety of facilities exist, usually outside health care provision; some offer detoxification, while others will only accept patients following detox. Used in patients where home environment is unsupportive of abstinence and there has been failure of previous treatment options.

Advice to all patients regarding relapse Returning to drinking is the most common outcome in patients. The stages of change model (p. 503) considers relapse to be at the beginning of a further process of change, but with increased knowledge as to future strategies to combat relapse. A relapse can be motivated by overconfidence or forgetting gains. A 'slip' does not mean a full-blown relapse is inevitable and all patients should have strategies to deal with relapse discussed and agreed 'ahead of time'.

Alcoholics anonymous (AA)

Alcoholics Anonymous (AA) is the best known and the most widespread of the voluntary self-help organisations for problem drinkers. It was founded in 1935 in the USA by Bill Wilson and Dr Bob Smith, themselves both problem drinkers. Currently there are ~3000 groups in the UK and ~88 000 groups worldwide. Associated organisations are Al-anon (for relatives of problem drinkers); Al-Ateen (for teenage children of problem drinkers); and Narcotics Anonymous (NA) (for addicts of illicit drugs).

AA views alcoholism as a lifelong, incurable disease whose symptoms can be arrested by lifelong abstinence. Many other groups will use a variant of the AA model—'12-step' programme. AA is a useful and effective intervention in many problem drinkers and all patients should be informed about AA and encouraged to consider attendance.

An AA meeting will generally follow a standard routine: there will be 10–20 people in each group, only first names are used; a rotating chairman will introduce himself with 'my name is X, and I am an alcoholic', then will read the AA preamble; a number of speakers are called from the floor who give an account of their stories and recovery if possible, leading to general discussion; the meeting ends with a prayer and is followed by informal discussions and contact between new members and sponsors who may offer emotional and practical support and perhaps a phone number. Open meetings are held where friends, family and interested professionals can attend. Closed meetings are for AA members only. *(See 'Useful addresses' for AA contacts in the UK and Ireland—p. 916.)*

The '12 steps'

1. We admitted we were powerless over alcohol—that our lives had become unmanageable.
2. Came to believe that a power higher than ourselves could restore us to sanity.
3. Made a decision to turn our will and our lives over to the care of God as we understood him.
4. Made a searching and fearless moral inventory of ourselves.
5. Admitted to God, to ourselves, and to another human being the exact nature of our wrongs.
6. Were entirely ready to have God remove these defects of character.
7. Humbly asked Him to remove our shortcomings.
8. Made a list of the persons we had harmed, and became willing to make amends to them all.
9. Made direct amends to such people wherever possible, except when to do so would injure them or others.
10. Continued to take personal inventory, and when we were wrong promptly to admit it.
11. Sought through prayer and meditation to improve our conscious contact with God as we understood Him, praying only for knowledge of His will for us and the power to carry that out.
12. Having had a spiritual awakening as a result of these steps, we tried to carry this message to alcoholics and to practice these principles in our affairs.

Maintenance interventions in alcohol misuse (2)—pharmacological methods

Aversive drugs

Disulfiram

Action Irreversible inhibition of acetaldehyde dehydrogenase (ALDH) which converts alcohol to carbon dioxide and water. If alcohol is taken, there is a build-up of acetaldehyde in the bloodstream causing unpleasant symptoms of flushing, headache, nausea and vomiting, and tachycardia.

Indication Can act as a helpful adjunct to therapy and allow the patient's relatives/employers regain confidence in their ability to remain abstinent.

Dose Prescribe once abstinence achieved. Starting dose: give 5 day's loading dose of 800 mg daily. Maintenance dose: 200 mg daily or 400 mg on alternate days (or 3 days/wk).

Side-effects Halitosis and headache. Rare reports of psychotic reactions and hepatotoxicity.

Notes:

• Patients should be counselled as to the nature and purpose of the drug and the likely side-effects if they drink.
• It is no longer recommended to give an alcohol 'challenge' to a patient newly started on disulfiram.
• Compliance is increased if the taking of the drug is monitored by another person (e.g. spouse).

Anti-craving drugs

Acamprosate

Action Believed to act through enhancing GABA transmission in the brain. Has been found to reduce alcohol consumption in animal models of alcohol addiction and patients taking it report diminished alcohol craving. In RCT, cohort treated with acamprosate showed an increased percentage remaining abstinent and a doubling of time to first relapse.

Indications Patients who wish to remain abstinent from alcohol.

Dose Once abstinence achieved: 666 mg tds.

Side effects GI upset, pruritis, rash, altered libido.

Notes:

• Discontinue if patient returns to regular drinking or relapses more than once while on the drug.
• Has no role in assisting with controlled drinking.
• Has no aversive action if alcohol is taken.
• Has no addictive potential itself.

Naltrexone

Action Antagonises the effects of endogenous endorphins released by alcohol consumption. It is believed that this diminishes both the desirable 'high' experienced on taking alcohol and the loss of control reported by most dependent drinkers.

Indications In motivated sub-groups of alcohol-dependent patients it appears to be effective in reducing total alcohol consumed and number of drinking days.

Dose Once abstinence achieved, give 50 mg od.

Side effects GI upset, feeling anxious/'on edge', headache, fatigue, sleep disturbance, 'flu-like' symptoms.

Notes:
- Does not have an aversive or dependence-producing effect.
- Not currently licensed in the UK for treatment of alcohol dependence.

Alcohol misuse disorders (1)

Acute intoxication The symptoms of alcohol intoxication will vary depending on the blood alcohol concentration (BAC), individual alcohol tolerance, and to some extent the setting in which the alcohol is taken. In general, as BAC rises from mild intoxication (BAC < 100 mg%) to moderate intoxication (BAC 100–200 mg%) to severe intoxication(BAC > 200 mg%) a characteristic syndrome of acute intoxication is observed. Initial symptoms are elevated mood, disinhibition and impaired judgement, followed by slurred speech, unsteady gait, nystagmus, ataxia, aggressiveness, lability of mood and impaired concentration, and eventually sopor and coma.

'At-risk drinking' There are reported benefits to health (lowered risk of coronary artery disease and strokes) associated with low levels of alcohol consumption as compared with those who are abstinent (the 'j-shaped curve'). Above this low level, health risks increase with increasing alcohol consumption. It is therefore arbitrary at which point drinking is considered 'at risk'. Patient and situational factors are important (e.g. any alcohol consumption while driving or in pregnancy carries increased risks; for patients with established alcohol-related organ damage any consumption is risky).

Harmful drinking (DSM-IV—alcohol abuse) Non-dependent drinking which continues despite established harm to the patient's physical or mental health secondary to the alcohol consumption. ICD-10 diagnosis considers only physical and mental health harm, not harm related to social sanction.

Alcohol dependence Harmful use of alcohol + established dependence syndrome (p. 502). Usually daily, stereotyped drinking pattern with increased tolerance, withdrawal features on abstinence, and 'relief drinking', (i.e. further drinking to alleviate the effects of withdrawals).

Pathological intoxication ('mania à potu') This is a medically and legally disputed syndrome which was not included in DSM-IV due to lack of empirical evidence. It is described as an idiosyncratic reaction to a small amount of alcohol characterised by severe agitation, belligerence, and violent behaviour followed by collapse, profoundly deep sleep, and amnesia for the events which followed the alcohol consumption. It is a very dubious diagnosis which is mainly sought after by defence lawyers, as most legal systems do not regard normal self-induced intoxication as a valid defence. There is of course a strong association between alcohol and violent crime. Careful re-examination of the history will usually demonstrate significant quantities of alcohol have been consumed.

Alcohol-induced amnesia ('blackouts') This term refers to transient amnesic episodes related to periods of intoxication. Characteristically the patient will report a 'gap' in their memory lasting several hours with global or partial amnesia for their actions during that time. The patient's behaviour as reported by witnesses is usually characteristic of their normal behaviour when intoxicated. This amnesia seems to be a failure of recall rather than initial registration and represents a reversible form of brain damage. Its occurrence is not predictive of longer-term cognitive impairment. It occurs in the later stages of a drinking career, if at all, and tends to recur once established. Two forms are described:

- *'En bloc'*—dense amnesia with well demarcated start and finish points.
- *Partial*—episodes with indistinct start and end point with islands of preserved memory and variable degrees of recall.

There is some degree of state-dependent recall in blackouts and a return to intoxication may aid recall. Because of the potential confusion of the term blackout with periods of LOC, the term *'alcoholic palimpsest'* is to be preferred.

Alcohol misuse disorders (2)

Alcoholic hallucinosis This is a substance-induced psychotic illness which is a rare complication of prolonged heavy alcohol abuse. The sufferer experiences hallucinations—usually auditory—in clear consciousness and while sober. The auditory hallucinations may begin as elemental hallucinations (e.g. bangs or murmurings) before, with continued alcohol use, being experienced as formed voices, most usually derogatory in nature. There may be secondary delusional elaboration.

- **Differential diagnosis** Transitory hallucinatory or illusionary experiences while intoxicated, delirium tremens, psychotic illnesses.
- **Course** In ~95% of patients there is rapid resolution of these symptoms on ceasing alcohol consumption but the symptoms rapidly recur on restarting drinking. In ~5% there are prolonged symptoms (<6 months after abstinence) and an emergence of more typical schizophrenic symptomatology.
- **Management** Persisting symptoms may be treated with anti-psychotic medication.

Alcohol-induced psychotic disorder with delusions Long recognised but only recently included in DSM-IV. Development of persecutory or grandiose delusions after long history of heavy drinking. No other features of delirium tremens. Resolves on abstinence.

Delirium tremens (p. 516).

Alcohol-related cognitive impairment The majority (50–60%) of heavy drinkers display some degree of cognitive impairment on cognitive testing while sober. There is impairment in short-term memory, long-term memory recall, new skill acquisition, ability to 'task-shift' and a decline in visuospatial ability greater than decline in language ability. CT/MRI examination of the brains of heavy drinkers reveals cortical atrophy (mainly white matter loss), and ventricular enlargement. Degree of structural abnormality is poorly correlated with degree of functional impairment.

Alcoholic dementia A potentially reversible, generalised dementia in which there is progression with continued drinking and arrest of decline and possible functional improvement on abstinence. There is cortical atrophy and ventricular enlargement (predominantly white matter loss). The changes correlate with total lifetime drinking and length of drinking history and occur earlier in women than men. Mechanism is believed to be a direct toxic effect of alcohol on neuronal tissue, with head injury, episodes of hypoglycaemia, and nutritional deficits contributing factors in some cases.

Wernicke-Korsakoff syndrome (pp. 530–1)

Pathological jealousy (Othello syndrome) This is a monosymptomatic delusional disorder (see p. 231) seen most commonly secondary to current or previous alcohol abuse. The form is a primary delusion in which the content is that the patient's spouse or partner has been or is being unfaithful. Delusional evidence may be provided to back up this belief and the patient may go to great lengths to obtain 'evidence' (e.g. following her, planting tape recorders, examining discarded clothing). There is a significant association with violence and even homicide towards the supposedly unfaithful partner.

Management
- Abstinence from alcohol with addition of anti-psychotic medication.
- It may be necessary for the couple to separate and advice to this effect may have to be given to the at-risk partner.

Psychiatric comorbidity

Anxiety and depressive disorders Symptoms such as generalised anxiety, panic attacks, and low mood are very frequently reported in alcohol abusers. Many patients with alcohol problems also merit diagnoses of depressive illness (~50%) or anxiety disorder (~75%). The phenomenology of these disorders is similar to that found when the disorders occur in isolation. The difficulty is deciding the sequence of events, as in some cases the alcohol problem is secondary to the patient 'self-medicating' with alcohol in order to relieve primary anxiety or depressive symptoms. Nonetheless, chronic alcohol use will act as a direct depressant, its secondary effects will produce depressogenic life events (e.g. loss of job) and alcohol-related effects such as 4 a.m. waking due to withdrawals or weight loss related to nausea may masquerade as, or mask, biological depressive features.

Patients may emphasise the primacy of the mood or anxiety features and seek their resolution before tackling the alcohol problem. Generally a primary mood or anxiety disorder diagnosis should not be made in the presence of continuing alcohol misuse and psychological or pharmacological treatment for mood disorder is unlikely to be effective. The correct course is to initiate detox if indicated and to reassess mood/anxiety symptoms after 4 weeks of abstinence, treating residual symptoms at this point. Only a minority will require formal treatment. An undiagnosed depressive illness preceding the alcohol problem is more common in women. Alcohol problems can also arise as a result of self-medication of agoraphobia and social phobia.

Suicide Classically quoted as lifetime risk of 10–15% in dependent drinkers. Now estimated at ~4% lifetime risk of suicide in those with alcohol problems. Psychiatric comorbidity is important, as is social isolation, physical ill health, and repeated failed attempts at abstinence.

Schizophrenia High rates of alcohol and substance use found in schizophrenic patients (~20%). Increased risk of violence and TD development. Alcohol is an easily available temporary treatment for some of the distressing symptoms of psychotic illness

Drug misuse Comorbid alcohol and drug misuse can be to enhance effects (e.g. euphoriant effect of alcohol and cocaine combined) or to minimise unpleasant side-effects (e.g. alcohol to relax after taking stimulants), or as a substitute when the primary drug is unavailable. Comorbid drug misuse is associated with poorer outcome. Some comorbidity can have an iatrogenic component where there is mixed abuse or substitution of benzodiazepines for alcohol. This can result from inappropriate prescribing of anxiolytics, misdiagnosis of alcohol problems as anxiety disorders, and repeated unsupervised withdrawals with hoarding of tablets. Aim to limit new prescriptions, review diagnosis in patients with treatment-resistance anxiety disorders, and avoid short-acting benzodiazepines (e.g. lorazepam).

Wernicke-Korsakoff syndrome

Wernicke encephalopathy and Korsakoff psychosis represent the acute and chronic phases of a single disease process—Wernicke-Korsakoff syndrome—which is caused by neuronal degeneration secondary to thiamine deficiency, most commonly seen in heavy drinkers.

Wernicke encephalopathy

Clinical features Acute onset of tetrad of: 1) acute confusional state; 2) ophthalmoplegia; 3) nystagmus; 4) ataxic gait. Associated features of: peripheral neuropathy, resting tachycardia, and evidence of nutritional deficiency. Ophthalmoplegia is most commonly 6th nerve palsy (paralysis of lateral gaze). The classical tetrad may not all be present in an undoubted case.

Aetiology Occurs secondary to thiamine (vitamin B_1) deficiency. Heavy drinkers are especially vulnerable due to poor intake (alcohol is calorie rich but vitamin poor), reduced absorption, and impaired hepatic storage. Other rare causes of thiamine deficiency are starvation, post-gastric resection, anorexia nervosa, and hyperemesis gravidarum.

Pathology Haemorrhages and secondary gliosis in periventricular and periaqueductal grey matter involving the mammiliary bodies, hypothalamus, mediodorsal thalamic nucleus, colliculi and tegmentum of midbrain.

Treatment

- Give high potency parenteral B_1 replacement—intramuscular *Pabrinex®*, 2 ampoules twice daily for 3–7 days. (N.B. Associated with allergic reactions: facilities for treatment of anaphylaxis must be available.) Avoid carbohydrate load until thiamine replacement is complete (e.g. do not rehydrate with glucose solutions).
- Treat immediately diagnosis is made or strongly suspected. In addition, consider treating all those at high risk (alcohol-dependent patients with poor nutrition) prophylactically with parenteral vitamins.
- All patients with symptoms of Wernicke encephalopathy and those at high risk should have parenteral vitamins as above. All other patients undergoing detox, or being assessed for alcohol problems should receive oral replacement—thiamine 100 mg tds for one month.
- Assess and treat for alcohol withdrawal syndrome (pp. 518–19).

Prognosis

- Untreated the acute phase lasts ~2 weeks with 84% of cases developing features of Korsakoff psychosis. Mortality of ~15% in untreated cases.
- With treatment, the ophthalmoplegia and confusion resolve within days, but the ataxia, neuropathy, and nystagmus may be prolonged or permanent.

Korsakoff psychosis

Clinical features Absence or significant impairment in the ability to lay down new memories, together with a variable length of retrograde amnesia. Working memory (e.g. ability to remember a sequence of numbers) is unimpaired as is procedural and 'emotional' memory. Thus the affected individual may be able to go with a psychologist to an interview room, perform adequately on working memory testing, show evidence of a new skill (e.g. mirror writing) they practised the day before, and yet later have no memory of ever having been in that room or having seen that psychologist before (although, on returning to the room, they may be more relaxed on subsequent occasions, due to state-related emotional memories). Confabulation for the episodes of amnesia may be prominent.

Aetiology Most commonly due to thiamine deficiency secondary to heavy alcohol use. Rarer causes are head injury, post-anaesthesia, basal/temporal lobe encephalitis, carbon monoxide poisoning, and thiamine deficiency secondary to other causes.

Pathology Pathological features are those of Wernicke encephalopathy. The presumed mechanism is disconnection of a mammillothalamic pathway crucial for memory formation.

Treatment
- Continue oral thiamine replacement for up to 2 years.

Prognosis
- 25% of cases show some degree of memory improvement over time with the remainder largely unchanged.
- The degree of impairment is directly related to the degree of memory impairment which may be incompatible with independent living.

Medical complications of alcohol misuse

Hepatic

- **Alcoholic liver disease (ALD)** is the most common cause of liver damage in the developed world. Presents as fatty change, alcoholic hepatis, and, finally, as cirrhosis.
  - Fatty change seen in >90% of heavy drinkers, can emerge after single heavy bout, may be asymptomatic, or may present as lethargy, malaise, painful, swollen liver, and obstructive jaundice. Reverses with abstinence.
  - Alcoholic hepatitis—40% of heavy drinkers.
  - Cirrhosis—up to 30% of heavy drinkers after 10–30 years. Predisposed to by genetic variation (reduced alcohol oxidation and increased acetaldehyde accumulation), female sex (less first pass metabolism and lower body water content for alcohol dispersal), comorbid hepatitis B or C infection.

Gastro-intestinal

- Gastritis/gastric erosions with consequent haematemesis.
- Metaplasia of lower third of the oesophagus (Barrett's oesophagus).
- Mallory-Weiss oesophageal tears secondary to vomiting.
- Peptic ulceration.
- Chronic diarrhoea.
- Chronic pancreatitis (alcohol is most common cause) with chronic fluctuating abdominal pain and steatorrhoea.

Cancers

- Hepatocellular, oesophagus, stomach, mouth, tongue, and pharynx.

Cardiovascular

- Hypertension.
- Dilated cardiomyopathy.
- Cardiac arrhythmias (esp. atrial fibrillation).
- CVA.
- Non- or very light drinkers have higher risk than light drinkers even after controlling for smoking, hypertension, etc. (i.e. 'the J shaped curve' for mortality); no specific drink type (i.e. not red wine); mechanism may be increase in protective HDL and reduced platelet adhesion.

Respiratory

- Tuberculosis.
- Klebsiella and streptococcal pneumonia.
- Increased vulnerability is related to decreased immunity, poor nutrition, and self neglect.

Neurological

- Wernicke-Korsakoff syndrome (pp. 530–1).
- Peripheral neuropathy.
- Central pontine myelinolysis (pseudobulbar palsy + quadriplegia).
- Marchiafava-Bignami disease (corpus callosum degeneration).
- Cerebellar degeneration.

- Optic atrophy.
- Alcoholic myopathy.

Genito-urinary
- Erectile problems.
- Hypogonadism in men.

Other
- Foetal alcohol syndrome (p. 710).
- Gout.
- Osteoporosis.
- Impaired absorption and diminished intake of specific vitamins and food overall.
- Contribution to accidents particularly RTA.
- Exacerbating factor in violent crime and assaults.
- Diminished compliance with treatment for other medical and psychiatric disorders.

Illegal drugs

In the UK, community surveys indicate that one third of adults have tried illegal drugs in their lifetime, with 10% having used them in the previous year. The rates for those aged under 25 are higher, with 50% lifetime use and 33% in the previous year. At all ages males have higher rates of drug use than females ($\male:\female=3$–4:1). Cannabis is the most commonly used illegal drug, while community rates for the other drugs of abuse are low. Users show a variable pattern of consumption with episodic and situational use for drugs with low dependence potential and a tendency to continuous dependent use for more 'addictive' drugs. Among some users, particularly those in the dance scene, polydrug use is the norm with individuals consuming more than 10 different drugs. Use of illegal drugs is commoner in the young, in the lower socio-economic classes, and in those with psychiatric illness. At any one time <33% of dependent users will be in contact with treatment services; mean length of dependent use before seeking help is 9 years.

There are as many patterns of drug use as drug user and individual patient assessment is mandatory; nonetheless a number of patterns of use of illegal drugs can be recognised:

- **Experimental use** Use of drug in order to explore effects. Common among young and heavily driven by drug availability and drug use among peers. Very common for 'softer' drugs, (e.g. cannabis, volatile chemicals), rarer for more 'hard' drugs, (e.g. heroin).
- **Situational use** Drug use limited to certain situations, (e.g. parties, raves). Mainly drugs with stimulant/hallucinogenic properties.
- **Recreational use** Regular but non-dependent use. May be limited in time by period of life (e.g. ending at the end of university life) or may progress to dependent use.
- **Polydrug use** Non-dependent use of variety of drugs. One drug may be taken to potentiate the effects of another or to manage unpleasant after effects of drug use. Risks can be additive or multiplicative.
- **Dependent use** Use of a drug for which a dependence syndrome (p. 502) has developed. Continued use may be motivated more by the desire to avoid withdrawals than by positive drug effects which may have diminished due to the development of tolerance. Tendency is for the use of the dependent drug to predominate, with other drugs being taken only if the primary drug is unavailable.
- **Dual diagnosis use** Drug users who also suffer from a major mental illness. An important group for therapeutic intervention.

Categories of drugs of abuse

- **Opiates** e.g. heroin, dihydrocodeine, methadone, codeine, buprenorphine, pethidine.
- **Depressants** e.g. benzodiazepines barbiturates, alcohol, GHB.
- **Stimulants** e.g. amphetamine, cocaine, MDMA.
- **Hallucinogens** e.g. LSD, PCP, mushrooms, ketamine.
- **Others** e.g. cannabis, volatile substances, anabolic steroids.

Street slang associated with drug misuse

Street drug name	Conventional name
Acid	LSD
Adam	MDMA
Angel dust	PCP
Billy	Amphetamine
Blow	Cannabis
Brown	Heroin
C, Charlie, Coke	Cocaine
Crack	Freebase cocaine
Dope	Cannabis
Downers	Depressant drugs
E, Ecstasy, Eccies	MDMA
GBH, Grievous bodily harm	GHB (gammahydroxybutyrate)
Gear	Heroin
Grass, Hash	Cannabis
Jellies	Temazepam
Marijuana	Cannabis
Mushies	Psilocybin mushrooms
Poppers	Volatile nitrates
Roids	Anabolic steroids
Roofies	Rohypnol
Skag	Heroin
Skunk	Potent form of cannabis
Smack	Heroin
Snow	Cocaine
Special K	Ketamine
Speed	Amphetamine
Sulph	Amphetamine
Uppers	Stimulant drugs
Vallies	Diazepam
Vitamin K	Ketamine
Whizz	Amphetamine

Slang term	Meaning
Backtrack	Allow blood to flow back into IV syringe and then reinject
Chasing	Consume heroin by heating on foil and inhaling the fumes
Cold turkey	Withdrawal symptoms (referring to the piloerection)
Cooking up	Melting down heroin prior to injection
Fix	The required regular dose of drug in a dependent user
Gouching	Apparent somnolence following heroin use
Jag up	To inject drugs IV
Juggling	Selling drugs to finance one's own dependency
Junkie	An individual dependent on a drug
Mainline	To inject drugs IV
Nodding, On the nod	Apparent somnolence following heroin use
Rattling	Suffering from withdrawals
Score	Obtain drugs
Script	Legitimate prescription for drugs
Shooting gallery	Place where individuals meet to use drugs IV
Skin popping	To inject drugs sub-dermally
Sorted	Having obtained sufficient drug for one's own needs
Spliff	Cannabis cigarette
Tab	Dose of LSD impregnated onto paper
Works	Syringe and needles

Opiates

The opiates are a group of chemicals derived from the opium poppy (papaver somniferum); synthetic compounds with similar properties are called opioids. They have potent analgesic properties and as such have wide legitimate uses in medicine. They are widely abused for their euphoriant and anxiolytic properties. Heroin is the most frequently abused opiate.

Heroin Illicit heroin is sold as a brown or white powder in 'bags' or 'wraps', costing £50–£100 per gram, with a typical dependent user taking 0.25–2.0 g per day. It is most commonly consumed by smoking ('chasing'), but is also taken orally, occasionally snorted, and parenterally by IV, IM, or subcutaneous routes. Street supplies are of variable purity (25–50% by volume); occasionally, a particularly pure batch is associated with a series of deaths and ODs from users used to a less concentrated form.

In common with other opiates, heroin binds to specific receptors for which there are endogenous ligands (endorphins). There are overall cortical inhibitory effects with diminished pain sensation. After consumption effects are virtually immediate with euphoria amounting to ecstasy, intense relaxation, and untethering from worries and cares.

Although recreational use is not unknown, the tendency is for progression to dependent use and this is the most usual pattern by the time of presentation to treatment services. An established dependent user may move from smoking to occasional or regular IV use to potentiate effects. Users develop tolerance with regular use and there is cross-tolerance to other opiates. Dependent patients may describe limited euphoriant effects, with the drug being mainly taken to avoid unpleasant withdrawals.

Acute medical problems associated with heroin use by any route include nausea and vomiting, constipation, respiratory depression, and loss of consciousness with aspiration (the cause of many fatalities). Injected use adds risks of local abscesses, cellulitis, osteomyelitis, bacterial endocarditis, septicaemia, and the transmission of viral infections (Hepatitis B and C, HIV). Opiate dependency develops after weeks of regular use and is associated with an unpleasant (but not generally medically dangerous) withdrawal syndrome (p. 500).

Interventions Give harm reduction advice to users who continue to use opiates: do not use opiates while alone; do not use in combination with other drugs; avoid IV route; if injecting, give safe injecting advice (opposite). Consider managed detox (p. 554) or transfer to maintenance prescribing (pp. 554–5) in established dependence.

Other opiates These include dihydrocodeine, morphine, methadone, pethidine, buprenorphine, and codeine. They may be taken in their pre-prepared tablet or liquid form or prepared for injection. Their acute and chronic risks are similar to heroin.

Safer injecting advice
If using heroin it is safest to avoid IV use which has the greatest risk of overdose and other complications. If using heroin IV:
• Use new sterile needles and syringes on each occasion (give details of local needle exchange services if available)
• Use sterile water (water from running cold kitchen tap is closest)
• Never share needles, syringes, spoons, or filters with another user
• Rotate injection sites
• Avoid injecting into neck, groin, or breast
• Avoid injection into infected areas
• Ensure that the drug is completely dissolved before injecting
• Always inject with, not against the blood flow
• Do not take heroin while alone

It is safest to use new sterile needles and syringe on each occasion. Failing this, rather than use dirty equipment, flush both needles and syringes several times with thin bleach, then several times with clean water.

Depressants

Drugs of this group produce their effects by generalised or specific cortical depression. They include the benzodiazepines, alcohol, and the barbiturates. They can be taken for their pleasurable anxiolytic and relaxant properties alone, or as a way of counteracting unpleasant side-effects of other drugs of abuse (e.g. to 'come down' after stimulant use).

Benzodiazepines A class of chemicals initially synthesised in the 1950s. Largely replaced barbiturates in clinical practice as they did not cause fatal respiratory depression. They have therapeutic uses as anxiolytics, hypnotics, anti-convulsants, and muscle relaxants. Problems of dependency arising from long-term use became recognised in the 1980s leading to a fall in their legitimate prescription, but did nothing to diminish their popularity as drugs of abuse. All benzodiazepines have similar effects and are distinguished by their length of action: short-acting (e.g. temazepam, oxazepam), medium-acting (e.g. lorazepam, alprazolam), long-acting (e.g. diazepam, nitrazepam, chlordiazepoxide).

Benzodiazepines are taken orally, or less commonly by injection. There is hepatic metabolism to active compounds, some with long half-lives. They enhance GABA transmission and produce marked anxiolytic and euphoriant effects. Tolerance develops rapidly (with cross tolerance to all drugs in the benzodiazepine group), so requiring increasing doses to achieve similar effects.

Acutely they cause forgetfulness, drowsiness, and impaired concentration and coordination with consequent risk of accidents. Use by injection is associated with the same infective risks as IV heroin (p. 538). An additional problem seen in IV benzodiazepine users is limb ischaemia secondary to intravenous use of melted tablet contents. Chronic use is associated with impaired concentration and memory and depressed mood, all of which are more severe in the elderly. Benzodiazepine dependency develops after 3–6 weeks of regular use. There is a withdrawal syndrome (p. 500) which can be complicated by seizures and delirium.

Interventions Harm reduction advice to user as for opiates (p. 538), specifying safe injecting advice (p. 539) if using via IV route. Consider managed detox or transfer to maintenance prescribing (p. 556) in established dependence.

Flunitrazepam (Rohypnol) A short-acting potent benzodiazepine seen particularly in dance settings with intoxicant and (probably apocryphal) aphrodisiac effects. As it can produce impaired judgement and anterograde amnesia and is tasteless in solution it has been implicated in cases of 'date rape'.

Gamma-hydroxy-butyrate (GHB) A synthetic compound originally developed as an anaesthetic which is a probable intrinsic neurotransmitter. Particularly seen in dance settings usually in combination with other drugs or alcohol. Produces a sense of dissociation, euphoria, and intoxication. Taken as liquid, 5–10 mg dosage with effects coming on in 15–30 minutes and lasting several hours. Side-effects of nausea and vomiting, seizures, and respiratory depression. Dependence rare but reported.

Barbiturates Group of compounds used as hypnotics/anxiolytics in clinical practice prior to the introduction of the benzodiazepines. Now rarely prescribed and rarely seen as drugs of abuse. They act by facilitating GABA neuro-transmission. There is rapidly increasing tolerance to their anxiolytic effects in regular use but not to the associated respiratory depression.

Stimulants

These drugs potentiate neuro-transmission and increase cortical excitability producing effects of increased alertness and endurance, diminished need for sleep, and a subjective sense of well-being. They include cocaine (and crack cocaine), amphetamines, 3,4, methylenedioxymethamphetamine (MDMA or ecstasy), and caffeine.

Cocaine The mild stimulant/euphoriant effects of the chewed leaves of the coca shrub have been known to the people of South American for thousands of years, but in its refined form cocaine is a potent and highly addictive drug. Cocaine hydrochloride is refined to a white powder which may be inhaled ('snorted') or dissolved and injected. The main route of intake is by inhalation as it undergoes rapid 'first pass' liver metabolism. The user forms the powder into 'lines' and inhales via rolled paper tube (classically, a high denomination banknote). Each line contains ~25 mg cocaine. Freebase ('crack') cocaine (produced by alkalinisation, which produces the hydrochloride-free ion form) has a lower vaporisation temperature than the hydrochloride and can be smoked. In terms of rapidity of action and peak blood levels this compares with IV use.

Cocaine acts as a local anaesthetic at the mucous membranes. It has widespread effects in potentiating dopaminergic, serotinergic, and noradrenalinergic neurotransmission by blocking neuro-transmitter reuptake. Its actions begin a few minutes after consumption. There is increased energy, increased confidence, euphoria, and diminished need for sleep but with rapid fall-off in effects due to rapid metabolism, leading to repeated use. There are very intense effects from freebase cocaine use with rapid and intense 'high' with subsequent dysphoria. Cocaine is usually taken in an opportunistic way, sometimes in association with other stimulant drugs.

Acute harmful effects include arrhythmias, intense anxiety, hypertension → CVA, acute impulsivity, and impaired judgement. Chronic harmful effects include necrosis of nasal septum, foetal damage ('crack babies'), panic and anxiety disorders, persecutory delusions, and psychosis. It is not associated with classical dependence but a minority of users will consume in a regular 'compulsive' pattern.

Interventions Harm reduction advice (including safe injecting advice, p. 539, if appropriate). No role for substitute prescribing in managing withdrawal or for maintenance prescribing.

Amphetamines A group of compounds synthesised in the late 19th Century with current legitimate uses in child psychiatry (p. 578) and in narcolepsy (p. 402). Sold as 5 mg tablets or as white powder (~£10 per gram). The powder may be swallowed, inhaled, or dissolved and injected. Use is usually situational or recreational, although very regular use with dependence is recognised. There is chemical similarity to noradrenaline and dopamine, producing similar pharmacological effects to cocaine, but its slower metabolism gives a longer duration of action.

Acute harmful effects include tachycardia, arrhythmias, hyperpyrexia. irritability, post-use depression, and quasi-psychotic state with visual, auditory, and tactile hallucinations. Dependency is not seen but marked psychological addiction occurs, particularly in situations associated with drug use. Anxiety and depressive symptoms are frequently seen in users; their proper assessment requires a period of abstinence.

Interventions Harm reduction advice (including safe injecting advice, p. 539, if appropriate). No role for substitute prescribing in managing withdrawals. Very limited role for maintenance prescribing of dexamphetamine sulphate in the management of chronic, primary, heavy IV users (specialist instigation only).

MDMA (Ecstasy) This compound was synthesised in 1914. and initially was occasionally used as a adjunct to psychotherapy. Initially legal, it became widely used in the mid 1980s in association with house, rave, and techno music. It is taken orally as 50–200 mg tablet. A typical pattern of use is two or more tablets taken at weekends.

MDMA causes serotonin release and blocks reuptake. It has structural similarities to mescaline and amphetamine, therefore has both hallucinogenic and stimulant properties, these effects appearing ~30 minutes after ingestion. The initial 'rush' period of intoxication lasts ~3 hours and is characterised by a feeling of increased camaraderie and 'closeness' to others, a pleasurable agitation relieved by dancing, and decreased fatigue.

Acute harmful effects include increased sweating, nausea and vomiting, and diminished potency despite increased libido. Deaths have occurred associated with dehydration and hyperthermia (a toxic reaction similar to serotonin syndrome appears to exist (p. 870)). Chronic harmful effects include possible neuro-toxicity, hepatotoxicity, and possible chronic cognitive impairment. There is tolerance to its effects but dependence does not occur. 'Hangover' effects develop 24–48 hours after ingestion including fatigue, anorexia, and depressed mood (which may be severe).

Interventions Harm reduction advice regarding maintaining hydration and avoiding overheating during use. No role for substitute prescribing in managing withdrawal or for maintenance prescribing. For all stimulant drugs there may be a problem of assessing other aspects of mental state, particularly affective and psychotic features while chaotic use continues. In selected patients, inpatient assessment will be indicated to allow this.

Hallucinogens

Hallucinogens (or psychedelics) are a heterogeneous group of natural and synthetic substances which produce altered sensory and perceptual experiences. They include: lysergic acid diethylamide (LSD), phenylcyclidine (PCP), magic mushrooms, ketamine, mescaline, 2,5-di-methoxy 4-methylamphetamine (DOM), and dimethyltriptamine (DMT).

Lysergic acid diethylamide (LSD) A compound synthesised by Hofman while working at Sandoz pharmaceuticals in 1944. He reported the hallucinatory experiences which followed his initial, accidental ingestion. The drug also occurs naturally in seeds of the 'Morning Glory' plant. It became strongly associated with 1960s culture when its use was at its peak. There was early experimentation with its role in psychotherapy but there is no current legitimate use. It is very soluble and intensely potent (effective dose ~250 micrograms). It is sold impregnated onto paper, in tablets, or as a powder.

LSD is a indolealkylamine with structural similarity to serotonin. There are direct and indirect effects on serotinergic and dopaminergic transmitter systems. It is not now thought to provide a good model for endogenous psychosis. Its actions are very markedly situation-and expectation-dependent. Effects develop 15–30 minutes after ingestion and last up to 6 hours. There is initial euphoria; a sense of detachment; a sense of novelty in the familiar and a sense of wonder at the normal; visual distortions and misperceptions; synaethesia; and distorted body image. Somatic effects include dizziness and tremors.

Acute harmful effects are behavioural toxicity (i.e. harm related to acting on beliefs such as having the ability to fly) and 'bad trips' (i.e. dissociation, fear of incipient madness, frightening perceptions). There is no risk of overdose and physiological dependence and withdrawals do not occur. Chronic harmful effects include flashbacks (p. 92) even many years after consumption, post-hallucinogenic perceptual disorder, persistent psychosis, and persistent anxiety/depressive symptoms.

Interventions Harm-reduction advice directed towards maintaining a safe environment during use and avoiding behavioural toxicity—do not use alone, use accompanied by non-user if possible. For all hallucinogens, acute psychotic features should in general be managed by admission, maintenance of a safe environment, symptomatic treatment of agitation (e.g. with benzodiazepine), with expectation of resolution. Continuing psychotic features should be managed as for acute schizophrenia, (p. 198).

Phenylcyclidine (PCP) A hallucinogen rarely seen in the UK except as a contaminant of other drugs. May be smoked, snorted, taken orally, or more, rarely, parenterally. There is direct binding to opioid and aspartate excitatory receptors as well as serotinergic and cholinergic effects producing acute effects of confusion, visual sensory distortions, aggression, and sudden violence (which may be severe). Intoxication may give way to longer psychotic states.

Magic mushrooms About a dozen varieties of hallucinogenic mushrooms grow in the UK, the best known being the 'Liberty Cap' (*Psilocybe semilanceata*). They may be eaten raw or cooked, dried or prepared as a drink. Possession and consumption of mushrooms is not an offence unless they have been processed or prepared for illicit use. Small doses cause euphoria, while larger doses (>25 mushrooms) cause perceptual abnormalities similar to LSD. They are not associated with dependence or withdrawal features and tolerance develops quickly making continuous use unlikely. Harmful effects include nausea and vomiting, dizziness, diarrhoea and abdominal cramps, behavioural toxicity, and risk of accidental consumption of toxic fungi.

Ketamine A compound structurally similar to phencyclidine used as veterinary anaesthetic and in battlefield surgery. It is a unique anaesthetic as it does not produce RAS depression, instead it prevents cortical awareness of painful stimuli. It is taken illicitly as a sniffed powder, mean dose ~100 mg. Small amounts lead to a sense of dissociation, larger amounts to LSD-like synaesthesia and hallucinations, associated with nausea, ataxia, and slurred speech. Rare late effects are flashbacks, psychosis, and amnesic syndromes.

Other drugs

Cannabis This is the most commonly used illegal drug, with only a small minority of its users ever using another illegal drug. It has been used for centuries as a pleasurable mind-altering substance and as a medication for a wide variety of ailments. Clinical trials are underway to clarify its role in the treatment of chronic pain. Its illegal use is of interest to psychiatrists because of its association with other drugs of abuse (as a 'gateway drug') and because of its exacerbating effect on chronic psychotic illnesses.

Cannabis is produced from the dried leaves, flowers, stems, and seeds of the weed *Cannabis Sativa*. It may be distributed as herbal material ('grass' or marijuana), as a resin ('hash'), or as cannabis oil. Cannabis may be smoked in cigarettes, alone, or mixed with tobacco; the resin form may be eaten directly or incorporated into foodstuffs (e.g. cakes). These various forms contain at least 60 psychoactive cannaboids, the most important of which is 9-delta-tetrahydrocannibinol (THC). The dried herb contains ~5% THC by weight; resin ~10%; and cannabis oil ~15%. A particularly potent form of cannabis ('skunk') is becoming increasingly available.

Usage pattern is very variable, from infrequent situational use to daily heavy use; the latter at highest risk of harmful effects and most likely to take other drugs. There is a specific cannaboid receptor and a naturally occurring agonist at this receptor—'anandamide'. The role of this endogenous system has yet to be defined. In addition, cannabis shows both weak opiate-like and weak barbiturate-like effects. The drug is metabolised to both active and inactive metabolites and absorption of cannabis metabolites into fat mean that urine tests remain positive for up to 4 weeks after regular use has ceased.

The effects of intoxication are apparent within minutes if the drug is smoked, peaking in ~30 minutes and lasting 2–5 hours. The effects of orally consumed cannabis are slower to begin and more prolonged. The immediate effects include mild euphoria ('the giggles'), a sense of enhanced well-being, subjective sense of enhanced sensation, relaxation, altered time sense, and increased appetite ('the munchies'). Physically there is mild tachycardia and variable dysarthria and ataxia.

Acute harmful effects include mild paranoia, panic attacks, and accidents associated with delayed reaction time. Cannabis is normally smoked with tobacco, therefore all of the health risks associated with tobacco will also apply. The tendency of cannabis smokers to inhale deeply and to retain the smoke in the lungs for as long as possible will exacerbate this risk. There are no reports of fatal overdose. Chronic harmful effects include dysthymia, anxiety/depressive illnesses, the disputed *amotivational syndrome* (possibly representing a combination of chronic intoxication in a heavy user and a long half-life). The drug is not usually associated with physical dependency but there is a mild but characteristic withdrawal syndrome in the previously heavy regular user who stops suddenly, consisting of insomnia, anxiety, and irritability. Cannabis use can precipitate an episode of or relapse of schizophrenia. In addition, in regular users it is associated with dose-related paranoid ideation and other psychotic features.

Interventions As an illegal drug there are no set guidelines on safe use. Clinical experience suggests that irregular use can be free from major problems. Abstinence is indicated in those with major mental illness and continuing cannabis use may expose those recovering from more serious drug problems to dealers and the drugs sub-culture.

Volatile substances Simple hydrocarbons such as acetone, toluene, xylene, and butane have intoxicant properties. These chemicals are found in a variety of common products including glue, solvents, lighter fuel, paint stripper, fire extinguishers, aerosols, paints, petrol, typewriter correcting fluid, and nail varnish remover. They are rapidly absorbed when deeply inhaled or by sniffing propellant gases or aerosols. They cause non-specific increased permeability of nerve cell membranes and produce euphoriant effects, disinhibition, slurred speech and blurred vision, and visual misperceptions.

Acute harmful effects include local irritation, headache, cardiac arrhythmias, acute suffocation by bag or laryngeal oedema, unconsciousness, aspiration, and sudden death. Chronic harmful effects include liver and kidney damage, memory/concentration impairment, and probable long-term cognitive impairment. There is a withdrawal syndrome similar to alcohol in very heavy regular users.

Interventions Education of users and 'at risk' groups. Most use will be experimental with few going on to regular use. Legal controls on substance availability.

Anabolic steroids These prescription-only medicines (e.g. nandrolone and stanozolol) have limited legitimate uses in the treatment of aplastic anaemia and osteoporosis. They can be abused by athletes and body builders seeking competitive advantage or, more rarely, for their euphoriant effects alone. They produce increased muscle mass and strength, with increased training time and reduced recovery time as well as euphoriant effects and a sense of increased energy levels. (Other drugs misused by athletes include thyroxine, growth hormone, diuretics, erythropoietin, and amphetamine.)

Use of anabolic steroids is associated with physical health problems including hypertension, hypogonadism, gynaecomastia, amenorrhoea, liver damage, impotence, and male pattern baldness; and with mental health problems including acute emotional instability (sometimes known as 'roid rage'), increased aggressiveness, persecutory/grandiose delusions, depressive illness, and chronic fatigue. If injected they can also be associated with infection risks (p. 538). There is no withdrawal syndrome.

Interventions Education of risks through coaches, teachers, etc. Effective monitoring of individual sports with out-of-season testing.

Assessment of the drug user

In most cases an assessment of a patient's history of drug use will form part of a routine psychiatric interview. In addition, all doctors should consider the possibility of, and be prepared to ask about, comorbid drug misuse when interviewing patients for other reasons. The more detailed assessment described here is appropriate for patients in whom drug use is the primary focus of clinical concern and who are being assessed for entry into a treatment programme. The detailed assessment of a patient with drug use problems will usually be carried out over more than one consultation. There are only a few circumstances (such as an opiate-dependent patient presenting as an acute medical emergency), where treatment should be considered before full assessment. History should cover the following topics:

Background information Name, address, next of kin, GP, names of other professionals involved (e.g. social worker, probation officer).

Reasons for consultation now Why has the drug user presented now, (e.g. pressure from family, pending conviction, 'had enough', increasing difficulty injecting)?. What does the user seek from the program? In females, is there a possibility of pregnancy?

Current drug use Enquire about each drug taken over the previous 4 weeks. Describe the frequency of use (e.g. daily, most days, at weekends); and the number of times taken each day. Record the amount taken and the route. Ask the user about episodes of withdrawal. Include alcohol, tobacco, and cannabis. If there is IV use, inquire about needle or other equipment sharing.

Lifetime drug use Record the age at first use of drugs and the changing pattern of drug use until the most recent consultation. Enquire about periods of abstinence or stability and the reasons for this (e.g. prison, relationship, treatment programme).

Complications of drug use Overdoses—deliberate or accidental. History of cellulitis, abscesses, or phlebitis. Hepatitis B and C and HIV status if known.

Previous treatment episodes Timing, locus, and type of previous drug treatment. How did the treatment attempt end? Was the treatment helpful?

Medical and psychiatric history All episodes of medical or psychiatric inpatient care. Contact with hospital specialists. Current health problems. Relationship with GP.

Family history Are there other family members with drug or alcohol problems? Family history of medical or psychiatric problems.

Social history Current accommodation. How stable is this accommodation? Sexual orientation and number of sexual partners. Enquire about safe sex precautions. Describe the user's relationships—sexual, personal, and family. Note how many of these individuals currently use drugs.

Forensic history Previous or pending convictions. Periods of imprisonment. Enquire about continuing criminal activity to support drug use (remind the patient about confidentiality).

Patient's aims in seeking treatment What is the patient's attitude to drug use? What treatment options do they favour?

MSE Observe for history or objective signs of depressed mood or suicidal thoughts or plans. Inquire directly about generalised anxiety and panic attacks (a benzodiazepine user may be self medicating a neurotic condition). Inquire directly about paranoid ideas and hallucinatory experiences and the directness or otherwise of their relationship with drug use.

Physical examination General condition. Weight. Condition of teeth. Signs of IV use (examine particularly arms for signs of phlebitis, abscess, or old scarring). Examine for enlarged liver. Signs of withdrawals on assessment.

Urine screening This is essential. Several specimens should be taken over several weeks. Repeated absence of evidence of a drug on screening make its dependent use unlikely. Occasionally, testing errors do occur so do not take action (e.g. stopping maintenance prescription) on the basis of the results of a single sample.

Blood testing FBC, LFT, discuss with patient the need for HIV and Hepatitis screening.

Urine drug testing	
Substance	**Duration of detectability**
Amphetamines	48 hours
Benzodiazepines	
Ultra-short-acting (e.g. Midazolam)	12 hrs
Short-acting (e.g. Triazolam)	24 hrs
Intermediate-acting (e.g. Temazepam)	40–80 hrs
Long-acting (e.g. Diazepam)	7 days
Cocaine metabolites	2–3 days
Methadone (maintenance-dosing)	7–9 days (approximate)
Codeine/morphine	48 hrs
(Heroin is detected in urine as the metabolite morphine)	
Cannabis	
Single use	3 days
Moderate use (4 times per week)	4 days
Heavy use (daily)	10 days
Chronic heavy use	21–27 days
Phencyclidine (PCP)	8 days (approximate)

Planning treatment in drug misuse

The longer-term goal of treatment will be eventual abstinence from drugs, but this may not be an achievable short-or medium-term goal in an individual case. Immediate treatment aims are therefore: to reduce drug related mortality and morbidity; to reduce community infection rates; to reduce criminal activity, including the need for drug users to sell to others to finance their own habit; to optimise the patient's physical and mental health; and to stabilise where appropriate on an alternative substitute drug.

Make diagnosis Confirm drug use (history, signs of withdrawals, urine testing). Assess presence and extent of dependence. Assess severity of current problems and risk of future complications. Explore social, relationship, and medical problems. Assess stage of change (p. 503) and motivation. What are the short-term and medium-term aims of treatment?

Consider need for emergency treatment Where there is evidence of psychotic illness or severe depressive illness the patient may require inpatient assessment.

Engage in service Treatment of drug misuse cannot be carried out through 'one off' interventions. Patients should be engaged in the service by empathic and non-judgemental interviewing, availability of the service close to the point of need, and ability of the service to respond to change in a previously ambivalent patient. Substitute prescribing will be a strong motivator for engagement in some patients but should always also have a role in helping the patient achieve some worthwhile change.

Decide treatment goals and methods After assessment and diagnosis the doctor should discuss with the patient their thoughts about treatment options given the patient's drug history and local treatment availability. The doctor may have strong feelings about the appropriateness of a certain treatment but this will not be successful unless the patient agrees. Plans may include:

- **Return to dependent use as previously** Where individuals present in withdrawals, without other medical surgical or psychiatric reasons for admission, and where there is no history of complicated withdrawal, and where there has been no previous involvement in treatment services, it is inappropriate to prescribe. The individual should not receive replacement medication. They should be offered the opportunity to attend for further assessment.
- **Counselling and support** For non-dependent drug use particularly episodic use this may be the appropriate course. Give drug information and harm-reduction advice, possibly coupled with referral to a community resource.
- **Detoxification** (pp. 554, 556) Where there is drug dependence and the patient wishes abstinence, then a plan for detox is considered. This may be community-based, with psychological support, symptomatic medication, or reducing substitute medication, or as an inpatient. Consideration should be given to support after detox. How is abstinence to be maintained?

- **Supported detox without prescription** Some individuals can withdraw from drugs of dependence without use of a prescription. This may occur particularly where other changes in a person's life (e.g. change of area, break from dependent partner) facilitate abstinence. Unsupported detox without any medical help is frequently reported by users.
- **Supported detox with symptomatic medication** Here, in addition to the support mentioned above, the individual is prescribed other, non-replacement drugs to ameliorate withdrawal symptoms (e.g. lofexidine in opiate withdrawal).
- **Conversion to substitute drug with aim of detox** Here the aim is to convert the individual's drug use from street-bought to prescribed, Then, from a period of stability, attempt supervised reduction in dose, aiming towards abstinence.
- **Conversion to substitute drug with aim of maintenance** Here the aim again is to convert from street to prescribed drugs, with stabilisation via maintenance prescribing in the medium term. In a dependent user who does not feel that they can move to abstinence in the short term, maintenance prescribing to suitably selected patients is useful and associated with overall health benefits.

Address other needs The drug treatment service should consider part of its role as being a gateway to other services which the drug user may require but be reluctant or unable to approach independently. Patients with social, financial, or physical health needs should have these explored and the need for referral considered. Do not make such referrals without the knowledge and agreement of the patient. Review psychiatric symptoms which have been attributed to drug use to assess their resolution. Consider 'in-house' or specialist psychiatric treatment of residual anxiety/depressive symptoms.

Substitute prescribing (1)—principles

Withdrawal syndromes Any drug consumed regularly and heavily can be associated with withdrawal phenomena on stopping, even if not a classical withdrawal syndrome. The severity of withdrawal symptoms experienced by individual patients does not correlate well with their reported previous consumption and so it is best to rely on objective evidence of withdrawal severity. Clinically significant withdrawal phenomena occur in dependence on alcohol, opiates, and benzodiazepines and are occasionally seen in cannabis, cocaine, and amphetamine use. In general, drugs with short half-lives will give rise to more rapid but more transient withdrawals. Detoxification refers to the process of managed withdrawal from drugs of dependence which can be aided by psychological support, symptomatic prescribing, or by prescription of reducing doses of the same or similar drug.

Substitute prescribing In many circumstances the management of a drug user will include prescription of substitute medication. This may be to enable *detoxification* from a dependent drug, or *maintenance prescribing*—a move from unstable street use to prescribed dependent use to facilitate change now with abstinence later. The prescription of a drug should not occur in isolation but should be part of a comprehensive management plan, previously agreed with the patient and with relevant members of the multidisciplinary team. Prescribing for drug users should be guided by local procedures and practice, by the Home Office document 'Drug misuse and dependence—guidelines on clinical management' and by the British National Formulary.

Substitute prescribing may have the following indications

- To acutely reduce or prevent withdrawal symptoms. Where detoxification is planned, a first step can be the conversion of all opiate or benzodiazepine use to a single prescribed drug, which can then be reduced in a planned manner. Short-term prescription of a substitute drug may also be indicated to alleviate symptoms of withdrawal complicating the assessment of a dependent patient presenting with a medical or surgical emergency.
- To stabilise drug intake and reduce secondary harm associated with street drug use. In patients who are not considering detox in the short term, substitute prescribing can be a means of harm reduction (e.g. by reducing risk of accidental OD or by changing from IV to prescribed oral use). In addition, having a stable, legitimate supply can reduce the need to resort to criminal activity to fund drug use, reducing the secondary, wider social harms of drug use.
- To begin a process of change in drug-taking behaviour. A major aim in substitute prescribing is to fully supply the dependent drug and to move the patient away from extra, recreational drug use and chaotic, polydrug misuse. After stabilisation, the user should be encouraged to discontinue contact with dealers and friends who continue to use drugs in a chaotic fashion.
- To provide an incentive to continued patient contact and involvement with treatment services.

Substitute prescribing should only be considered where:
- There is objective evidence of current dependence. This should include a history of daily consumption, description of withdrawal symptoms, history of drug seeking to relieve or prevent withdrawals, and consistent presence of the drug on urine screening.
- The patient displays realistic motivation to change their drug use in a way which would be aided by prescription, (e.g. to cease IV heroin use on instigation of oral methadone prescription).
- The doctor believes the patient will cooperate with the prescription and that circumstances exist to allow adequate monitoring.

Assessing need for substitute medication

Before prescribing substitute medication for detoxification or maintenance the treating doctor should positively confirm dependence via:
- Positive history of daily use with features of dependence syndrome.
- Presence of drug in two urine specimens at least 1 week apart.
- Objective evidence of withdrawal features at assessment.

Writing a controlled drug prescription
- In doctor's own handwriting (some specialists have local exemption to this regulation but hand signature is always required).
- Patient's name, age, and current address.
- Name, concentration, and type of preparation required (e.g. methadone, 1 mg in 1 ml, sugar-free suspension).
- Dose and frequency.
- Total quantity of drug to be dispensed in both words and figures (not required for temazepam).
- Signed and dated.

Substitute prescribing (2)—opiates

Opiate detoxification

Opiate withdrawal In an opiate dependent individual, withdrawal symptoms appear 6–24 hours after the last dose and typically last 5–7 days, peaking on the 2nd or 3rd day. The withdrawal following discontinuation of the longer-acting methadone is more prolonged with symptoms peaking on the 7th day or so and lasting up to 14 days. *Symptoms of opiate withdrawal:* sweating; dilated pupils; tachycardia; hypertension; piloerection ('goose flesh'); watering eyes and nose; yawning; abdominal cramping; nausea and vomiting; diarrhoea; tremor; joint pains; muscle cramps.

Symptomatic medication Several non-opiate, oral medications are effective in ameliorating symptoms of opiate withdrawal. Unlike opiates, they are not liable to abuse or diversion to the black market.

- *Lofexidine* Alpha-adrenergic agonist. Starting dose: 200 micrograms bd, increased in 200–400 microgram steps up to maximum of 2.4 mg daily given in 2–4 divided doses. Measure baseline BP and monitor BP while raising dose (risk of symptomatic hypotension). 10 day course, withdraw over 2–4 days.
- *Loperamide* For treatment of diarrhoea. 4 mg initial dose with 2 mg taken after each loose stool. Maximum daily dose:16 mg.
- *Metoclopramide* For nausea and vomiting. 10 mg dose, up to maximum of 30 mg daily
- *Ibuprofen* For headaches and muscle pains. 400 mg dose, up to maximum of 1600 mg daily.

Substitute prescribing Several opiates are used in detoxification regimes. Where it is planned to continue prescribing on a maintenance basis, currently methadone is the drug of choice.

- *Methadone* Long-acting synthetic opiate. Its half-life is 24 hours and it is therefore suitable for daily dosing (which can be supervised). At daily dose >80 mg it produces near saturation of opiate receptors, minimising the 'reward' of further consumption. It is prescribed as a coloured liquid, unsuitable for IV use, at concentration 1 mg/1 ml. A sugar-free form is available. Licensed for use in opiate withdrawal and maintenance.
- *Buprenorphine* A partial opiate agonist. Licensed for treatment of drug dependence. Available in once-daily sublingual preparation. 8 mg ~ = 30 mg methadone. Believed to produce less euphoria at higher doses than methadone. Abuse potential as tablet can be prepared for injection.
- *Dihydrocodeine* Short-acting opiate. Not licensed for use in drug dependence. Occasional use in reduction regimes in patients already on a stable dose of street dihydrocodeine or in final stages of dose reduction in patients on doses of methadone <15 mg daily. Need for 2–4 times daily doses means that all dosage cannot be supervised.

Opiate maintenance

In maintenance prescribing, the aim is to prevent under-dosing (risk of use of street opiates, withdrawal symptoms) and overdosing (sedation, more drug available than required with diversion to the black market). There is research evidence[1] that a methadone script reduces street usage, criminality, and drug-related mortality. For outpatient initiation of methadone maintenance, arrange to review the patient in the morning with them having consumed no opiates for the previous 24 hours. Assess withdrawals and dispense methadone as follows:

- None or mild → no prescription. Review following day.
- Moderate (aches, dilated pupils, yawning) →10–20 mg methadone.
- Severe (vomiting, piloerection, hypertension) → 20–30 mg methadone.

Review after 4 hours and repeat dose if severe withdrawals continue, up to 30 mg. Review daily over the first week with dose increments of 5–10 mg daily if indicated. Methadone reaches a steady state 5 days after the last dose change. Arrange regular review after first week, making subsequent increases by 10 mg on each review up to ~120 mg. Stabilisation may take up to 6 weeks to achieve. For maintenance monitoring, see p. 558.

Dose reduction After stabilisation and complete abstinence from street opiates, a decision should be made as to whether the aim is dose reduction or maintenance prescribing. Rapid reduction regimes reduce the dose over 14–21 days (perhaps using the above symptomatic drugs as adjuncts). Usually reduction is more gradual. Slow reduction is over 4–6 months, reducing by ~5–10 mg each fortnight. In reduction regimes, make the largest absolute cuts at the beginning and make smaller, more gradual cuts as the total dose falls (i.e. aim to keep the percentage drop in dose similar). In general do not carry out reduction against the wishes of the patient as it is better to carry on a maintenance script rather than return to street use. Occasionally 'tread water' then restart reduction.

Opiate relapse prevention In previously dependent opiate users who have successfully completed detox, the opiate antagonist *naltrexone* may be used as an aid to relapse prevention. Taken regularly it will prevent the rewarding, euphoriant effect of opiate consumption.

Naltrexone Prescribed to aid abstinence in formerly dependent patients who have been drug free for >7 days. Starting dose 25 mg, increased to 50 mg daily. Total weekly dose may be given 3 days per week (e.g. to aid compliance, or to enable supervision), give 100 mg Monday and Wednesday and 150 mg on Friday. Naltrexone is also used in specialist inpatient facilities to facilitate rapid detox over 5–7 days.

Converting opiate dose to methadone dose

Drug	Daily dose	Methadone equivalent
Street heroin	0.5 mg–1 g	50–80 mg
Morphine	10 mg	10 mg
Dipipanone (Diconal)	10 mg	4 mg
Dihydrocodeine (DF118)	30 mg	3 mg
Pethidine	50 mg	5 mg
Codeine phosphate	30 mg	2 mg

1 Ward J Mattick R. Hall W (1997) *Maintenance treatment and other opioid replacement therapies.* Harwood Academic Press.

Substitute prescribing (3)— benzodiazepines

Benzodiazepine detoxification

Benzodiazepine withdrawal Chronic benzodiazepine use leads to development of dependence, with a characteristic withdrawal syndrome. The symptoms appear within 24 hours of discontinuing a short-acting benzodiazepine, but may be delayed for up to 3 weeks for the longer-acting preparations. *Symptoms of benzodiazepine withdrawal:* anxiety; insomnia; tremor; agitation; headache; nausea; sweating; depersonalisation; seizures; delirium.

Substitute prescribing As for opiates, benzodiazepine substitute prescribing should only be undertaken where there is clinical evidence of dependence, a clear treatment plan, and suitable patient monitoring in place. Substitute prescribing in benzodiazepine dependency uses the long-acting *diazepam*. In prescribing for patients with benzodiazepine dependency, convert all benzodiazepine doses to diazepam using the table opposite. The aim is to find the lowest dose which will prevent withdrawal symptoms (which may be well below the amount the patient has been taking). Divide the daily dose to avoid over sedation.

Benzodiazepine maintenance

Unlike methadone maintenance in opiate dependency, there is no evidence that long-term benzodiazepine prescription reduces overall morbidity. There is evidence that long term prescription of >30 mg diazepam daily is associated with harm. New prescriptions should be for 30 mg or less with patients already on higher doses reduced to this amount.

Dose reduction Cut dose by ~1/8th of total dose each fortnight. For low dose 2.5 mg fortnightly; for high dose 5 mg fortnightly. Review and halt or temporarily increase if substantial symptoms re-emerge. If patient is also opiate-dependent and on methadone, keep methadone stable while reducing benzodiazepine.

Conversion to equivalent diazepam dose

Drug	Dose
Diazepam	5 mg
Nitrazepam	5 mg
Temazepam	10 mg
Chlordiazepoxide	15 mg
Oxazepam	15 mg
Loprazolam	500 micrograms
Lorazepam	500 micrograms
Lormetazepam	500–1000 micrograms

Monitoring of maintenance prescribing

Detoxification and stabilisation on maintenance medication are often followed by rapid relapse despite successful completion. It is important to build monitoring of compliance into treatment strategies from the beginning.

Review Regular review of all patients on maintenance prescription is indicated at least monthly. At each review:

- Is dose sufficient? Is there evidence of withdrawals? Obtain feedback from pharmacist /community nurse.
- If dose insufficient? Consider small weekly increases in dose. Stop if evidence of intoxication.
- Confirm use of illegal drugs via history, urine testing, and observation of evidence of IV use.
- Plan movement towards goals.
- Consider intervention in mental health/other issues.
- Consider need for period of increased supervision.

Supervision of substitute prescribing The aim of supervised consumption is to ensure that the drug is being used as prescribed.

- Supervised consumption usually for initial minimum period of three months, taking into account work and child care issues.
- Consider ongoing supervised consumption (e.g. in pharmacy).
- Once-daily dosing with daily pick-up of drugs.
- No more than one week's prescription at a time.
- Advice re. children and methadone.
- Close liaison with pharmacist and GP.
- Thorough and clear records should be kept.
- No replacement of 'lost' prescriptions

Discontinuing a failing treatment Where there is persistent non-compliance with treatment and where attempts to improve compliance or modify treatment goals have failed then the maintenance should be discontinued.

- Discontinue via reduction regime
- Offer involvement with other services
- Inform GP and pharmacist

Psychotic illnesses and substance misuse

The association of substance misuse and psychotic features is a common and problematic one in clinical practice. The key to management is accurate diagnosis. Psychotic symptoms represent underlying psychiatric abnormality in this group of patients as in any other. There is not a general finding of 'low-grade' psychotic features in substance users and apparent psychotic features should not be attributed to effects of substance use without further inquiry.

Psychotic features during drug intoxication Substances with hallucinogenic or stimulant activity can produce psychotic features during acute intoxication. This is not consistent and varies by drug dose and setting. These are characterised by a rapidly changing pattern of symptom type and severity and include visual and other hallucinations, sensory distortions/illusions, and persecutory and referential thinking. They are characteristically rapidly fluctuating hour by hour and show resolution as the drug level falls.

Psychotic features during withdrawal In patients with physiological dependency on alcohol, benzodiazepines, or cocaine, withdrawals may be complicated by delirium in which variable psychotic features may be prominent. These will occur in the context of the general features of delirium (p. 734). There may be fluctuating visual or tactile hallucinations and poorly formed persecutory delusional ideas.

Residual psychotic illness (drug-induced psychosis) In some individuals, psychotic features continue after the period of acute intoxication and withdrawals has passed. These may be symptomatically more typical of primary psychotic illness and, once established, should be treated as for acute episodes of schizophrenia (p. 198).

Genuine comorbidity Many individuals with primary psychotic illnesses will misuse substances. In addition to the intrinsic risks of substance misuse, this carries risks in this group of diminished treatment compliance, risk of disinhibition leading to violence, and exacerbation of the primary illness. In view of the sometimes obvious (to others) causal link between drug use and relapse it is worth asking why patients persist in substance use. Reasons include:

- Endemic drug use within patient's environment, (e.g. home or social setting) or within other individuals with mental health problems.
- As means of self medicating distressing positive and negative symptoms (which may be improved by addressing these symptoms directly).

Legal issues related to drug and alcohol misuse

Fitness to drive It is the patient's responsibility to inform the DVLA of any 'disability likely to affect safe driving'. The DVLA regard drug misuse as a disability in this context. Group 1 licences cover motor cars and motor cycles, group 2 licences cover HGVs and buses. Decisions regarding licensing are made on a case-by-case basis; however, the DVLA's current guidelines are as follows:

- **Alcohol misuse:** loss of licence until 6-months (group 1) or 1-year (group 2) period of abstinence or controlled drinking has been achieved with normalisation of blood parameters.
- **Alcohol dependence:** loss of licence until 1-year (group 1) or 3-year (group 2) period of abstinence, with normalisation of blood parameters. Consultant referral and support may be required.
- **Dependency/persistent use of cannabis, amphetamines, MDMA, LSD and hallucinogens:** loss of licence until 6-months (group 1) or 1-year (group 2) period of abstinence. Medical assessment and urine screening may be required.
- **Dependency/persistent use of heroin, morphine, cocaine, methadone:** loss of licence until 1-year (group 1) or 3-year (group 2) period of abstinence. Independent medical assessment and urine screening prior to relicensing. A favourable consultant report may be required for group 1 and will be required for group 2. Subject to annual review and favourable assessment, drivers complying fully with a consultant-supervised methadone maintenance programme may be licensed.

Travel abroad Patients receiving a methadone prescription can travel abroad with a supply. Amounts up to 500 mg do not need a licence; amounts above 500 mg require a Home Office licence, obtained by application by the prescriber to the Home Office stating the patient's name and address, the strength, form, quantity, and daily amount of the drug prescribed, and the date of departure and return. In both cases the Home Office advises patients to carry a 'To whom it may concern' letter, indicating that the drug has been legitimately prescribed. This advice applies only to the right to take the drug out of the UK and return with any surplus. Travellers are advised to contact the embassy or consulate of the destination country prior to travel to ensure that import of methadone is allowed under local laws: countries' regulations vary widely.

Registration of drug addicts Compulsory registration of all drug addicts to the Home Office register of addicts ceased in 1997. Since then data have been collected on a regional basis via the anonymised regional drug misuse databases. Details regarding supply of forms in each area can be found in the BNF.

Drug testing and treatment orders (DTTOs) A form of community sentence introduced in the UK in 2000. The court makes an order requiring offenders with drug problems to undergo treatment and follow-up with a drug treatment service. This may be part of another community order or a sentence in its own right. The sentencing court monitors compliance via mandatory urine testing. Sentence plans may change in response to individual progress or problems. May last 6 months to 3 years.

Child and adolescent psychiatry

Introduction

The 'normal' and 'abnormal' child

The practice of child psychiatry involves the detection, evaluation, and care of children who have mental health needs. This may occur within formal specialist services or at a primary health care level, so it is essential that all individuals involved in the care of children have at least a basic understanding of normal and abnormal childhood experience and behaviour. Differentiating 'normal' from 'abnormal' can be difficult in young people since they are subject to developmental change and thus 'normality' evolves and varies according to differing age. Furthermore, what is normal may vary according to the family, social, religious, and cultural environment. Models of normal childhood experience and behaviour that are based solely on the norms of a particular society may be completely inappropriate in a different context. Having said this, there are a number of core 'norms' that transcend societal barriers, and likewise there are a number of core mental syndromes that have been shown to exist worldwide.

'Adaptive' and 'maladaptive' behaviours

Another principle that bears consideration in caring for the mental health needs of young people is the fact that *symptoms are not always abnormal*. An evolutionary perspective is useful here since it may be helpful to consider whether a specific experience or behaviour that manifests is adaptive or maladaptive. Is the symptom a normal response in a given situation that serves to successfully elicit caring behaviour from the parent or other caregiver? For example, a baby's persistent crying when hungry is adaptive and therefore 'normal' because it is 'designed' to elicit prompt feeding. Likewise, anxiety in a 2-year-old who is being separated from his/her parent into the care of a stranger is normal since, at this developmental stage, the child may perceive the attachment figure as the only source of safety. On the other hand, disabling separation anxiety in a 7-year-old is considered abnormal since the child has achieved a level of cognitive development at which he/she should have learned that many non-attachment figures might be considered 'safe'.

The barb in the arrow of childhood suffering is this: its intense loneliness, its intense ignorance.

Akhenaton (1354 BC), Egyptian king

If there is anything we wish to change in the child, we should first examine it and see whether it is not something that could better be changed in ourselves.

Carl Gustav Jung (1875–1961)

Assessment (1)—principles

The 'biopsychosocial approach'

Understanding and managing successfully the mental and behavioural problems of children depends upon the thoughtful consideration of all the biological, psychological, and social factors that may play a role in the generation of symptoms. It is important to remember that several factors may interact in a dynamic 2-way fashion, giving rise to symptoms. The 'biopsychosocial approach' is useful at all stages of the evaluation and intervention provided to a child.

The role of the multidisciplinary team

Child and adolescent (C&A) mental health care exemplifies the relevance of and need for a multidisciplinary approach. For medically trained professionals who are used to 'leading the team', C&A work may be at first a little bewildering. New trainees may find themselves at a loss as to the nature of their role within a team where social workers and psychologists may be better equipped to manage a specific case. But because young people are embedded within family, social, and educational systems, their problems cannot be medicalised and treated within an exclusively medical model. An holistic management plan for a child or adolescent presenting to health services might include the involvement of some or all of the following professionals:

- Psychiatrists and psychiatric nurses
- Psychologists and psychotherapists
- Occupational therapists, speech therapists, and physiotherapists
- Social workers, welfare agencies, and other statutory bodies
- Specialist paediatricians and neurologists
- Teachers and educational services
- Police services and the legal/court system

Children and families

When a young person comes into contact with mental health services he/she is more likely to have been referred for help than to have brought him or herself. This is important to remember, since 'the patient' may have no say in his/her referral and this may have implications for the therapeutic relationship. In addition, one is rarely dealing with the young person alone—young people are usually dependant upon caregivers, whether they are parents or other adults. Thus one is commonly confronted by a room full of people who may have differing experiences, motivations, and interpretations of the young 'patient's' problems and needs. The professional in this situation needs to be aware of the various dynamics and be vigilant in remaining objective and non-partisan. Sometimes a child's 'symptoms' are in fact the presenting symptoms of a family problem. Children may become anxious, depressed, or behaviourally disturbed as a result of marital conflict, parental illness, or dissocial behaviour, or other pathologies within the home. In these cases the challenge is to disentangle and identify the root causes of the child's symptoms. Likewise, families and other caregivers need to be actively included within the management plan for a child. With adolescents this may not always be the case.

Assessing children and their families

Flexibility is important when assessing children and their families. While a general system of assessment works in most cases, not all children have a standard 'nuclear family' arrangement. For example, some may live in foster homes or in children's homes. Older adolescents too, may have variable domestic situations, including being alienated from their families. Thus sensitivity to individual circumstances is mandatory. In general though, an assessment should include the components listed on pages pp. 570–1.[1,2]

1 Barker P (1988) *Basic Child Psychiatry*. Blackwell Science Ltd, Oxford.

2 Goodman R and Scott S (1997) *Child Psychiatry*. Blackwell Science Ltd, Oxford.

Assessment (2)—practice

Interviewing the family

- Where possible it is advisable to see the child or adolescent with all members of the family who live in the house. A good explanation to family members is to stress the importance of individual perspectives and experiences of the problem and the fact that each member can contribute to the solution.
- Establishing rapport or 'joining the family' is a primary objective of the initial interview.
- Define the problem/s and the desired outcome.
- Obtain the family history and construct a genogram.
- Developmental history of the child, parental relationship issues, and parental physical and mental health may best be obtained from parents alone, as it may be inappropriate discussing such information with children present.
- Observe family functioning and interactions. Note patterns of communication, degree of warmth, power dynamics, alliances, etc.

Interviewing the child alone

- Establishing rapport and gaining the child's confidence are primary objectives of the first interview. Young children should be invited to play, draw, etc.
- Begin with subjects well away from the presenting problem/s (e.g. interests and hobbies, friends and siblings, school, holidays).
- Progress to enquiring about child's view of the problem, worries, fears, sleep and appetite, mood, self-image, peer and family relationships, experiences of bullying or teasing, abuse, persistent thoughts, fantasy life, abnormal experiences, suicidality, etc. (It may take several interviews to obtain a full picture.)
- Observe: levels of activity and attention; physical and mental level of development; mood and emotional state; quality of social interaction.
- Physical examination—usually have a parent present.

Gathering other information

- Obtain consent to contact school for meeting or report from teachers, school psychologists, etc. Consider asking teacher to complete a checklist (e.g. Child Behaviour Checklist; Connors' Teacher Rating Scale).
- Consult other caregivers, medical professionals who have treated the child, and social agencies that have been involved with the child and/or family.
- Other rating scales (e.g. K-SADS; BDI).
- Psychological tests: may include IQ, personality and developmental assessments.
- Investigations: haematology; chromosome studies; EEG; CT; etc.

Formulation of the problem

- Consider aetiology in terms of constitutional, temperamental, physical, and environmental factors.
- Most symptoms fall into one (or several) of the following domains: emotional symptoms; conduct symptoms; developmental symptoms; relationship symptoms.
- Consider predisposing, precipitating, perpetuating, and protective factors.

Adolescence[1]

Adolescence is not just a blend of childhood and adulthood; it is a stage with unique biological and social characteristics of its own. Behavioural problems and disorders occurring during adolescence often represent exaggerations or unresolved versions of the normal development tasks of adolescence. Adolescence is a relatively new social phenomenon, since the age of puberty has steadily dropped while education has become prolonged over the last few centuries. This means that, particularly in the developed world, individuals achieve physical and sexual maturity before they assume adult roles.

Biological factors defining adolescence include the achievement of sexual maturity as well as the physical and cognitive changes resulting from hormonal shifts. These changes are sexually dimorphic but do not approach the extent of sexual dimorphism apparent in other primates.

Some of the psychological and social tasks of adolescence include:

- **Identity formation**—during adolescence the individual attempts to develop a strong sense of differentiated self; this includes a social identity, a sexual identity, a work identity, and a moral identity. (DSM-IV provides a coding for 'Identity Problem' under the rubric of *other conditions that may be a focus of clinical interest*.)
- **Self-determination**—there is a shift from accepting rules and boundaries imposed by others to setting them oneself; this involves substituting self-imposed control for externally imposed control.
- **Exploration vs. commitment**—the dual process of exploring ('keeping options open') versus making a commitment to particular options, choices, beliefs, etc. Premature commitment can lead to 'foreclosure' while prolonged exploration without commitment is sometimes called 'the psychosocial moratorium'.
- **Puberty rites**—some societies provide structured rituals to assist the adolescent with the transition from childhood to adulthood.

Disorders of adolescence

These are normally classified in terms of:
- Residual childhood problems (e.g. conduct disorder; separation anxiety disorder)
- Problems of adolescent transition (e.g. anorexia nervosa; parasuicide; substance misuse)
- Early adult disorders (e.g. bipolar disorder; schizophrenia)

Epidemiology of adolescent disorders

The Isle of Wight Study[2] remains a classic investigation of adolescent psychopathology. Findings include: 10% had psychiatric disorders; another 10% had feelings of misery and worthlessness (? depression); most had emotional or conduct disorders; half of 14-yr-olds with disorders already had the disorder at 10 yrs of age.

I would there were no age between ten and three-and-twenty, or that youth would sleep out the rest; for there is nothing in the between but getting wenches with child, wronging the ancientry, stealing, fighting.

Shakespeare: *The Winter's Tale* (Act III Scene 3)

1 Goodman R and Scott S (1997) *Child Psychiatry*. Blackwell Science Ltd, Oxford.

2 Rutter M, Graham P, Chadwick OF, Yule W (1976) Adolescent turmoil: fact or fiction? *J Child Psychol Psychiatry* **17**, 35–56.

An approach to behavioural problems

Five categories of behavioural problems:

- **Disruptive**—this includes oppositional, aggressive, destructive, disobedient, hyperactive, and substance abuse behaviours.
- **Anxious**—may manifest as clinginess, worry, fearfulness, shyness, avoidant behaviour, sleep problems, regressive behaviours (e.g. enuresis, encopresis, separation anxiety), somatisation, hyperactivity, ritualistic behaviours, etc.
- **Moody**—may manifest as irritability, sadness, crying, avoidant behaviour, regressive behaviours, 'acting out' (oppositional behaviours), poor weight gain, sleep problems, etc.
- **Social deficits**—manifests as playing alone, shyness, avoidant behaviours, no friends, unable to read social cues, relationship difficulties, inappropriate behaviours, language problems.
- **Developmental deficits**—may be deficits in language, motor function, milestones, etc.

N.B. Many 'symptoms' cross category boundaries, so it is important to gain as broad a view of the behavioural 'syndrome' as possible. It may also be that a dimensional view of childhood behavioural problems is more appropriate than rigid categorisation.

Differential diagnosis of various behavioural 'symptoms'

Since individual 'symptoms' can occur in more than one disorder, it is worth considering a differential diagnosis for the presenting behavioural symptom. It is also extremely important to differentiate a clearly maladaptive behaviour from one that is developmentally or situationally appropriate. 'Normal' behaviours also include those that form part of the child's expected testing and experimentation of the world. The child presenting with the following symptoms could have any of the listed conditions (which are discussed individually later in this section):

- **Hyperactive**—ADHD, oppositional and conduct disorders, anxiety, depression, mania, PDDs, substance abuse, sexual abuse.
- **Inattention**—ADHD, oppositional and conduct disorders, LD/PDDs, mood disorders, anxiety disorders, substance abuse, sexual abuse.
- **Separation problems**—attachment disorders, anxiety, depression, developmental problems, sexual abuse.
- **Social problems, avoidance**—depression, anxiety, social phobia, PDDs, sexual abuse.
- **Aggression, hostility**—oppositional and conduct disorders, ADHD, mania, psychosis, depression, anxiety, developmental disorders, LD/PDDs, substance abuse, sexual abuse.
- **Regressive behaviours**—depression, anxiety, developmental problems, LD/PDDs, substance abuse, sexual abuse.
- **Sexually inappropriate behaviours**—sexual abuse, conduct disorders, substance abuse, mania, psychosis, LD/PDDs, normal testing.
- **Somatisation**—anxiety, depression, LD/PDDs, psychosis, sexual abuse.

- **Tantrums**—oppositional and conduct disorders, ADHD, depression, anxiety, LD/PDDs, sexual abuse, physical problems, mania, psychosis.
- **Ritualistic behaviours**—normal, anxiety, OCD, LD/PDDs, psychosis.

Assessment of behavioural disorders—general principles

- **Identify the problem behaviour/s**—obtain a full description (from parents, child, teachers, etc.) of the problem behaviour/s. This should include the evolution of the behaviour, a chronology of the child's typical daily activities, the setting in which the behaviour occurs, the effects of it on family, school, relationships, etc, and attitudes of others to the behaviour/s. It is always appropriate to speak to the child alone (if possible) to establish his/her views, desires, and mental state.
- **Determine the parental strategy**—it is important to find out how the parents deal with the behaviour/s. This includes information about their expectations, philosophy of parenting, interpretation of the behaviour/s, moral, religious, and cultural views on parenting, etc. Also, how do the parents react or respond to the behaviour/s? How do they discipline or punish? What do they tolerate? Are they permissive or restrictive? Are they overprotective or uninvolved? Do they feel empowered or impotent, helpless, and incompetent as parents? How do they manage their frustrations, anger, etc? What coping mechanisms do they have?
- **Family history and dynamics**—as well as gathering a full family history of health, psychiatric problems, social and cultural circumstances, and support structures, it is also important to assess parental and sibling relationships, the presence of any significant stressors or losses, and how the problem behaviour interacts with family dynamics.
- **Social behaviour**—the evolution of the child's social behaviour, including social developmental, attachment behaviour, imaginary play, reading of social cues, relationships, and language use.
- **School behaviour**—attendance, changes in school, separation issues, socialisation, performance, peer and teacher interactions and responses, friendships, bullying, etc.
- **Child's health and development**—pregnancy, birth, and developmental milestones. Was the child planned, wanted? How did siblings react? How did parents and siblings cope? Any post-partum problems? Were there supports? Also, child's temperament, illnesses, treatment, etc.
- **Direct observation of parent-child interaction**—during the interview/s it is important to note how the child behaves and how parents respond and interact with the child. If siblings can be present their behaviour and interactions can also be evaluated. A home and/or school visit may add additional information about the behaviour in these settings.
- **Collateral information**—teachers, extended family, and social services may be able to provide important input and permission should be sought to contact and involve them where appropriate.

Attention deficit hyperactivity disorder (ADHD)

In recent years ADHD has become increasingly diagnosed and is the focus of both a great deal of research and an excess of media publicity. Many C&A mental health services have experienced a major increase in referrals for assessment for ADHD and doctors are under increasing pressure to prescribe stimulant medication for 'difficult kids'. The accepted definition of ADHD is: 'a persistent pattern of inattention and/or hyperactivity that is developmentally inappropriate'. DSM-IV specifies that at least some of the symptoms must have their onset before 7 yrs of age. (This is controversial, since studies have demonstrated that up to 90% of the 'inattentive' subtype may have a later onset[1].) Furthermore, the behaviour should occur in at least 2 settings and should persist for at least 6 months, to fulfil diagnostic criteria.

Clinical features (see opposite)

Epidemiology In the USA, incidence is estimated at 3–5%, while in the UK the figure of 1% is reported. There is a male predominance of 3:1.

Aetiology Genetics: 50% risk in MZ twins; 2x risk in siblings; ↑CD and substance abuse in parents; genes 5, 6, and 11 implicated. **Neurological** functional imaging shows frontal metabolism. **Neurotransmitters** DA and NA dysregulation in the prefrontal cortex. **Psychosocial** stress; family dysfunction; poor attachment; etc. **Evolutionary** 'response-ready' traits may have adaptive benefits. **Other** food additives, lead and alcohol exposure (little evidence).

Comorbidity ADHD is highly comorbid with 50–80% of children having a comorbid disorder: specific learning disorders (60%); CD and ODD (40%); substance abuse; depression; bipolar disorder[2] (**NB** Overlap in symptomatology).

Outcome Approximately 20% develop dissocial personality traits; 15–20% develop substance misuse problems; high rates of suicidality, poor self-esteem, unemployment. ADHD symptoms may persist into adulthood (20–30% with full ADHD syndrome and ~60% with 1 or more core symptoms). Impulsivity-hyperactivity remits early, while inattention often persists. Studies show a pattern of psychopathology, cognition, and functioning in adults similar to that in children and adolescents.[3]

Assessment

* Interview with parents, including full developmental, medical, and family history and assess family functioning.
* Interview with child: evaluate for physical or comorbid psychiatric disorder and assess attachment style and level of activity.
* Collateral information from school, agencies, etc. A school visit to observe behaviour in the classroom may be useful.
* Connor's Assessment Scale.

Treatment Effort should be made to provide psychological and social interventions before resorting to pharmacological treatment. Principles are:

- CBT methods, especially behavioural, are often effective
- Social skills training
- Parent management training
- Individual/family/group therapies
- Educational/remedial interventions
- Stimulants (e.g. Methylphenidate (Ritalin®); dextroamphetamine; pemoline)
- Other medications occasionally used are: desipramine; imipramine, and clonidine (NB specialist use only)

Clinical features of ADHD

- **Hyperactivity-impulsivity symptoms** include: fidgeting, moving, getting up and running about, climbing on desks, etc.; talking excessively; unable to play quietly; blurting out answers; jumping the queue; continually interrupting.
- **Inattention symptoms** include: cannot sustain attention; easily distracted; poor task completion; dislikes, can't organize, and makes mistakes with tasks that require attention; doesn't listen, is forgetful, and loses things for tasks.
- Very young children are often sensitive, have poor sleep, cry a lot, and are constantly active.
- Two groups are recognised anecdotally: the 'organic' group may have soft neurological signs, subtle motor and visuo-perceptual abnormalities, learning difficulties, and some degree of coordination problems; the 'dynamic' group commonly have a history of deprivation, poor attachment, stress and depression, and high levels of frustration.

---

1 Applegate B, Lahey BB, Hart EL, et al. (1997) Validity of the age-of-onset criterion for ADHD: a report from the DSM-IV field trials. *J Am Acad Child Adol Psychiatry* **36**, 1211–21.

2 Giedd JN (2000) Bipolar disorder and attention-deficit/hyperactivity disorder in children and adolescents. *J Clin Psychiatry* **61** (suppl 9), 31–4.

3 Biederman J, Faraone SV, Spencer T, et al. (1993) Patterns of psychiatric comorbidity, cognition, and psychosocial functioning in adults with attention deficit hyperactivity disorder. *AJP* **150**, 1792–8.

Methylphenidate (Ritalin®)

Mode of action

An indirect sympathomimetic that ↑ release of DA and NA.

Indications

ADHD and narcolepsy.

Clinical effects

↑ concentration and attention and ↓ impulsivity.

Side-effects

↓ Appetite and weight; nausea and vomiting; anxiety, insomnia, dysphoria, headaches; rarely tics, cardiac problems, and ↑ BP; high dose can cause psychosis or seizures. **Growth suppression** may be a long-term outcome of high doses over long periods without 'drug holidays'.

Prescribing practices

Vary, with higher doses in the USA (1 mg/kg) than in the UK (0.3 mg/kg).

Principles of prescribing (see NICE guidelines opposite)

- Start with 5–10 mg in morning; can add 5–10 mg at midday; late dose can cause insomnia
- Start low and titrate weekly
- Check weight, BP, and liver function regularly
- Monitor response (Connor's Rating Scale)
- May develop 'tolerance' over time; can get rebound hyperactivity as effect wears off (NB short t$\frac{1}{2}$ 1–2hrs); give 'drug holidays' over weekends

N.B. The 1990s saw increasing use and abuse of Ritalin worldwide. Concerns include the possibility of dependence, tardive tic disorders, and growth suppression. Vigilance should be exercised in correct diagnosis and prescription of ritalin.

NICE guidance on the use of methylphenidate (Ritalin®, Equasym®) for attention deficit/hyperactivity disorder (ADHD) in childhood

- Methylphenidate is recommended for use as part of a comprehensive treatment programme for children with a diagnosis of severe attention deficit/hyperactivity disorder (ADHD). 'Severe ADHD' is broadly similar to a diagnosis of hyperkinetic disorder (HKD), although in some cases treatment may be appropriate for children and adolescents who do not fit the diagnostic criteria for HKD but are experiencing severe problems due to inattention or hyperactivity/impulsiveness.
- Methylphenidate is not currently licensed for children under the age of six or for children with marked anxiety, agitation, or tension; symptoms or family history of tics or Tourette's syndrome; hyperthyroidism; severe angina or cardiac arrhythmia; glaucoma; or thyrotoxicosis. Caution is required in the prescribing of methylphenidate for children and young people with epilepsy, psychotic disorders, or a history of drug or alcohol dependence.
- Diagnosis should be based on a timely, comprehensive assessment conducted by a child/adolescent psychiatrist or a paediatrician with expertise in ADHD. It should also involve children, parents and carers, and the child's school, and take into account cultural factors in the child's environment. Multidisciplinary assessment, which may include educational or clinical psychologists and social workers, is advisable for children who present with indications of significant comorbidity.
- Treatment with methylphenidate should only be initiated by C&A psychiatrists or paediatricians with expertise in ADHD, but continued prescribing and monitoring may be performed by GPs, under shared care arrangements with specialists.
- Careful titration is required to determine the optimal dose level and timing. The drug should be discontinued if improvement of symptoms is not observed after appropriate dose adjustment.
- A comprehensive treatment programme should involve advice and support to parents and teachers, and could, but does not need to, include specific psychological treatment (such as behavioural therapy). While this wider service is desirable, any shortfall in its provision should not be used as a reason for delaying the appropriate use of medication.
- Children on methylphenidate therapy should receive regular monitoring. When improvement has occurred and the child's condition is stable, treatment can be discontinued at intervals, under careful specialist supervision, in order to assess both the child's progress and the need for continuation of therapy.

Conduct disorder (CD)[1,2]

Essence A repetitive and persistent pattern of behaviour in which the basic rights of others or major age-appropriate societal norms or rules are violated. These violations include aggression or cruelty to people and animals, destruction of property, deceitfulness or theft and serious violation of rules (e.g. truanting or running away). The term 'delinquent' is unfashionable and refers to the individual whose behaviour leads them into the criminal justice system—'young offender' is the modern term.

CD is important because it is common; it is the cause of great suffering in both the individual and in society; it is a risk factor for adult antisocial behaviour; and it is a major burden on public resources. In many countries it constitutes one of the major public mental health problems, making prevention strategies important (see opposite).

Epidemiology In North America CD is the most common reason for psychiatric evaluation in children and adolescents. It has an earlier onset and is more common in boys than in girls.

Aetiology A family history of antisocial behaviour or substance abuse, low CSF serotonin, low IQ, and brain injury are *biological factors* associated with risk for CD. *Psychosocial risk factors* include: parental criminality and substance abuse; harsh and inconsistent parenting; domestic chaos and violence; large family size; low socio-economic status and poverty; early loss and deprivation; lack of a warm parental relationship; school failure; social isolation; and exposure to abuse and societal violence.

Comorbidity ADHD; substance abuse; suicidality.

Clinical features (As above) Other common features: early sexual behaviour, gang involvement, low self-esteem, lack of empathy.

Course and outcome CD is often chronic and unamenable to treatment. Adult outcomes include: dissocial personality disorder; criminality; substance abuse; and mental disorders. However, less than 50% of CD cases have severe and persistent antisocial problems as adults.

Predictors of poor outcome are: early onset (before 10 yrs); low IQ; poor school achievement; attentional problems and hyperactivity; family criminality; low socio-economic status; and poor parenting.

Protective factors are: female gender; high intelligence; resilient temperament; competence at a skill; warm relationship with a key adult; commitment to social values; strong and stable community institutions; increased economic equality.

Assessment

- Clarify the purpose of the assessment (clinical, community, forensic).
- Obtain a full history with collateral from school, community, and legal system.
- Identify causal risk and protective factors.
- Assess for comorbidity and make a diagnosis (±psychometric testing).
- Formulate the problem and establish management plan (see opposite.)

Management of CD[3]

Multiple strategies are indicated:
- Ensure the safety of the child
- CBT problem-solving skills-in individual/group setting
- Parent management training-to improve social exchanges/stability
- Functional family therapy-combined CBT/systems approach
- Multi-systemic therapy-family-based, including school and community
- Medication-only for comorbid disorders (e.g. ADHD—p. 576)
- Academic and social support-referral to relevant agencies/groups

---

Prevention strategies and policy implications

- **Preschool child development programmes**—identifying parents and families at risk and instituting home visits and support
- **School programmes**—identify children at risk and institute classroom enrichment, home visits, and parent and teacher training
- **Community programmes**—identify children and adolescents through their involvement with social agencies and institute interventions such as enhanced recreation programmes, parent training and adult mentoring of youth
- **Social and economic restructuring** to reduce poverty and to improve family and community stability.

Oppositional defiant disorder (ODD)

Essence An enduring pattern of negative, hostile, and defiant behaviour, without serious violations of societal norms or the rights of others. Behaviour may occur in one situation only (e.g. home) and may lead to social isolation, depression, or substance abuse.

Epidemiology Onset is between 3 and 8 years old. More common in boys during childhood but equal rates in adolescence. A common condition affecting 15–20 % of C & As.

Aetiology Temperamental factors; sick or traumatised child; power struggle between parents and child (NB differentiate from normal autonomous 'struggle' of the young child and adolescent).

Outcome ¼ show no symptoms later in life but many progress to CD and/or substance abuse.

Management Same management principles as for CD (see above).

1 Bassarath L (2001) Conduct disorder: a biopsychosocial review. *Can J Psychiatry* **46**, 609–16

2 Waddell C, Lipman E, Offord D (1999) Conduct disorder: practice parameters for assessment, treatment, and prevention. *Can J Psychiatry* **44** (supp 2), 35s–39s.

3 Kazdin AE (2000) Treatments for aggressive and antisocial children. *Child Adolesc Psych Clinics N America* **9**, 841–58.

Pervasive developmental disorders (PDDs)[1]

Pervasive developmental disorders (PDDs) define a spectrum of behavioural problems commonly associated with autism. They frequently involve a triad of deficits in *social skills*, *communication/language*, and *behaviour*. The feature that all have in common is a difficulty with social behaviour. DSM-IV categorises PDDs as follows:

- Autism (pp. 584–5)
- Asperger's syndrome
- Rett's syndrome
- Childhood disintegrative disorder
- PDD-NOS

PDDs are characterised by either a lack of normal development of skills or the loss of already acquired skills. There is a gender bias with male > female predominance in all syndromes except Rett's syndrome (female predominance). Prevalence of PDD ranges from 10–20 cases per 10 000 individuals.

Asperger's syndrome (AS)[2]

Essence A syndrome first described by Hans Asperger in 1944 characterised by severe persistent impairment in social interactions, repetitive behaviour patterns, and restricted interests. IQ and language are normal or, in some cases, superior. Mild motor clumsiness (ICD-10) and a family history of autism may be present. Newton and Einstein may have had AS.

Epidemiology Male predominance. Prevalence may be as high as 1 in 300 as AS is almost certainly under-recognised.

'Autistic spectrum' There is some evidence that AS forms a spectrum with autism and high-functioning autism in terms of aetiology, pathology, and clinical presentation. Children with AS may have more striking autistic features before age 5, but later develop 'normally' in most spheres excepting social behaviour. Social deficits commonly manifest in adolescence or early adulthood when the individual experiences difficulty with intimate relationships. Psychiatric comorbidity is high with depression most common. BPAD and schizophrenia are more common than in the general population.

Rett's syndrome (RS)[3]

A genetic disorder (X-linked) of arrested neuro-development that affects almost exclusively females. Prevalence is 1 per 10–20 000. The first 6 months of life are normal, but between 6 and 18 months there is progressive head growth, loss of motor skills, loss of hand skills, stereotypies, abnormal hand movements, loss of social skills and language development. Seizures occur in 75% while spasticity, scoliosis, and respiratory difficulties are common outcomes. Developmental arrest plateaus and many may reach adulthood, although disability is great and prognosis poor.

Childhood disintegrative disorder (CDD)[4]

Rare, occurring in fewer than 5 in 10 000 children. Male predominance. There is normal development for 2–3 years, followed by a loss of acquired motor, language, and social skills between ages 3 and 4 years. Stereotypies and compulsions are common. Cause is unknown and prognosis is poor.

PDD-NOS

Also termed 'atypical autism', PDD-NOS is relatively common and encompasses sub-threshold cases where there are impairments of social interaction, communication, and/or stereotyped behaviour patterns or interest, but where full criteria for other PDDs are not met.

Did Newton and Einstein have AS?

Isaac Newton may well have had AS. He hardly spoke, was so engrossed in his work that he often forgot to eat, and was lukewarm or bad-tempered with the few friends he had. If no one turned up to his lectures, he gave them anyway, talking to an empty room. He had a nervous breakdown at 50, brought on by depression and paranoia.

As a child, Albert Einstein was a loner, and repeated sentences obsessively until he was seven years old. He became a notoriously confusing lecturer. In spite of this, he made intimate friends, had numerous affairs, and was outspoken on political issues.

1 Shaw JA (1999) Practice parameters for the assessment and treatment of children and adolescents who are sexually abusive of others. American Academy of Child and Adolescent Psychiatry Working Group on Quality Issues. *J Am Acad Child Adolesc Psychiatry* **38** (12 supp), 32s–54s.

2 Gillberg C (1998) Asperger syndrome and high-functioning autism. *BJP* **172**, 200–9.

3 Schneider JH and Glaze DG (2002) www.emedicine.com

4 Bernstein BE (2007) www.emedicine.com

Autism[1]

Essence Autism was first described by Maudsley in 1867 and named 'infantile autism' by Leo Kanner in 1943. It is a syndrome that has engendered controversy in terms of its definition, relationship to other syndromes (e.g. schizophrenia), and aetiology. It is characterised by a triad of symptoms:
- Abnormal social relatedness
- A qualitative abnormality in communication or play
- Restricted, repetitive, and/or stereotyped behaviour, interests, and activities

In addition, 70% have mild to moderate LD. The remaining 30% with normal IQ are classified as either **high-functioning autism** (with language difficulties) or **Asperger's syndrome** (with normal language). NB This last point is controversial and many would consider AS not to be classified as a form of autism. In general terms, 1–2% of those with autism have a 'normal' life; 5–20% have a 'borderline' prognosis (i.e. varying degrees of independence); but 70% are totally dependent upon support.

Epidemiology The onset of symptoms is typically before age 3. Male: female ratio is 3–4:1. Prevalence is 5–10 per 1000 individuals.

Aetiology The cause is unknown but a number of hypotheses exist: genetic (↑ in Down's syndrome and fragile X); obstetric complications; toxic agents; pre/postnatal infections (↑ with maternal rubella); autoimmune (anecdotal MMR-not proven);↑ association with neurological disorders (e.g. tuberous sclerosis)

Pathophysiology MRI: some have ↑brain size; ↑lateral and 4th ventricles; frontal lobe and cerebellar abnormalities. **Pathology:** abnormal purkinje cells in cerebellar vermis; abnormal limbic architecture. **Biochemistry:** ⅓ have ↑ serum 5HT; some have ↑ β-endorphin immunoreactivity.

Clinical features
- **Abnormal social relatedness:** impaired non-verbal behaviour; poor eye contact; impaired mentation; failure to develop peer relationships; reduced interest in shared enjoyment; lack of social or emotional reciprocity and empathy; attachment to unusual objects.
- **Abnormal communication or play:** delay or lack of spoken language; difficulty in initiating or sustaining conversation; stereotyped and repetitive (or idiosyncratic) language; mixing of pronouns; lack of developmentally appropriate fantasy, symbolic, or social play.
- **Restricted interests or activities:** encompassing preoccupations and interests; adherence to non-functional routines or rituals; resistance to change; stereotypies and motor mannerisms (e.g. hand or finger flapping or body rocking); preoccupation with parts of objects.
- **Neurological features:** seizures; motor tics; ↑ head circumference; abnormal gaze monitoring; ↑ ambidexterity.
- **Physiological features:** unusually intense sensory responsiveness (e.g. to bright lights, loud noise, rough textures); absence of typical

response to pain or injury; abnormal temperature regulation; ↑ paediatric illnesses.
- **Behavioural problems:** irritability; temper tantrums; self-injury; hyperactivity; aggression.
- **'Savants':** a minority may have 'islands of precocity' against a background of LD (i.e. isolated abilities).

Differential diagnosis Other PDDs; childhood schizophrenia; LD; language disorders; neurological disorders; sensory impairment (deafness or blindness); OCD; psychosocial deprivation.

Assessment of autism

- A multidisciplinary approach is required, involving psychiatrists, psychologists, paediatricians, neurologists, speech therapists, OT, and primary care teams.
- Full clinical evaluation: including physical and mental state as well as specific developmental, psychometric, and educational assessments.
- Rating scales: Autism Behaviour Checklist (ABC); Childhood Autism Rating Scales (CARS); Autism Diagnostic Interview-Revised (ADI-R); Autism Diagnostic Observation Schedule (ADOS).

Treatment strategies for autism

- Educational and vocational interventions: special versus mainstream
- Behavioural interventions: includes behaviour modification, social skills training, and CBT methods
- Family interventions: education; support; advocacy
- Speech and language therapy; OT; physiotherapy; dietary advice; etc.,
- Pharmacotherapy: symptom management (e.g. antipsychotics, for stereotypies); SSRIs for compulsive and self-harming behaviours and depression/anxiety
- Treat medical conditions (e.g. epilepsy, GIT problems)

---

1 Brasic JR (2002) www.emedicine.com

Language and learning disorders (LLDs)[1]

DSM-IV groups together a number of LLDs that share the following:
- Performance significantly below that expected for IQ or age
- A discrete developmental disability in the absence of LD
- Commonly present as emotional or behavioural problems
- 50% have a comorbid psychiatric disorder and many have other LLDs
- Most show strong evidence of heritability

Reading disorder ('dyslexia')

Difficulty with reading, in most cases involving a deficit in phonological-processing skills. 4% of school-age children. Male predominance. There is often a family history of dyslexia. 20% have comorbid ADHD or CD. Management includes 1:1 remedial teaching and parent involvement improves long-term outcome.

Disorder of written expression

Often coexists with dyslexia and manifests as difficulties with spelling, syntax, grammar, and composition. Occurs in 2–8% of school-age children with a 3:1 male predominance. Difficulties may first emerge with the shift from narrative to expository writing assignments.

Mathematics disorder

Female predominance and occurs in 1–6% of school-age children. Often associated with visuo-spatial deficits and attributed to right parietal dysfunction.

Language disorders

Includes **expressive** and **receptive language disorders, phonological disorder** and **stuttering**. There are delays or difficulties in language use that are not attributable to sensory or motor deficit or environmental deprivation, in excess of that based on scores of non-verbal intelligence. These disorders are highly heritable and may relate to impaired rapid temporal processing of auditory information. Male predominance and occurs in 5–10% of school-age children. Treatment includes speech therapy.

Stuttering[2]

A disturbance in the normal fluency and time patterning of speech. Usually struggle with initial syllables. Male predominance of 3:1. Most children grow out of it but stuttering affects 1–2% of adults. Majority of cases are developmental but occasionally there are acquired cases (e.g. head injury). **Aetiology:** genetic; incomplete cerebral dominance; hyperdopaminergic state. **Management:** speech therapy; antipsychotics (risperidone); (SSRIs) may have some effect).

1 AACAP (1998) Practice parameters for the assessment and treatment of children and adolescents with language and learning disorders. *J Am Acad Child Adolesc Psychiatry* 37 (10 supp), 46s–62s.

2 Costa D and Kroll R (2000) Stuttering: an update for physicians. *CMAJ* 162, 1849–55.

Enuresis

Essence Voluntary or involuntary voiding of urine, usually at night, in a child of 5 years or older. More common in males than females. Approximately 3–7% of 7-year-olds. Enuresis commonly results in low self-esteem and often becomes a focus for family conflict.

Aetiology Genetic—75% have a family history of enuresis; generalised developmental delay; poor potty training; psychosocial stressors (e.g. birth of a sibling, hospitalisation, starting school, domestic conflict); comorbid psychopathology (e.g. depression); organic causes.

N.B. Very important to exclude organic cause: UTI; obstructive uropathy; neurological problems; diabetes mellitus; seizures; drug side-effects.

Course Distinguish between 1° (never dry) and 2° (previously dry) enuresis.

Management Behavioural modification is the mainstay and includes:
- Restrict fluids at night
- 'Night lifting'
- Record-keeping (e.g. starcharts)
- Mattress alarm
- Rewards
- Imipramine—anticholinergic effect of increasing sphincter tone. 80% have some improvements but tolerance may develop after 6 weeks. NB Potential hazards of TCAs in children.

Encopresis

Essence Voluntary or involuntary soiling of stool in inappropriate places or in a child of 4 years or older. More common in males than females. Approximately 5% of children over 4 years of age.

Aetiology Regression under stress; power struggle with parents; child is preoccupied or distracted; organic causes. (Mechanism often involves retention/constipation with overflow.)

N.B. Very important to exclude organic cause: Hirschprung's disease; anal pathology; drug side-effects; neurological problems; nutritional disorders.

Course Usually stops by adolescence. Encopresis commonly results in low self-esteem, ostracism, and family over-involvement.

Management It is important to manage family stress and discord, educate parents about minimising shame (change pants often), and support the child psychologically. A paediatric referral is always indicated. Behavioural methods (see above) are the mainstay of treatment, but imipramine may offer some improvement.

Other behavioural disorders

Motor skills disorder

There are a number of conditions affecting children where the primary problem involves an impairment of motor function. This may manifest as a delay in developmental milestones and includes impairments of coordination, fine motor skills, and gross movement. Gross motor impairments suggest genetic aetiology while fine motor impairments suggest environmental causation. Treatment involves physiotherapy, OT, and educational assistance.

Sleep disorders

Classified as for adult sleep disorders (see pp. 388–425). The main syndromes that manifest in children and adolescents are: *nightmare disorder* (p. 418); *sleep terror disorder* (p. 415); and *sleepwalking disorder* (pp. 414–15). Management is the same as for adults.

Feeding and eating disorders of infancy and early childhood[1]

Pica This is a common condition where there is persistent (>1month) eating of non-nutritive substances at a developmentally inappropriate age (>1½ yrs). Common substances are: dirt, stones, hair, faeces, plastic, paper, wood, string, etc. It is particularly common in individuals with developmental disabilities and may be dangerous or life-threatening depending on the substance ingested. *Consequences* may include toxicity, infection, or GIT ulceration/obstruction. Typically occurs during 2nd and 3rd yrs of life, although young pregnant women may exhibit pica during pregnancy. *Hypothesised causes* include: nutritional deficiencies; cultural factors (e.g. clay); psychosocial stress; malnutrition and hunger; brain disorders (e.g. hypothalamic problem).

Rumination This is the voluntary or involuntary regurgitation and rechewing of partially digested food. Occurs within a few minutes postprandial and may last 1–2 hrs. Regurgitation appears effortless and is preceded by belching. Typical onset 3–6 months of age, may persist for several months and then spontaneously remit. Also occurs in older individuals with LD. May result in weight loss, halitosis, dental decay, aspiration, recurrent RTI, and sometimes asphyxiation and death (5–10% of cases). *Causes* include: LD; GIT pathology; psychiatric disorders; psychosocial stress. *Treatment* includes physical examination and investigations; behavioural methods; nutritional advice.

---

1 Ellis CR and Schnoes CJ (2002) *www.emedicine.com*

Attachment disorders

Normal attachment Attachment refers to the strong emotional bond that exists between a child and the primary caregiver. John Bowlby described the formation of healthy secure attachment from early infancy, as well as a normal pattern of *separation anxiety* commencing between 6 and 9 months, peaking between 12 and 18 months and decreasing during the 3rd year.

Disorders of attachment Insecure attachment manifests as *anxious*, *avoidant*, or *reactive* attachment and predisposes the child to other neurotic disorders later on.

Separation anxiety disorder

This represents increased and inappropriate anxiety around separation from attachment figures or home, which is developmentally abnormal and results in impaired normal functioning. It occurs in about 3.5% of children and 0.8% of adolescents.

Causes genetic vulnerability; anxious, inconsistent, or over-involved parenting; and regression during periods of stress, illness, or abandonment.

Symptoms anxiety about actual or anticipated separation from or danger to attachment figure; sleep disturbances and nightmares; somatisation; and school refusal (especially in adolescents).

Comorbidity depression; anxiety disorders (panic with agoraphobia in older children); ADHD; oppositional disorders; learning disorders; and developmental disorders.

Assessment full physical examination; attempt interview on own; parental interview including full developmental and family history; collateral from school if consented.

Treatment family/group therapies; CBT and play therapies; bridging back to school; SSRIs (e.g. fluoxetine, paroxetine).[1]

Reactive attachment disorder

This disorder reflects a disturbed pattern of social relatedness, is diagnosed before age 5 yrs, and may manifest as either *inhibited* or *disinhibited-* subtypes. *Causes*: deprivation and neglect, and this usually reflects a disturbance in the dyadic relationship between caretaker and child. *Contributing factors* include: caretaker may be young, isolated, inexperienced, and/or depressed; child may have difficult temperament and/or have a sensory impairment. It is more common in poverty-stricken and socially disrupted environments.

Symptoms failure to thrive; malnutrition; listlessness; vigilance; withdrawal; diffuse attachments in disinhibited subtype.

Differential LD; PDD; neurological disorders; psychosocial dwarfism.

Management hospitalise and secure protection if indicated; therapy focuses on caretaker-child dyad; involve social services.

Ethology and attachment

The history of attachment theory is closely allied to the development of ethology, the study of animal behaviour in its natural environment. Konrad Lorenz (an Austrian doctor) and Nico Tinbergen (a Dutch biologist) are recognised as the fathers of ethology, and shared the Nobel Prize in 1973 for their contributions to the field. Some of their most important discoveries were the identification of *imprinting, fixed action patterns* (FAPs), and *innate releasing mechanisms* (IRMs)—all of which have informed the understanding of infant attachment behaviour. Lorenz classically described imprinting in ducklings and Greylag goslings, the phenomenon where young animals form an immediate and irreversible social bond with the first moving object they encounter. The phenomena of FAPs and IRMs were first observed in the herring gull and the stickleback, and formed a basis for understanding the complex innate mechanisms that facilitate mother-infant bonding during the first weeks.

During the 1950s and 1960s, John Bowlby and Margaret Ainsworth used ethological principles to study the formation of healthy and abnormal attachment in children. Ainsworth developed the Strange Situation Procedure, an experiment that she used in several cultural settings to establish universal patterns of attachment. Healthy attachment was classically described as 'secure', while 'insecure' attachment encompassed 'anxious', 'resistant', and 'avoidant' types. These latter concepts are recognised in contemporary nomenclature under the diagnoses 'separation anxiety disorder' and 'reactive attachment disorder'. Bowlby also coined the term 'critical period' to describe the stage during which the infant is most responsive to developing secure attachment.

---

1 Bernstein BE (2002) *www.emedicine.com*

Anxiety disorders—overview[1,2]

Anxiety and fear are an inherent part of the human condition and in times of danger are often adaptive. As a result of changing developmental and cognitive abilities during childhood, the content of normal fears and anxieties shifts from concerns about concrete external things to abstract internalised anxieties. Anxiety disorders are characterised by irrational fear or worry causing significant distress and/or impairment in functioning and their relative prevalence reflects this shift in content. Thus specific disorders appear more common during specific stages of development.

Epidemiology Anxiety disorders are among the most common psychiatric disorders in youth. Prevalence rates range from 5–15% with 8% requiring clinical treatment. Age of onset varies for each disorder but range from 7 to 12 yrs. Separation anxiety disorder and specific phobia usually have onset in early childhood, Generalised anxiety disorder occurs across all age groups, while obsessive-compulsive disorder, social phobia, and panic disorder tend to occur in later childhood and adolescence.

Aetiological factors Genetic vulnerability; temperament that exhibits 'behavioural inhibition' (timidity, shyness, and emotional restraint with unfamiliar people or situations); anxious attachment; negative life events; dysregulation of 5HT and NA systems.

Organic causes of anxiety *Medical conditions:* hyperthyroidism; cardiomyopathy; arrythmias; respiratory and neurological diseases. *Substances:* alcohol; caffeine; cocaine; amphetamines; cannabis; SSRIs; LSD; ecstasy; etc.

Assessment

- Physical examination and interview with child
- Interview with parents including developmental and family history
- Rating scales: K-SADS; Hamilton Anxiety Rating Scale; DISC; CBCL

Treatment principles

- CBT is supported by a number of controlled studies as the psychological treatment of choice for paediatric anxiety disorders. Focuses on relaxation training, exposure and response prevention, and cognitive restructuring.
- Psycho-education and parent training.
- Psychodynamic therapies include group, family, and individual/play techniques.
- Pharmacological: SSRIs are first-line agents, but there are some data supporting specialist use of buspirone, alprazolam, and clonazepam in older children and adolescents with resistant symptoms.

1 Labellarte MJ, Ginsburg GS, Walkup JT, Riddle MA (1999) The treatment of anxiety disorders in children and adolescents. *Biological Psychiatry* **46**, 1567–78.

2 Dadds MR and Barrett PM (2001) Practitioner review: psychological management of anxiety disorders in childhood. *J Child Psychol Psychiat* **42**, 999–1011.

Generalised anxiety disorder

Essence Characterised by developmentally inappropriate and excessive worry and anxiety on most days about things not under one's own control. Severe enough to cause distress and/or dysfunction. Children are often perfectionist and self-critical. Most common anxiety disorder of adolescence with approximately 4% prevalence in this group. More common in females during adolescence. Only ⅓ seek treatment.

Symptoms Excessive worry; restlessness, irritability and fatigue; poor concentration; sleep disturbances; muscle tension. In *children*: somatic symptoms (headache; stomach pains or 'irritable bowel'; rapid heart beat; shortness of breath); nail biting and hair pulling; and school refusal.

Comorbidity Very high rates—up to 90%. Other anxiety disorders, depression, conduct disorders, and substance abuse are most common.

Management CBT; SSRIs; benzodiazepines (see p. 356 for overview).

Panic disorder/agoraphobia[1]

Essence Recurrent, unexpected **panic attacks** are the hallmark of this disorder, together with a period during which the child is concerned about having another attack and the possible consequences of an attack and exhibits significant behavioural changes related to the attacks. These latter features are referred to as **anticipatory anxiety**. The first attack must be uncued. A panic attack is described as a discrete period of increased fear peaking at about 10 minutes and lasting about ½ to 1 hr.

Symptoms Sweating, flushing, trembling, palpitations and tachycardia, chest pain, shortness of breath and choking, nausea and vomiting, dizziness, paraesthesia, depersonalisation and derealisation, and a fear of dying. N.B. In **young children** somatic symptoms predominate rather than classic symptoms. Agoraphobia may or may not coexist with the disorder, but is usually present. The essential feature is anxiety about being in a situation in which escape would be difficult or help unavailable should a panic attack occur. This leads to avoidance of places or situations and may result in school refusal and separation anxiety.

Epidemiology Panic disorder has an estimated prevalence of 3–6% and is more common in females post-puberty. Peak onset is 15–19 yrs.

Comorbidity Depression, substance abuse, and other anxiety disorders (especially social phobia) are most common.

Management Exclude organic causes (pp. 344–5); CBT; SSRIs; benzodiazepines (see pp. 348–9 for details).

1 Larsen LH (2002) www.eMedicine.com

Social phobia and selective mutism

Essence

Social phobia (SP) is extremely common and often undiagnosed and is the 3rd most common mental health disorder in America. It is characterised by marked fear of one or more social or performance-related situations where the person is exposed to scrutiny and in which embarrassment may occur. Exposure to social situations usually causes an anxiety reaction (may be a panic attack) that is distressing and recognised as inappropriate. Thus situations are either avoided or endured with discomfort. This may lead to agoraphobia and in severe cases school refusal.

Selective mutism (SM) primarily affects children and often manifests at school when the child cannot speak when called upon by teachers. The child may designate a friend or family member to serve as an interpreter and whispers in that person's ear in order to communicate.

Epidemiology SP is most common in adolescents with an estimated prevalence of 5–15% as opposed to only 1% in children. SM is seen in less than 1% of children in community settings and may represent SP with early onset. SP is more common in girls and the average age of onset for both genders is 12 yrs. Family studies demonstrate a 2x increased risk for SP in the relatives of SP probands, while twin studies show a 3x increased risk in monozygotic twins.

Comorbidity High rates of other anxiety disorders (especially GAD, simple phobia, and panic disorder) in approximately 30–60% cases, with mood disorders (20%) and substance abuse also frequent comorbidly.

Prognosis Although the prognosis for treated SP is fair to good, comorbid conditions may persist and hinder educational and social progress. Those who experience symptoms in 2 or more situations have a poorer outcome than those experiencing symptoms in a single situation only.

Management High levels of clinician awareness in diagnosing SP; individual and family assessments; K-SADS rating scale; CBT; SSRIs; moclobemide (specialist use only).

Simple phobias[1,2]

Essence Excessive fear of an object or situation with distress and phobic avoidance. There may be anticipatory anxiety and exposure can precipitate a panic attack.

Causes Familial pattern in some cases; paired conditioning and sensitisation.

Epidemiology Very common (10% in some studies); $♀:♂ = 2:1$.

Comorbidity Depression; substance abuse.

Subtypes Animal phobias; natural environment phobias (especially 5–10 yr-olds); blood/infection/injury phobias; situational phobias (e.g. lifts, closed spaces); other.

Management CBT is the mainstay, including relaxation training and graded exposure.

1 Velting ON and Albano AM (2001) Current trends in the understanding and treatment of social phobia in youth. *J Child Psychol Psychiat* **42**, 127–40.

2 Bernstein BE (2002) *www.eMedicine.com.*

Post-traumatic stress disorder[1,2]

Essence A syndrome characterised by a triad of symptoms: intrusive re-experiencing of a traumatic event; avoidance; and hyperarousal. Recognised in children since the 1980s. Symptoms variable in young children, but similar to adult pattern in older children.

Traumatic event Require exposure to a trauma with response involving fear, helplessness, or disorganized, agitated play (in young children).

Epidemiology Prevalence varies according to age, but develops in approximately 3–6% of children exposed to a trauma. Most exposed do not develop the disorder and those that are affected usually have a pre-existing vulnerability (i.e. 'an unnatural response to an unnatural event').

Clinical presentation in young children (Scheeringa criteria[3]):
- Compulsive repetitive play representing part of the trauma and failing to relieve anxiety
- Recurrent recollections of the event
- Nightmares, night terrors, and difficulty going to sleep
- Constriction of play
- Social withdrawal
- Restricted affect
- Loss of acquired developmental skills especially language regression and toilet training
- Decreased concentration and attention
- New aggression
- New separation anxiety

Depression is common in older children and adolescents.

Comorbidity Common in PTSD with depression, anxiety disorders, and substance abuse frequent in adolescents. Behavioural disorders common in young children.

Clinical assessment
- Interview with child (drawing and play methods useful in young child).
- Interview with parents including developmental and family history and account of the trauma.
- Instruments include K-SADS-PL and the Children's Post-Traumatic Stress Reaction Index.

Treatment (see p. 370)
- CBT focusing on psychoeducation and managing anxiety symptoms.
- Group treatments in case of mass trauma (N.B. debriefing controversial).
- SSRIs may be indicated for severe anxiety or depressive symptoms.

Terr classification of childhood trauma*

Type 1
Classic single, acute, traumatic event; the most common form in children.

Symptoms:
- full, detailed memories
- 'omens' or 'cognitive reappraisal'
- misperceptions

Type 2
Follows longstanding or repeated exposure to extreme external events, (e.g. chronic abuse).

Symptoms:
- denial and psychic numbing
- self-hypnosis, depersonalization, and dissociation
- rage, self-harm, and/or extreme passivity

Common outcomes include: borderline, antisocial, and narcissistic personality disorder or dissociative identity disorder.

* Terr L (1991) Childhood traumas: an outline and overview. *AJP* **148**, 10–20.

1 Perrin S, Smith P, Yule W (2000) The assessment and treatment of post-traumatic stress Disorder in children and adolescents. *J Child Psychol Psychiat* **41**, 277–89.

2 Yule W (2001) Posttraumatic stress disorder in the general population and in children. *J Clin Psychiatry* **62** (suppl 17), 23–8.

3 Scheeringa MS and Gaensbauer TJ (2000) Post-traumatic stress disorder. In *Handbook of Infant Mental Health*. Zeanah CH (ed.). The Guildford Press.

Obsessive–compulsive disorder (OCD)[1,2]

Essence (see p. 358) OCD is characterised by recurrent obsessions and/or compulsions that cause impairment in terms of time (>1hr/day), distress, or interference in functioning.

Epidemiology Prevalence in adolescents 1–3.6%. May occur as early as 5 yrs of age and mean age of onset is 10 yrs. Male predominance (3:2) in childhood, with equal gender distribution in adolescence. Mild *subclinical* obsessions and compulsions are common in the general population (4–19%). Although 50% of all cases have their onset by age 15, paediatric OCD is usually recognised only when severe, often years after onset. Often a chronic course with 50–70% still symptomatic after 5 years.

Aetiology Increased incidence in 1st degree relatives and in monozygotic twins; possible autoimmune process; reduced volume of caudate nucleus; hyperactive orbitofrontal circuits (SPET); 5HT receptor dysfunction.

Symptoms Contamination fears with ritualised washing and avoidance; repetitive doubting and checking (e.g. locks); repetitive counting, arranging, or touching.

Differential diagnosis Normal developmental rituals; Tourette's/tic disorder; Sydenham's chorea; PANDAS (see opposite); OCD 'spectrum' disorders (see p. 358); trichotillomania; OC personality disorder; psychotic disorders; side-effects of stimulants; rarely, basal ganglia disease.

Comorbidity 70% have at least one comorbid disorder. Includes other anxiety disorders, OCD spectrum disorders, ADHD, conduct disorders, developmental disabilities, substance abuse, eating disorders, and mood disorders.

Clinical assessment

- Full physical including neurological examination
- Psychiatric interview with the child
- Symptom rating and monitoring of severity over time: Children's Yale-Brown Obsessive Compulsive Scale (CY-BOCS)
- Interview with parents including full developmental and family history

Treatment approaches

- CBT, especially graded exposure and response prevention. Shown to reduce relapse.
- Pharmacological: 1st line agents include SSRIs (fluoxetine and sertraline) and clomipramine. Augmentation with clonazepam, haloperidol, and risperidone. Maintenance therapy for at least 1–2 years. Relapses common and long-term treatment advised after 2 relapses. (See p. 621 for dosages.)
- Psycho-education: important for both parents and child.

PANDAS[3] (paediatric autoimmune neurological disorder associated with streptococcus) An autoimmune syndrome associated with OCD and/or tic disorder, with pre-pubertal onset, characterised by episodic exacerbations of symptoms in association with evidence of Group A β haemolytic streptococcal infection.

1 Rapoport JL, Inoff-Germain G (2000) Treatment of obsessive-compulsive disorder in children and adolescents. *J Child Psychol Psychiat* **41**, 419–31.

2 AACAP (1998) Practice parameters for the assessment and treatment of children and adolescents with obsessive-compulsive disorder. AACAP. *J Am Acad Child Adolesc Psychiatry* **37** (10 supp), 27s–45s.

3 Swedo SE, Leonard HL, Garvey M, *et al* (1998) Pediatric autoimmune neuropsychiatric disorders associated with streptococcal infections: clinical description of the first 50 cases. *AJP* **55**, 264–71.

(Gilles de la) Tourette's syndrome

Essence Characterised by multiple motor and one or more vocal tics, present for at least a year, causing distress and impaired function.
- Facial tics are often the initial symptoms, but tics involving the neck, shoulders, and upper extremities are also common.
- Vocal tics range from meaningless sounds to clear words and *coprolalia* (expletives).
- Typically, tics vary over time with more complex tics emerging after some years.
- Frequency of tics wax and wane, with exacerbations often related to physical and emotional stress.

Epidemiology Mean age of onset is 7 years and $\male:\female$ = 3:1. Prevalence is approximately 5/10 000.

Aetiology Genetic factors—autosomal dominant and polygenic common (with increase in monozygotic twins and 1° degree relatives); dopamine system (antipsychotics reduce symptoms), basal ganglia implicated; Post-infectious (see PANDAS above).

Comorbidity OCD and ADHD common; also other tic disorders, LD, depression, anxiety, impulse and conduct disorders.

Management Psychoeducation; CBT; medication if tics are disabling and non-responsive to other therapies—haloperidol (pimozide, sulpiride, and clonidine for specialist use).

Other tic disorders

Chronic motor or vocal tic disorder More common that Tourette's syndrome, with a better long-term outcome.

Transient tic disorder Motor and/or vocal tics are present transiently for less than one year.

Depression in children and adolescents

Both major depressive and dysthymic disorders are common, familial, and recurrent in young people, and usually persist into adulthood. These disorders seem to be manifesting at earlier ages with successive cohorts, and comorbidity is high (approx. 50–70%). They are commonly associated with poor psychosocial, family, and academic function. Risk of suicide is high and so early detection and treatment are a priority.

Major depressive disorder

Epidemiology *Prepubescent*: prevalence up to 3% with 1:1 gender ratio. *Adolescent*: prevalence approx. 8% for males and 14% for females. Notably, during the last 50 years, there has been a steady increase in the risk for depression in children and adolescents.

Risk factors Family history/parent with mood disorder; loss of a parent or parental divorce; abuse; negative life events; family conflict; etc.

Clinical features
- *Young children* Apathy, poor feeding, failure to thrive, separation anxiety, irritability, aggression, tantrums, hyperactivity, somatisation, regressed behaviour (enuresis, soiling, etc).
- *Older children* Somatisation, school refusal, poor school performance, and sleep disturbance are common. Also 'acting out' vs. 'regression'.
- *Adolescents* Melancholia, low self-esteem, substance abuse, suicidal acts, school refusal, behavioural problems, biological symptoms, psychotic symptoms.

Note: 20% with an MDE will later manifest bipolar disorder. Risk factors include: psychosis; psychomotor retardation; family history of BPD; pharmacologically induced hypomania.

Comorbidity Dysthymia and anxiety disorders (50–80%); substance abuse (20–30%); disruptive disorders; somatisation; suicide (see p. 606).

Differential Medical conditions; substances; adjustment disorders; other psychiatric disorders.

Dysthymic disorder

Epidemiology 0.5–1.5% in children and 1.5–8% in adolescents.

Clinical features and course
- Depressed mood or irritability for at least 1 year.
- Other features are:poor energy and concentration; low self-esteem; feel unloved; anger; anxiety.
- High comorbidity (esp. MDD) and protracted course (3–4 years).

Management of depression[1]

Assessment

- Initial conjoint interview with parents/family and child.
- Physical examination and interview with child (play techniques may be useful with young child). NB. Check for comorbid problems. May require several interviews to develop rapport and ensure a full assessment. Evaluate suicide risk at every stage.
- Interview with parents to assess developmental and family history.
- Collateral from teachers, GP, social services, etc.
- Rating scales include Beck Depression Inventory and Child Depression Inventory, but are more useful for symptom screening, assessing severity, or monitoring improvement than for diagnosing depression.
- Laboratory investigations as indicated.

Treatment

- Establish therapeutic alliance and provide education to child and family.
- **Psychotherapy** is a reasonable initial treatment in mild to moderate depression. This may be individual, group, or family therapy and the mode should be decided individually in each case. Factors such as patient preference, availability of resources and expertise, and family context may influence choice. CBT is one of the most researched techniques, but IPT, behaviour therapy, psychodynamic therapy, and supportive therapy are used.
- **Pharmacotherapy**
  - SSRIs are regarded as 1st line therapy. Best evidence for use of fluoxetine. Starting dose: 5 mg/day for 4 weeks; then review.
  - TCAs are not supported by trials and have been associated with cardiac toxicity. However, individual cases may respond better to TCAs than to SSRIs. NB Check ECG, BP, Resting pulse, and weight prior to commencing a TCA. Starting dose: 1.5 mg/kg/day in children; 25–50 mg/day in adolescents. (Repeat ECG prior to increasing dose.)
  - Combination treatment should be considered in all cases (i.e. psychotherapy + medication). Also multidisciplinary involvement (e.g. social worker, OT).

Maintenance treatment

- **Psychotherapies** are particularly useful in maintenance phase and have been shown to reduce relapse.
- **Pharmacotherapy**: there are no studies of maintenance therapy in depressed C&A so similar principles should be used as for adults. Multiple episodes, complicated episodes (e.g. psychosis), and chronic symptoms are indications for maintenance. 2 or 3 episodes—maintenance for 1–3 years; >3 episodes, psychosis, or treatment resistance—consider longer treatment. Therapy should be continued at the dose required for remission.

---

1 AACAP (1998) Practice parameters for the assessment and treatment of children and adolescents with depressive disorders. *J Am Acad Child Adolesc Psychiatry* **37** Supp 10, 63S–83S.

Suicide and suicidal risk in young people[1]

Epidemiology Overall increase during the 20th Century, suicide now represents the 3rd cause of death in adolescents (12% of mortality in this group); represents 2% of child deaths. More prevalent in males than females.

2 important points:
- Completed suicide is only the tip of the iceberg of suicidal behaviour/ideation.
- There is a very strong association between depression and suicidality.

5 factors common to children and adolescents who attempt suicide:
- Life stressors
- Impulsivity
- Can't tolerate negative affect
- Cognitive distortions
- Hopelessness

Risk factors for suicide Mood disorder; other comorbid psychiatric disorder (e.g. substance use, anxiety, disruptive and personality problems); previous suicidal behaviour; family history of mood disorder or suicidal behaviour; exposure to family violence, to trauma, or abuse; availability of lethal agents (e.g. guns); poor parent-child communication; school problems; negative life events.

Management
- **Consider the need to hospitalise**—either to remove a child from a bad environment, or to observe closely for risk, or to intervene if risk is high. Factors indicating hospitalisation include:
  - Young child
  - Toxic environment
  - Runaway
  - Previous attempt
  - Serious attempt
  - Serious lethal method
  - Comorbid psychiatric disorder
- **Outpatient**—involve the family; commence treatment for psychiatric disorder (N.B. consider risk of overdose); follow-up regularly.

Prevention
General measures include:
- Screening and treating psychiatric disorders
- Crisis lines/access to help
- Education of parents, the public, and the media
- Intervene in cluster situations (e.g. several suicides in a school)
- Gun control

A pathway to suicidal behaviour

Predisposing factors	e.g. previous attempt; psychiatric disorder
↓	
Precipitating factors	e.g. 'domino effect' (suicide in community or in the media)
↓	
Opportunity	e.g. access (e.g. to a gun); privacy
↓	
Attempt	

Gun control and adolescent suicide (a U.S. perspective)

Accessibility to firearms, particularly handguns, influences the rate of teen suicides. Firearms are the most common method of suicide by youth. The increase in the rate of youth suicide (and the number of deaths by suicide) over the past four decades is largely related to the use of firearms as a method. Handguns were used in nearly 70% of teen suicides in 1990, up 20% since 1970. The most common location for the occurrence of firearm suicides by youth is the home. A home with a handgun is almost ten times more likely to have a teen suicide than a home without. There is a positive association between the accessibility and availability of firearms in the home and the risk for youth suicide. The risk conferred by guns in the home is proportional to the accessibility (e.g. loaded and unsecured firearms) and the number of guns in the home. If a gun is used to attempt suicide, a fatal outcome will result 78% to 90% of the time. Public policy initiatives that restrict access to guns (especially handguns) are associated with a reduction of firearm suicide and suicide overall, especially among youth.

Youth Suicide by Firearms Task Force

1 Flisher AJ (1999) Annotation: mood disorder in suicidal children and adolescents: recent developments. *J Child Psychol Psychiat* **42**, 439–49.

Bipolar disorder in children and adolescents[1,2]

Epidemiology BPD is rare in prepubescent children but rates of diagnosis are increasing. Adults with BPD report onset in childhood in only 0.5% of cases. Males predominate in childhood cases, while gender rates are equal in adolescents. Prevalence in adolescents is approximately 1%. (NB. Rates may be underestimated as 70% of initial presentations are a depressive episode). Familial factors are important with a 4 times greater risk of mood disorder in offspring of parents with BPD.

Clinical presentation Standard ICD-10 and DSM-IV criteria apply but several differences in C&A presentation should be noted:
- Manic children typically present with *atypical* or *mixed* features (e.g. irritability, labile mood, rapid cycling course and behavioural problems).
- Behavioural problems include: school problems, fighting, substance abuse, and sexual behaviour.
- The course is often non-episodic and chronic.
- There is wide developmental variability in presentation.
- Normal childhood imaginative play, boastfulness, overactivity, exuberance, and grandiosity may be mistaken for symptoms of BPD.
- Adolescent presentation may be bizarre, mood-incongruent, and/or paranoid. Schneiderian 1st rank symptoms occur in 20% cases.
- N.B. Early onset BPD is misdiagnosed as schizophrenia in ~50%.
- There is a high degree of symptom overlap between ADHD, ODD, and BPD in C&A.

Comorbidity ADHD (70%), substance abuse (40%), ODD (40%), anxiety disorders (30%), borderline PD, Tourette's syndrome (8%), bulimia nervosa (3%).

Outcome Early onset BPD has a poor outcome with 50% showing long-term decline in function. There is commonly a family history, suggesting that this is a highly genetic form of BPD. The course is often chronic and less responsive to treatment, with atypical and rapid-cycling features especially difficult to treat. Suicide risk is high with rates of completed suicide approximately 10%.

Management
- A full evaluation is required with collateral from family and school. Important factors include: +ve family history of mood disorder; the pattern of mood change; comorbid conditions; suicide risk.
- Clinical examination to exclude medical cause (e.g. hyperthyroidism).
- Admission to child or adolescent unit is preferable, for the purposes of observation, treatment, and safety.
- Psychological therapies include patient and family education, behavioural methods, and supportive therapy.

1 James A and Javaloyes A (2001) The treatment of bipolar disorder in children and adolescents. *J Child Psychol Psychiat* **42**, 439–49.

2 Giedd JN (2000) Bipolar disorder and attention-deficit/hyperactivity disorder in children and adolescents. *J Clin Psychiatry* **61** (suppl 9), 31–4.

Treatment guidelines for early-onset BPD (see p. 312)

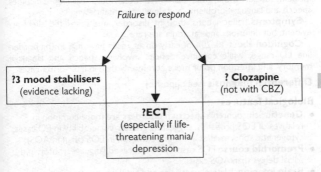

Classic mania

Lithium
0.8–1.2 mmol/L

**Classic mania
or
Dysphoric mania**
Sodium valproate
60–100 μg/ml

**Rapid cycling
mania**
Sodium valproate
60–100 μg/ml
Carbamazepine
7–10 μg/ml

Agitated
Add benzodiazepine

Psychotic
Add atypical antipsychotic

Lithium plus sodium valproate *or*
Lithium plus carbamazepine *or*
Sodium valproate plus carbamazepine

Failure to respond

?3 mood stabilisers
(evidence lacking)

?Clozapine
(not with CBZ)

?ECT
(especially if life-
threatening mania/
depression

Schizophrenia in children and adolescents[1,2]

Background and definitions Historically, rare cases of schizophrenia in children were noted as early as Kraepelin and were distinguished from autism and other PDDs. However, by the 1970s, 'childhood schizophrenia' included a broad spectrum of early-onset psychoses including infantile autism. Then, beginning with DSM-III, the distinction was again recognised with the same diagnostic criteria used in both adult and childhood-onset schizophrenia. Current research supports the notion of continuity between childhood and adult-onset disorder, with appropriate developmental adjustments in the former. Current classification (DSM-IV) recognises both 'early-onset schizophrenia' (EOS) with onset before age 18 and 'very early-onset schizophrenia' (VEOS) with onset before 13 yrs.

Epidemiology VEOS is extremely rare and the rate of onset then increases sharply during adolescence, peaking during late adolescence and early adulthood. There is a 2:1 male predominance during childhood, but this evens out with increasing age.

Clinical presentation Clinically, early-onset disorder resembles poor-outcome adult schizophrenia in that it is a chronic severe illness with a poor prognosis. The majority of cases have *premorbid* abnormalities, including social withdrawal, disruptive behaviour, learning difficulties, speech and language problems, and developmental delays.

    Symptoms hallucinations, thought disorder, and restricted affect are evident, but delusions and catatonia are rare.

    Cognition about 10–20% of early-onset cases have IQs in the borderline LD range, while cognitive deficits involving speech and language, memory, and attention occur more commonly than in later-onset cases.

Differential diagnosis (see opposite)

Biological features

- **Genetic** Schizophrenia-spectrum disorders are more common in relatives of EOS probands, suggesting greater vulnerability in EO cases; cytogenetic abnormalities are more common in EOS (than in AOS).
- **Premorbid course** EOS cases have increased language, motor, and social delays than AOS cases.
- **Brain imaging** ↑ lateral ventricles and total grey matter volume compared with AOS; similar functional deficits to AOS.
- **Obstetric complications** similarly implicated as in AOS.

Course and outcome

- EOS has a more insidious onset and poorer long-term outcome than AOS.
- Onset before 15 yrs is associated with lower IQ, ↑ cognitive deficits, and ↑ negative symptoms.
- Onset before 21 yrs results in ↑ social deficits in adulthood and only 20% have a favourable long-term outcome.
- EOS also seems to be associated with a poorer treatment response.

- Approx. 30% receive a later diagnosis of schizo-affective disorder or BPAD.

Management The principles of management are similar to that in AOS. However, several points are important:
- The emphasis should be upon early detection and intervention. This may include screening of high-risk individuals.
- Avoid depot and sedating antipsychotics—atypicals are commonly used as first-line agents in EOS.
- Psychosocial treatments should include family work and focus on psychoeducation, social skills, and problem-solving strategies and CBT methods. Therapies should address age-appropriate developmental tasks.

Psychosis in children and adolescents

Psychotic illnesses are rare in young children and present a particular challenge in both diagnosis and management. Very young children under 6 yrs have preoperational cognitions and thus 'reality testing' is blurred by a range of normal fantasy material. Imagined friends, transient hallucinations under stress, and loose associations may all occur as part of the normal spectrum of childhood experience.

Differential diagnosis There are many causes of psychotic symptoms in children and adolescents. This means that the assessment of a child with symptoms requires extreme care and thoroughness.

Possible causes include:
- Normal experience
- Organic conditions (e.g. TLE, thyroid disease, brain tumour, SLE, and substance misuse disorders)
- Mood disorders
- PDD/Autism
- OCD
- Schizophrenia
- Language disorders
- Dissociative disorders
- Culture-bound syndromes

---

1 AACAP (2000) AACAP official action. Summary of the practice parameters for the assessment and treatment of children and adolescents with schizophrenia. *J Am Acad Child Adolesc Psychiatry* **39**, 1580–2.

2 Nicolson R, Lenane M, Hamburger SD, et al. (2000) Lessons from childhood-onset schizophrenia. *Brain Research Reviews* **31**, 147–56.

Substance abuse in children and adolescents[1]

Substance abuse is increasingly common in young people. It may occur in a number of different contexts. These include:

- Experimentation
- Educational pressures
- Entanglements (e.g. relationship break-ups)
- Employment (unemployment)
- Extrication (from bad domestic situations)

Risk factors

- Biological vulnerability
- Personality traits (high novelty-seeking and low harmavoidance)
- Comorbid psychiatric disorders
- Parental problems (poor communication and rolemodelling, antisocial behaviour, substance abuse)
- Socio-economic deprivation
- Peer involvement (e.g. increasing association with the 'rave' culture)

Comorbidity Conduct disorders; ADHD; depression; poor cognitive, social, and emotional development.

Management

- Early identification of high-risk children (e.g. parents are substance abusers)
- Treat comorbid psychiatric disorders (N.B. antidepressant is contra-indicated if comorbid stimulant abuse)
- CBT methods
- Involve the family early on
- Legal and social interventions

1 Gilvarry E (2000) Substance abuse in young people. *J Child Psychol Psychiatry* **41**, 55–80.

Child abuse (1)—general issues[1]

In recent decades there has been growing awareness that the abuse of children can take many forms. All forms of child abuse involve the elements of power imbalance, exploitation, and the absence of true consent. They may concern acts of commission or acts of omission. Lord Clyde[2] suggested, 'Abuse is the wrongful application of power by someone in a dominant position'. The management of child abuse involves many professionals including police, social workers, educationalists, and health workers. Thus a multidisciplinary approach is required in order to fully assess the extent or risk of abuse and to provide the appropriate interventions. Working with child abuse is stressful and may invoke strong feelings and opinions (e.g. regarding the relative cost to the child of investigation versus non-investigation).

Categories of abuse

Physical abuse Where there is physical injury to the child and it is known, admitted, or reasonably suspected that the injury was inflicted by a carer or member of the same household; or where a carer knowingly fails to prevent injury or acted without due regard for the safety of the child; or where the nature of the injury is inconsistent with the account of how it occurred. (Includes Munchausen syndrome by proxy—see opposite).

Physical neglect Persistent or severe exposure of a child to danger or the persistent failure to fulfill the child's basic needs (food, sleep, nappy changing, clothing, warmth, shelter, or medical needs) which is likely to result in serious impairment of the child's health and development. This may also occur when an adult carer persistently pursues or allows a child to follow a lifestyle inappropriate to the child's developmental needs or which jeopardises his/her health. Leaving a child unattended or inadequately supervised may also qualify as physical neglect.

Non-organic failure to thrive Failure to meet expected weight and growth norms or developmental milestones, which does not have a basis in an hereditary or medical condition.

Emotional abuse Failure to provide for the child's basic emotional needs such as to have a severe effect on the behaviour and development of the child. This may include persistent coldness, hostility, or rejection by the caregiver and can be seen as the 'willful destruction or significant impairment of a child's confidence'. Other types of abuse are likely to result in emotional abuse.

Sexual abuse Any child below the age of consent will be deemed to have been sexually abused when any person, by design or by neglect, causes that child to be involved in any activity that might reasonably be expected to lead to the sexual arousal or gratification of that or any other person, including organised networks. This definition holds whether or not there has been genital contact and whether or not the child is said to have initiated the behaviour.

Abuse by young people or children

This involves activities between children/young people of a sexual or physical nature where one or more of the following characteristics is present: lack of true consent; inequalities in power (such as age, developmental stage, or size); actual or threatened coercion. A distinction must be made between behaviour normally expected between young people/ children and that which is clearly of an abusive nature.

Munchausen's syndrome by proxy

(Factitious or induced illness syndrome—FIIS)

- Part of a factitious syndrome that is manifest by a person feigning or inducing illness in a child (or others) in order to obtain medical attention.
- A form of *child abuse* in that it subjects the child to emotional abuse, unnecessary medical procedures, hospitalisation or other treatments that are harmful to the child.
- Can be very difficult to detect as the perpetrating (and colluding) adult/s often deny and disguise their behaviour.
- It is essential for professionals to be alert to it, especially where a child repetitively presents for medical attention.

Undetected, this form of abuse can result in very serious consequences (including fatality) for the child.

---

1 Adapted from the NHS Child Protection Guidelines of the Social Work Department, Lothian Health, Edinburgh, Scotland.

2 Report of enquiry into the removal of children from Orkney in February 1991.

Child abuse (2)—alerting signs

The following are signs that may alert one to abuse, but it is important to remember that other causes may exist, and also that these behaviours should be viewed within the context of other information at one's disposal.

Signs of possible physical abuse

- unexplained injuries or burns, especially if recurrent
- improbable excuses given for injuries
- refusal to discuss injuries
- untreated injuries or delay in reporting them
- excessive physical punishment
- limbs kept covered in hot weather; avoidance of swimming, PE, etc.
- fear of returning home
- aggression towards others
- running away

(N.B. 'Injuries' may occur for other reasons such as: genuine accidents; haematological disorders; Mongolian blue spots (normal in some darker skinned people); skin conditions such as impetigo or naevi; rare bone diseases; swelling of eye due to tumour; undiagnosed birth injury such as fractured clavicle.)

Signs of possible physical neglect

- constant hunger
- poor personal hygiene
- constant tiredness
- poor state of clothing
- frequent lateness or non-attendance at school
- untreated medical problems
- low self-esteem
- poor peer relationships
- stealing

Signs of possible non-organic failure to thrive

- significant lack of growth
- weight loss
- hair loss
- poor skin or muscle tone
- circulatory disorders

Signs of possible emotional abuse

- low self-esteem, continual self-deprecation
- sudden speech disorder
- significant decline in concentration
- socio-emotional immaturity
- rocking, head-banging, or other neurotic behaviour
- self-mutilation
- compulsive stealing
- extremes of passivity or aggression
- running away
- indiscriminate friendliness

Signs of possible sexual abuse
Behavioural

- lack of trust in adults or over-familiarity with adults
- fear of a particular individual
- social isolation, withdrawal, and introversion
- sleep disturbances (nightmares, irrational fears, bed wetting, fear of sleeping alone, needing a nightlight)
- running away from home
- girls taking over the mothering role
- reluctance or refusal to participate in physical activities or to change clothes for activities
- low self-esteem
- drug, alcohol, or solvent abuse
- display of sexual knowledge beyond child's years
- unusual interest in genitals of adults, children, or animals
- expressing affection in inappropriate ways
- fears of bathrooms, showers, or closed doors
- abnormal sexualised drawing
- fear of medical examinations
- developmental regression
- poor peer relations
- over-sexualised behaviour
- eating disorders
- compulsive masturbation
- stealing
- psychosomatic complaints
- sexual promiscuity

Physical/medical

- bruises, scratches, or other marks to the thighs or genital area
- itch, soreness, discharge, unexplained bleeding from the rectum, vagina, or penis
- pain on passing urine or recurrent urinary tract infection
- recurrent vaginal infection
- venereal disease
- stained underwear
- unusual genital odour
- soiling or wetting in children who have been trained
- discomfort/difficulty walking or sitting
- pregnancy, particularly when reluctance to name father

Child abuse (3)—assessment, management, and psychiatric outcome

Principles of assessment and management of child abuse

- Early detection in children at high-risk or presenting with alerting signs
- A multi-disciplinary approach is essential with early consultation across disciplines
- Maintain confidentiality where necessary and possible
- Assessment should be measured, sympathetic, and above all child-centred
- Attempt to engage and involve parents/carers at all stages and keep them informed in all but the most exceptional circumstances
- Evaluate the child's physical, emotional, cognitive, and sexual development, as well as the child's position in the family
- Evaluate the family in terms of: degree of social isolation and support; levels of stress; emotional maturity of the parents; parental relationship; role of non-abusing parent; and family dynamics
- Consider extra-familial factors such as: deficiencies in support services; failure of inter-professional communication; socio-political environment
- Important to clarify the family's perception of the problem and to gain their cooperation with changes/interventions required
- Remove/hospitalise child if there is an immediate risk of, or ongoing, abuse
- Consider whether siblings are at risk
- Involve social services early
- Consider whether police involvement is required immediately or whether there is time for a measured multidisciplinary response
- Balance the benefits/costs of non-intervention versus that of intervention
- Above all, put the needs of the child first

Psychiatric outcome of chronic abuse

Children who are abused have an extremely high rate of psychiatric disorders, both during the abuse and later on.

Some of the most common disorders associated with previous abuse:

- PTSD
- dissociative disorders
- conversion disorders
- borderline personality disorder
- depression
- paraphilias
- substance abuse

Prescribing in children and adolescents[1,2]

Principles

- They are not small adults! This is particularly important in regard to the dynamics and kinetics of drugs. Some drugs are metabolised faster while others more readily cross the BBB. Susceptibility to side-effects also varies with age (e.g. children are more likely to develop dystonias and less likely to develop akathisia with neuroleptic treatment).
- Due to variability in drug response according to weight, dosage is calculated in mg/kg rather than at fixed doses.
- Medication should be considered as just one component of treatment—it should be accompanied by psychological, social and educational interventions.
- Drugs are often prescribed for *symptoms* rather than *syndromes* (e.g. stimulants for hyperactivity in PDDs).
- Drug trials in children are problematic both ethically and practically, so there is inadequate data regarding safety and efficacy for many psychotropics. Thus clinicians are often faced with ethical decisions regarding the use of drugs not licensed for use in these age groups.

1 Taylor D, Paton C, Kerwin R (2003) *The Maudsley Prescribing Guidelines, 7th Ed.* Martin Dunitz: London.

2 Riddle MA, Kastelic EA, Frosch E (2001) Pediatric psychopharmacology. *J Child Psychol Psychiat* **42**, 73–90.

Guidance for specific psychotropics

Indication	Suggested dosage range for children and adolescents
Psychotic disorder	1st line: atypical antipsychotics • Risperidone 2–4 mg/day • Olanzapine 2.5–15 mg/day • Quetiapine 100–400 mg/day • Amisulpride 100–400 mg/day 2nd line: typical antipsychotics • Haloperidol 0.5–5 mg/day • Chlorpromazine 10–100 mg/day *Clozapine*—start with 12.5 mg/day; increase to maximum of 500 mg/day
Aggression/acute behaviour disturbance	• Risperidone 0.25–2 mg/day • Amisulpride 50–300 mg/day • Haloperidol 0.02–0.08 mg/kg/day
Depression/anxiety	• Fluoxetine 10–20 mg/day • Sertraline 25–100 mg/day • Citalopram 10–20 mg/day N.B. Paroxetine in C&As is now specifically contraindicated, due to increased risk of suicide.
Nocturnal enuresis	• Desmopressin 20–40 µg nocte intranasally • Imipramine 0.5–1 mg/kg nocte (N.B. ECG prior to therapy)
Mania/bipolar disorder	• Lithium 30 mg/kg/day (N.B. short half-life in children) • Sodium valproate 500–2000 mg/day • Carbamazepine 100–600 mg/day

Forensic psychiatry

Introduction

'Forensic' comes from the latin 'forensis' (the forum or court). The scope of forensic psychiatry can be broadly defined as those areas where psychiatry interacts with the law. Although all psychiatrists may be involved, from time to time, in forensic work, forensic psychiatrists in the UK are specifically involved in the assessment and management of mentally disordered offenders and other patients with mental disorders who are, or have been potentially or actually, violent. Provision of forensic services varies across the country and forensic psychiatrists work in a variety of settings (e.g. high-security hospitals; medium-secure units; low-secure wards and sometimes open wards; outpatients, day hospitals, and within community teams; prisons).

This section on forensic psychiatry concentrates on mentally disordered offenders. A separate section (Legal and ethical issues) covers mental health legislation and other non-criminal legal matters. The practice of forensic psychiatry is dependent on legislation, the criminal justice system, and local service provision. Hence, although some aspects have fairly wide applicability (e.g. the relationship between mental disorder and offending), many aspects (e.g. legal provisions for mentally disordered offenders) are specific to a particular jurisdiction. We have tried to cover the main legal jurisdictions of the British Isles (England and Wales, Scotland, Northern Ireland, and the Republic of Ireland) in some detail. (The names of these jurisdictions will be abbreviated to E&W, Scot, NI, and RoI respectively.)

The other problem with legislation is that it changes over time, and as we write this we are in a time of particular upheaval.

- In England and Wales, the Mental Health Bill 2002 and Mental Incapacity Bill 2003 have been published. The former is the subject of much controversy and at the time of writing seems to have been stalled.
- In Scotland, the Mental Health (Care and Treatment) (Scot) Act 2003 has been passed, and will probably be implemented in 2005. It replaces the Mental Health (Scot) Act 1984 and amends the provisions for mentally disordered offenders under the Criminal Procedure (Scot) Act 1995. The Criminal Justice (Scot) Act 2003 also amends the latter, but we await its implementation. The Adults with Incapacity (Scot) Act 2000 is in the early stages of implementation.
- In Northern Ireland, reform of the Mental Health (NI) Order 1986 and services for mentally disordered offenders are currently under consideration.
- In the Republic of Ireland, the Mental Health Act 2001 has replaced its predecessor dating back to 1945, and is currently being implemented. Procedures for mentally disordered offenders are set to change with the publication of the Criminal Law (Insanity) Bill 2002.

With all these changes it is difficult to present useful up-to-date information. In this section, provisions for mentally disordered offenders are those contained in the most recently passed Acts. Bills may be mentioned, but it is unclear at present what these will be like when they become Acts. The information presented is therefore up-to-date at the time of writing, but may be superseded relatively soon.

The following abbreviations are used to refer to legislation:

MHA 1983	Mental Health Act 1983
MH(NI)O 1986	Mental Health (Northern Ireland) Order 1986
MH(CT)(S)A 2003	Mental Health (Care and Treatment) (Scotland) Act 2003
CP(S)A 1995	Criminal Procedure (Scotland) Act 1995

Other legislation will be referred to in full, or abbreviations used in tables or boxes will be explained where they arise.

The criminal justice system[1,2,3]

The criminal justice process
The following outlines the chain of events that may happen following the commission of an offence:

Offence reported to police → police record offence → police investigate offence → police find suspect → police charge suspect → report to prosecutor → decision of prosecutor to prosecute → initial court appearance (remanded on bail or in custody) → trial → conviction → sentence (community, prison, fine, discharge, mental health disposal).

Most offenders will not go through all these stages (e.g. by pleading guilty an offender may go from initial court appearance directly to sentencing). At various stages there may be specific provisions for mentally disordered offenders (see p. 668 for overview and pp. 670–1 for details).

Prosecution
E&W Following report by police *Crown Prosecution Service* decides whether individual should be prosecuted; headed by *Director of Public Prosecutions*; service divided into areas and further into branches each headed by *Chief Crown Prosecutor*. Some minor offences prosecuted by police.

Scot *Lord Advocate* responsible for prosecuting serious crimes; heads the *Crown Office* in Edinburgh; most of work carried out by 'advocates-depute'. *Procurators fiscal* prosecute less serious crime locally.

NI Department of the *Director of Public Prosecutions* for NI. Director discharges his functions under the superintendence of the Attorney General.

RoI *Director of Public Prosecutions* responsible for prosecution.

Criminal Courts
E&W

Magistrates' Court All adult defendants appear here first—decision made to remand on bail or in custody; hear all summary (minor) cases and some indictable (serious cases); maximum sentence 6 months' imprisonment; magistrates are mainly lay justices of the peace with some legally qualified stipendiary magistrates in some urban areas.

Crown Court Deal with more serious indictable offences—cases are committed by the Magistrates Court for trail &/or sentencing; deal with appeals from Magistrates Court; 6 regions or 'circuits'; trials heard by judge and jury (12 adults); sentencing by judge.

Youth Court Juvenile offenders (aged 10–17 years); magistrates with special training hear cases; serious cases committed to Crown Court.

Court of Appeal (Criminal Division) Usually 3 judges; hears appeals by defendant against conviction or sentence; hears appeals by the Crown against sentence; can increase or reduce sentence.

Queen's Bench Division of the High Court (Divisional Court) Appeals on points of law and procedure.

House of Lords Hears appeals against decisions of the above court; Law Lords deliver opinions; only points of law of general public importance.

Scot
District Court Minor cases heard by lay justices of peace (maximum sentence 60 days' imprisonment) or (only in Glasgow) stipendiary magistrates (similar powers to sheriff).

Sheriff Court 6 sheriffdoms, each headed by Sheriff Principal; summary (sheriff alone) or some solemn (sheriff and jury) cases heard; maximum sentence 3 months' (summary) or 3 years' (solemn) imprisonment.

High Court of Justiciary (Criminal Trials) Hears serious cases; judge and jury (15 adults); unlimited sentencing powers; Edinburgh, Glasgow, and on circuit in other towns and cities.

High Court of Justiciary (Court of Criminal Appeal) Cases heard by 3 or more judges; no appeal to House of Lords.

NI
Essentially as for E&W.

Diplock Courts (judge sitting alone) for indictable scheduled (mainly terrorist) cases.

RoI
District Court Legally qualified justices; summary (up to 6 months' imprisonment) and some indictable (up to 12 months' imprisonment) cases heard.

Circuit Court Cases heard by judge and jury; indictable cases and appeals from District Court.

Central Criminal Court (High Court) Cases heard by High Court judge and jury; serious indictable cases

Special Criminal Court Only scheduled offences (mainly terrorist cases); cases heard by 3 judges.

Court of Criminal Appeal 1 justice of the Supreme Court and 2 of the High Court hear appeals from 3 above courts.

Supreme Court Chief Justice and High Court justices hear appeals from the above court.

1 Grounds A (1995) The criminal justice system. In *Seminars in Practical Forensic Psychiatry* (eds. Chiswick D and Cope R). London: Gaskell.

2 Bailey S (1990) Lawyers, legislation, the administration of the law and legal aid. In *Principles and Practice of Forensic Psychiatry* (eds. Bluglass R and Bowden P). Edinburgh: Churchill Livingstone.

3 Nichcison G (1990) The courts and law in Scotland. In *Principles and Practice of Forensic Psychiatry* (eds. Bluglass R and Bowden P). Edinburgh: Churchill Livingstone.

Crime[1–4]

A crime is an act that is capable of being followed by criminal proceedings. It is a man-made concept defined by the rules of the state and modified by legislation, therefore there are differences between countries and across time in the same country. Age of criminal responsibility: England, Wales, and NI-10 years; Scot-8 years; RoI-7 years.

Classification of crime

- **Crimes against the person** Offences of interpersonal violence: minor assault, homicide; sexual offences: indecent exposure, rape; robbery
- **Crimes of dishonesty** Burglary; theft and handling stolen goods; fraud and forgery
- **Criminal damage** Property damage; arson
- **Car crime**
- **Drug crime** Use, possession, supplying
- **Other**

Crime rates The table on p.00 shows the annual number of officially recorded crimes in the countries of the British Isles. From the British Crime Survey only about half of crime is reported to the police (and officially recorded), of which between 25–50% is cleared up by the police.
- Theft, burglary, criminal damage, and car crime are the most common.
- Violent crimes are uncommon; sex offences and robbery are rare.

Who commits crimes? Young males aged 10–20 yrs account for 50% of crime. Females ~20% of offenders. Peak age: males 14–17 yrs; females 12–15 yrs.

What are the 'causes' of crime? The following factors are associated with offending. They interact, and causality cannot be assumed.
- **Genetic factors** MZ more concordant than DZ twins for officially recorded and self-reported offending. In adoption studies children are more similar to biological than adoptive parents.
- **Intelligence** Low intelligence associated with offending.
- **Personality** Impulsivity and lack of empathy.
- **Family** Childhood factors linked to later offending: poor parental supervision, erratic/harsh discipline, marital disharmony and parental separation, parental rejection, low parental involvement, antisocial parents, and large family size. Offenders who marry non-offending spouses reduce their rate of offending.
- **Peers** Most delinquent acts are committed with others. Offending with others versus alone decreases with age. Close relationship between delinquent activities of friends. Offenders are unpopular in non-offending groups but popular in offending groups.

1 Simmons J (2002) *Crime in England and Wales 2001/2002.* London: Home Office.

2 Scottish Executive (2002) *Recorded Crime in Scotland 2001. Statistical Bulletin—Criminal Justice Series* (CrJ/2002/1). Edinburgh: Scottish Executive.

3 NI Office (2002) *A Commentary on Northern Ireland Crime Statistics 2001.* Belfast: NI Office, Statistics and Research Branch.

4 An Garda Siochana (2002) *Year 2001 Crime Statistics(Annual Report).* Dublin: An Garda Siochana.

- **Schools** No clear evidence that school factors influence offending. The following are not related to delinquency rates: age and state of buildings, number of children, amount of space, pupil/teacher ratio, academic emphasis, teacher turnover, number of outings. High punishment and low praise associated with delinquency—but is this cause or effect? Alternative placements and approaches to disruptive and delinquent pupils may reduce delinquency compared with mainstream education.
- **Socio-economic deprivation** Poverty and poor housing associated with later offending. Employment protective.
- **Ethnicity** Higher rates of offending in Afro-caribbean than in white males. Lower rates in Asian males. Is association due to socio-economic deprivation, discrimination, different rates of arrest?
- **Alcohol and substance misuse** See mental disorder and offending (p. 645).

Crime statistics for the British Isles

The following table is based on offences officially recorded by the police for 2001 (Scot and RoI) and 2001–2 (E&W and NI). Different jurisdictions use different categories and definitions so comparisons between jurisdictions should be made very cautiously. Numbers of crimes with percentage of total for that jurisdiction in parentheses.

	E&W	Scot	NI	RoI
Violence against the person	650154 (11.7)	19523 (4.6)	26104 (18.8)	3876 (4.5)
Sexual offences	49612 (0.9)	5987 (1.4)	1431 (1.0)	1939 (2.2)
Robbery	121375 (2.2)	4228 (1.0)	2222 (1.6)	2880 (3.3)
Theft	2267055 (41.0)	169454 (40.0)	41720 (30.0)	45652 (52.7)
Burglary	878535 (15.9)	44868 (10.7)	17143 (12.4)	24015 (27.7)
Fraud and forgery	317399 (5.7)	17410 (4.1)	8619 (6.2)	3492 (4.0)
Criminal damage	1064470 (19.3)	94924 (22.5)	39953 (28.8)	1407 (1.6)*
Drug offences	121332 (2.2)	36175 (8.6)	1108 (0.8)	2380 (2.7)
TOTAL	5527082 (100.0)	421093 (100.0)	138786 (100.0)	86663 (100.0)

*Only arson for RoI

Homicide

Definition Homicide is the killing of a person by another.

Types of homicide
Legal classification:
- **'Lawful'**: *Justifiable* (e.g. on behalf of State); *excusable* (e.g. accident).
- **'Unlawful'**: *Murder*—mandatory life sentence; *manslaughter/culpable homicide* discretion in sentencing (imprisonment, community, mental health disposal, discharge); *infanticide*—(not in Scot) sentencing as for manslaughter; *death by dangerous driving*.

The traditional 'psychiatric' classification:
- **'Normal' homicides**—no psychiatric disorder
- **'Abnormal' homicides**—psychiatric disorder

However, this is determined by whether the individual was found insane, convicted of infanticide, or found to be of diminished responsibility— therefore it is really a legal classification.

Homicide rates 882 recorded homicides in E&W in 2001–2, 106 in Scot (2001), 55 in NI (2001–2), 74 in RoI (2001). Rates per million population per year for 1997–9: E&W 15, Scot 20, NI 31, RoI 13.5, European Union average 17.0, USA 62.6, South Africa 564.9.

Victims of homicide Usually male (70%); 60–80% known to offender; 30–50% related or partner; 15% children (highest risk under 1 year old) usually killed by parent (75%); less than 5% parent (matricide > patricide); 40–50% of females killed by partner or ex-partner; males more commonly killed by acquaintances (25% E&W, 60% Scot) and strangers (37% E&W, 20% Scot).

Perpetrators of homicide Predominantly male (80–90%); using sharp implement (most common 30–40%), kicking/punching, strangulation (more common with female victims), or blunt force; anger, jealousy, revenge, or threat of separation are usual motives; often involving alcohol, or sometimes drugs.

Mental disorder and homicide Minority of homicide offenders are mentally disordered. Alcohol and drug dependence most common, then personality disorder. Schizophrenia, delusional disorder, and depression may be relevant in a few cases. E&W: 5–10% of cases result in diminished responsibility, infanticide, or insanity; half of these result in a hospital disposal. Scot: 4% of cases result in hospital disposal.

Psychiatric assessment in homicide cases As with other offences need to assess mental state both currently and at time of offence. In most jurisdictions murder carries a mandatory punishment (life imprisonment in the main jurisdictions of the British Isles). To achieve a hospital disposal the offender has to be found insane or of diminished responsibility (does not apply in Ireland). See p. 678.

Homicide inquiries In E&W independent inquiries following homicides committed by people in contact with mental health services have been mandatory since 1994. They have been criticized for being inefficient, costly, misleading, unsystematic, and unjust. A systematic national approach has been made in the National Confidential Inquiry[1]. The main issues to be highlighted include: need for training in risk assessment and management; better means of documentation and recording, particularly *risk* information; addressing non-compliance and disengagement from services; managing comorbid alcohol and drug misuse; access to help for families at times of concern; appropriate use of mental health legislation; policies on management of personality disorder; addressing stigma; culture of blame.

Legal aspects of homicide in different jurisdictions

E&W

Murder Offender of sound mind and discretion, and had malice aforethought (intent to cause death or grievous bodily harm). Intent assumed if reckless, knowing that death or serious harm was virtual certainty.

Manslaughter Homicide unlawful, but circumstances do not meet full criteria for murder or there are certain mitigating factors, such as:
(1) immediate severe provocation
(2) abnormality of mind (diminished responsibility under section 2 (1) Homicide Act 1957; see p. 679)
(3) suicide pact (section 4 (1) Homicide Act 1957).

Infanticide (see p. 678)

Scot

Murder Homicide committed with wicked recklessness or intent.

Culpable homicide Equivalent of manslaughter. Provocation, diminished responsibility are recognised, but no legal category for suicide pacts.

No officially recognized crime of infanticide, such cases are usually prosecuted as culpable homicide.

NI

Murder, manslaughter, infanticide—as for E&W.

RoI

Murder defined as an intentional act to kill (narrower than E&W definition).

Manslaughter, infanticide—as for E&W, but no diminished responsibility. N.B. Diminished responsibility will probably be introduced under Criminal Law (Insanity) Bill 2002.

---

1 Appleby L (2000) Safer services: conclusions from the report of the National Confidential Inquiry. *Advances in Psychiatric Treatment* **6**, 5–15.

Violence (1)—theoretical background[1,2]

Definition Violence is an act that causes injury or harm. The term may cover a range of acts from the killing of another person to verbal abuse, and may also be used to cover acts causing damage to property including arson. In this section the focus is on acts of physical assault on others. Property damage and arson are considered on p. 640, and sexual offences on p. 636.

Types of aggression Various have been described in terms of the determinants, biological substrate, goals, and characteristics of the aggressive act. Broadly they fall into three groups:

- **Instrumental aggression** Aggression as a means to attain a goal, usually planned and not associated with increased arousal (e.g. violence used to carry out a robbery or control the victim of a sexual assault). A related term from animal studies is *predatory aggression*—aggression used by predatory animals when hunting food (aka *interspecific aggression*.) *Sadistic aggression* is a form of instrumental aggression used to achieve sexual and/or emotional pleasure through control and/or inflicting harm on a victim.

- **Expressive aggression** (aka *affective aggression, reactive aggression, hostile aggression, angry aggression, fear-induced aggression, irritable aggression, indiscriminate aggression.*) Aggression with the primary goal of harming the victim in response to feelings of hostility towards the victim; emotional arousal in the perpetrator (due to fear, frustration, anger, resentment) and usually impulsive (although may be planned) (e.g. violence in response to discovery of infidelity or in response to being threatened). A related term from animal studies is *defensive aggression*—aggression used when threatened.

- **Aggression seen in social interactions** (a form of expressive aggression, aka *intraspecific aggression*) e.g. intermale aggression, territorial aggression, and maternal aggression.

Although some acts of aggression clearly fall into one of these, many combine features of both e.g. aggression may be used to subdue the victim of a sexual assault (instrumental) and also as an angry reaction to the victim striking back (expressive).

Theories of aggression

- **Biological** Ethological studies of lower animals suggest aggression functions to ensure population control; selection of the strongest for reproduction and social organisation; low levels of 5-HT activity and cholesterol associated with aggression; modest genetic contribution; limbic and frontal areas important in determining aggression; testosterone may facilitate aggression.

- **Psychodynamic** *Freud:* aggression initially seen as response to frustration, later as an instinct; hostile character traits may be caused by fixation at/regression to oral or anal stage. *Ego psychologists:* aggressive instinct needs to be sublimated or displaced. *Neo-Freudians:* emphasised socio-cultural origins of aggression. *Attachment theory:* emphasises early relationships and the impact of their disruption on adult interaction.

- **Learning theory** Rewarding/reinforcing contingencies important, leading to the development and maintenance of aggressive responses to certain stimuli or in order to attain goal (material gain, escape from aversive stimulus). *Frustration aggression hypothesis:* frustration leads to aggression depending on the perceived value of the blocked goal and the degree of frustration (depends on degree of prior reinforcement or punishment); punishment may inhibit aggression, but may itself be frustrating or provide model for aggression. *Observational learning* (modelling).
- **Cognitive** Learning theories seen as too simple and cognition important; cognitive distortions about victims may facilitate aggressive behaviour; appraisal of arousal and context important in determining occurrence of aggression; causal attributions and moral evaluations of self and others may facilitate or reduce aggression.
- **Social** *Social structure theory:* poor socio-economic standing stifles pursuit of financial and social success, so seek success through deviant methods. *Social process theory:* socialisation process through contact with institutions and social organisations steers individual towards violence. *Neutralisation theory:* neutralisation of personal beliefs and values as person drifts between conventional and offending behaviour. *Social control theory:* direct (e.g. through punishment) and indirect (e.g. through social affiliation) control prevents violence. *Labelling theory:* an original deviant act (primary deviance) results in stigmatisation and labelling, leading to hostility, alienation, and resentment in the individual and further deviant behaviour (secondary deviance).

1 Mackintosh J (1990) Theories of violence. In *Principles and Practice of Forensic Psychiatry* (eds. Bluglass R and Bowden P). Edinburgh: Churchill Livingstone.

2 Gunn J (1993) Non-psychotic violence. In *Forensic psychiatry: clinical, legal and ethical issues* (eds. Gunn J and Taylor P). Oxford: Butterworth-Heinemann.

Violence (2)[1,2]

Causes of a violent act

Violent acts involve a perpetrator, a victim, and contextual factors. There will usually be an interplay between factors related to these three. Many of the background factors associated with offending generally (see p. 628) are associated with violence, although violent offenders are usually young adults rather than teenagers. The specific factors of importance in determining the occurrence of aggressive acts are the same as those needing to be considered in assessing the risk of violence (see pp. 646–7).

Types of violent offences

The range of recognised violent offences (excluding sexual offences) is shown opposite. The seriousness of an assault may be determined by chance factors such as the availability of medical care and the physical health of the victim. Other ways of categorising violent offences are in terms of the victims and circumstances: domestic/spousal abuse, child abuse (see p. 614), elder abuse.

Rates of violence

Per 10 000 of the adult population there were 676 assaults and 84 robberies in E&W compared with 458 assaults and 54 robberies in Scot in 1999 as estimated from the British Crime Survey 2000 (i.e. number of actual incidents rather than number of officially recorded offences). The total numbers of officially recorded violent offences are shown opposite.

Psychiatric assessment and management

The clinical assessment of a person who has been violent or who appears to be at risk of violence involves a thorough psychiatric history and mental state examination and an assessment of risk (see pp. 646–7). If the person is facing criminal charges then a report may have to be prepared considering the issues set out on pp. 666–7. Management of risk is described on p. 647. The acute management of violent patients is described on p. 896.

Domestic violence

1 in 4 women experience domestic violence during their lifetimes. Women are victims of 70% of domestic violence. In over 10% of cases serious injuries occur (e.g. broken bones, loss of consciousness). May be a contributory factor in 25% of suicide attempts and in 75% of cases children witness the violence. Accounts for 25% of violent crime in Britain (which will be an underestimate).

Elder abuse

Prevalence (from US figures) 3–5% of the elderly subject to violence, neglect, or emotional abuse, particularly females. Perpetrators are usually son or daughter, perhaps under stress, with alcohol or drug problems and unable to cope with looking after victim.

1 Cordess C (1995) Crime and mental disorder I. Criminal behaviour. In *Seminars in Practical Forensic Psychiatry*(eds. Chiswick D and Cope R). London: Gaskell.

2 Gunn J (1993) Non-psychotic violence. In *Forensic psychiatry: clinical, legal and ethical issues* (eds. Gunn J and Taylor P). Oxford: Butterworth-Heinemann.

Recorded violent offences

The following figures are the violent offences recorded by the police in each of the jurisdictions in the British Isles in 2001 (Scot and RoI) or 2001–2 (E&W and NI). Note that different jurisdictions have different ways of defining and classifying violent offences.

E&W (2001–2)

Homicide	886
Attempted murder	858
Threat or conspiracy to murder	13648
Child destruction	0
Causing death with vehicle	407
Wounding	16537
Endangering railway passenger or life at sea	18
Other wounding	212059
Possession of weapons	28740
Harassment	113677
Cruelty to or neglect of children	3048
Abandoning child under 2	49
Child abduction	583
Procuring illegal abortion	6
Concealment of birth	3
Assault on a constable	30010
Common assault	231625
TOTAL VIOLENCE AGAINST THE PERSON	**650154**
Robbery*	121375

Scot (2001)

Serious assault (includes homicide)	7296
Handling an offensive weapon	8671
Robbery	4228
Other	3556
TOTAL NON-SEXUAL CRIMES OF VIOLENCE	**23751**
Petty assault*	54870

NI (2001–2)

Homicide	55
Attempted murder	164
Threat or conspiracy to murder	740
Causing death with vehicle	23
Wounding/assault occasioning actual bodily harm	6507
Aggravated assault	941
Common assault	13971
Police assault	1563
TOTAL VIOLENCE AGAINST PERSON	**26104**
Robbery*	2222

RoI (2001)

Homicide:

Murder	52
Murder—attempt	2
Abortion	0
Manslaughter	6
Infanticide	0
Murder—threats	14
Procuring or assisting abortion	0
TOTAL HOMICIDE	**74**

Assaults:

Assault causing harm	3114
Coercion	4
Harassment	276
Poisoning	4
Assault/obstruction/resisting peace officer	236
Endangerment	41
False imprisonment	46
Abduction	81
TOTAL ASSAULTS	**3082**
Robbery*	2880

* Indicates offences not officially categorised as violent offences in the relevant jurisdiction.

Sexual offences (1)

Offences range from prostitution and indecent exposure to rape. Other types of offences (e.g. homicide, assault, robbery, theft, and burglary) may have a sexual component, but are not officially recognised as sexual offences. Sex offending, sexual deviation (p. 464), and inappropriate sexual behaviour (a range of sexual behaviours which cause offence and/or harm to others) are overlapping but distinct concepts. A man who commits a sexual offence against a child may or may not be a paedophile and a man who exposes himself may or may not be an exhibitionist. A 17-year-old male who has sexual intercourse with his 15-year-old girlfriend is committing a sexual offence, but will neither have a sexual deviation or be displaying sexually inappropriate behaviour. Here the focus will be on indecent exposure and contact sexual offences against adults and children.

Types of sexual offences and offenders The range of officially recognised sexual offences is set out on p. 639. Legal classifications change and a legal label says nothing about the nature of the actual incident. Various typologies (based on the nature of the act, the motivation of the offender, the characteristics of the offender, and the characteristics of the victim) lack validity, reliability, and practical utility.

Indecent exposure The most common sexual offence. Classification:

- *Exhibitionists* Inhibited men, often previous unremarkable character, with sudden powerful urge to display genitals, who make little attempt to avoid capture and who make no further erotic or obscene gestures/attempt any contact with victim.
- *Disinhibited*—by alcohol, stress, or psychiatric disorder.
- *Aggressive, impulsive, and antisocial*—a small minority.

Most do not reoffend. A small number may progress to more serious sexual offences. Rates of further indecent exposure: first time offenders 20%, previous sexual offences—60%, previous sexual and non-sexual offences—70%. Factors which may indicate risk of escalation to more serious offences are as set out below for sexual offences generally.

Rape and other sexual assaults on adults Usually perpetrated by men against women and, less often, other men. Female perpetrators uncommon. Typologies lack validity, but may be classified as: *aggressive, sexual,* or *sadistic*. Most rapists are young males from poor social and educational backgrounds who have a history of other offending. A small number of these offenders are sexual sadists. Sadistic fantasy is common in men, but sadistic sexual offending is rare—features which may be associated with acting out sadistic fantasies are social isolation, coexisting other paraphilias, lack of empathy, disinhibition (by alcohol, drugs, stress, or psychiatric disorder). 15% of rapists reoffend sexually and 20% go on to commit non-sexual violent offences.

Rape and other sexual assaults on children Female children are victimised more than males.

- *Intra-familial abuse (incest)* is usually perpetrated by fathers or step-fathers against daughters. Family pathology (dysfunctional families with generational blurring) often mixed with pathology in the perpetrator (alcohol misuse, personality disorder, paedophilia—but only in a minority).

- *Extra-familial* abuse is less common. Adolescent offending is associated with poor social skills, physical unattractiveness, and isolation from peers. Adult offenders are more likely to have paedophilic sexual fantasies than adolescent offenders and intra-familial offenders. In some cases offending against children reflects general antisocial tendencies or the expression of repressed paedophilic impulses in susceptible men disinhibited (by alcohol, stress, or psychiatric disorder). Many offenders become skilled at targeting and grooming victims to gain their trust. A very rare minority have sadistic paedophilic fantasies. Cases of sexually motivated killing of children are extremely rare.

Rates of sexual offences Rates of recorded sexual offences are shown on p. 639. Many sexual offences are not reported.

Rates of sexual reoffending Extra-familial child offenders > offenders against adults > incest offenders.

Internet offences There are an increasing number of cases of people arrested for using and/or distributing child pornography over the internet. Many of these people would probably not have been identified as sexual offenders previously.

Sexual offences (2)

Characteristics of sex offenders A heterogeneous group—possible relevant factors: deviant sexual fantasy, sexual dysfunction, abnormal personality (impulsivity, lack of empathy, inhibition, social anxiety), relationship difficulties (poor social skills, social isolation), alcohol or drug misuse, denial and minimisation of offending, cognitive distortions (regarding sex, women, or children), problems with assertiveness and control of anger, previous histories of victimisation.

Mental disorder and sex offending The most common mental disorders found in sex offenders: personality disorder, paraphilias, alcohol and substance misuse; severe mental illness is rare. Sex offenders with psychosis share many of the features of other sex offenders and offending is rarely due to specific psychotic symptoms. Disinhibition due to mania or organic disorders may lead to, usually minor, sexual offences. Most sex offences committed by people with LD are associated with lack of sexual knowledge, poor social skills, and inability to express a normal sex drive appropriately. A few more serious and persistent LD offenders may share characteristics of other sex offenders.

Assessment of sex offenders Full psychiatric history and MSE—emphasis on the nature of the incident(s), psychosexual history, and previous offences, utilising sources of information other than the accused. It may be difficult to build up a full picture of a person's sexual fantasies and activities. Some centres (mainly in North America) use penile plethysmography (measuring the extent of penile erection in response to various stimuli).

Risk assessment (pp. 646–7) Consider the following factors: sexual deviation; personality disorder; mental illness; substance misuse; relationship problems; employment problems; previous offences (sexual and non-sexual); previous supervision failure; frequency, types, and escalation in sexual offending; physical harm to victims and use of weapons; denial/minimisation and cognitive distortions; future plans and attitudes towards intervention.

Management of sex offenders Some mentally disordered offenders require treatment in hospital (esp. those with mental illness or marked LD). In psychotic sex offenders it is usually important to address factors common to other sex offenders. Those with personality disorders, paraphilias, and substance misuse are normally dealt with by the criminal justice system. Within the criminal justice system, both in prison and the community, group CBT programmes have been developed. A small number of sex offenders receive psychodynamic treatment at specialist clinics. Medications such as anti-androgens, anti-gonadotrophins, and SSRIs may be used in a few offenders.

Specific legal provisions The Sex Offenders Act 1997 requires sex offenders to register their address with the police. The Crime and Disorder Act 1998 enables courts to impose Sex Offender Orders on convicted sex offenders who are not registered under the Sex Offender Act and whose behaviour gives cause for concern. The order requires the offender to register with the police and to desist from behaviour that has been identified as indicative of future risk. The same Act allows courts to impose extended sentences on sex offenders. The extended sentence comprises a custodial element with an 'extended' period of supervision post-release for up to 10 years.

Recorded sexual offences

Sexual offences recorded by the police in each of the jurisdictions in the British Isles in 2001 or 2001–2. Note that different jurisdictions have different ways of defining and classifying sexual offences.

E&W (2001–2)

Buggery	354
Indecent assault on a male	3613
Gross indecency between males	163
Rape of a female	9008
Rape of a male	735
Indecent assault of a female	21765
Unlawful sexual intercourse with a girl <13	170
Unlawful sexual intercourse with a girl <16	1336
Incest	93
Procuration	130
Abduction	263
Bigamy	74
Soliciting or importuning by a man	1648
Abuse of position of trust	408
Gross indecency with a child	1665
TOTAL OFFENCES	**41425**
Indecent exposure (recorded with other offences)	8187

Scot (2001)

Rape	589
Assault with intent to rape	164
Indecent assault	1154
Lewd and libidinous practices	1557
Indecent exposure	808
Incest	34
Homosexual acts	133
Sexual intercourse with a girl <16	179

Prostitution offences	1328
Other crimes of indecency	41
TOTAL CRIMES	**5987**

NI (2001–2)

Rape	252
Attempted rape	40
Buggery	27
Indecent assault of female	286
Indecent assault of female child	308
Indecent assault of male	34
Indecent assault of male child	55
Homosexual acts	5
Indecent exposure	333
Indecent conduct towards a child	23
Other sexual offences	32
TOTAL OFFENCES	**1431**

RoI (2001)

Sexual assault	1048
Sexual offence involving mentally impaired person	10
Gross indecency	33
Buggery	36
Unlawful carnal knowledge	78
Rape (section 4)	66
Bestiality	2
Aggravated sexual assault	18
Indecency	150
Rape of a female	335
Incest	16
Brothel keeping	5
Prostitution	142
TOTAL OFFENCES	**1048**

Other offences[1]

Arson

Arson (fire-setting in Scot) is considered to be a serious offence due to its potential to threaten life and cause massive destruction. Only a small proportion (less than 20%) of arson offences lead to prosecution.

Classification As with sex offenders and other offenders typologies are fraught with problems. The following groups have been described (but they are not mutually exclusive): insurance fraud, covering evidence of crime, politically motivated, gang activity, revenge/anger, cry for help, desire for power, desire to be hero, fascination with fire, sexual excitement, suicide, psychiatric disorder.

Psychiatric disorder Alcohol/substance misuse and personality disorder are the most frequent; less common are psychosis, organic disorders, and learning disability (previously highlighted association due to studies of patients in secure hospitals). Pure 'pyromania' is rare—features are usually seen in individuals with personality disorders.

Assessment Full psychiatric assessment with detailed examination of current and previous offences.

Management Treatment of mental disorder if present; specific psychological interventions have been proposed but little evidence; important to take steps to prevent access to matches and lighters if ongoing risk in hospital setting.

Outcome Rates of further arson 2–20%, rates of any reoffending 10–30%. No specific indicators of risk.

Other damage to property

Acts of vandalism are common, especially in adolescence. There is little psychiatric literature on criminal damage excluding arson.

Stalking

Stalking is not a specific offence, although the recent *Protection from Harassment Act 1997* and *Malicious Communications Act 1998* have introduced legislation of specific relevance for E&W. Stalking is a pattern of intrusive behaviour (unwanted contacts and communications), which implicitly or explicitly threatens a victim and leads to considerable fear. Behaviours include threats, assaults, sending gifts, initiating legal action, and making complaints. Figures from USA indicate that 8% of women and 2% of men have been stalked at some point. Many cases not reported to police. Most cases involve males stalking women with whom they have had a relationship previously.

Classification Problems as with other typologies. Psychotic v non-psychotic; previous relationship v no previous relationship. A typology based on motivation and context: *rejected* (pursues ex-intimate in hope of reconciliation and/or vengeance), *intimacy seekers* (believe they love victim and that victim reciprocates), *incompetent suitors* (intrudes seeking a date or brief sexual encounter), *resentful* (seeking revenge for actual or perceived slight), *predatory* (prelude to sexual assault).

Psychiatric disorder Commonly personality disorder (narcissistic/borderline/antisocial/paranoid, sometimes schizoid or dependent) and alcohol/drug misuse. May be psychotic: various types of delusions may be involved, primary erotomania is rare.

Assessment Diagnosis of any mental disorder and assessment of relationship with victim.

Management Clinical management may include treating mental disorder, understanding what is sustaining behaviour, confronting denial/minimization/justification, enhancing empathy, addressing social and interpersonal deficits, managing alcohol and drug misuse. But no clear evidence available to guide management.

Outcome Research from USA. About half cease within a year and a quarter last 2–5 years. 25% of cases result in violence and 2% in homicide.

Crimes of dishonesty

Burglary, theft, and fraud are common offences which are rarely associated with psychiatric disorder. *Shoplifting* has attracted some clinical attention. About 5% of shoplifters suffer from significant mental disorder (personality disorder, substance misuse, depression, schizophrenia, dementia). Pure kleptomania is extremely rare (see p. 386).

Drug offences

Mental disorder rarely an issue.

Car crime

Impaired ability to drive may be caused by a number of disorders (see p. 828). Occasional rare cases of people disinhibited by mania or impaired by dementia who cause serious injury or death. However, mental disorder is rarely an issue in car crime.

1 Mullen, PE et al (2001) The management of stalkers. *Advances in Psychiatric Treatment* **7**, 335–42.

Mental disorder and offending (1)—overview

What is the relationship between mental disorder and offending?

Mental disorder is common and offending is common, so it would not be surprising to find an individual with both. But is the relationship more than coincidental? When looking at studies of this relationship one needs to consider:

- The nature of the sample studied (community v institutional; clinical v epidemiological; pre-treatment v post-treatment; offenders v non-offenders)
- The criteria used to define mental disorder (legal v clinical v operationalised) and the method used to determine its existence (case notes v interviews; clinically trained v lay interviewers)
- The criteria used to define offending (types of officially recorded offences included; inclusion of unreported or unprosecuted 'offences') and the method used to detect offences (official records v self-report v third-party report).

Most of the research has focused on violence. The following are the main conclusions to be drawn from current evidence.

- People with mental disorder as a broad group are no more or less likely to offend than the general population.
- Some specific mental disorders do increase the risk of a person acting violently, particularly alcohol and drug-related disorders and personality disorders (especially those with predominant cluster B characteristics).
- Schizophrenia has a modest association with violence, but the overwhelming majority of people with schizophrenia are never violent, being more likely to be victims than perpetrators of violence.
- In people with mental disorders the factors most strongly associated with offending are the same as for non-mentally disordered offenders: male gender, young age, substance misuse, disturbed childhood, socioeconomic deprivation.
- When considering an offence perpetrated by a person with mental disorder, one should bear in mind that, as with any offence, there is interplay between the perpetrator, the victim, and the situational circumstances. Although mental disorder may play a part it is rarely the only factor that leads to an offence.

Mental disorder and offending (2)— specific disorders and offending[1,2,3]

Schizophrenia

The life-time risk of violence in people with schizophrenia is about 5 times that in the general population. People with schizophrenia account for less than 10% of all violent crime in Britain. The factors most commonly associated with violence in people with schizophrenia are those associated with violence in people without psychosis. Alcohol and drug misuse are particularly important. Specific symptoms may be important but clearly are not enough in themselves, otherwise virtually every person with schizophrenia would be violent. Threat control-override symptoms (delusions regarding being threatened or being controlled) have been found to be associated with violence, but again, most patients with these symptoms are never violent. The role of command auditory hallucinations is unclear. When people with psychosis are violent the victim is more likely to be known to them (particularly relatives) than when violence is committed by non-psychotic individuals.

Delusional disorders

Delusional disorders are probably over-represented among patients detained in secure psychiatric hospitals, however the research on the association between delusional disorders and violence is difficult to interpret as the samples are usually selective and uncontrolled, and in many studies patients with delusional disorders are lumped in with patients with other psychoses, especially schizophrenia. Increased risk of violence has been reported to be associated with persecutory delusions, misidentification delusions, delusions of jealousy, delusions of love, and querulous delusions. Jealousy may be dangerous whether it is delusionally based or not. In some cases it is difficult to differentiate between pre-morbid personality disorder (perhaps with paranoid and/or narcissistic features) and delusional disorder. The relevant beliefs are probably no less risky if they are over-valued ideas than if they are delusional.

Affective disorders

Affective disorders have a far less strong relationship with offending and violence than schizophrenia. Mania commonly leads to minor offending due to grandiosity and disinhibition, but rarely leads to serious violence or sexual assaults. Depression is very rarely associated with violence or offending. Extended suicide (also known as altruistic homicide), in which a depressed parent (usually the father) kills members of their family before attempting and perhaps succeeding in killing themselves, is extremely rare and impossible to predict. In some cases it occurs in depressive psychosis associated with nihilistic delusions, but more commonly there is a history of marital breakdown in people who are depressed and suicidal but not psychotic. A historical association between shoplifting and depression has been highlighted, but is probably insignificant.

Alcohol and substance-related disorders

Alcohol and drug-related problems are more strongly linked to offending and violence than any other mental disorders. A number of aspects of alcohol and substance misuse may be relevant: direct effects of intoxication or withdrawal; funding the habit; the personal and social consequences of dependence; the neuropsychiatric sequelae of prolonged misuse; the social context (peer group, socio-economic deprivation, childhood mistreatment), and personal characteristics (impulsivity and sensation seeking), which may lead to substance misuse, may also be associated with offending.

Personality disorders

Personality disorder is more strongly related to offending and violence than mental illness. Personality disordered offenders are heterogeneous: only a small number are psychopathic (see p. 448). Various aspects of personality disorder may be related to offending: impulsivity, lack of empathy, poor affect regulation, paranoid thinking, poor relationships with others, problems with anger and assertiveness.

Learning disability

Offending occurs more often in people with milder forms of learning disability than in those with severe learning disability. Offences are broadly similar to those in non-learning disabled offenders and are associated with family and social disadvantage. Evidence for increased rates of sex offending and fire-raising is based on highly selected patient samples in secure hospitals and is therefore questionable. In some learning disabled offenders poor social development, poor educational achievement, gullibility, and impaired ability to communicate may be important factors. Profound and severe learning disability may be associated with disturbed behaviour, including aggression, but would rarely come to the attention of the criminal justice system.

Organic disorders

Aggression is well recognised in dementia, but rarely leads to serious violence. Delirium and brain injury may lead to aggression. In head injury cases it may be difficult to differentiate the effects of the head injury from pre-morbid personality. Epilepsy is twice as common in offenders as in the general population, but this is probably due to shared environmental and biological disadvantages that predispose individuals to both. Violence resulting from epileptic activity is extremely rare.

1 Higgins J (1995) Crime and mental disorder II. Forensic aspects of psychiatric disorder. In *Seminars in Practical Forensic Psychiatry* (eds. Chiswick D and Cope R). London: Gaskell.

2 Walsh E, Buchanan A, Fahy T (2002) Violence and schizophrenia: examining the evidence. *BJP* **180**, 490–5.

3 Chiswick D (1998) The relationship between crime and psychiatry. In *Companion to Psychiatric Studies* (eds. Johnstone EC, Freeman CPL, Zealley AK). Edinburgh: Churchill Livingstone.

Assessing risk of violence[1,2,3]

Context Risk of violence to others is assessed by psychiatrists in a range of situations, (e.g. acute assessments in casualty, allowing patients leave; court reports, determining whether a patient should progress from a secure setting).

Types of violence risk assessment
- *Clinical* Traditionally carried out in an unstructured manner, perhaps guided by the research literature. Clinical risk assessment criticised due to lack of reliability, validity, and transparency.
- *Actuarial* (e.g. VRAG): Statistical approaches based on multivariate analyses of factors in samples of forensic patients or prisoners to determine which predict further violence. Variables predictive of recidivism given weightings and combined to give score. From this score a probability of recidivism can be calculated. Criticised as factors identified invariably historical unchangeable attributes. Considered by some to be inflexible and unable to inform risk management.
- *Structured clinical* (e.g. HCR-20): Intermediate approach. Combines historical factors of actuarial approach with dynamic factors in structured way. Clinically the consideration of each factor is more important than the actual scores, so act as useful aide memoirs. The approach here is based on this method.

Information Sources of information determined by nature and context of assessment, using as many sources of information as possible: records (psychiatric, general practice, social work, prison, school, criminal), interviews (patient, relatives, staff), psychometric (e.g. PCL-R).

Factors to consider (based on HCR-20)
- **Historical** *Previous violence* (convicted and non-convicted, nature, motivation, victims, context); *relationships* (lack of relationships, unstable relationships); *employment* (poor employment record, disciplinary problems); *substance misuse; mental illness* (noting its relationship to previous aggression); *personality disorder* (dissocial, emotionally unstable, paranoid, psychopathy); *childhood problems* (behavioural disturbance, mistreatment); *previous difficulties with supervision* (absconding, lack of attendance, lack of compliance).
- **Current (internal)** *Symptoms* (delusions, hallucinations); *threats* (towards particular victim or group); *fantasies* (violence, sexual); *attitudes* (pro-criminal, minimisation, denial); *impulsivity; insight* (into illness, into personality, into previous violence and precursors); *response to treatment* (pharmacological and psychosocial); *plans* (realistic).
- **Current (external)** *Weapons; access to victims; support* (formal and informal); *destabilisers* (alcohol, drugs, homelessness, victimisation); *stress* (relationship problems, debt, life events).

1 Quinsey VL, Harris GT, Rice ME et al (1998) *Violent offenders: appraising and managing risk.* Washington DC: American Psychological Association.

2 Webster CD, Douglas KS, Eaves D, Hart SD (1997) *HCR-20 Assessing risk for violence* (version 2). Vancouver: Simon Fraser University.

3 Royal College of Psychiatrists (1996) *Assessment and Management of Risk of Harm to Other People. Council Report CR53.* London: Royal College of Psychiatrists.

Formulation Anchored by historical factors with current factors indicating immediate/short-term risk. Risk of what, to whom, when, under what circumstances? Acknowledge uncertainties and information gaps. Emphasise context(s) in which person may be at increased/decreased risk. If using actuarial methods: are they applicable to this person/risk? Are normative values from an appropriate sample?

Communication The assessment must be communicated in an appropriate and understandable way to others. It must also be documented. Use of scores, percentages, or terms such as low, medium, or high should be explained.

Risk management The factors identified in the risk assessment should indicate areas to be addressed in management. They may point to the need for specific treatments (pharmacological or psychological), supervision, support, or detention.

Risk assessment instruments

A number of risk assessment instruments have been developed. Some are structured clinical methods, while others are actuarial. The following list indicates the type of risk assessed and whether the tool is actuarial or structured clinical in nature. Most of these tools require specific training and all require familiarity with the tool and the risk being assessed. There is no consensus as to which tools should be used and when, and some argue that risk assessment tools should not be used at all.

Historical, clinical and risk 20—(HCR-20)	Violence/structured clinical
Violence risk appraisal guide (VRAG)	Violence/actuarial
Psychopathy checklist—revised (PCL-R)	Violence/actuarial
Risk assessment, management, and audit systems (RAMAS)	Violence/structured clinical
Risk assessment guidance framework (RAGF)	Violence/structured clinical
Offender assessment system (OASys)	Violence/structured clinical
Reconviction prediction score (RPS)	Violence/actuarial
Risk of reconviction (ROR) score	Violence/actuarial
Offender group reconviction scale (OGRS)	Violence/actuarial
Risk of sexual violence protocol (RSVP) (previously SVR-20)	Sex offending/structured clinical
Sexual offending risk appraisal guide (SORAG)	Sex offending/actuarial
Rapid risk assessment of sex offender recidivism (RRASOR)	Sex offending/actuarial
Static 99	Sex offending/actuarial
SONAR	Sex offending/actuarial
Matrix 2000 (previously structured anchored clinical judgement (SACJ)	Sex offending/actuarial
Spousal assault risk assessment (SARA)	Spouse abuse/structured clinical

Secure hospitals and units[1]

Within the health service there are psychiatric hospitals and units that offer varying degrees of security. The terms high, medium, and low security are used to categorise these services, and give some indication of the level of risk that can be managed within a particular unit. However, there are no clear definitions of these levels of security; different units at the same security level may operate in very different ways; there is blurring between the different levels; and rather than thinking of patients in terms of level of security required it is better to consider a particular patient's risk, how this should be managed, and how a particular unit may or may not be able to manage the risk. The network of secure services for a particular area vary considerably from region to region.

Security does not just rely on the physical barriers and monitoring, although these are important. Knowing patients well (from studying their backgrounds and interacting with them) and developing good relationships with them contribute to 'relational security'. Multidisciplinary risk assessment and management are also important.

High security hospitals

There are five high security hospitals in the British Isles:

• **English special hospitals**—Ashworth, Broadmoor, and Rampton Hospitals. Serve E&W and are each part of a local NHS Trust. Each has about 500 beds.

• **State Hospital (Carstairs)**. Serves Scot and NI. Managed by a special health board. About 250 beds.

• **Central Mental Hospital (Dundrum)**. Serves the RoI. Managed by the Eastern Health Board. About 80 beds.

Patients admitted from prisons, courts, or less secure hospitals. Patients must be detained under mental health or criminal procedure legislation. Majority of patients have committed offences, but a substantial minority are transferred from other hospitals where they are unmanageable. Patients should pose a grave immediate danger to the public. Admissions are usually for several years.

Medium secure units

Medium secure units are not as virtually escape-proof as high security hospitals but are more secure than locked wards. Vary in size from 30–100 beds. Each region in E&W has one or more medium secure units; in Scot medium secure units are developing with one open so far; there are no such units in NI or the RoI. Patients are admitted from prisons, courts, and less secure units, and also from high security hospitals. Admissions are not usually for more than 2 years. Patients may move on to low security, open wards, or the community, being managed by general or forensic services depending on • local service provision, patients' backgrounds, and clinical needs.

Some specialist units have developed for personality disordered patients, learning disabled patients, women, and adolescents.

The State Hospital, Carstairs and the Central Mental Hospital, Dundrum admit many patients who would be admitted to medium secure units in E&W due to the under-development of local secure forensic provision in Scot, NI, and the RoI.

Low security units

Low secure units and wards have locked doors but do not usually have a secure perimeter. Some regional forensic services have a combination of low and medium secure wards; in areas of Scot and NI there are low secure forensic wards without medium secure units. Psychiatric intensive care units (PICUs) are low secure short-stay wards primarily for the care of acutely disturbed general psychiatry patients. In a few areas they also take patients from courts, prisons, and more secure units, but they are not well-suited to providing longer-term assessment or treatment.

Referring a patient to secure forensic services

- A comprehensive assessment should be made and details of this should be sent with the referral.
- Particular attention should be given to the risk the person poses (p. 646) and why this risk cannot adequately be managed in less secure services.
- Patients should meet the criteria for compulsory detention in hospital under relevant legislation.

---

1 Kennedy, HG (2002) Therapeutic uses of security: mapping forensic mental health services by stratifying risk. *Advances in Psychiatric Treatment* **8**, 433–43.

Police liaison (1)

Prevalence of psychiatric disorder

2–5% of people held in custody by the police suffer from mental disorder. About 1–2% suffer from severe mental illness.

Liaison and diversion

- **Diversion** of people with mental disorders from the criminal justice system to health care can operate at any stage of the criminal justice process. The term is often used to refer to **early diversion**, the transfer of mentally disordered people from police custody or at their first court hearing.
- **Diversion schemes** operate in some areas whereby a specific service is provided to the police and/or courts to help identify and divert mentally disordered individuals. These schemes may also be known as police or court *liaison schemes*.
- **Police or court liaison** is the process or system by which mental health services provide assessment and/or diversion for people with mental disorder at an early stage of the criminal justice process.
- In some areas there are formal diversion schemes, but from area to area there are differences.

In many cases where a person is diverted, the police, prosecutor, or court will discontinue the criminal justice process. This will be particularly appropriate in most cases where individuals with mental disorder will have committed relatively minor offences. However, diversion does not necessitate this, and where appropriate, particularly where more serious offences have been committed, a prosecution may be pursued in parallel with diversion for care and treatment.

Powers allowing police to take a person to a place of safety

- The police have powers under mental health legislation to convey a person who they believe is suffering from mental disorder to a place of safety. (Specific powers are set out opposite.)
- The purpose of these powers is to allow for a psychiatric assessment.
- The use by the police of these powers does not oblige mental health services to admit the person.

Arrest and detention in custody

Where an offence has been committed a mentally disordered offender may be arrested and taken into police custody.

- **Issues to be addressed when assessing a person in police custody**:
  - Is there evidence of mental disorder?
  - Is treatment in hospital required? If so how urgently?
  - What is the nature of the alleged offence and is there any evidence of a serious risk to others?
  - Is the person fit to remain in police custody?
  - Is the person fit to be interviewed by the police? Do they require an appropriate adult?
  - Would they be fit to plead if they appeared in court? (see p. 672)

- **Options following assessment if person appears to be mentally disordered:**
  - admission to hospital informally or under mental health legislation
  - treatment in the community
  - recommend admission on remand following first court appearance
  - recommend further assessment on remand in custody or on bail following first court appearance.
- **Fitness to remain in police custody** There are no legal criteria to determine whether a person is 'fit to remain in police custody'. A person may be unfit to remain in police custody due to physical illness or mental disorder. Where a person is mentally disordered such that there would be a serious immediate risk to their own health if they remained in the police cells, then they would be unfit to remain in police custody, and should usually be admitted to hospital.

Powers allowing the police to take a mentally disordered person to a place of safety

E&W Section 136 MHA1983 allows the police to apprehend a person who appears to be mentally disordered found in a public place, and convey them to a place of safety where they may be detained for up to 72 hours. The place of safety should be a mental health setting, but often a police station is used. The purpose of section 136 is to allow for the person to be assessed by mental health services. Following the assessment the person may be diverted to mental health services (informally or under compulsion), arrested and taken into police custody, or released.

Scot Section 297 MH(CT)(S)A2003 allows similar provisions in Scot, but detention may only be for up to 24 hours.

NI Article 130 MH(NI)O1986 allows similar provisions in NI, but detention may only be for up to 48 hours.

RoI Under the section 12 MHA2001, if a garda has reasonable grounds for believing that a person is suffering from a mental disorder and that, because of the disorder, there is a serious likelihood of the person causing harm to himself/herself or another person, the garda may take the person into custody. If necessary, the garda may use force to enter the premises where it is believed that the person is. The garda must then go through the normal application procedure for involuntary detention in an approved centre. If the garda's application is refused, the person must be released immediately. If the application is granted, the garda must remove the person to the approved centre.

N.B. *In E&W, Scot, and NI these powers do not allow the police to enter premises if they want to remove a person who appears to be suffering from mental disorder. Under these circumstances powers are available under s135 MHA1983, s293 MH(CT)(S)A2003, and article 129 MH(NI)O1986.*

Police liaison (2)[1,2,3]

Police interviews—fitness, false confessions, and appropriate adults

Mental disorder may affect a police interview by: impairing the ability of a person to communicate; leading to the person giving unreliable evidence or making a person vulnerable to becoming distressed. In some cases mental disorder may be so severe that a person is unfit to be interviewed.

- There is no legal basis for **fitness to be interviewed** but the following issues may be relevant:
  - Does the detainee understand the police caution after it has been fully explained to him or her?
  - Is the detainee fully orientated in time, place, and person and does he or she recognise the key persons present during the police interview?
  - Is the detainee likely to give answers which can be seriously misconstrued by the court?
- Where a person is mentally disordered and fit to be interviewed, an **appropriate adult** should be present during the police interview. Appropriate adult schemes operate differently in the different jurisdictions of the British Isles (see below).
- **False confessions** have been at the heart of some notorious miscarriages of justice. Three types are recognised:
  - Voluntary (the person voluntarily presents and confesses to a crime he has not committed)
  - Coerced compliant (persuasive interrogation leads to a person confessing to an offence he knows he has not committed)
  - Coerced internalised (amnesia or subtle manipulation by the interrogator leads to the person believing he has committed a crime which he has not).

Appropriate adults

- **E&W** The Police and Criminal Evidence Act (PACE) 1984 and its Codes of Practice provide a statutory basis for appropriate adults. Appropriate adults should be requested by the police where a detained person is under 16 or is deemed to be 'vulnerable' (perhaps due to mental disorder). The appropriate adult may be a relative or carer.
- **Scot** No statutory basis for appropriate adult schemes. Schemes operate to provide appropriate adults, who should not be a relative or carer, and who should be requested by the police when they are interviewing any mentally disordered person. These schemes do not cover children.
- **NI** Similar statutory basis as E&W.
- **RoI** No specific provisions.

1 Gudjonnson GH (1993) *The psychology of interrogations, confessions and testimony.* Chichester: Wiley.

2 Birmingham L (2001) Diversion from custody. *Advances in Psychiatric Treatment* **7**, 198–207.

3 Pearse J and Gudjonnsen G (1996) How appropriate are appropriate adults? *Journal of Forensic Psychiatry* **7**, 570–80.

Court liaison

Broadly covers all aspects of psychiatric assessments for courts, but here is used narrowly to refer to psychiatric assessment at an early (usually the first) court appearance. The terms 'liaison' and 'diversion' in relation to police and courts are described on p. 650. Preparation of court reports and giving evidence in court are covered on pp. 662–7.

Some areas have court liaison or diversion schemes, aimed at identifying people with mental disorders at an early stage of the court process and diverting them to appropriate mental health services where necessary. Some screen all detainees, but most rely on referrals from criminal justice staff when mental disorder is suspected. In many schemes the first assessment is by a CPN who then refers the person on if necessary. Back up from psychiatrists is necessary for those cases where admission, particularly under compulsion, may be necessary.

Features of successful court liaison schemes

- 'owned' by mainstream general or forensic services
- staffed by senior psychiatrists
- nurse-led and closely linked to local psychiatric services
- good working relationships with courts and prosecution
- good methods for obtaining health, social services, and criminal record information
- access to suitable interview facilities
- use of structured screening assessments
- direct access to hospital beds
- ready access to secure beds
- access to specialised community facilities
- integrated with police and prison liaison schemes

In many areas there are no dedicated schemes. Under these circumstances it is important that it is clear to the police, courts, social services, and health services how an urgent assessment may be obtained if necessary.

Issues to be addressed when assessing a person at an early court appearance

- Is there evidence of mental disorder?
- Is assessment and/or treatment in hospital required?
- If so, how urgently?
- What is the nature of the alleged offence and is there any evidence of a serious risk to others?
- Is the person fit to plead? (see p. 672)

Options following assessment if person appears to be mentally disordered

- admission to hospital informally or under mental health legislation
- treatment in the community

- recommend admission on remand (see p. 668)
- recommend further assessment on remand in custody or on bail

In many cases it will be appropriate for the criminal justice process to be discontinued. However, where serious offences are alleged it would usually be appropriate, if diversion is necessary, for the person to be remanded in hospital (see pp. 668–9).

Prison psychiatry (1)—overview

Introduction
The average daily population of prisons in the UK is almost 50 000. Prisons in the UK are either local prisons (accommodating remand prisoners and prisoners serving sentences of less than 2 years) or training prisons (taking prisoners serving sentences of more than 2 years). In practice a number of prisons perform both functions. Security varies depending on the categories of prisoners held. All prisoners are categorised solely on security considerations: 'A' (the highest category requiring maximum security) to 'D' (the lowest category, suitable for open conditions). Most female prisoners are kept in separate prisons.

The prison remand
A person accused of committing an offence may be held on remand in prison whilst awaiting trial and/or sentence. Courts should not remand a person in custody unless there is a good reason not to grant bail. Mentally disordered offenders are more likely to be remanded in custody than other offenders perhaps because: they are more likely to be homeless; they are considered less likely to comply with bail; they are perceived as more dangerous because of their mental disorder; there are a number of statutory objections to bail for mentally disordered defendants even where the offence is not punishable by imprisonment; and even though remands in custody for reports are discouraged there is a lack of hospital or specialist bail facilities.

The prison sentence
A prison sentence is imposed on an offender by a judge. He will consider a number of factors, including any mitigating or aggravating circumstances. The sentence may serve one or more of the following functions: punishment, deterrence, reparation, incapacitation, rehabilitation. In certain circumstances there may be a mandatory prison sentence (e.g. a life sentence for murder). Most prisoners serving determinate sentences are released before the end of their sentence and subject to a period of supervision and/or recall. The exact nature of this depends on the nature of the offence and the length of the sentence imposed. Life-sentenced prisoners have a tariff (time to serve as punishment) set by the judge; when this has been served release is a decision for the Home Secretary advised by the parole board (for mandatory life-sentenced prisoners in E&W) or for the parole board (for discretionary life-sentenced prisoners in E&W and for all life-sentenced prisoners in Scot).

Mental disorder in prisoners
The prevalence of mental disorder in the prison population is high, especially in remand and female populations. Psychotic disorders: 2–10%; affective/neurotic disorders: 6–59%; alcohol-related disorder: 22–63%; drug-related disorder: 20–73%; personality disorder: 10–75%. It has been estimated that 23–55% of prisoners have psychiatric treatment needs, with 2–5% requiring transfer to psychiatric hospital.

Mental health services in prison

Traditionally the prison medical service has been separate from the main-stream health service. Health screening occurs on reception to prison but is cursory and ineffective. Officially prisons should give prisoners access to the same quality and range of health care services as the general public receives from the NHS. Psychiatrists from the health service provide sessions or may visit for a particular case. Prisons may have mental health nurses who provide assessment, monitoring, and support for prisoners and advice to other staff. Some prisons have multi-disciplinary mental health teams. In E&W greater partnership between the NHS and the prison service is proposed in the provision of mental health services to prisoners.

Prison psychiatry (2)—the role of the psychiatrist[1,2]

Psychiatrists may be asked to assess prisoners for the following reasons:
- To provide court reports (see p. 662)
- To provide assessment and treatment at the request of a prison medical officer
- For statutory purposes (e.g. preparing reports for the parole board)

When arranging to see a prisoner, a psychiatrist should make an appointment which will fit in with the prison routine. There will usually be only 2–3 hours in the morning or afternoon when there is access to prisoners. The psychiatrist will have to wait to be escorted by prison staff.

Assessment of prisoners

Prisoners should be seen on their own unless prison staff or other sources indicate this would be unwise. It may be difficult to get relevant information about the prisoner's day-to-day functioning and presentation from prison staff, although attempts should be made to do this. Ask the prisoner for a relative's telephone number and permission to speak to them. The prison medical file may not contain all the necessary information, and in some cases other prison records should be examined. History taking, MSE, and information gathering should proceed as with any other psychiatric assessment. Short cuts and sloppy practice should not be allowed to creep into psychiatric practice in prison.

Options in the management of mentally disordered prisoners

If a psychiatrist assesses a prisoner and finds that they are mentally disordered he may:
- Treat the person in prison
- Arrange for the person to be transferred to mental health services, either by arranging direct transfer from prison (see p. 671) or by recommending a mental health disposal through the courts if the prisoner has not been sentenced yet.

No prison, or prison medical centre, is recognised as a hospital under mental health legislation. Therefore compulsory treatment under the Mental Health Act cannot be given. All prisoners with severe mental illness should be transferred to hospital for treatment. Legal provisions for transferring prisoners to hospital are set out on p. 669. Similar provisions for remand prisoners are discussed on p. 668 and listed on pp. 670–1 for each jurisdiction.

Treatment in prison
- Medication, monitoring, and modest psychological treatment (supportive psychotherapy perhaps utilising some cognitive-behavioural or psychodynamic techniques) may be offered to prisoners with mental disorders who do not require treatment in hospital.
- Various treatment programmes to address offending behaviour have been developed in prisons. These are run by the prison service and do not involve mental health services. Programmes are available for areas

such as sexual offending, anger management, alcohol and substance misuse, problem solving.
- Some prisons specialise in treating certain mentally disordered prisoners—e.g. HMP Grendon in England offers therapeutic community treatment for personality disordered prisoners who volunteer to be transferred there; there is a 17-bed psychiatric unit at HMP Maghaberry in NI.

Suicide in prison

Suicide is the most common mode of death in prisons. The rate is approximately 9 times that in the general population. The most common means is by hanging. Remand prisoners, young offenders, and those with histories of substance misuse and violent offences are at particular risk.

Many factors probably contribute to the increased rate of suicide in prisons, including:
- histories of psychiatric disorder
- previous self-harm
- alcohol and substance misuse
- social isolation

These are compounded by:
- uncertainty
- powerlessness
- bullying
- isolation

The task of identifying prisoners who are at risk is extremely difficult as those who kill themselves share the same vulnerabilities and stresses with many other prisoners who do not.

A major factor that may reduce suicide rates is improvement in prison conditions. Isolation of prisoners at risk in strip cells still occurs although it is becoming less frequent and is against official guidance.

---

1 Birmingham L (2003) The mental health of prisoners. *Advances in Psychiatric Treatment* **9**, 191–201.

2 Chiswick D and Dooley E (1995) Psychiatry in prisons. In *Seminars in Practical Forensic Psychiatry* (eds. Chiswick D and Cope R). London: Gaskell.

Legal provisions for transfer of prisoners to hospital

Sentenced prisoners

E&W

Section 47 MHA1983 allows for the transfer of a mentally disordered sentenced prisoner to hospital. There must be reports from two registered medical practitioners addressing what category of mental disorder the person suffers from and whether this is of a nature or degree to warrant hospital detention. The reports are submitted to the Secretary of State who decides whether or not to grant a 'transfer direction'.

Section 49 MHA1983 allows the Secretary of State to add a 'restriction direction' to a transfer direction, which has the same effect as a restriction order under section 41 (see p. 671) and may last as long as the sentence the person was serving. In practice section 47 is rarely made without section 49.

Scot

Section 136 MH(CT)(S)A2003 sets out similar provisions for Scot. There must be reports from two medical practitioners (one approved) addressing whether the prisoner has a mental disorder, that the mental disorder is 'treatable', that the person would be at risk or pose a risk to others, and that the transfer is necessary. The reports are submitted to the Scottish Ministers who decide whether or not to grant a 'transfer for treatment direction'. All transferred prisoners are treated as restricted patients for the duration of the prison sentence that they are serving.

NI

Article 53 MH(NI)O1986 sets out similar provisions for NI. Two medical practitioners (one appointed for the purposes of part II by the Mental Health Commission) must submit reports to the Secretary of State. The issues are similar to E&W, except the mental disorder must be mental illness or severe mental impairment. The order is called a 'transfer direction'. Article 55 allows the addition of a 'restriction direction' as in E&W.

RoI

The law in this area is complex and obscure.

Section 8 Criminal Justice Act 1960 confirms provisions under section 2 and section 3 of the Criminal Lunatics (Ireland) Act 1838 and section 13 of the Lunatic Asylums (Ireland) Act 1875, allowing for the transfer of insane prisoners from prison to hospital. Transfer to the Central Mental Hospital is allowed under Central Lunatic Asylum (Ireland) Act 1845. Two doctors must certify insanity and the Minister of Justice must authorise the transfer.

Section 17 Criminal Justice Administration Act 1914 allows the transfer of a prisoner to the Central Mental Hospital for assessment or treatment on a 'hospital order' authorised by a Minister of Justice. The prisoner does not need to be certified and this is therefore an informal measure.

In practice, forms issued by the Minister for Justice, Equality, and Law Reform are used. Criminal Law (Insanity) Bill 2002 does not contain provisions for the transfer of prisoners (which would therefore remain unchanged); this has been criticised by several bodies, and such provisions will probably be included.

Prisoners awaiting trial or sentence

E&W

Section 48 MHA1983 is similar to section 47 but provides for transfer of unsentenced prisoners. Other differences from section 47: the person must have mental illness or severe mental impairment (cannot be used for psychopathic disorder or mental impairment) and there must be urgent need for treatment. This section also enables the transfer of civil prisoners and people detained under immigration legislation.

Scot

Section 52 CP(S)A1995 provisions ('assessment orders' and 'treatment orders'), as described on p. 670, may be used for prisoners awaiting trial or sentence. The necessary medical recommendations are made to the Scottish Ministers who then apply to a court for the person to be admitted to hospital, in the same way as for a hospital remand made at any court appearance.

NI

Article 54 sets out similar provisions for NI as section 48 MHA1983 for E&W. Again, one of the two doctors must be approved under part II by the Commission. The prisoner may not be transferred to the State Hospital, as it is in another jurisdiction and the court process has not been completed.

RoI

Provisions are as set out above for sentenced prisoners.

Court reports and giving evidence (1)

A psychiatrist may be required to provide reports and give evidence in criminal and civil proceedings; the following deals with reports in criminal proceedings.

Introduction Reports may be requested by the prosecution, the court, or by a solicitor. The assessment should be objective and professional, and should not be influenced by which 'side' has made the request.

The clinical issues The clinical issues will involve those that psychiatrists usually assess: diagnosis, treatment needs, prognosis, etc. However, specific attention needs to be given to how these clinical issues interact with the legal issues in question. What is the relationship between any psychiatric disorder and past, present, and future offending? How might treatment or the natural course of the disorder impact on the likelihood of further offending? What impact might the current mental state have on the person's ability to participate in the court process?

The legal issues The request for psychiatric assessment should indicate the legal issues towards which the psychiatrist should direct the assessment. However in many cases the instructions are not specific. The main issues to consider are usually:

- Fitness to plead (see p. 672)
- Responsibility (see pp. 676–9)
- The presence of mental disorder and whether assessment and/or treatment under compulsion (or otherwise) is required (see pp. 668–9)
- The risk the person poses (may be relevant in whether a restriction order is imposed, in determining if disposal should be to a secure unit or special hospital, or perhaps in determining the nature of the sentence imposed; see p. 669).

Before the interview

- Comprehensive background information should usually be provided by those requesting the report. Unfortunately this is often lacking. Ideally one should have the opportunity to examine: document specifying the charges, police summary, witness statements, records of interviews with the accused, records of previous offences, other reports. Sometimes tape recordings of interviews, photographic or video evidence may be available.
- Arrangements should be made to interview the person in prison (if they have been remanded in custody), as an outpatient (if they have been remanded on bail), or in hospital (if they have been admitted to hospital). The psychiatrist should be given reasonable time to complete the assessment and produce a considered report. If there is insufficient time then this should be stated in the report and any opinion given should be qualified.

The interview
- Check the person's correct name and details. Introduce yourself and state who has requested the report.
- Make it clear that the interview is not confidential and that the information in the report will be seen by others.
- Clarify that the person has understood this, and seek their consent to prepare the report.
- If the person refuses to be interviewed then this should be respected and reported to the person requesting the report.
- Ask the person's permission to contact a relative and/or their GP for further information.
- Follow the usual format for a psychiatric assessment.
- Enquiry about the circumstances of the offence and the person's understanding of the court process will need to be made in addition.
- More than one session may be necessary in some cases.
- Physical examination and investigations should be performed if indicated.

After the interview
Further information may be gathered from the following sources:
- Interviews with relatives or staff (health care, prison, or social services):
- Health (psychiatric or general practice), prison, social work, or educational records.
- In some cases specific psychometric testing by a psychologist may be necessary (e.g. where a person appears to be learning disabled).

Court reports and giving evidence (2)[1–4]

The report

- The various strands of the assessment should be brought together in the report.
- The report should be clear, concise, well structured, and jargon-free.
- Technical terms (e.g. schizophrenia, personality disorder, delusions, hallucinations, thought disorder) should be explained if they are used.
- If a number of sources of information have been used, indicate where the particular factual information in the report has come from, particularly when there are inconsistencies (e.g. 'according to …', 'he stated that …').
- The main body of the report should present the information gathered; the opinion should present the conclusions concerning the relevant issues and lead to the recommendations.
- The opinion and recommendations should confine themselves to psychiatric issues. Punitive sanctions, such as imprisonment, should never be recommended.

There is no set format for a report, just as there are different ways of presenting history and mental state. A suggested structure is given on pp. 666–7.

What will happen to the report?

- The report becomes the property of whoever requested it.
- Defence reports may or may not be produced in evidence in a particular case; prosecution reports must be revealed to the defence.
- Copies of the report should not be sent by the psychiatrist to others (such as the patient's GP, another psychiatrist, or a probation officer) without the consent of both the person examined and the person who commissioned the report.
- A psychiatric report may come to be included in various records (health, prison, probation), and may in the future be used for reference or in further legal proceedings.

Giving evidence

In most cases a psychiatrist will not be required to give oral evidence. However under some circumstances this will be the case: a report requires clarification, the court finds it difficult to accept the opinion, there are conflicting reports, in specific circumstances where oral evidence is obligatory (e.g. where a restriction order is under consideration). If you are requested to attend court:

- Clarify with the court when you should attend.
- Prepare in advance by examining the papers and re-reading your report.
- Consult references and anticipate questions.
- Present in a smart, confident, professional manner and be punctual.
- Counsel may request a conference before the court sits.
- Have a brief interview with the accused in the court cells if he has not been seen for sometime and particularly where fitness to plead may be an issue.

When called to give evidence you will be asked to take the oath, and then will be questioned by the barrister or solicitor who called you. You will then be cross-examined by the 'other side' before being re-examined. You may take notes with you, but ask the judge before referring to them. Speak clearly and slowly, and explain technical terms. Address the judge. If counsel's questioning is not allowing you to get the appropriate information across, then ask the judge if you may clarify your response.

A note on addressing the judge:

- **E&W**—High Court 'My Lord' or 'My Lady'; local judge 'Your Honour'; Magistrate's Court 'Sir' or 'Madam'.
- **Sc**—High Court and Sheriff Court 'My lord' or 'Sir' and 'My lady' or 'Ma'am'.
- **NI**—as E&W.
- **RoI**—'Your Lordship', 'Judge', or 'Sir'.

1 Bluglass R (1995) Writing reports and giving evidence. In *Seminars in Practical Forensic Psychiatry* (eds. Chiswick D and Cope R). London: Gaskell.

2 Bluglass R (1990) The psychiatrist as an expert witness. In *Principles and Practice of Forensic Psychiatry* (eds. Bluglass R and Bowden P). Edinburgh: Churchill Livingstone.

3 Chiswick D (1990) The psychiatric report: Scotland. In *Principles and Practice of Forensic Psychiatry* (eds. Bluglass R and Bowden P). Edinburgh: Churchill Livingstone.

4 Grounds A (1993) Psychiatric reports for legal purposes in the United Kingdom. In *Forensic psychiatry: clinical, legal and ethical issues* (eds. Gunn J and Taylor P). Oxford: Butterworth-Heinemann.

Suggested format for criminal court report

- The following sets out a comprehensive list of the matters that may be set out in a report.
- Not all of the issues will be relevant in every case. For example:
  - Where there is little information available and the recommendation is for further assessment, then the report may be relatively brief, focusing on the issues of relevance to the making of any relevant order.
  - Where the person has been convicted, consideration of fitness to plead, insanity at the time of the offence, and diminished responsibility (in murder cases) is irrelevant.
  - Where a report is updating a previous report prepared in the same case relating to the same offence (or alleged offence) or is recommending the extension of an order, then the report may be relatively brief, as long as it addresses whether the person fulfils the criteria for that order and why extension is necessary.

Preliminary information

- At whose request the assessment was undertaken, circumstances of assessment (place, time, any constraints on assessment such as inadequate time to complete assessment due to prison routine).
- Sources of information used (interview with the person, interviews with others, documents examined).
- The person's capacity to take part or refuse to take part and understanding of the limits of confidentiality.
- If any important sources of information could not be used, there should be a statement as to why this was the case.

Background history family history; personal history; medical history; psychiatric history; recent social circumstances; personality; forensic history.

Circumstances of offence or alleged offence

Progress since offence or alleged offence: particularly where there has been a considerable period of time since the (alleged) offence.

Current mental state

Opinion

- Fitness to plead
- Presence of mental disorder currently and whether the criteria for the relevant order are met
- Presence of mental disorder at the time of the offence:
  - The relationship between any mental disorder and the offence (this is still relevant even if the person has been convicted as it may affect the choice of disposal)
  - Whether the person was insane at the time of the offence
  - In murder cases, whether there are grounds for diminished responsibility

- Assessment of risk:
  - The risk that the person might pose of re-offending
  - The relationship between this risk and any mental disorder present
  - Does the person require to be managed in a secure setting (medium secure unit, high security hospital)
- What assessment or treatment does the person require?
  - Does the person need further assessment? (Where? Does the person need a period of inpatient assessment and at what level of security? Why? What issues remain to be clarified?)
  - Does the person require treatment? (What treatment do they need and where?)
- State any matters that are currently uncertain and the reasons they remain uncertain

Recommendation

- Should the court consider using any particular order (and if so what arrangements have been made for the person to be received in hospital or elsewhere under this order)
- Whose care will the person be under

Consider whether an alternative order may be appropriate if circumstances change so that the order recommended above cannot be acted on e.g.
- If the person is or is not found to be insane
- If the person is or is not convicted

Medical practitioner's details: name; current post; current employer; qualifications; whether fully registered with the GMC; approved under relevant mental health legislation; a statement that the report is given on soul and conscience (in Scot); statements as to whether the medical practitioner is related to the person and has any pecuniary interest in the person's admission to hospital or placement on any community based order (if a mental health disposal is being recommended); the medical practitioner should sign the report.

Overview of the pathways of mentally disordered offenders through the criminal justice and health systems

The following gives an overview of the criminal justice process, and how at each stage mental disorder may lead to certain courses of action being taken. Different procedures are available in the 4 main jurisdictions of the British Isles (see also pp. 670–1 for a summary of the legal provisions for each jurisdiction). The numbers appearing in superscripts below give an indication as to which procedures are not applicable in all 4 jurisdictions: 1. E&W and Scot only; 2. Not in RoI; 3. Scot only.

Arrest and police custody
After being apprehended an individual may be diverted to mental health services informally or under civil procedures. Police may also have specific powers allowing them to take mentally disordered individuals for assessment by psychiatric services.

Pre-trial
- At a pre-trial court appearance a mentally disordered individual may be remanded to hospital for assessment and/or treatment[2]. With more minor offences criminal proceedings may be taken no further and an individual may receive care from mental health services either informally or using compulsory measures under mental health legislation.
- If an individual is remanded in prison, but appears to be mentally disordered, procedures may allow for the transfer of that person to hospital.
- If an individual is remanded on bail, conditions may be attached so that they are required to be assessed and/or treated by psychiatric services.

Trial
- If a person's mental state is such that they cannot participate in the court process then they may be found unfit to plead and would subsequently only be liable to receive a mental health disposal.
- Mental disorder may affect a person's legal responsibility for their actions:
  - Automatic behaviour (automatism) may lead to complete acquittal or acquittal on the grounds of insanity.
  - A severe mental disorder may be such that a person is held not to be legally responsible for their actions and they are acquitted on the grounds of insanity (also known as not guilty by reason of insanity). Following such a finding they would only be liable to receive a mental health disposal.
  - In murder cases, mental disorder may lead to diminished responsibility, reducing the offence to manslaughter, thus avoiding the mandatory life sentence and allowing flexibility in disposal (which may be a penal or mental health disposal).
  - Despite the presence of mental disorder at the time of trial and/or at the time of the offence, a mentally disordered offender may plead

or be found guilty. Mental disorder may then be taken into account when sentence is passed.

Post-conviction/pre-sentence

* Procedures may allow a mentally disordered offender to be assessed in hospital after conviction but prior to sentencing[2].
* Individuals remanded in prison awaiting sentence may be transferred to hospital if they appear mentally disordered, as at the pre-trial stage[2].

Sentencing

Following conviction a mentally disordered offender may receive a mental health disposal[2]:

* A compulsory order to hospital
* A compulsory order to hospital with special restrictions in more serious cases
* A compulsory order to hospital with a prison sentence running in parallel[1]
* A compulsory order in the community[3]
* Other community disposals

They may alternatively, despite the presence of mental disorder, receive a penal disposal either in prison or the community. During a prison sentence if a person appears to be mentally disordered they may be transferred to hospital.

1 E&W and Scot only.

2 Not in RoI.

3 Scot only.

Legal provisions for procedures relating to mentally disordered offenders

	E&W	Scot	NI	RoI
Police				
Detention of mentally disordered person found in public place	s136 MHA1983	s297 MH(CT)(S)A2003	a130 MH(NI)O1986	s12 MHA2001
Detention of mentally disordered person in private premises	s135 MHA1983	s293 MH(CT)(S)A2003	a129 MH(NI)O1986	s12 MHA2001
Pre-trial				
Remand to hospital for assessment	s35 MHA1983	s52B-J CP(S)A1995	a42 MH(NI)O1986	—
Remand to hospital for assessment	s36 MHA1983	s52K-S CP(S)A1995	a43 MH(NI)O1986	—
Transfer of untried prisoner to hospital	s48 MHA1983	s52B-J P(S)A1995 or s52K-S CP(S)A1995	a54 MH(NI)O1986	*
Trial				
Criteria for fitness to plead	R v Prichard	HMA v Wilson Stewart v HMA	R v Prichard	R v Prichard (s3 CL(I)B2002)
Procedure relating to a finding of unfitness to plead	s2–3 and sch 1–2 CP(IUP) A1991	s54–57 CP(S)A1995	a49 and 50A MH(NI)O1986	Lunacy(Ireland) Act 1821, Juries Act 1976 (s3CL(I)B2002)
Criteria for insanity at the time of the offence	M'Naghten Rules	HMA v Kidd	CJ(NI)A1966	Doyle v Wicklow County Council
Procedure relating to a finding of insanity at the time of the offence	s1&3 and sch 1–2 CP(IUP) A1991	s54 and 57 CP(S)A1995	a50 and 50A CJ(NI)O1996	Trial of Lunatics Act 1883 (s4CL(I)B2002)
Criteria for diminished responsibility	s2 Homicide Act 1957	Galbraith v HMA	CJ(NI)O1996	— (s5 CL(I)B2002)
Post-conviction but pre-sentence				
Remand to hospital for assessment	s35 MHA 1983	s52B-J CP(S)A1995 s200 CP(S)A1995	a42 MH(NI)O1986	—

	E&W	Scot	NI	RoI
Remand to hospital for treatment	s36 MHA1983	s52K-S CP(S)A1995	a43 MH(NI)O1986	—
Interim hospital/ compulsion order	s38 MHA 1983	s53 CP(S)A1995	—	—
Transfer of untried prisoner to hospital	s48 MHA1983	s52B-J CP(S)A1995 or s52K-S CP(S)A1995	a54 MH(NI)O1986	*
Sentence				
Compulsory treatment in hospital under MHA	s37 MHA1983	s57A CP(S)A1995	a44 MH(NI)O1986	—
Restriction order	s41 MHA1983	s59 MHA1983	a47 CP(S)A1995	— MH(NI)O1986
Hybrid order (hospital disposal with prison sentence)	s45A-B MHA1983	s59A CP(S)A1995	—	—
Compulsory treatment in community under MHA	—	s57A CP(S)A1995	—	—
Guardianship	s37 MHA1983	s58(1A) CP(S)A1995	a44 MH(NI)O1986	—
Intervention order for incapable adult	—	s60B CP(S)A1995	—	—
Psychiatric probation order	sch2 (p5) Powers of Criminal Courts (Sentencing) Act 2000	s230 CP(S)A1995	sch1(p4) CJ(NI)O1996	—
Post-sentence				
Transfer of sentenced prisoners to hospital	s47 MHA1983	s136 MH(CT)(S)A2003	a53 MH(NI)O1986	*
Restriction direction for transferred prisoner	s49 MHA1983	**	a55 MH(NI)O1986	—

Notes:
a = article; p = paragraph; s = section; sch = schedule; CJ(NI)A1966 = Criminal Justice (NI) Act 1966; CJ(NI)O1996 = Criminal Justice (NI) Order 1996; CL(I)B2002 = Criminal Law (insanity) Bill 2002; CP(IUP)A1991 = Criminal Procedure (Insanity and Unfitness to Plead) Act 1991; CP(S)A1995 = Criminal Procedure (Scot) Act 1995; MHA1983 = Mental Health Act 1983; MHA2001 = Mental Health Act 2001; MH(CT)(S)A2003 = Mental Health (Care and Treatment) (Scot) Act 2003; MH(NI)O1986 = Mental Health (NI) Order 1986;- = no such procedure in this jurisdiction; (…) = proposals in CL(I)B2002 for RoI are in parentheses;- * = procedure may involve various old pieces of legislation, ** = all s136 MH(CT)(S)A2003 transfer directions in Scot are restricted.

Fitness to plead (1)—assessment

Essence If a person's mental disorder is such that they cannot participate adequately in the court process, then it has long been held that it is unfair for the person to be tried. If this is the case the court finds the person unfit to plead (also known as insanity in bar of trial (in Scot) and incompetent to stand trial) and the trial does not proceed.

Legal criteria The details of these vary in different jurisdictions, but broadly cover the same issues. (See opposite)

Clinical assessment of fitness to plead

The assessment of fitness to plead is concerned with the current mental state and ability of an accused. This involves:

• Making a diagnosis of mental disorder
• Determining the impact of this disorder on the abilities covered in the legal criteria.

Clinicians should be aware that the mental state of an individual may change and therefore if some time has elapsed between a clinical examination and the accused's appearance in court then a brief re-examination may be necessary.

Diagnoses that may be relevant:

Dementia and other chronic organic conditions, delirium, schizophrenia and related psychoses, severe affective disorders (mania and depression), LD.

Features of an individual's mental state due to their disorder to be taken into consideration:

• Ability to communicate (schizophrenic thought disorder, manic flight of ideas, depressive poverty of speech, dysphasia of dementia)
• Beliefs (e.g. the individual may have delusions that they have a divine mission and that the court process is irrelevant to them)
• Comprehension (may be impaired in dementia, acute confusion, or learning disability)
• Attention and concentration (may be impaired in any of the conditions listed above)
• Memory (as noted above amnesia for the alleged offence is irrelevant, but short-term memory failure due to organic impairment may be such to make following proceedings in court impossible).

In some cases suggestions may be made as to how the communication and understanding of the accused may be facilitated. However such suggestions must be practicable in court.

In most cases psychiatric evidence is unanimous and followed unquestioningly in court. A recommendation that an individual is unfit to plead should be reserved for cases where this is beyond doubt. In borderline cases certain measures (such as a hospital remand) may allow further assessment and treatment to clarify the issue. Where the index offence is relatively minor it may be appropriate for charges to be dropped and for civil detention to be initiated. In such cases prosecutors are usually keen to take this course.

Fitness to plead—legal criteria for finding

E&W: *R v Prichard (1836) 7 C&P 303*

'Whether he can plead to the indictment ... [&] ... whether he is of sufficient intellect to comprehend the course of proceedings on trial, so as to make a proper defence—to know that he might challenge any of you [the jury] to whom he might object—and to comprehend the details of evidence ...'

Scot: *HMA v Wilson 1942 JC 75*

'... a mental alienation of some kind which prevents the accused giving the instruction which a sane man would give for his defence or from following the evidence as a sane man would follow it and instructing his counsel as the case goes, along any point that arises.'

Similar criteria set out recently: *Stewart v HMA* (No. 1) *1997 JC 183*

'The question for [the trial judge] was whether the appellant, by reason of his material handicap, would be unable to instruct his legal representatives as to his defence or to follow what went on at his trial. Without such ability he could not receive a fair trial.'

The test excludes amnesia for the circumstances of the alleged offence.

NI: As for E&W

RoI: Currently as for E&W, but proposals for statutory definition under s3(2) Criminal Law (Insanity) Bill 2002:

'An accused person shall be deemed unfit to be tried if he or she is unable by reason of mental disorder to understand the nature or course of the proceedings so as to: (a) plead to the charge, (b) instruct a legal representative, (c) make a proper defence, (d) in the case of a trial by jury, challenge a juror to whom he or she might wish to object, or (e) understand the evidence.'

Fitness to plead (2)—procedures

What happens after a person is found unfit to plead?

A person who is unfit to plead may not be subject to penal sanctions. Traditionally the person would be detained indefinitely in a secure hospital with special restrictions on discharge until they recovered to the extent that they could be tried (although the person would rarely go back for trial even if they recovered!). This unsatisfactory arrangement is still the case in the RoI. In E&W, Scot, and NI, following a finding of unfitness to plead, there is a trial of facts where the court determines if the person did the act charged. If the facts are found the person may be subject to one of a range of mental health disposals depending on their mental state, their needs, and the risk they might pose. See following for details.

Proceedings following a finding

E&W

- Proceedings set out in the Criminal Procedure (Insanity and Unfitness to Plead) Act 1991.
- Following a finding of unfitness to plead there is a *trial of facts* held to determine whether on the balance of probability it is likely that the person committed the offence.
- If this is not found to be the case the defendant is discharged; if it is found to be the case the person may be subject to one of the following disposals:
  - Hospital order (almost identical to s37 MHA1983)
  - Hospital order with restriction order (almost identical to s37 and s41 MHA1983)
  - Guardian order (almost identical to s37MHA1983)
  - Supervision and treatment order (similar to psychiatric probation order)
  - No order
- If the person had been charged with murder then there is a mandatory hospital order with an unlimited restriction order.

Scot

- Proceedings set out under s54—57 CP(S)A1995.
- Following a finding of *insanity in bar of trial* there is an 'examination of facts'.
- Whilst awaiting this the person may be placed in prison, on bail, or in hospital under a temporary compulsion order.
- At the 'examination of facts' a determination is made as to whether on the balance of probability it is likely that the person committed the offence.
- If this is not found to be the case the defendant is discharged; if it is found to be the case the person may be subject to one of the following disposals:
  - Compulsion order (almost identical to s57A CP(S)A1995) in hospital or the community
  - Compulsion order in hospital with a restriction order (almost identical to s57A and s59 CP(S)A1995)

- Interim compulsion order (almost identical to s53 CP(S)A1995)
- Guardianship order or intervention order (identical to such orders under the Adults with Incapacity (Scot) Act 2000;
- Supervision and treatment order (similar to a psychiatric probation order)
- No order
- In Scot there is no longer a mandatory restriction order in murder cases. The interim compulsion order is to be used in all cases where the person appears to pose a considerable risk to others; following assessment, if the person is determined to pose a high risk according to the criteria set out under section 210E CP(S)A1995, then the mandatory disposal is a compulsion order to hospital with a restriction order.

NI

- Articles 49 and 50A MH(NI)O1986 set out almost identical procedures as for E&W.

RoI

- A finding of *unfitness to plead* currently leads to a High Court order for indefinite detention at the Central Mental Hospital. Any application for discharge or parole must be approved by the Minister for Justice.
- Proposals under the Criminal Law (Insanity) Bill 2002 are that:
  - If a person is found unfit to be tried, and the court is satisfied that there is a reasonable doubt that he committed the act alleged, it will acquit him and no further action under criminal proceedings will be taken.
  - If that is not the case, then following a finding of unfitness to be tried the person must be examined by a doctor to determine if they meet the criteria for detention under the Mental Health Act 2001; this may occur via a 28-day period of assessment in a designated centre.
  - If the person does meet such criteria then they are detained in a designated centre until they are fit to be tried or they no longer require detention in hospital. The designated centre may be a prison or hospital.

Fitness to stand trial

Fitness to stand trial is a separate issue from fitness to plead. It concerns whether a person is so unwell (either mentally or physically) that they are unable to appear in court or appearing in court would be detrimental to their health. In most circumstances an individual who was unfit to stand trial due to mental disorder would be unfit to plead.

Criminal responsibility (1)

If a person was mentally disordered at the time of an offence this may affect their legal responsibility for their actions. The relevant legal issues are:
- insanity at the time of the offence
- automatism
- diminished responsibility (pp. 678–9)
- infanticide (p. 678)

Insanity at the time of the offence

In some cases the court may find that a person's mental condition was such that they cannot be held responsible for their actions; they are then acquitted on the grounds of insanity (also known as insanity at the time of the offence, not guilty by reason of insanity, or guilty but insane [the present term in the RoI]). For legal criteria, see opposite page.

Automatism

- If an individual commits an offence when his body is not under the control of his mind (e.g. when asleep) he is not guilty of the offence.
- Legally this is called an *automatism*. (NB This is different from the clinical concept of automatism occurring during a complex partial seizure.)
- In **E&W** two legal types of automatism are recognised: insane and sane (*automatism simpliciter*). The distinction is based on whether the behaviour is likely to recur:
  - **Insane automatism**—due to an *intrinsic* cause (e.g. sleepwalking, brain tumours, epilepsy) results in an acquittal on the grounds of insanity.
  - **Sane automatism**—due to an *extrinsic* cause (e.g. confusional states, concussion, reflex actions after bee stings, dissociative states, night terrors, and hypoglycaemia) results in a complete acquittal.

N.B. The distinction is less important now that there is a flexible range of disposals available for those found insane.

- In Scot (until recently) **sane automatism** was not recognized—it is now recognised only in cases where an *external factor* is shown to have caused the accused's dissociated state of mind.

What happens after a person is acquitted on the grounds of insanity?

- Disposal after an acquittal on the grounds of insanity is identical to that following a finding of unfitness to plead with the facts found in E&W, Scot, and NI; and that following a finding of unfitness to plead in the RoI. (See opposite).

Insanity at the time of the offence—legal criteria

E&W: M'Naghten Rules of 1843 (West and Walk 1977)

'Every man is presumed to be sane, until the contrary be proved, and that to establish a defence on the grounds of insanity it must be clearly proved that at the time of committing the act the accused party was labouring under such a deficit of reason from disease of the mind to not know the nature and quality of the act; or that if he did know it, that he did not know that what he was doing was wrong'.

Also:

'If the accused labours under a partial delusion only [meaning an isolated delusional belief or system, rather than a partially held delusion or over-valued idea], and is not in other respects insane, he should be considered in the same situation as to responsibility as if the facts with which the delusion exists were real'.

Scot: HMA v Kidd 1960 JC 61

'... in order to excuse a person from responsibility on the grounds of insanity, there must have been an alienation of reason in relation to the act committed. There must have been some mental defect ... by which his reason was overpowered, and he was thereby rendered incapable of exerting his reason to control his conduct and reactions. If his reason was alienated in relation to the act committed, he was not responsible for the act, even although otherwise he may have been apparently quite rational.'

NI: Criminal Justice (NI) Act 1966

A defendant who is found to have been 'an insane person' at the time of the alleged offence shall not be convicted. *'Insane person'* means *'a person who suffers from mental abnormality which prevents him —*
1. *from appreciating what he is doing; or*
2. *from appreciating that what he is doing is either wrong or contrary to law; or*
3. *from controlling his own conduct'*

Mental abnormality is defined as *'an abnormality of mind which arises from a condition of arrested or retarded development of mind or any inherent causes or is induced by disease or injury'.*

RoI: Currently to be found guilty but insane the rules are similar to the M'Naghten Rules with the addition of an alternative strand (Doyle v Wicklow County Council (1974) IR 55), that he:

'...was debarred from refraining from committing the damage because of a defect of reason due to his mental illness.'

Proposals under s4(1) Criminal Law (Insanity) Bill 2002:

'Where an accused person is tried for an offence and, in the case of the District Court or Special Criminal Court, the court or, in any other case, the jury finds that the accused person committed the act alleged against him or her and, having heard evidence relating to the mental condition of the accused given by a consultant psychiatrist, finds that—(a) the accused person was suffering at the time from a mental disorder, and (b) the mental disorder was such that the accused person ought not to be held responsible for the act alleged by reason of the fact that he or she—(i) did not know the nature and quality of the act, or (ii) did not know that what he or she was doing was wrong, or (iii) was unable to refrain from committing the act, the court or the jury, as the case may be, shall return a special verdict to the effect that the accused person is not guilty by reason of insanity.'

Criminal responsibility (2)

Diminished responsibility

- In **murder cases**, a person's mental condition may be such that although they cannot be fully absolved of responsibility they are found to be of diminished responsibility (known as impaired mental responsibility in NI).
- Diminished responsibility does not currently apply in the RoI although proposals for its introduction are contained in the Criminal Law (Insanity) Bill 2002.
- A finding of diminished responsibility does not result in acquittal, but in conviction for the lesser offence of manslaughter (or culpable homicide in Scot).

For legal criteria, see opposite page.

Infanticide

- In cases involving the killing of a child aged under 12 months by the mother she may be convicted of infanticide instead of murder if the court is satisfied that the balance of her mind was disturbed by reason of her not fully having recovered from the effect of giving birth to the child, or by reason of lactation consequent upon the birth (Infanticide Act 1938 for E&W, Infanticide Act (NI) 1939, Infanticide Act 1949 for RoI).
- These criteria set a lower threshold than those for diminished responsibility.
- Disposal in such cases is flexible, as with manslaughter.
- This defence is not available in Scot where diminished responsibility would be used instead in such cases.

What happens following a finding of diminished responsibility?

- A person is convicted of manslaughter (or culpable homicide in Scot) instead of murder.
- There is therefore no mandatory sentence of life imprisonment and the court may pass any sentence it sees fit: penal sanctions in the community or prison, or any of the mental health disposals available following conviction (see pp. 670–1).

Diminished responsibility—legal criteria

E&W: *Section 2 Homicide Act 1957 states*

'When a person is party to the killing of another, he shall not be convicted of murder if he was suffering from such abnormality of mind (whether arising from a condition of arrested or retarded development of mind or any inherent causes or induced by disease or injury) as substantially impaired his mental responsibility for his acts and omissions in doing or being a party to the killing.'

In **R v Byrne (1960) 44 Cr App R 246** 'abnormality of mind' was interpreted widely:

'... a state of mind so different from that of ordinary human beings that the reasonable man would term it abnormal. It appears to us to be wide enough to cover the mind's activities in all its aspects, not only the perception of physical acts and matters and the ability to form a rational judgement whether an act is right or wrong, but also the ability to exercise will-power to control physical acts in accordance with that rational judgement.'

Scot: these were recently set out in **Galbraith v H MA Advocate 2001 SCCR 551**. The conclusions of the court were:

'In essence, the judge must decide whether there is evidence that, at the relevant time, the accused was suffering from an abnormality of mind which substantially impaired the ability of the accused, as compared with a normal person, to determine or control his acts.'

'Psychopathic personality disorder' and voluntary intoxication are excluded. The effect of a finding of diminished responsibility is that the accused is found guilty of culpable homicide rather than murder.

NI: **Criminal Justice Act (NI) 1966** defines the defence of '*impaired mental responsibility*':

'Where a party charged with murder has killed or was party to the killing of another, and it appears to the jury that he was suffering from mental abnormality which substantially impaired his mental responsibility for his acts and omissions in doing or being party to the killing, the jury shall find him not guilty of murder but shall find him guilty (whether as principal or accessory) of manslaughter.'

RoI: Not currently available. Proposals under **s5(1) Criminal Law (Insanity) Bill 2002**:

'Where a person is tried for murder and the jury or, as the case may be, the Special Criminal Court finds that the person—(a) committed the act alleged, (b) was at the time suffering from a mental disorder, and (c) the mental disorder was not such as to justify finding him or her not guilty by reason of insanity, but was such as to diminish substantially his or her responsibility for the act, the jury or court, as the case may be, shall find the person not guilty of that offence but guilty of manslaughter on the ground of diminished responsibility.'

Assessing 'mental state at the time of the offence'

Clinical examination

- Necessitates the reconstruction of the circumstances of the offence and in particular the mental state of the accused at that time.
- Along with interviewing the accused it is extremely helpful to peruse witness statements, police reports, and transcripts of police interviews (or if possible, to view videotaped interviews).
- Other important sources to help with 'retrospective' assessment:
  - Relatives, or other persons, who knew the defendant at the time.
  - Any psychiatric assessment carried out soon after the offence (if the police or court were sufficiently concerned about their mental state).
  - Any records of contact with psychiatric services at the time, and the views of relevant staff who were involved in these contacts.

Putting the legal criteria into clinical terms

For insanity at the time of the offence:

- The accused should have been suffering from a severe mental disorder which was the overwhelming factor in determining the occurrence of the offence.
- There should be a clear relationship between the offence and the symptoms of the mental disorder.
- However it should be noted that the criteria for insanity at the time of the offence in Scot, NI, and the RoI are broader than not knowing what one is doing or that it is wrong, and encompass an inability to control one's actions due to mental disorder (see criteria on p. 677).
- Diagnoses that may be relevant: dementia and other chronic organic disorders (including those secondary to alcohol or drug misuse); delirium (including delirium tremens); schizophrenia and related psychoses; severe affective disorders with psychotic symptoms; severe LD.

NB In most successful cases the diagnosis is a psychotic disorder, and delusions or hallucinations are directly relevant to the behaviour constituting the offence.

For diminished responsibility:

- The accused should have evidently been suffering from an 'abnormality of mind' (i.e. a mental disorder not severe enough to deem them 'insane', but of sufficient degree to substantially impair their ability to determine or control their actions; see criteria on p. 679).
- Diagnoses that may be relevant: any of the diagnoses listed above for insanity, as well as: non-psychotic affective disorders; acute stress reactions, adjustment disorders, and post-traumatic stress disorder; personality disorders (not primary dissocial personality disorder in Scot); sexual deviation (not in Scot); mild to moderate LD and pervasive developmental disorders (including autistic spectrum disorders).
- Other conditions that have been successful in gaining a diminished responsibility verdict are 'pre-menstrual syndrome' and 'battered spouse syndrome'.

Learning disability

Introduction

More than any other specialty in psychiatry, learning disability (LD) presents a multi-faceted, complex discipline, encompassing everything from molecular genetic diagnostic techniques to provision of adequate social supports. Confronted by multiple physical, psychiatric, social, occupational, communication, and educational problems (to name but a few), it is all too easy to feel overwhelmed. However, LD can be one of the most rewarding specialties: dealing with children, adolescents, adults, the elderly, families, and carers; utilising a multidisciplinary approach through collaboration with other health care professionals, psychologists, teachers, and community services; significantly impacting upon the quality of life of both patients and their family/carers.

There are great variations in the range and quality of services or the LD population in different geographical areas (meaning that 'local knowledge' is essential). With the closure of large institutions, there are fewer specialist inpatient services. This means that work will be concentrated in the community, with differing degrees of support, and often in liaison with adult services when admission to hospital is required (see p. 696). When involved with specialist inpatient units, the clinician's role may be more managerial than 'hands on', except when admission is for assessment of behavioural or psychiatric problems.

The role of the LD psychiatrist includes:
- Establishing the reason for developmental delay in infants and young children (see p. 694).
- Establishing the nature and extent of specific learning difficulties and the statement of special educational needs for children of school age.
- Assessing longer-term social care needs particularly in advance of transitional stages (e.g. adolescence, later life—see p. 720.)
- Assessing behavioural problems (see p. 718) or possible psychiatric problems (see p. 714) in children or adults.
- Ensuring physical problems, sensory impairments, or other disabilities are not overlooked and facilitating access to general medical services and other specialist assessments.

A structured approach is essential because of the complexity of needs in many people with LD (see p. 690). The ultimate aim of the process of assessment is to determine need and to inform what types of intervention and/or treatment may be effective (and to the benefit) of the person concerned (i.e. social, educational, psychological, medical, or psychiatric). The process ought to be open and transparent, with clear communication between the clinical team, the person with the problem (when possible), and family/carers. All too often problems arise when expectations are unrealistic, or where there are misunderstandings about the actual role of particular members of the clinical team. The clinician may act as a focal point in the collation and dissemination of information, being a 'fixed point' for the family/carers who may be somewhat 'at sea' with the dizzying array of professionals involved in the care of the child or adult with LD.

Historical perspective

The Mental Deficiency Act (1913) and The Elementary Education (Defective and Epileptic Children) Act (1914) were turning points in the management of those diagnosed as 'mentally defective' or 'feebleminded' (by 'duly qualified' medical practitioners) in the UK, requiring local authorities to provide suitable care in special institutions or the guardianship of families, and educational placements in special schools or classes. These 'segregation' acts moved those with LD from home, asylum, or workhouse, to special institutions, with the aim of providing for their special needs and the hope of social treatments (through education and training). This addressed the social concerns of the day, by scapegoating the 'feebleminded' as the cause of everything from social problems (e.g. poverty, alcoholism, unemployment, promiscuity, illegitimacy) to racial, and even imperial, decline. Defining 'idiots', 'imbeciles', and the 'feebleminded' by their ability to look after themselves (rather than by intelligence) led to 'moral insanity' (e.g. having an illegitimate child, habitual drunkenness) being used as grounds for committal to an institution.

Progress was being made in classifying 'defectives', but most medical authorities believed causation was inherited (a 'neuropathic trait'). This fed directly into prevalent eugenic notions of preventing 'racial decline' by segregation, with physical stigmata (e.g. facial characteristics) seen as 'proof' that appearance (esp. 'racial characteristics') and mental health were inter-related. Nowadays, such ideas seem simplistic (like the practice of phrenology at the time), but the notion that the Caucasian races were 'more civilised' had significant influence at the turn of the 20th century. Some doctors even advocated compulsory sterilisation 'to protect social health, but permit liberty'. It would take decades, and two world wars, before social, political, and scientific pressure finally dismantled these firmly held ideas.

Impetus came from concerns about large institutions, forms of treatment, and rights of the mentally handicapped. In the 1960s, official enquiries found evidence of abuse, malpractice, and neglect. Alarm among social reformers about the conditions in institutions was fuelled by Erving Goffman's *Asylums*. Efforts were made to reduce stigma by replacing older labels with less pejorative terms, (e.g. 'mental subnormality', 'mental retardation', 'mental handicap' for 'mental deficiency', 'idiot', 'imbecile'; 'trisomy 21' or 'Down's syndrome' for 'mongolism'; 'congenital hypothyroidism' for 'cretinism'). In 1968, ICD-8 (WHO) classified 'mental retardation' according to *severity* of intellectual impairment (by IQ assessment) and social factors. The 1970s/80s saw major policy changes, emphasising integration with mainstream resources and education, away from institutions and to the community. Many people with LD moved from hospitals to purpose-built hostels or 'group homes'.

Understanding of the aetiology of LD expanded from the 1950s onwards, with Lionel Penrose's *Biology of Mental Defect* in 1949, and the discovery of the genetic basis of Down's syndrome by Jérôme Lejeune in 1959. By the 1970s most standard textbooks recognised multiple aetiologies (genetic and environmental), separating pre-, peri-, and post-natal causes. Karyotyping, identifying metabolic abnormalities, and isolating infectious agents, allowed for laboratory diagnoses, rather than reliance on clinical observation.

Pharmacological treatments of epilepsy, behavioural disturbance, movement disorders, and psychiatric comorbidity; dietary treatments of metabolic disturbances; behavioural and cognitive approaches; improved assessment/management of social/occupational functioning, communication problems, and educational needs have allowed rational management of LD. Problems still exist (e.g. inadequacy of funding for community care/resources, unequal distribution of specialist services), but the outlook for people with LD in this, the 21st century, is more promising than it was at the turn of the last.

Classification

In the UK, the preferred term 'learning disability' (deemed to be the least pejorative) is used interchangeably with the internationally agreed term 'mental retardation' (used in both ICD-10 and DSM-IV). ICD-10 defines 'mental retardation' as 'a condition of arrested or incomplete development of the mind, characterised by impairments in cognition, language, motor and social abilities'.

Both ICD-10 and DSM-IV also agree on the use of the terms *mild, moderate, severe,* and *profound* to describe the degree of mental retardation, with arbitrary 'cut-offs' varying only slightly:

IQ range for categories	ICD-10	DSM-IV
Mild	50–69	50–55 to 70
Moderate	35–49	35–40 to 50–55
Severe	20–34	20–25 to 35–40
Profound	Below 20	Below 20–25

ICD-10 guidelines

Mild Delay in acquiring speech, but eventual ability to use everyday speech; generally able to independently self-care; main problems in academic settings (i.e. reading, writing); potentially capable of working; variable degree of emotional and social immaturity; problems more like the normal population. Minority with clear organic aetiology, variable associated problems (autism, developmental disorders, epilepsy, conduct disorders, neurological and physical disabilities).

Moderate Delay in acquiring speech, with ultimate deficits in use of language and comprehension; few acquire numeracy and literacy; occasionally capable of simple supervised work. Majority have an identifiable organic aetiology, a substantial minority have associated problems (autism, developmental disorders, epilepsy, conduct disorders, neurological and physical disabilities).

Severe Similar to moderate, but with lower levels of achievement of visuospatial, language, or social skills. Marked motor impairment and associated deficits.

Profound Comprehension and use of language very limited; basic skills limited at best; organic aetiology clear in most cases; severe neurological and physical disabilities affecting mobility common; associated problems (atypical autism, pervasive developmental disorders, epilepsy, visual and hearing impairment) more common.

DSM-IV additional features:
- Onset before age 18.
- Deficits/impairments in present adaptive functioning in at least 2 areas from:
  - Communication
  - Self-care
  - Home living

- Social/interpersonal skills
- Use of community resources
- Self-direction
- Functional academic skills
- Work
- Leisure
- Health
- Safety

'Subcultural' LD

Although the concept of 'psychosocial' causation (due to physical and emotional neglect) is controversial, it is true to say that mild or borderline intellectual impairment is more common in families of lower socio-economic status. This is best viewed as a cultural norm, and individuals generally have no, or only minor, impairments in adaptive functioning (i.e. lack of disability or handicap—see p. 688). Generally the intellectual ability of family members is also in the borderline range, dysmorphic characteristics are less likely, and other impairments or disabilities are unusual. This is in contrast to biological causation where impairments are more significant, there is no difference in socio-economic status, parents and sibling are usually of normal intelligence, and dysmorphic features are more common.

Impairments, disabilities, and handicaps

It is often confusing when terminology is used interchangeably. This is especially true for learning disability or mental retardation when they are inaccurately used as diagnostic terms. In fact, they both describe a constellation of impairments with associated disability and handicap, the aetiology of which may be known (e.g. Down's syndrome) or unknown (e.g. childhood disintegrative disorder). The WHO[1] has proposed a system of classification which helps define needs and direct interventions/treatments, without making specific aetiological assumptions:

Impairment
- Any loss or abnormality of psychological, physiological, or anatomical structure or function.
  - A deviation from some norm in an individual's biomedical status.
  - Characterised by losses or abnormalities that may be temporary or permanent.
  - Includes the existence or occurrence of an anomaly, defect, or loss in a limb, organ, tissue, or other structure of the body, or a defect in a functional system or mechanism of the body, including the systems of mental functioning.
  - Is not contingent upon aetiology.

Disability
- Any restriction or lack (resulting from impairment) of ability to perform an activity in the manner or within the range considered normal for a human being.
  - Concerned with compound or integrated activities expected of the person or of the body as a whole (e.g. tasks, skills, and behaviours).
  - Includes excesses or deficiencies of customarily expected activities and behaviour, which may be temporary or permanent, reversible or irreversible, and progressive or regressive.
  - The process through which a functional limitation expresses itself as a reality in everyday life.

Handicap
- A disadvantage for a given individual, resulting from impairment or disability that limits or prevents the fulfilment of a role that is normal for that individual.
  - Places value on this departure from a structural, functional, or performance norm by the individual or his/her peers in their cultural context.
  - Is relative to other people and represents discordance between the individual's performance or status and the expectations of their social/cultural group.

- A social phenomenon, representing the social and environmental consequences for the individual stemming from his/her impairment or disability.

1 World Health Organisation (1980) International classification of impairments, disabilities, and handicaps (10th revision). *World Health Organisation*, Geneva.

The process of assessment—a structured approach

When a person with LD presents to services because of a particular problem (e.g. 'challenging behaviour', see pp. 716–7), the task for the clinician is to determine the underlying *cause*, which will include predisposing, precipitating, and perpetuating factors. Causation may in fact be multifactorial, and because of this a structured approach is best. Some aspects of assessment may be well documented (e.g. the aetiology of the LD), particularly when the patient is an adult. Any 'diagnostic formulation' should always take note of previous assessments and highlight what further assessments may be helpful.

- **Intellectual impairment** Assessed using standardised tests (e.g. Wechsler scales).
- **Severity of LD** ICD-10 or DSM-IV criteria (see p. 686).
- **Disabilities** Assessments of functioning (e.g. Vineland Adaptive Behaviour Scales, American Adaptive behaviour Scales, Hampshire Assessment for Living with Others (HALO)).
- **Handicap** Assessment of quality of life and life experiences (e.g. Life Experiences Checklist).
- **Aetiology of LD** See **Assessing causation p. 694**.

Other aspects of assessment will include:

- **Full physical examination** As this may identify undiagnosed problems, which the patient may be unable to communicate.
- **Mental state examination** See **Psychiatric comorbidity in the LD population p. 714**, which may go unrecognised and untreated. This includes temperament, usual behaviour patterns, current medication.
- **Communication difficulties** Which may include formal speech and language assessment.
- **Environmental and social factors** Which may be contributing to the problem.

Current support network

Assessment will involve not only talking to the patient, but also gathering information from previous documentation (including current treatments / previous diagnoses), family/carers, other support services, and teachers. The aim is to view the current problem in the light of past experiences, known problems, and current situational factors. A longitudinal approach is advised (i.e. does the current presentation reflect a recurrent problem, is it part of progressive functional decline, or does it represent a new, unidentified problem/unmet need?). It is useful to document the current supports received by the patient, and any important contacts for future reference.

Needs' assessment

Should it be the case that the persons' needs have changed, then there may be a statutory responsibility to undertake a formal 'needs' assessment', taking into account the wishes of the person (if they have capacity to make the kinds of decisions required) and others involved in care provision. This includes social care, educational, and health care needs.

Aetiology

A specific cause for LD can be identified in about 80% of severe and 50% of mild cases. About 50–70% of cases will be due to a prenatal factor, 10–20% perinatal, and 5–10% postnatal. The identification of aetiological factors is important because it allows for discussion of the risk of recurrence in future pregnancies. A known cause can allow for discussion of likely disabilities, possible cognitive impairments, and prognosis. This can be useful for planning supports/services, access to education, and optimising environmental factors (see **Needs and priorities, p. 690**).

Modern classifications of aetiological factors are based on timing of the event:

Genetic causes

- Autosomal chromosome disorders (e.g. Down's syndrome, pp. 700–1)
- Sex chromosome disorders (see p. 702)
- Deletions and duplications (see pp. 704–5)
- Autosomal dominant (p. 706) and recessive (pp. 706–7) conditions
- X-linked recessive (p. 708) and dominant (p. 709) conditions
- Presumed polygenic conditions (e.g. neural tube defects, pervasive developmental disorders)
- Mitochondrial disorders, maternally inherited (e.g. MERRF myoclonic epilepsy with ragged red fibres).

CNS malformations of unknown aetiology About 60% of all CNS malformations do not have a known genetic or exogenous cause. The types of malformation seen indicate the timing of the causative event, but not its nature (see opposite).

External prenatal factors (see **Non-genetic causes of LD, p. 710**) Particularly in the early stages (during blastogenesis or organogenesis). Infection; exposure to medication, alcohol, drugs, and toxins; maternal illness (diabetes, hypothyroidism, hypertension, malnutrition), and gestational disorders.

Perinatal factors Occurring around the time of delivery. Neonatal septicaemia; pneumonia; meningitis/encephalitis; other congenital infections; problems at delivery (asphyxia, intracranial haemorrhage, birth injury); other newborn complications (respiratory distress, hyperbilirubinaemia, hypoglycaemia).

Postnatal factors Occurring in the first years of life. CNS infections, vascular accidents, tumours; causes of hypoxic brain injury (e.g. submersion); head injury (e.g. RTAs, child abuse); exposure to toxic agents; psychosocial environment (i.e. deprivation).

Other disorders of unknown aetiology (see p. 711) e.g. cerebral palsies, epilepsy, autistic spectrum disorders, childhood disintegrative disorders.

Types of malformation and the timing of the causative event

Timing (in gestation)	CNS event	Malformation
3–7 weeks	Dorsal induction	Anencephaly, encephalocele, meningomyelocele, other neural tube closure defects
5–6 weeks	Ventral induction	Prosencephalies and other faciotelencephalic defects
2–4 months	Neuronal proliferation	Microcephaly or macrocephaly
3–5 months	Neuronal migration	Gyrus anomalies and heterotopias
6 months	Neuronal	Myelination
(to 1st year of life)	organisation	Disturbed connectivity (dendrite/ synapse formation)
		Disturbed proliferation of oligodendrocytes and myelin sheets

Assessment of causation

This requires comprehensive history taking from the parents (examination of prenatal records), and a careful physical examination of the child.

Factors in the history

- **Family history** Parents: ages; consanguinity; medical history; any previous pregnancies (including abortions, stillbirths). Wider family: any history of LD; specific cognitive impairments; congenital abnormalities; neurological or psychiatric disorders.
- **Gestational history** General health and nutrition; maternal infections; exposure to medication, drug and alcohol use, toxins, radiation; chronic medical conditions; history of pre-eclampsia, abnormal intrauterine growth, or foetal movements.
- **Birth of child** Gestational age; multiple pregnancy (birth order); duration of labour; mode of delivery; any complications; any placental abnormalities. Examination of birth records (Apgar scores, weight, length, head circumference).
- **Neonatal history** Need for special care (respiratory distress, infections, hypoglycaemia, hyperbilirubinaemia), baby checks (physical examination, Guthrie test).
- **Childhood history** Weight gain, growth pattern, feeding pattern, sleeping pattern, early developmental milestones. History of childhood illnesses (esp. CNS infections or seizures, metabolic/endocrine disorders) and accidents. General systemic enquiry.

Physical examination

- Look for evidence of any dysmorphic features and note whether these are seen in close relatives, (e.g. skin—pigmentation, dermatoglyphics; facial features; musculoskeletal abnormalities).
- Full physical examination of all systems including neurological examination for localising signs.
- If suggested by the history/examination, ophthalmological and audiological examinations should be arranged.

Investigations

- Standard routine tests will include FBC, U&Es, LFTs, TFTs, glucose, infection screening (blood and urine), and serology (ToRCH—toxoplasmosis, rubella, cytomegalovirus, herpes simplex virus; HIV).
- Where dysmorphic features are evident, or physical signs indicate, arrange X-rays of skull, vertebrae, chest, abdomen, hands, feet, and long bones; cardiac/abdominal ultrasound.
- If metabolic disorder is suspected (e.g. progressive course) arrange screening tests of blood and urine.
- If genetic disorder suspected arrange for karyotyping (G-banding, high resolution banding, fluorescence *in situ* hybridization—FISH) or other more specific genetic tests (e.g. FraX DNA testing).
- Other more detailed investigations may include neurophysiological tests (EEG, evoked potentials), neuroimaging (cranial ultrasound, CT/MRI, functional imaging), (neuro)pathological examination (fibroblast culture; biopsies—muscle, skin, rectum).

Overview of management approaches (1)—considerations and choices

Cautionary notes

- Attributing 'treatment success' to a particular intervention may miss the 'real' reason for improvement e.g. return of familiar carer, more structured environment (if admitted to specialist centre), or treatment effects on 'undiagnosed' primary condition (e. g. anticonvulsant used for aggressive behaviour may actually be treating underlying epilepsy).
- Many conditions may run *relapsing-remitting* courses, leading to erroneous conclusions about effectiveness of an intervention, which only become clear when symptoms return *despite* treatment.
- Improvement (or worsening) of symptoms may reflect *normal* maturational processes or, conversely, further pathological degeneration.
- Because of the wide variation in aetiology (genetic, environmental, psychological, social) and the complexity (and variable degree) of cognitive impairments, most trials of treatment are by nature empirical. Most management plans will inevitably be *individually* tailored and the current 'evidence base' for many treatment modalities is limited.
- Issues of *consent to treatment* should be seriously considered in a population who may have varying degrees of *capacity* (see Ethics and the law section, pp. 820–3).

A therapeutic environment

Provision of care and support should always be within an appropriate setting. Support may be: **general** (care provided by usual carers, schools, community teams) and/or **specific** (addressing particular needs e.g. special education, parental support groups, physical or psychiatric problems, maladaptive behaviours). Although, in general, every effort will be made to sustain a 'normal' environment (i.e. remaining at home, integration into 'mainstream' schools, use of local community resources), often more specialised environments are necessary (see below).

Factors influencing management choices

- The nature of the problem (i.e. biological, psychological, social).
- The degree and aetiology of the LD.
- Comorbid physical conditions (which may restrict choice of medication).
- Situational factors (i.e. practicalities of instituting various treatment options, supports, ability to monitor progress).

Admission to specialist environments

Sometimes disabilities or problems may be too severe or too complex to manage with standard community resources:

- The degree of LD or the specific cognitive impairments require well-structured, predictable environments that cannot be provided elsewhere.
- The degree of physical impairment requires more intensive specialist nursing, or a safer environment where medical care is close at hand (e.g. severe treatment-resistant epilepsy).

- The severity of behavioural problems prohibits management at home (e.g. abnormally aggressive or disinhibited behaviour which constitutes a serious risk of harm to themselves or others).
- The person requires treatment for a comorbid psychiatric disorder, which has failed to respond to initial treatment.

Other reasons may include:

- Respite placements to allow individuals and their families some relief from the intensity of long-term care.
- Assessment of complex problems—to disentangle environmental from illness factors, or where treatment requires close monitoring.
- 'Crisis' admissions due to an acute breakdown of usual supports.

Overview of management approaches (2)—treatment methods

Behavioural treatments

May be used to help teach basic skills (e.g. feeding, dressing, toileting), establish normal behaviour patterns (e.g. sleep), or more complex skills (e.g. social skills, relaxation techniques, assertiveness training). Behavioural techniques may also be used to alter maladaptive patterns of behaviour (e.g. inappropriate sexual behaviour, phobias).

Cognitive therapies and CBT

For borderline, mild, or moderate LD, cognitive approaches may be adapted to the level of intellectual impairment. These may be effective in the teaching of problem-solving skills, the management of anxiety disorders and depression, dealing with issues of self-esteem, anger management, and treatment of offending behaviours (e.g. sex offenders).

Psychodynamic therapies

May be helpful in addressing issues of emotional development, relationships, adjustment to life events (e.g. losses, disabilities, and bereavement). The range of approaches varies from basic supportive psychotherapy, to more complex group and family therapies.

Pharmacological treatments

Cautions

- Comorbid physical disorders (e.g. epilepsy, constipation, cerebral palsy) increase the need to closely monitor adverse effects.
- Atypical responses such as increased (or reduced) sensitivity, and 'paradoxical' reactions are more common, hence low doses and gradual increases in medication are advisable.
- The evidence base for many drug treatments is lacking and many claims for efficacy are at best based on small, open, uncontrolled trials.

Antipsychotics

For the treatment of comorbid psychiatric disorders (e.g. schizophrenia and related psychosis) and acute behavioural disturbance. May also be effective in managing autistic spectrum disorders, self-injury, social withdrawal, ADHD, and tic disorders.

Antidepressants

Effective for the treatment of depression, OCD, and other anxiety disorders. They have also been used in the management of violence, self-injury, 'non-specific' distress, and other compulsive behaviours.

Anticonvulsants

There is some evidence for the use of anticonvulsants in the treatment of episodic dyscontrol (e.g. carbamazepine), but this may be due to better control of underlying epilepsy.

Lithium
Aside from the treatment of bipolar affective disorder and augmentation of antidepressant therapy, lithium may have some utility in reducing aggressive outbursts.

β-Blockers
May be useful in conditions of heightened autonomic arousal (e.g. anxiety disorders) which may be at the root of aggressive behavioural disturbance.

Stimulants (e.g. methylphenidate)
For the treatment of ADHD (see pp. 576–8).

Opiate antagonists (e.g. naltrexone)
May be effective in the treatment of repetitive self-injury.

Anti-libidinal drugs (e.g. cyproterone acetate and medroxyprogesterone, which reduce testosterone levels) Used in the treatment of sexual offending (see p. 467).

Down's syndrome[1]

Down's syndrome is the most common genetic cause of LD. It is due to trisomy of chromosome 21. Its main features are LD and associated characteristic facies and habitus. Although Down's syndrome is diagnosed at birth, LD only becomes evident at the end of the first year of life, with subsequent delayed developmental milestones. The IQ in adults is most often below 50 (range: low to high/moderate LD). Those who survive into their 40s and 50s show pathological brain changes similar to Alzheime's disease (AD).

Aetiology Risk factors for giving birth to a child with Down's syndrome: being aged over 40yrs; having a previous child with the syndrome; and Down's syndrome in the mother (although pregnancy is rare). Incidence per 1000 living births is approx. 0.5 for a woman under 25, 0.7 under the age of 30, 5 under 35, 25 under 40, and 34.6 over the age of 45. Despite this, most children with Down's syndrome (70–80%) are born to mothers under the age of 35 (due to the higher number of pregnancies in younger women).

Genetics Full **trisomy 21** (non-disjunction) in ~95% of cases. **Robertson translocations** in ~5% (of which ~45% show fusion—usually 14 and 21, also 13/15/22 and 21 described). **Mosaicism** (a mixture of normal and trisomic cell lines) ~2–5%: IQ can be in the 70s and physical features may be less marked.

Clinical features

- **General** Short stature (mean 1.4–1.5m), overweight (~30%), muscular hypotonia.
- **Head and neck** Brachycephaly and reduced AP diameter, maxilla reduced more than mandible, underdeveloped bridge of nose, eyes close together, Brushfield's spots—grey or very light yellow spots of the iris, epicanthic fold, low-set ears, high-arched palate, protruding tongue, instability of atlanto-axial joint, narrowed hypopharynx (may lead to sleep apnoea).
- **Congenital heart defects** (~50%) e.g. ASD, VSD, mitral valve disease, patent ductus arteriosus.
- **Congenital GI abnormalities** Oesophageal atresia, Hirschprung disease, umbilical and inguinal hernia.
- **Hands** Short broad hands with a single palmar crease (simian crease), syndactyly (webbed fingers), clinodactyly (incurving of fingers), and altered dermatoglyphics.
- **Eye defects** Strabismus ~20%, myopia ~30%, blocked tear ducts, nystagmus, late-life cataracts, keratoconus.
- **Hearing defects** Structural anomalies may lead to recurrent otitis media, sensorineural deafness.
- **Immunological abnormalities** Raised IgG and IgM, lowered T-lymphocytes.
- **Endocrine abnormalities** Thyroid dysfunction (hypothyroidism ~20%), diabetes.
- **CNS abnormalities** Reduced brain weight ~10–20%, reduced gyri, cortical thinning, underdeveloped middle lobe of cerebellum, reduced

neuronal numbers in cerebellum/locus coeruleus/basal forebrain, reduced cholinergic neurones, neuropathological changes similar to AD (in those over 40yrs), epilepsy (5–10%).

Sexual development

- **Males**: normal course; delayed puberty; problems with spermatogenesis (unless mosaic).
- **Females**: normal onset of menstruation; fertile, but problems with ovulation and follicular growth; early menopause.

Psychiatric comorbidity Associated with ~18% of children and ~30% of adults with Down's syndrome (usually depression ~10%; less commonly bipolar affective disorder, OCD, Tourette's disorder, schizophrenia, increased risk of autism).

1 James Langdon Down remarked in his original observations on 'mongolism' (1866) that he was surprised it had not been described earlier. In fact, the first description of this syndrome was made in 1838 by Esquirol (1772–1840), with similar observations reported by Séguin (1812–1880) in 1844. The typical phenotype has also been noted in paintings dating from the Middle Ages. In 1959 the chromosomal abnormality leading to Down's syndrome was found by the French human geneticist Jérôme Lejeune (1926–1994). In doing so, Lejeune became the first researcher to elucidate the genetic mechanism of an inherited disorder.

Sex chromosome disorders

Turner's syndrome Sex chromosome monosomy; karyotype 45, XO (i.e. phenotypically female); LD rare.

Trisomy X Sex chromosome trisomy; karyotype 47, XXX; 1:1000 female births. **Clinical features** Slight increase in height, ~70% have learning disorder (usually mild), some evidence of reduced fertility (children have normal karyotypes), possibly increased incidence of schizophrenia.

Klinefelter's syndrome Sex chromosome trisomy; karyotype 47, XXY; 1:1000 male births (50% due to paternal and 50% maternal nondysjunction). **Clinical features** Variable degree of development of secondary sexual characteristics with hypogonadism, scant facial hair (90%), gynaecomastia (50%). Taller than average (~4cm), asthenic body build, median IQ ~90 with skewed distribution—most in 60–70 range, uncertain association with psychiatric disorders.

XYY male Sex chromosome trisomy; karyotype 47, XYY; 1:1000 male births. **Clinical features** Controversial suggestion of higher incidence in prison populations, IQ may be slightly lower than average, behavioural problems commonly seen.

Deletions and duplications

α-Thalassaemia mental retardation Small deletion; karyotype 16pter-p13.3 (cryptic terminal deletion). **Clinical features** LD.

Angelman ('Happy puppet') syndrome Microdeletion (60–75% of cases); karyotype 15q11-q13; 1:20 000–30 000; a contiguous gene syndrome (the complement of PWS) with 80% due to deletion of maternally derived chromosome 15, 2% uniparental disomy (UPD)—i.e. inheritance of 2 genes from the same parent (paternal), the remainder due to direct mutations. **Clinical features** Ataxia (jerky limb movements, gait problems); epilepsy (86%); paroxysms of laughter; absence of speech; facial features (blond hair, blue eyes, microcephaly, flattened occiput, long face, prominent jaw, wide mouth, widely-spaced teeth, thin upper lip, mid-facial hypoplasia); severe/profound LD; other behaviours (hand flapping, tongue thrusting, mouth movements); other problems (URTIs, ear infections, obesity).

Crit du chat Partial monosomy; karyotype 5p- (varies from deletion of a small band at 5p15.2 to the entire arm of 5p); usually sporadic, occasionally inherited; 1:20 000–50 000. **Clinical features** 'Cat-like' cry (possibly due to abnormal laryngeal development), microcephaly, rounded face, hypertelorism, micrognathia, dental malocclusion, epicanthic folds, low-set ears, hypotonia, severe/profound LD. Puberty occurs normally and some may survive to adulthood.

Di George (Velo-cardio-facial) syndrome Microdeletion; karyotype 22q11.2; incidence 1:5000.**Clinical features** ~50% have LD (mild: 2/3; moderate: 1/3), cardiac abnormalities (75%: Fallot tetralogy, VSD, interrupted aortic arch, pulmonary atresia, truncus arteriosis), facial features (microcephaly, cleft palate/submucous cleft, small mouth, long face, prominent tubular nose, hypoplasia of adenoids—nasal speech, bulbous nasal tip, narrow palpebral fissure, minor ear abnormalities, small optic discs/tortuous retinal vessel/cataracts), hypocalcaemia (60%—seizures, short stature, hearing problems, renal problems, inguinal/umbilical hernia), hypospadias (10% of males), long, thin hands (hypotonia and hyperextensible fingers), associated behavioural and psychiatric disorders (including schizophrenia, blunted/inappropriate affect).

Miller-Dieker syndrome Microdeletion; karyotype 17p13.3. **Clinical features** Lissencephaly, profound LD.

Prader-Willi syndrome (PWS) Microdeletion; karyotype 15q11-q13; 1:10 000–1:20 000; the complement of Angelman syndrome; 75% deletion of paternally derived chromosome 15, 25% UPD (maternal). M:F = 4:3. **Clinical features** *Neonates* Hypotonia, sleepiness, unresponsiveness, narrow bifrontal diameter, triangular mouth (feeding difficulties and swallowing problems), strabismus, acromicria (shortness of extremities). *Childhood/adolescence* Short stature, hypogenitalism (cryptorchidism, micropenis; amenorrhoea), behavioural disorders (over-eating and obesity, self-injurious behaviour), mild-moderate LD, speech abnormalities, sleep disorders. **Associated features** Small hands and feet, cleft palate, almond-shaped eyes, strabismus, incurved feet, clubfoot, congenital hip dislocation (abnormalities of the knee and ankle), scoliosis. **Other physical**

problems Diabetes, GI problems (obstruction, duodenal ulcer, rectal prolapse, gall stones), heart disease, respiratory (asthma, cor pulmonale), renal calculi, hearing deficits, hypothermia.

Rubenstein-Taybi syndrome Microdeletion of the gene encoding human cAMP-regulated enhancer binding protein; karyotype 16p13.3; incidence 1:125 000. **Clinical features** LD and dysgenesis of the corpus callosum. **Other features:** broad thumbs and great toes; persistence of foetal finger pads; facial features (short upper lip, pouting lower lip, maxillary hypoplasia, beaked nose, slanted palpebral fissure, long eyelashes, ptosis, epicanthic fold, strabismus, glaucoma, iris coloboma); cardiac problems (pulmonary stenosis and hypertension, mitral vale regurgitation, patent ductus arteriosus); propensity to keloid formation; genitourinary features (hypoplastic kidneys, cryptorchidism, shawl scrotum); GI problems (constipation, megacolon); collapsible larynx (leading to sleep apnoea); epilepsy (25%); behavioural problems (sleep problems, stereotypies e.g. rocking, self-injurious behaviour).

Smith-Magenis syndrome Rare—incidence 1:50 000; deletion in 17p11.2. **Clinical features** Moderate LD; facial features (brachycephaly, broad face, flattened mid-face, strabismus); myopia; short broad hands; upper limb deformity; insensitivity to pain. **Behavioural problems** 'Self-hugging' posturing, aggression, self-injury, hyperactivity, severe sleep problems, other autistic features.

Williams syndrome Small deletion; karyotype 7q11.23 (possibly gene for elastin or protein kinase—LIMKI); 1:55 000 live births; may also be related to excessive maternal vitamin D intake. **Clinical features** Hypercalcaemia (in ~50%) with supravalvular aortic stenosis and unusual facies. *Neonates* May be irritable, have feeding problems and failure to thrive. *Childhood* Growth retardation, 'elfin' facial features, hoarse voice, premature wrinkling and sagging of the skin, cardiovascular anomalies (e.g. supravalvular aortic stenosis), urinary tract abnormalities (asymmetrical kidneys, nephrocalcinosis, bladder diverticuli, urethral stenosis), pulmonary artery stenosis, mild to moderate LD (verbal often better than visuospatial and motor abilities). Often there is abnormal attachment behaviour (manifest as anxiety, poor peer relationships, hypersensitivity, or conversely as social disinhibition, excessive friendliness).

Wolf-Hirschhorn syndrome Partial monosomy; karyotype 4p-. **Clinical features** Severe LD; many survive to adulthood.

Autosomal dominant conditions

This group of disorders is also termed the **phakomatoses**—a variety of conditions with neurocutaneous signs.

Neurofibromatosis Caused by a number of genetic conditions, 1:40 000; variable association with LD.

Von Hippel-Lindau syndrome A rare genetic condition associated with angiomatous tumours in various areas of the body and LD.

Sturge-Weber syndrome Not inherited, but associated with 'port wine stains', angiomas of the meninges in the temporal and occipital areas, with LD, epilepsy, and hemiparesis.

Tuberous sclerosis (TSC) Occuring in 1:7000–10 000; M = F. **Clinical features** Varying degree (usually severe) of LD (50%), seizures (e.g. 'Salaam attacks' and other types, in 90%), hamartomas of the CNS (including the retina) as well as ependymomas and astrocytomas, facial angiofibroma, adenoma sebaceum, depigmented skin patches ('ash leaf spots' in 96%), shagreen patches, depigmented naevi, subcutaneous nodules, 'café-au-lait' spots, fibromas of the nails, pitted tooth enamel, hypoplasia, and occasionally tumours of the heart (rhabdomyeloma, hamartoma), kidney problems (Wilm's tumour, renal cysts), olfactory hamartomas, hypertension, and aortic aneurysm. **Subtypes** *TSC1*: 1:12 000; associated with a gene (for hamartin—believed to be tumour-suppressant) near the ABO blood group locus on chromosome 9 (9q34—40% of cases). *TSC2*: associated with a gene for tuberin (a guanosine triphosphatase-activating protein also believed to be tumour-suppressant) on chromosome 16 (16p13.3-); more psychiatric and behavioural problems. *TSC 3*: a rare translocation of a gene on chromosome 12.

Autosomal recessive conditions

These conditions include some of the lysosomal storage diseases e.g. mucopolysaccharide storage—Hurler syndrome, Sanfillipo disease (see below), sphingolipid storage*—Tay-Sachs disease, Niemann-Pick disease (sphingomyelins), glucoprotein storage—sialidosis; phenylketonuria; and rare disorders such as Laurence-Moon syndrome and Joubert syndrome (see below).

Phenylketonuria A *preventable* cause of severe LD, due to deficiency of phenylalanine hydroxylase (long arm of chromosome 12), leading to phenylalaninaemia and phenylketonuria; prevalence 1:15 000; diagnosed postnatally ('Guthrie test'). **Clinical features** Fair hair/skin and blue eyes (lack of pigment—tyrosine deficiency), neurological signs (stooped posture, broad-based gait, increased tone and reflexes, tremor, stereotypes movements). **Behavioural problems** Hyperactivity, temper tantrums, perseveration, echolalia. **Management** Supervised early dietary restriction of phenylalanine. **Prognosis** Even with dietary treatment, lower than average IQ.

Sanfillipo disease Due to disorders of the breakdown of heparan sulphate, of which there are 4 subtypes (types A–D). Prevalence 1:25 000–325 000. **Clinical features** Severe LD, claw hand, dwarfism, hypertrichosis, hearing loss, hepatosplenomegaly, biconvex lumbar vertebrae, joint stiffness. **Behavioural problems** Restlessness, sleep problems, challenging behaviour. **Aetiology** *Type A* (most severe, most common) mapped to 17q25.3 (heparan sulphate sulphatase).*Type B* 17q21 (N-acetyl-α-D-glucosaminidase).*Type C* on chromosome 14 or 21 (acetyl-CoA-α-glucosaminide-N-acetyltransferase). *Type D* 12q14 (N-acetyl-α-D-glucosamine-6-sulphatase). **Prognosis** Poor, many die between 10–20yrs of respiratory tract infections.

Hurler syndrome Due to deficiency in A-L-iduronidase (4p16.3); incidence 1:76 000–144 000. **Clinical features** Progressive LD (eventually severe/profound), skeletal abnormalities (short stature, kyphosis, flexion deformities, claw hand, long head, characteristic facial appearance), hearing loss, respiratory and cardiac problems, hepatosplenomegaly, umbilical/inguinal hernia. **Prognosis** Poor, some survive to 20s; may benefit from allogenic bone transplantation.

Laurence-Moon syndrome Associated with multiple loci (11q13, 11q21, 15q22, 3p13); prevalence 1:125 000–160 000 (higher in Bedouins of Kuwait and Newfoundland). Also known as **Laurence-Moon-Biedl syndrome** (incorporating Bardet-Biedl syndrome which shares clinical features, but additionally there is central obesity and polydactyly). **Clinical features** Mild-moderate LD, short stature, spastic para-paresis, hypogenitalism (most males are infertile), night blindness (due to red cone dystrophy), NIDDM, renal problems (diabetes insipidus, renal failure).

Joubert syndrome Exceptionally rare, no loci identified, but recessively inherited. **Clinical features** Severe LD, characteristic hyperpnoea ('panting like a dog'), cerebellar dysgenesis, hypotonia, ataxia, tongue protrusion, facial spasm, abnormal eye movements, cystic kidneys, syndactyly/polydactyly. **Behavioural problems** Self-injury. **Prognosis** Poor—no specific treatments.

X-linked recessive conditions

These include other **lysosomal storage diseases** e.g. mucopolysaccharide storage—**Hunter syndrome** (see below); trihexosylceramide storage—**Fabry disease** and other extremely rare conditions such as **Lesch-Nyhan syndrome** and **oculocerebrorenal syndrome of Lowe**.

Hunter syndrome Caused by iduronate sulphatase deficiency (mapped to Xq27-28); incidence 1:132 000–280 000 (more common in male Ashkenazi Jews: 1:34 000). Only 20% have complete depletion of iduronate sulphatase and two subtypes are recognised: **Type A** Progressive LD and physical disability, with death before age 15yrs. **Type B** Milder form, with minimal intellectual impairment and better prognosis. **Clinical features** Dyostosis (dwarfism, grotesque facies 'gargoylism', degenerative hip disease, joint stiffness, claw hand, pes cavus, cervical cord depression), eye defects (retinitis pigmentosa, papilloedema, hypertrichosis), umbilical/inguinal hernia.

Lesch-Nyhan syndrome An extremely rare X-linked recessive condition, due to a mutation in HPRT gene (hypoxanthinephosphoribosyl transferase) on the short arm of chromosome Xq26-27, with a nearly total loss of the enzyme leading to hyperuricaemia. Prognosis is poor and most affected individuals die in early adulthood. **Clinical features** Children appear healthy at birth, dystonias become apparent around 3–4 mths with delayed developmental milestones, later there is development of spasticity, choreoform movements and transient hemiparesis (which may be misdiagnosed as cerebral palsy), variable degree of LD (usually severe), microcephaly is common, ~50% develop epilepsy. **Behavioural problems** Around age 2 yrs (sometimes not until adolescence) self-mutilating behaviours may be seen (biting of lips, inside of mouth, fingers). Sometimes there is an episodic pattern, and some may show a reduction in frequency and severity after age 10yrs. May be associated with verbal and physical aggression. There is no clear cause for this behaviour—CNS findings include reduction in dopamine in the basal ganglia and at synaptic terminals (but not in the cell bodies of the substantia nigra), with other monoaminergic systems apparently intact. **Management** Even treating hyperuricaemia does not appear to reduce behavioural problems; however there is some evidence for use of SSRIs.

Oculocerebrorenal syndrome of Lowe Very rare X-linked recessive condition (Xq24-26); incidence 1:200 000. **Clinical features** Moderate-severe LD (up to 25% have normal IQ), short stature, hypotonia, epilepsy (~30%), eye problems (e.g. congenital cataracts), renal problems (tubular dysfunction). **Behavioural problems** Temper tantrums, hand-waving movements, self-injury (~70%—esp. in early adolescence).

X-linked dominant conditions

Fragile X syndrome

The most common inherited cause of LD, affecting ~1:4000 males and 1:8000 females, with X-linked dominant transmission. Penetrance is low, but greater in males than females (due to the 'protective' effects of the second normal X chromosome in females). Gene sequence has been cloned[1] and designated FMR-1. The syndrome is associated with a large sequence of triplet repeats $(CGG)_n$ at a fragile site on the X chromosome (Xq27.3). In affected males 'n' > 230–1000+, in transmitting males and obligate females n = 43–200, and in the general population n = 6–54 (mean 30).

Clinical features Variable, subtle, and often cannot be detected before adulthood. May include: large testicles and ears, smooth skin, hyperextensible fingers, flat feet, mitral valve prolapse, inguinal and hiatus hernia, facial features (long, narrow face with underdevelopment of the mid-face, macrocephaly), epilepsy (~25%), variable LD (borderline to profound), behavioural features appear to be similar to those seen in ADHD and autism: hand flapping / waving, repetitive mannerisms, shyness, gaze avoidance, poor peer relationships, communication difficulties (e.g. delayed language development, conversational rigidity, perseveration, echolalia, palilalia, cluttering and overdetailed/circumstantial speech), psychiatric problems (e.g. mood and personality disorders). NB General domestic and daily living skills may be excellent. *Brain imaging:* reduced posterior cerebellar vermis, enlarged hippocampus and caudate nuclei, enlarged ventricles.

Other disorders with 'fragile' sites

Two other fragile sites have been found on the X chromosome. The original 'fragile X' site has hence been designated 'FRAX A'. FRAX E, caused by FMR-2 mutation is also associated with mild LD, with an incidence of 1:100 000, and 200–1000 triplet repeats. FRAX F has not (yet) been associated with any disorder. Another fragile site has been located on chromosome 16 (FRA 16) associated with a large GCC triplet expansion—but no specific clinical disorder.

Aicardi syndrome

Rare (only 200 reported cases—all female); dysgenesis of the corpus callosum and cerebrum, with severe LD; prognosis poor (often death in infancy).

Clinical features Microcephaly, facial asymmetry, low-set ears, eye lesions (chorioretinal lacunae), hypotonia, scoliosis, epilepsy.

Behavioural problems 25%—aggression, lack of communication, tiredness/sleep problems, self-injurious behaviour.

---

1 Verkerk AJ, Pieretti M, Sutcliffe JS, et al (1991) Identification of a gene (FMR-1) containing a CGG repeat coincident with a breakpoint cluster region exhibiting length variation in fragile X syndrome.*Cell* **65**, 905–14.

Non-genetic causes of LD

Congenital hypothyroidism

A treatable cause of mental and growth retardation due to loss of thyroid function; incidence 1:3500–4000, but now screened for neonatally and treated early with thyroxine. If untreated, leads to typical clinical picture of lethargy, difficulty feeding, constipation, macroglossia, and umbilical hernia.

Foetal alcohol syndrome (FAS)

One of the major causes of LD, incidence 0.2–3 per 1000 live births. 10–20% of cases of mild LD may be caused by maternal alcohol use. Important factors include: level of drinking, bingeing, other drug use (including smoking), genetic variation, and low socio-economic status. May be due to the effects of alcohol on NMDA receptors, which may alter cell proliferation.

Clinical features *Perinatal problems* Signs of alcohol withdrawal (irritability, hypotonia, tremors, seizures); *Facial features* Microcephaly, small eye fissures, epicanthic folds, short palpebral fissure, small maxillae and mandibles, underdeveloped philtrum, cleft palate, thin upper lip; *Growth deficits* Small overall length, joint deformities; *CNS features* High incidence of mild LD, associated behavioural problems (hyperactivity, sleep problems), optic nerve hypoplasia (poor visual acuity), hearing loss, receptive and expressive language deficits; *Other physical abnormalities* ASD, VSD, renal hypoplasia, bladder diverticuli.

Other toxins

e.g. cocaine, lead, bilirubin, coumarin anticoagulants, phenytoin.

Infective agents

ToRCH, syphilis (treponema pallidum), HIV, and other causes of meningitis and encephalitis.

Hypoxic damage

Secondary to placental insufficiency, pre-eclampsia, birth trauma, severe prematurity, 'small for dates' babies (foetal growth retardation), or multiple pregnancy.

CNS and skull developmental abnormalities

Micro-and macrocephalies, spina bifida, hydrocephalus, craniostenosis, callosal agenesis, lissencephalies, holoprosencephalies.

Disorders of unknown aetiology

This includes a broad range of disorders associated with LD, but for which a clear aetiology is as yet undetermined e.g. **cerebral palsies, epilepsy, autistic spectrum disorders** (see pp. 584–5), **childhood disintegrative disorders** (see below), and other clearly defined syndromes with a suspected (but not yet proven) genetic basis (e.g. **Cornelia de Lange syndrome**—see below).

Rett syndrome

Exclusively affecting girls, incidence 1:10 000–15 000.

Clinical features Normal development up to 18–24mths, followed by development of abnormal involuntary movements (hand flapping and hand wringing), often with autistic features (may be misdiagnosed). By age 5yrs up to 72% have epilepsy, and general progression is to spasticity of the limbs, plateauing for a short time (associated with improved social skills), before further motor deterioration with marked spasticity, rigidity, muscle wasting, contractures, and deformities. *Behavioural problems* Low mood, anxiety (with marked distress—often situation-specific), self-injury (40–50%), sleep problems (often involving laughing).

Aetiology Unknown, may be associated with MECP2 gene at Xq28.

Prognosis Characteristic progression to severe disability with moderate to severe LD.

Disintegrative disorder

Clinical features Characterised by normal development until the age of ~4yrs, followed by profound regression with disintegration of behaviour, loss of acquired language and other skills, impaired social relationships, and stereotypies.

Aetiology Unknown, but may follow minor illness or viral encephalitis (e.g. measles).

Prognosis Poor, with development of severe LD.

Cornelia de Lange syndrome (Brachmann-de Lange syndrome)

Usually IQ is below 60 (range 30–86), prevalence 1:50 000–100 000, mode of inheritance unknown (possibly autosomal dominant).

Clinical features Hypertrichosis (hirsuitism, synophyrs, long eyelashes), facial features (depressed nasal bridge, eye abnormalities, prominent philtrum, thin lips, down-turned mouth, anteverted nostrils, bluish tinge around eyes/nose/mouth, widely-spaced teeth, high-arched palate, low-set ears, micrognathia, short neck), limb deformities (esp. upper limbs), cryptorchidism/hypoplastic genitals (males), small umbilicus, low-pitched cry, small nipples. Associated with GI problems, congenital heart defects, visual and hearing problems, skin problems, epilepsy, and death in infancy.

Behavioural problems Expressive language deficits, feeding difficulties, sleep disturbance, self-injury, temper tantrums, mood disorders, and autistic features.

Epilepsy and LD

Epilepsy represents a particular diagnostic challenge when it occurs in people with LD. It may begin at any age, presentations may change over time, and multiple forms may occur in the same individual. The prevalence of epilepsy is ~40% in the hospitalised LD population and is higher in severe (30–50%) than mild (15–20%) LD

Common pitfalls

- Epilepsy may be misdiagnosed in patients with LD, particularly when there is a history of sudden unexplained aggression, self-mutilation, and other 'bizarre' behaviours, including abnormal or stereotyped movements, fixed staring, rapid eye blinking, exaggerated startle reflex, attention deficits, or unexplained intermittent lethargy. (If antiepileptic medication has been previously prescribed for these kinds of presentations, consider careful withdrawal with close monitoring.)
- Non-epileptic (pseudo) seizure disorder can also occur in patients with epilepsy.
- Epilepsy-related behaviours may also be confused for psychiatric problems e.g. hallucinations in simple (somatosensory) partial seizures; psychosis-like episodes during complex partial seizures (esp. temporal or frontal lobe); or post-ictal confusion.

Diagnosis

- **History and examination** May be difficult to obtain accurate information, often relying on third-party information (home video may be useful). Try to exclude other differential diagnoses (e.g. infection, trauma, hypoglycaemia, hyperventilation, withdrawal from drugs or alcohol, over-sedation, localising signs of intracranial pathology, evidence of movement disorders). Also conduct a MSE, focusing on observed behaviours, identification of any stressors (esp. if anxiety-provoking).
- **Investigations** Baseline laboratory tests—FBC, U&Es, LFTs, glucose. Consider EEG and CT/MRI (in complex cases video-EEG monitoring may be very useful), PET or SPECT (to detect areas of hypometabolism).

Co-occurrence

- Epilepsy is commonly associated with numerous causes of LD e.g. Down's syndrome (5–10%), fragile X (25%), Angelman syndrome (90%), Rett syndrome (90%). This may be due to shared aetiologies such as alterations in neuronal development and function, or co-associated brain lesions (haemorrhage, ischaemia, neoplasm, vascular malformation).
- Frequent epileptic seizures may lead to (or worsen) permanent loss of intellectual functioning (e.g. 'acquired epileptic aphasia'/Landau-Kleffner syndrome, progressive partial epilepsies such as epilepsia partialis Kozhevnikov or Rasmussen syndrome type 2) emphasising the need for early diagnosis and treatment to prevent often fatal progression.

Epilepsy syndromes in infancy and childhood

Infancy *Early infantile epileptic encephalopathy* due to congenital or acquired abnormal cortical development; early myoclonic epileptic encephalopathy possibly due to metabolic disorders; infantile spasms/West syndrome[1] due to intrauterine infections (toxoplasmosis, CMV, rubella), Down's syndrome, tuberous sclerosis, progressive degenerative disorders, or intracranial tumours; severe myoclonic epilepsy.

Childhood A variety of other myoclonic epilepsy syndromes are recognised: Lennox-Gastaut syndrome, myoclonic-astatic epilepsy (Doose syndrome), progressive myoclonus epilepsies (Baltic or Lafora disease), Northern epilepsy.

Treatment

NB *This is essentially the remit of the neurologist, not the psychiatrist— liaison with other specialists is vital.*
Choice of treatment will depend upon a number of factors:

- Accurate classification of the type of seizures / epilepsy syndrome
- Possible drug interactions
- Minimising side-effects (esp. cognitive impairment)

Points to note:

- Behavioural problems may be associated with antiepileptic drugs, and may be more common in patients with brain injury or LD (e.g. phenobarbitone, primidone, benzodiazepines, vgabatrin).
- Communication difficulties may make assessment of side-effects more difficult.
- For intractable epilepsy, neurosurgery may be an option, but is not without significant ethical considerations.

Prognosis

There is wide variation in outcome; however up to 70% of patients with LD can achieve good control of their epilepsy without major side-effects.

1 West syndrome is the triad of infantile spasms, mental retardation, and hypsarrhythmia (characteristic EEG finding of chaotic intermixed high-voltage slow waves and diffuse asynchronous spikes).

Psychiatric comorbidity in the LD population

Although originally thought to be mutually exclusive, it is now clear that psychiatric disorders do occur more frequently in the LD population than the general population. Confusion of primary and secondary handicap may lead to underdiagnosis. The lack of longitudinal studies makes any prediction of outcome speculative at best.

Schizophrenia

Clinical features Age of onset tends to be earlier (mean 23yrs), with few differences in symptomatology, except in severe LD where there may be unexplained aggression, bizarre behaviours, mood lability, or increased mannerisms and stereotypies.

Aetiology Genetic factors are important (associated with FHx). Co-association suggests possible contiguous gene deletions, or one underlying genetic condition presenting with multiple clinical presentations.

Bipolar affective disorder

Prevalence is estimated to be greater than the general population (2–12%), with difficulty in making the diagnosis in severe LD. Symptom 'equivalents' may include: hyperactivity, wandering, mutism, temper tantrums.

Depressive disorder

Clinical features Biological features tend to be more marked, with diurnal variations. Suicidal thoughts and acts may occur in borderline-moderate LD, but are less frequent in severe LD (need to exclude other ritualistic self-injurious behaviours). Other causes of mood disturbance (e.g. perimenstrual disorders) should also be considered.

Other disorders

Anxiety disorders May be difficult to distinguish from depression, except where there are situational features.

OCD Reported to be more prevalent in LD. Differential diagnosis: ritualistic behaviours, tic disorders, behavioural manifestations of autism/Asperger disorder.

ADHD Often a prominent feature in children with LD (up to 20%). Stimulants may help in mild LD with clear symptoms, but has no clear efficacy in severe-profound LD.

Personality disorder Difficult to define, but prevalence is estimated in ~20% of mild-moderate LD patients who are inpatients.

Behavioural disorders and 'challenging' behaviour

Behavioural disorders are over-represented in LD populations, ranging from minor antisocial behaviours to seriously aggressive outbursts. Prevalence estimates are 7% of the LD population: 14% for inpatients (esp. 25–29yr-olds), and 5% for those in the community (esp. 15–19yr-olds).

Studies of behavioural disorders in the LD population identify 6 relatively consistent groupings of the types of pathological behaviours[1] which may create a significant burden for parents/carers:

- Aggression-antisocial
  - *Antisocial behaviours* Shouting, screaming, general noisiness; anal poking/faecal smearing (may reflect constipation); self-induced vomiting/choking; stealing.
  - *Aggressive outbursts* Against persons or property.
  - *Severe physical violence* Rare.
  - *Self-injurious behaviour* Skin picking, eye gouging, head banging, face beating (more common in severe/profound LD; prevalence 10% overall, 1–2% most sever.)
- Social withdrawal
- Stereotypic behaviours (some of which may be *self-injurious*)
- Hyperactive disruptive behaviours
- Repetitive communication disturbance
- Anxiety fearfulness

When these behaviours are particularly severe, they are often termed **'challenging'** (see opposite).

Associated factors

Assessment of behavioural problems should cover a number of interrelated domains:

- **Cognitive functioning** Severity of intellectual impairment, language ability, memory (visual/verbal), performance of specific tasks (e.g. complex motor tasks), social comprehension.
- **Temperament** Particularly high emotionality, high activity, poor sociability.
- **Physical problems** e.g. epilepsy, cerebral palsy, cardiac problems, GI problems, visual/hearing impairment.
- **Medication** Particularly psychotropic drugs may produce or mask cognitive, behavioural, or emotional problems. Sometimes a 'drug holiday' may be helpful to assess how medication contributes to the presentation.
- **Psychological factors** *Primary reinforcers* e.g. food, drink, pain (often undetected). *Secondary reinforcers* e.g. praise, environment, aversive stimuli.
- **Communication difficulties** Frustration of normal forms of communication.
- **Adverse experiences** Common to the general population, and also particular to the LD population e.g. experience of institutions, social rejection, neglect, and emotional, physical, or sexual abuse.

- **Environmental factors** Living conditions, stability and continuity of day-to-day activities (NB Most common precipitants: multiple short-term residential placements; multiple changes in care staff.) The quality of the care environment may be directly responsible for behavioural problems and assessment should include factors such as: social relationships, specific environmental stressors, consistency of care, and lack of stimulation.
- **Comorbidity** Psychiatric disorders may complicate the presentation of behavioural problems e.g. *ADHD* (see p. 576); *conduct disorder/ oppositional defiant disorder* (see p. 581); *tic disorders* (see p. 602); *anxiety disorders* (see pp. 344–57)—fears/phobias, separation anxiety (see p. 590), PTSD (see p. 368), OCD (see p. 538); *depressive disorder* (see pp. 246–51); *bipolar disorder* (see pp. 304–11); *pervasive developmental disorders* (see p. 582). Identification and appropriate treatment may significantly improve behavioural problems.
- '**Behavioural phenotypes**' (see below).

Criteria for clinically significant 'challenging behaviour'

- At some time the behaviour has caused more than minor injuries to themselves or others, or destroyed their immediate living or working environment.
- At least weekly behaviours requiring intervention by staff; placed them in physical danger; caused damage that could not be rectified; caused at least 1hr of disruption.
- Behaviour has caused over a few minutes' disruption at least daily.

Qureshi H (1994) The size of the problem.
In: Emerson E, McGill P, Mansell J (Eds)
Severe mental retardation and challenging behaviours: designing high quality services
Chapman and Hall, London.

'Behavioural phenotypes'

Many genetic causes of LD are associated with characteristic patterns of behaviour. Recognising these 'behavioural repertoires' may help in diagnosis and management, and forms the basis for ongoing research into the genetic basis of some behavioural problems. Examples include: **Down's syndrome** (oppositional, conduct, and ADHD); **fragile X syndrome** (autism, ADHD, stereotypies e.g. hand flapping); **Lesch-Nyhan syndrome** (self-mutilation); **Prader-Willi syndrome** (OCD, multiple impulsive behaviour disorder e.g. hyperphagia, aggression, skin picking); **Smith-Magenis syndrome** (severe ADHD, stereotypies—'self-hugging', severe self-injurious behaviours, insomnia); **Williams syndrome** ('pseudomature' language ability in some; initially affectionate and engaging; later anxious, hyperactive, and uncooperative).

1 Einfeld SL, Aman M (1995) Issues in the taxonomy of psychopathology in mental retardation. *J Autism Dev Disord.* **25**, 143–67.

Behavioural disorders—assessment and principles of management

At all stages in assessment and management, it will be essential to involve parents, carers, and other allied professionals (e.g. teachers) both as sources of information and in implementing any proposed interventions.

Assessment

- Exclusion of psychiatric disorder.
- Exclusion of physical disorder (and assessment of general state of health).
- Assessment of physical impairments (vision, hearing, etc.)
- Assessment of communication difficulties (including formal speech and language assessment).
- Assessment of specific cognitive impairments (including formal psychological testing).
- Identification of environmental and social factors.
- Use of behavioural diaries (by carers/staff) 'ABC's—: antecedents, behaviours, consequences.

Management

Following assessment, *specific* factors should be addressed—psychiatric/physical causes, reduction of stimuli/reinforcers, modification/removal of environmental factors, social issues.

Approaches may involve:

- **Educational interventions** Both for families/carers (to improve understanding) and for patients (to ensure educational needs are being appropriately met in a suitable setting).
- **Social interventions** To address unmet needs at home, with family/carers, or widen access to other services or facilities (to provide opportunities for social interaction and improve support networks).
- **Facilitating communication of needs** Addressing impairments of hearing, vision, and language (including use of pictures, sign language, electronic speech devices).
- **Behavioural interventions** Modification of behaviour using operant conditioning (e.g. removal of aversive stimuli, rewarding 'good' behaviour, use of appropriate attention—'neutral' response to attention-seeking behaviours), secondary reinforcers, modelling, 'positive programming'.
- **Cognitive approaches** At an appropriate level for degree of cognitive impairment and language abilities—may range from counselling on specific issues to simple imitation of relaxation/breathing techniques.
- **Pharmacotherapy** Including specific comorbid conditions (e.g. ADHD—stimulants; OCD—SSRIs; antidepressant treatment; tic disorders—antipsychotics; epilepsy—anticonvulsants). Sometimes a trial of antipsychotic treatment may be useful for serious aggression, hyperactivity, or stereotypies (often depot; caution in epilepsy; increased risk of EPSEs). Other options for aggression, agitation, or self-injurious behaviours (mainly empirical evidence): anticonvulsants, lithium, β-blockers, buspirone. For self-injurious behaviours alone there is some evidence for opiate antagonists (e.g. naltrexone).

- **Physical interventions** (i.e. restraint): from splints and headgear to isolation (to protect individual and others from injury/damage to property).

Any intervention should be closely monitored to ensure compliance, acceptability, and therapeutic response. In the case of medication, side-effects should be minimised and if treatment is deemed ineffective drugs should be carefully withdrawn (to avoid secondary problems).

Critical periods of changing needs

Adolescence

This may be a difficult transitional period; issues that may require attention include:

- **Engaging with adult services** Loss of the additional support provided by supported mainstream, or special schools, may lead to problems if there is not a smooth transition to adult services. Where appropriate (or available) this may include moving to *social educational/ day centres*. Some countries have specific legislation to ensure that needs are identified early (e.g. 'transitional planning' from the age of 14 under the UK Education Act 1993).

- **Social/economic independence**
  - *Employment* Depending on the level of disability, this may be in *sheltered employment, workshops*, or *supported open employment*. Despite changing attitudes, there are considerable barriers to finding work in the open job market, although for some this may be worth pursuing.
  - *Living arrangements* Loss of additional social supports may actually increase the burden of care shouldered by the family. For some, the wish for independence or the lack of family support may be best met with *small group homes* where support may be tailored to individual needs.

- **Health and mental health needs**

- **Sexual relationships** Societal views may find it difficult to accept the fact that people with LD have 'normal sexual desires', which can be more of a problem for families/carers than the individuals themselves. Nonetheless, issues raised by appropriate sexual relationships will include consideration of contraception, understanding of the responsibilities of parenthood, issues of commitment and marriage. Many people, particularly with mild LD, are capable of being successful parents and provide a stable environment for children with appropriate support.

Later adulthood

- **Changing health needs** With increasing age, health needs may be unrecognised or there may be failure to access services. Despite issues of capacity and consent to medical treatment, everyone has a right to high standards of medical care, and this ought not to be neglected.

- **Changing mental health needs** These may relate to changing symptomatology over time, altered tolerance of medication, and additional specific age-related cognitive impairment (e.g. due to chronic intractable epilepsy, early onset Alzheimer's disease in Down's syndrome).

- **Ageing carers** The ability of carers to continue to provide the same level of care for their children ought to be considered *before* a crisis is reached. This requires an ongoing assessment of supports. Increasing reliance on carers may also lead to social isolation, and it is prudent to raise the issue of planning for the future at an early stage. Issues of bereavement may complicate support arrangements due to the consequent life changes (e.g. may need to move out of the family home and entail learning to be with new carers and people who will have problems of their own). There may be cultural differences in preferences and expectations, and these should be sympathetically addressed.

Family issues

Having a child with LD is a major, unexpected blow to any family. Individual responses vary, but the majority of parents do adapt well to the situation and show remarkable resilience and resourcefulness. Depression is quite common in parents and should not be overlooked. Important positive factors include: having a good relationship with their partner and the support of relatives and friends. Needs and priorities will vary over time and should be identified early and addressed collaboratively with the involvement of parents and other carers in any key decisions (see opposite).

Early impact

Prenatal diagnostic screening can place parents in the unexpected position of having to make difficult choices even *before* the birth of their child. Advice and counselling are a necessary and important part of the screening process, and should not be ignored even when testing is regarded as 'routine'. The mistaken assumption that screening 'guarantees' a healthy child may lead to even greater feelings of disappointment and anger, magnified further by anxious times after the birth, with a baby in a special care unit. Although some conditions can be diagnosed at birth, often parents only realise there is a problem when their child fails to reach developmental milestones, or develops seizures after an apparently 'normal' infancy. Often the response is one of bereavement (see p. 366) or guilt, and parents may need support to 'work through' their feelings.

The importance of diagnosis

Clear diagnosis is essential and may greatly relieve the anxieties of many parents who may blame themselves for their child's problems. It may allow access to specific supports including parent groups and education regarding what the future may hold (i.e. usual course, associated problems, prognosis). For inherited conditions, the issue of further genetic counselling/testing of family members needs to be addressed. Provision of clear information allows individuals to make informed decisions about being tested and to weigh the risks of having other affected children.

The effect on other family members

Although it was previously thought that having a child with LD impacted adversely on other unaffected siblings (often leading to the removal of the child from the family), there is little evidence that this is the case and worries about long-term damage appear unfounded. In fact, brothers and sisters of individuals with LD appear to be drawn to the caring professions and many end up working as doctors, nurses, teachers, or providing support for children with special needs. Grandparents may be a useful supportive resource for parents, but may also need to come to terms with their own feelings of having a disabled grandchild.

The 'burden of care'

For carers, informal support may actually be more valuable than formal (professional) support. Frequent appointments or regular home visits may be more disruptive than helpful. Developmental delay brings with it associated problems (e.g. longer time until the child can walk, achieve continence, acquire language/communication skills, establish a normal sleep pattern). The social, financial, and psychological impact on carers should be acknowledged and appropriate help and support provided. For infants and children, schooling may be both a benefit (in terms of learning social skills, support/respite for parents, and close contact with teachers/other parents) and a burden (particularly if necessary specialist schooling is not locally available). Transitional periods (e.g. adolescence/ early adulthood) are accompanied by parental anxieties as well as changes in how needs are met (see **Critical periods of changing needs**, pp. 720–1). Advance planning will go some way to alleviate increased carer stress. Carers may also be concerned about what will happen to their child when they are no longer able to care for them and the open discussion of these issues, with provisional planning, may help avert crises (see also **Ageing carers**, p. 720).

Needs and priorities

- Early, accurate diagnosis.
- Informative genetic advice to parents and other family members.
- Access to high-quality primary (and secondary) health care.
- Advice and access to appropriate help and support (practical help, financial assistance, social and educational needs).
- Help and advice with any communication problems (communication aids, learning of sign language).
- Consideration of the needs of carers (education, support groups, respite care).
- Provision of specialist and domiciliary help with specific behavioural problems.
- 'Safety net' of open access to increased support when necessary.
- Acknowledgement that needs will change over time (and planning for this—see pp. 720–1).

Liaison psychiatry

Introduction

Liaison psychiatry is concerned with the diagnosis and management of psychiatric and psychological illness in general medical populations. It is unique among the psychiatric sub-specialties in that it concerns itself not with a particular subset of disorders, or treatment of patients of a particular age range, but patients within a particular clinical setting. The development of a distinct sub-specialty of liaison psychiatry is in some ways a result of the separation of psychiatric specialists from their medical and surgical colleagues and practices. There are after all no liaison surgeons; general surgeons merely attend general medical wards as required and give advice to the treating team or take over the patient's care.

The sub-speciality is a relatively recent innovation and dates in its current form since the 1960s. Motivations to its development were the low rate of outside referral in proportion to prevalence of the disorders in the population under review and increasing medical specialisation leading to lack of confidence and competence with psychiatric/psychological problems. The role of the liaison psychiatrist will be defined, more than the other sub-specialties, by custom and practice in the hospital concerned.

The main workload will in general include:
- Diagnosis of new psychiatric illness in general patients.
- Management of pre-existing psychiatric illness in general patients.
- Somatic presentation of psychiatric illness.
- Psychiatric and emotional complications of physical illness.
- Management of medically unexplained or functional illnesses.
- Management of behavioural disturbance.
- Assessment following attempted suicide and deliberate self-harm.
- Assessment of alcohol and drug abuse.
- Problems related to childbirth and the puerperium.
- Issues related to capacity and legal powers.

The sub-specialty referred to as liaison psychiatry in the UK is, in most of the rest of the world, referred to as 'consultation-liaison psychiatry'. This longer name better describes the two related approaches of practitioners in this field. The *consultation* aspect of the job covers episodic referrals made for advice on diagnosis, prognosis, need for further investigations, or management. It may include patients where the request is to consider taking over care. The *liaison* aspect refers to a closer relationship with a unit, with involvement in unit planning, staff support, policy development, and training as well as involvement in individual clinical cases. The balance between the liaison and consultation aspects of the job will depend on the specialty concerned, and the hospital type.

Presentations of psychiatric illness on the general wards

While working in liaison psychiatry you can expect to see a wide variety of disorders and presentations. Many of these will not be unique to the general setting, and their management is described in other sections of this book. Some common referrals are:

- Adjustment disorder p. 364
- Depressive illness pp. 246–51
- Patients presenting after parasuicide pp. 730–3
- Alcohol problems pp. 504–33
- Drug problems pp. 534–60
- Acute confusional state p. 734
- Psychiatric aspects of organic conditions pp. 130–1
- Medically unexplained symptoms pp. 736–9
- Behavioural disturbance pp. 896–7
- Assessment of dementia pp. 132–3
- Post-partum illnesses p. 756
- Illnesses specific to women pp. 434–7
- Questions regarding capacity p. 822
- Issues of consent to/refusal of treatment pp. 820–3

Working in the general hospital

Liaison psychiatry is unusual in that you will work as a psychiatrist based in a general hospital. This can bring its own difficulties and challenges as well as rewards. Firstly you will be operating 'on enemy territory' to some extent. General hospital doctors in the various specialties will have their own ideas about psychiatry, as well as about the indicated treatment in each case (which may differ from yours). Nonetheless it is well to remember that you have a range of skills and knowledge that will be useful and are not shared by other members of staff. You should rely on these and your own judgement, backed up by senior colleagues, in difficult situations.

When you come to working in a general hospital you may feel initially overwhelmed. There are many new disorders, altered presentations of familiar disorders, a new tempo of working, and patients suffering medical conditions about which you may know very little. Liaison psychiatry takes a variety of types of referral and they will vary by the type of hospital, the population served, and the specialty mix within the hospital. The person receiving the referral should take details of the patient, their GP, their treating team, and the nature of the problem, including its urgency. It is helpful to clarify what questions the treating team want addressed. It is also important to clarify that the patient understands that psychiatric referral has been made and agrees to this.

Where the situation is not an emergency, it can be useful to review any psychiatric or departmental records for previous contacts, prior to assessing the patient. A discussion with the GP may also be helpful. On arrival on the ward, review the medical record of this and previous admissions and speak to a senior member of the treating team. Clarify the patient's diagnosis and any investigations or treatments planned. Discuss the patient with the nursing staff—they may have useful information regarding the patients symptoms around the clock and their mood day to day. Arrange a private room for the interview if at all possible.

Introduce yourself to the patient as a psychiatrist or psychological medicine specialist. Explain your role, which may be misunderstood by the patient, who my feel you are there to 'see if I'm crazy'. Stating that the medical team are concerned about some of the patient's symptoms and they want a specialist in these symptoms to give them some advice is often an acceptable phrasing for patients. If a definitive psychiatric diagnosis is possible, write this clearly in the notes, along with a provisional management plan and any treatment recommendations. Clarify in the notes if further psychiatric review is planned and when, and which symptoms should cause them to seek an earlier review. If at all possible, discuss your findings with the medical team face to face.

Parasuicide assessment

Parasuicide is a deliberately undertaken act which mimics the act of suicide but does not result in death. Psychiatric assessment of such patients is mandatory once their medical condition allows. The involvement of mental health professionals in the assessment of patients following para-suicide relates to the following observations:

- In this population of patients, roughly 1% will die by completed suicide in the 24 months after the initial parasuicidal act, with the risk highest in the weeks following the original act. This represents a mortality by suicide 50–100 times that of the general population.
- The rates of completed suicide are significantly raised in all mental disorders excepting mental handicap and dementia. Studies examining completed suicides in patients with mental illness show inadequate doses of therapeutic drug treatment, increased drop-out rate from follow-up, and increased presence of untreated comorbidity.
- Clear risk factors exist for completed suicide (see below) and the closer the parasuicidal patient approximates to these demographics, the greater the relative risk. However, the absolute risk is low and estimate of the risk in a particular case relies on assessment of the individual act and the mental state.

Assessment The initial management of the patient following overdose or other deliberate self harm will be by specialist toxicologists or general medical/surgical specialists. Early psychiatric assessment may be required for advice regarding detainablity, behavioural disturbance, drug/alcohol withdrawal, or delirium, but assessment of the parasuicide itself should be deferred until conscious level is full. The history should focus on the act itself, the patient's mental state and recent life events, and past medical/psychiatric history. It may be easier to assess these in reverse order moving from the factual history towards the emotive descriptions of the parasuicidal act itself after building rapport.

Features of act

- **Method** ~90% of parasuicides are by self-poisoning with self-cutting making up most of the remainder. Use of method likely to be fatal (e.g. jumping, hanging) is indicative of clear intent to die.
- **Patient's belief in the lethality of the method** Did the patient *believe* that that combination of tablets was likely to be fatal? Serious suicidal intent is associated with medically trivial overdoses—and vice versa.
- **Length of planning** Was the act impulsive—'on the spur of the moment', or planned in advance—and for how long?
- **Triggers** Was there a clear precipitant (e.g. row with partner)? Were they intoxicated at the time? Was there any direct 'gain' (e.g. patient in custody at the time of act)?
- **Final acts** Was there a suicide note? Did they make any other 'acts of closure' (e.g. setting affairs in order, arranging for the care of children)?
- **Precautions to avoid discovery** Where did the act take place? Would they have anticipated being found? Did they signal or tell their intentions to another? Was anyone else actually present at the time?
- **Previous similar acts** Is this act a repeat of a previous non-fatal act? Are there any different features?

- **Actions after act** What did they do after the act? How did they end up coming to hospital?

Mental state

- **Attitude now to survival** Are they relieved or disappointed to be alive? Do they have ongoing wish to die? How do they feel about the future and what plans (if any) do they have?
- **Affective symptoms** Current affective symptoms. Recent symptoms of low mood, anhedonia, and hopelessness. Biological depressive features.
- **Substance misuse problems** Evidence for current drug or alcohol misuse or dependence.
- **Other mental disorder** Enquire directly about other symptoms of mental disorder as directed by the history.
- **Risk to others** Is there any evidence of intent to harm anyone else? Did the parasuicidal act put anyone else at risk?

Personal and past medical/psychiatric history

- **Recent life events** Describe recent loss or change of events (e.g. bereavements, job loss, relationship break-up).
- **Current life situation** State of current significant relationships. Type and security of job and accommodation. Presence of legal/criminal problems.
- **Previous or current psychiatric diagnoses** Clarify with hospital records if further details required or if significant history.
- **Physical health problems** Again clarify with records or GP if required.

Risk factors for completed suicide

- Socio-demographic factors
  - Male sex
  - Elderly
  - Single, divorced, or widowed
  - Living alone, poor social support
  - Unemployed or low socio-economic class
- Personal/mental health factors
  - Previous parasuicide or DSH
  - Any mental disorder (greatest risk in major depression and anorexia nervosa, then functional psychosis, then neurotic and personality disorders)
  - Dependence on alcohol or drugs
  - Recent inpatient psychiatric treatment
  - Concurrent physical disorder
  - Recent bereavement

Management after parasuicide

Reasons for act Only a minority of patients presenting after parasuicide have evidence of clear intent to die. Assessment will reveal a mixture of the following types of case:

- Those whose intent was unequivocally to die but were prevented by discovery, chance, or overestimation of the lethality of the method.
- Those who were ambivalent whether they lived or died, 'letting the chips fall as they may'.
- Those whose act was impulsive and 'in the heat of the moment' in response to an immediate stressor.
- Those whose actions were designed to communicate distress—the classical 'cry for help'.
- Those whose actions were manipulative in nature and designed to provoke changed behaviour from others.
- Those attempting to escape from intolerable symptoms or an intolerable situation.
- Those whose intent is later unclear even to themselves.

There may initially be diagnostic confusion with the following groups: 1) deliberate overdoses of drugs taken for intoxicating effect; 2) deliberate self-harm (e.g. wrist cutting) which is a repetitive, ritualistic action whose intent is to relieve tension, not to kill or seriously injure; 3) accidental overdoses of prescribed or OTC medication. 1 and 2 may merit psychiatric evaluation in their own right and 3 should be examined carefully for evidence of post hoc rationalisation of a parasuicide.

Assessment aims By the end of assessment you should aim to answer the following questions:

- **Is there ongoing suicidal intent?** Evidenced by: continuing stated wish to die; ambivalence about survival; sense of hopelessness towards future; clear intent to die at time of act.
- **Is there evidence of mental illness?** Diagnosed in the normal way. Most common diagnoses are depressive illness and alcohol misuse. Be alert to comorbid substance misuse and to the combination of an acute stressor on the background of a chronic condition.
- **Are there non-mental health issues which can be addressed?** Many patients will reveal stressors such as: family or relationship difficulties; emotional problems (particularly relating to previous abuse; school or employment problems; debt; legal problems; problems related to immigration). They can be usefully directed to appropriate local services.

Management

- **Ongoing suicidal intent** In many cases this will be managed by admission to a psychiatric ward, on a compulsory basis if necessary.
- **Mental illness**
  - *Patients already known* to mental health services Here close liaison with the usual team is required to agree a joint management plan.
  - *New diagnoses* Here the focus should be on integrating with an appropriate service for follow-up, rather than necessarily starting new treatments. The type of appropriate follow-up depends on the

type of disorder (e.g. GP review for moderate depressive illness, referral to alcohol services for alcohol abuse). Short-term community outreach from liaison psychiatry can 'bridge' the patient to the general services. Try to ensure follow-up is as soon as possible, even if non-urgent, as otherwise non-attendance is very high.

  • *Admission required* For both new and established mental illnesses, admission will sometimes be indicated after parasuicide even where there is no ongoing suicidal intent. This may be due to seriousness of condition (e.g. new psychotic illness) or to allow for a period of inpatient assessment of mental state. It should not simply be in order to defer or devolve the decision about discharge—ask yourself what will have changed to mean discharge in a few days will be safer than now.

• **Other issues** With the patient's permission discuss the case with an appropriate agency (e.g. abuse counselling service, school counsellor). Clarify the appropriateness of the referral and referral method and feed these back to the patient.

• **In all cases** Discuss and agree management plan with patient. In most cases discuss with GP (mandatory if GP input is required). Consider provision of emergency crisis card giving details of emergency psychiatric service and telephone contact for emergency counselling/support services.

Frequent attenders A small minority of patients attend emergency services repeatedly with parasuicidal acts or deliberate self harm without suicidal intent. A management plan for such patients should be agreed on a case-by-case basis. The aim should be to avoid 'rewarding' maladaptive behaviours, (e.g. by repeated admissions providing 'time-out' from stressful situations), while providing appropriate support and treatment.

Acute confusional state (delirium)

Essence A stereotyped response of the brain to a variety of insults, very commonly seen in hospital inpatients. It is a clinical syndrome of fluctuating global cognitive impairment associated with behavioural abnormalities. Like other acute organ failures it is more common in those with chronic impairment of that organ.

Epidemiology Extremely common in medical and surgical inpatients (10–20%). Particularly vulnerable include: elderly; pre-existing dementia; blind or deaf; very young; post-operative (especially cardiac); burn victims; alcoholic and benzodiazepine dependent; serious illness particularly multiple. Carries significant mortality as well as morbidity to patient and others and is a cause of delayed discharge.

Clinical features

- Impaired level of consciousness with reduced ability to direct, sustain, and shift attention.
- Global impairment of cognition with disorientation, and impairment of recent memory and abstract thinking.
- Disturbance in sleep/wake cycle with nocturnal worsening of symptoms.
- Psychomotor agitation and emotional lability.
- Perceptual distortions, illusions, and hallucinations—characteristically visual.
- Speech may be rambling, incoherent, and thought disordered.
- There may be poorly developed paranoid delusions.
- Onset of clinical features is rapid with fluctuations in severity over minutes and hours (even back to apparent normality).

Differential diagnosis Mood disorder; psychotic illness (new major mental disorder very much less likely than delirium in a hospitalised patient, particularly if elderly); post-ictal; dementia (characteristically has insidious onset with stable course and clear consciousness—clarify functional level prior to admission).

Aetiology The cause is frequently multi-factorial and the most likely cause varies with the clinical setting in which the patient presents.

- **Intracranial** CVA; head injury; encephalitis; primary or metastatic tumour; raised ICP.
- **Metabolic** Anaemia; electrolyte disturbance; hepatic encephalopathy; uraemia; cardiac failure; hypothermia.
- **Endocrine** Pituitary, thyroid, parathyroid or adrenal diseases; hypoglycaemia; diabetes mellitus; vitamin deficiencies (thiamine, B12, folate, nicotinic acid).
- **Infective** UTI; chest infection; wound abscess; cellulitis; SBE.
- **Substance intoxication or withdrawal** Alcohol; benzodiazepines; anticholinergics; psychotropics; lithium; antihypertensives; diuretics; anticonvulsants; digoxin; steroids; NSAIDs.
- **Hypoxia** Secondary to any cause.

Course and prognosis Delirium usually has a sudden onset, usually lasts less than 1 wk, and resolves quickly. There is often patchy amnesia for the period of delirium. Mortality is high (estimated to be up to 50% at 1 yr). May be a marker for the subsequent development of dementia.

Assessment
- Attend promptly (situation only tends to deteriorate and behaviorally disturbed patients cause considerable anxiety on medical wards).
- Review time-course of condition with nursing and medical staff and review notes—particularly medicine kardex and blood results.
- Establish pre-morbid functional level (e.g. from relatives or GP).

Management 4 main principles of management:
- Identify and treat precipitating cause.
- Provide environmental and supportive measures (below).
- Avoid sedation unless severely agitated or necessary to minimise risk to patient or to facilitate investigation/treatment.
- Regular clinical review and follow-up (MMSE useful in monitoring cognitive improvement at follow-up).

Environmental and supportive measures in delirium

- Education of all who interact with the patient (doctors, nurses, family, etc.).
- Reality orientation techniques. Firm clear communication—preferably by same staff member. Use of clocks and calendars.
- Create an environment that optimises stimulation (e.g. adequate lighting) reduce unnecessary noise; mobilise patient whenever possible.
- Correct sensory impairments (e.g. hearing aids; glasses).
- Optimise patient's condition—attention to hydration, nutrition, elimination, pain control.
- Make environment safe (remove objects with which patient could harm self or others).

Brown TM and Boyle MF (2002) Delirium. *BMJ* **325**, 644–7.

Sedation in delirium

- Use single medication.
- Start at low dose and titrate to effects.
- Give dose and reassess in 2–4 hours before prescribing regularly.
- Avoid PRN medication if possible.
- Review dose regularly and taper and stop ASAP.
- Consider:
  - Haloperidol 0.g–1mg up to max of 4mg daily
  - Lorazepam 0.5mg–1mg up to max of 4mg daily
  - Risperidone 1mg–4mg up to max of 6mg daily

Medically unexplained symptoms (1)—introduction

It is increasingly recognized that a substantial proportion of patients presenting to primary care, or to any hospital specialty will have symptoms for which, after adequate investigation, no cause can be found. Non-specific symptoms without underlying organic pathology are very common and usually transient. Where they become prolonged enough to merit medical attention they may present to any speciality, with presentations such as pain, loss/disturbance of function, and altered sensation.

Symptom 'meaning' The 'problem' of Medically Unexplained Symptoms (MUS) arises, in part, from the different meanings symptoms hold for patient and doctor. Patients present to doctors with illness (symptoms and behaviours); doctors diagnose and treat disease (pathology and other recognised syndromes). The patient wants explanation and treatment for their symptoms and the route to this is a generally through being given a diagnosis. If there is no recognised diagnosis available the doctor may respond with 'there's nothing wrong', expecting to be met with pleasure. The patient however is baffled—there *is* 'something wrong' and the symptoms are still there. The doctor may then undertake a number of courses of action: continue to investigate in the hope of finding something; treat the patient anyway as a therapeutic trial; refer to another specialty; or dismiss the patient.

Psychiatric role The role of psychiatry in the assessment and management of these patients has changed substantially over recent years (hopefully for the better). Formerly patients were referred 'at the end of the line', often after prolonged, inconclusive tests and unsuccessful interventions. Patients often misinterpreted (and resented) the referral as suggesting that symptoms were 'all in your mind', or were feigned. Psychiatrists sometimes took an overly narrow view of their role and responsibility, unhelpfully dismissing patients as having 'no psychotic or depressive illness', or colluding with patient's desire for a 'clean bill of mental health' in order to return to treatment seeking behaviour. We are currently at an early stage of our understanding of medically unexplained illnesses. While no specialty has 'all the answers' in the management of this patient group, psychiatry can offer: experience of the presentation of MUS across the hospital specialties; ability to assess and treat the frequently comorbid depressive/anxiety symptoms; and a tolerance for diagnostic uncertainty and ability to take a long-term view of improvements.

Misdiagnosis A frequently expressed concern doctors hold about this group of patients is the risk of 'getting it wrong', (often associated with poorly formed worries about litigation). A long-held belief was that, despite repeated negative findings, all such patients (or a majority), would eventually be found to suffer from an organic disease which would, in retrospect, account for their symptoms. This concern was largely based on older, poorly conducted studies with significant methodological flaws. Recent follow-up studies suggest that the misdiagnosis rate for functional illness is 5–10%, (e.g. comparable to other medical and psychiatric diagnoses such as idiopathic epilepsy and schizophrenia). This improvement has followed both the development of modern imaging and investigatory techniques, and the use of operational diagnostic criteria for psychiatric diagnosis.

Iatrogenic harm A problem common to all members of this group of disorders is the potential for iatrogenic harm. These patients often accrue considerable morbidity and even mortality due to excess negative investigations, irradiation, operative procedures, etc. Those disorders associated with chronic pain carry the risk of iatrogenic opiate dependency. Often at the later stages of the patient's illness this secondary morbidity is more problematic than the original symptoms. A major positive intervention in these patients is therefore the avoidance of iatrogenic harm.

Medically unexplained symptoms (2)—clinical presentations

Classification Patients presenting with somatic symptoms for which no adequate physical cause can be found make up a large and heterogeneous group in all clinical settings, from primary to tertiary care. Our lack of full understanding of this group of disorders is reflected in the confusing and disputed classification system adopted. Our modern concepts arose from the concept of 'hysteria'—of repressed emotions being expressed as physical symptoms. There are differences between ICD-10 and DSM-IV in the classification of this group of disorders and each classification contains a number of disputed and unsatisfactory categories. One difficulty has been the residual old labels still in use; another has been the confusion of names indicating symptom and disorder; a third has been the substantial overlap between the syndromes described.

Somatisation This is the experience of psychological distress as physical symptoms. Its distinction from other symptoms seen in functional illness is shown opposite. Somatisation is a symptom of various disorders commonly seen in liaison psychiatry and may occur: 1) as a normal accompaniment of physical illnesses; 2) as a common presentation of depressive illness; 3) as a core component of illness ('somatic syndromes'); 4) as part of a longstanding pattern of behaviour ('somatisation disorder').

1) As a normal accompaniment of physical illness

Complaint of symptoms and help-seeking behaviour is adaptive. All illnesses have emotional components which deserve attention. Both doctor and patient may be more comfortable dealing with specialty-appropriate symptoms (e.g. a patient presenting with pain post-radiotherapy may be articulating a desire for reassurance that the tumour has not reoccurred). While some doctors may be reluctant to deal with the emotional context of illness, patients may have worries and express these as somatic complaints. These should often be understood as part of the emotional reaction to illness, not dismissed as 'functional overlay'. Their appropriate treatment is via consultation with the responsible clinician. Psychological factors may (positively or negatively) influence outcome in treatment of physical illnesses by their effects on advice seeking, treatment compliance, and perceived quality of life.

2) As a common presentation of depressive illness

Somatic complaints are common presentations of affective illnesses, with this prevalence increased in certain sub-groups (e.g. elderly, children, certain immigrant populations). Conversely, anxiety and depressive symptoms are a common finding in both the physically ill and those with somatisation.

3) As a core component of the illness (the 'somatic syndromes')

These conditions are usually reported as individual clinical syndromes; however, several factors are common to them all. There is presentation by the patient with symptoms which are suggestive of an underlying organic illness; these symptoms cause distress; there is no identifiable organic illness which is sufficient to explain the symptoms; and the causation is attributed to psychological factors which may be more or less apparent. A variety of presentations are seen across the medical and surgical specialties:

GI medicine—irritable bowel syndrome
Gynaecology—chronic pelvic pain
Rheumatology—fibromyalgia
Cardiology—atypical chest pain
ENT—globus hystericus
Neurology—tension headache, pseudo-seizures

4) Part of a longstanding pattern of behaviour
Somatisation disorder (pp. 742–3).

Causative mechanisms Currently unclear, but the following may play a part: patient psychological factors; patient's health beliefs; affective state; underlying personality; degree of autonomic arousal; increased muscle tension; effects of hyperventilation; effects of disturbed sleep; effects of prolonged inactivity; impaired ability to filter afferent stimuli.

Functional symptoms

- *Somatisation:* the experience of bodily symptoms with no, or no sufficient psychical cause, with presumed psychological causation.
- *Hypochondriasis:* the belief that one has a particular illness despite evidence to the contrary—an overvalued idea.
- *Conversion:* the process by which thoughts or memories unacceptable to the conscious mind are repressed from conscious expression and 'converted' into physical symptoms, sometimes with symbolic meaning to the patient.
- *Dissociation:* the separation of unpleasant emotions and memories from consciousness with subsequent disruption to the normal integrated function of consciousness.
- *Dysmorphophobia:* the belief that one has a significant deformity—an overvalued idea.
- *Pain:* an unpleasant sensory or emotional experience associated with actual or potential tissue damage.
- *'Functional overlay':* symptoms 'over and above' those thought to be appropriate given the extent of the (undoubted) organic illness.

Medically unexplained symptoms (3)—management principles

Accepting cases for assessment Psychiatrists should be reluctant to accept patients for assessment of MUS where significant doubt still exists in the treating doctor's mind as to the diagnosis (e.g. where significant further investigations are planned). They should also be reluctant to be put in the position of 'last hurdle' before an otherwise planned intervention (e.g. 'I'll perform your operation if the psychiatrist gives the go-ahead').

Management principles Definitive treatments validated by RCT evidence are not currently available for MUS. In addition, these patients present a heterogenous group, in terms of presentation, 'psychological mindedness', and severity. Nonetheless the following principles may be helpful. Management should include: 1) thorough assessment; 2) confident diagnosis; 3) clear explanation; 4) minimisation of iatrogenic harm; 5) empirical use of potentially beneficial treatments; and 6) consideration of involvement in treatment trials.

Assessment

* Prior to the consultation, obtain the full hospital case records for all specialties. Discuss the case with the GP and obtain copies of GP records if available. Clarify whether the patient is seen in other hospitals or health care services and aim to obtain these records. Establish whether there are any pending investigations and what the patient has been told about their presumed diagnosis.
* At the interview: establish full details of current symptoms; circumstances of symptom onset; and 'life context' of symptom development.
* Explore their illness beliefs: specific worries about cause and possible prognosis; ask the patient to describe their understanding of their symptoms and what they feel they may represent.
* Full details of past medical history (may be reticent—'no problems before current symptoms' or overly dramatic); what were they told at the time by the doctors treating them?
* Remember to explore possible psychiatric differential diagnoses—full mental state as normal, even if no symptoms spontaneously mentioned.
* Observe patient in waiting room/onward/entering and leaving room—be alert to inconsistencies in symptoms.

Diagnosis

* *A positive and confident* diagnosis is crucial.
* Be willing to make organic and non-organic diagnosis (e.g. where there is undoubted organic disease but also significant MUS morbidity).
* Acknowledge the patient's distress and disability; a diagnosis of MUS should not mean to the patient that you believe that there is 'nothing wrong with them'.

Explanation

* Terminology in this field is variable, imprecise, and potentially offensive (e.g. supratentorial, hysterical). The terms 'functional illness' or 'medically unexplained illness' are generally acceptable to patients.

- Begin with a clear explanation summing up what is (and what is not) wrong: 'You are suffering from a functional, not structural, problem of your nervous system. This is a common problem which we have seen in many other patients.' Various analogies may be used as appropriate (e.g. computer hardware vs. software problem; piano working but out of tune).
- Emphasise what can and cannot be done: 'We can help train the body to function normally again', 'We might not be able to pinpoint the exact cause'.
- Allow the patient to query what you have said (you should have allowed sufficient time at the end of the interview). Allow carers/relatives to become involved in this exploration of your explanation.
- Copy your clinic letter to the GP and the hospital professionals caring for patient. Consider, in certain situations, copying the letter to patient.

Minimise iatrogenic harm

- In all MUS patients, be aware of the risk of iatrogenic harm and justify any risks taken by benefit to the patient, over and above the gratification of seeming to give the patient 'what they want'.
- Accept that there may be a chronic illness which can be managed but not 'cured'.
- Appropriately investigate *genuinely new* symptoms.
- In planning further investigations in patients with MUS, proportionately greater weight should be placed on objective rather than subjective change.
- Clear verbal, written (and in some cases, face to face) communication between all involved professionals is especially crucial in this group of patients: everyone should 'know what's going on'.
- Accept that there will be a proportion of severe cases who are unable to leave sick role and who must be managed by changing how the system responds to them.

Empirical use of potentially beneficial treatments

- Often there is improvement in patient perception of symptoms following confident diagnosis and explanation.
- All patients with prominent depressive/anxiety symptoms should have these treated in the normal way.
- Consider empirical trial of antidepressant medication even where affective features are not prominent.
- Consider use of physiotherapy to aid regaining of functional loss.
- Consider referral for assessment for formal psychotherapy.
- Consider referral to other resource (e.g. pain management).

Involvement in treatment trials

- Little is known about the course of these disorders over time and less about appropriate treatments: consider patients for involvement in research.

Somatisation disorder

A chronic disorder of multiple medically unexplained symptoms, affecting multiple organ systems presenting before the age of 40. It is associated with significant psychological distress, functional impairment, and repeated presentations to medical services. Full blown somatisation disorder or 'Briquet's syndrome' probably represents the severe end of a continuum of abnormal illness behaviour (pp. 6–7).

Clinical features Patients will have long, complex medical histories ('fat-file' patients), although at interview may minimise all but the most recent symptomatology. Symptoms may occur in any system and are to some extent suggestible. The most frequent symptoms are non-specific and atypical. There may be discrepancy between the subjective and objective findings (e.g. reports of intractable pain in a patient observed by nursing staff to be joking with relatives). Symptoms are usually concentrated in one system at a time but may move to another system after exhausting diagnostic possibilities in the previous. Life revolves around the illness as does family life.

Diagnosis is usually only suspected after negative findings begin to emerge as normal medical practice is to take complaints at face value. Key diagnostic feature is multiple, atypical, and inconsistent medically unexplained symptoms in a patient under the age of 40. There is excessive use of medical service and alternative therapies. Chronic cases will have had large numbers of diagnostic procedures and surgical or medical treatments. High risk of iatrogenic harm and iatrogenic substance dependence. Hostility and frustration can be felt on both sides of the doctor-patient relationship. There may be 'doctor-shopping' and 'splitting' of the attitudes of staff caring for them. Psychological approaches to treatment are hampered by on-going investigations of ever rarer diagnostic possibilities and by the attribution of symptoms to fictitious but 'named' medical entities.

Two-thirds of patients will meet criteria for another psychiatric disorder, most commonly major depressive or anxiety disorders. There is also association with personality disorder and substance abuse. They characteristically deny emotional symptoms or attribute them directly to physical handicaps—'the only reason I'm depressed is this constant pain'.

Aetiology Observable clinical association with childhood illnesses in the patient and a history of parental anxiety towards illness. Increased frequency of somatisation disorder in first degree relatives. Possible neuropsychiatric basis to the disorder with faulty assessment of normal somatic sensory input. Association with childhood sexual abuse.

Epidemiology Lifetime prevalence of ~0.2%. Markedly higher rate in particular populations. ♀:♂ ratio 5:1. Age of onset is childhood to early 30s.

Differential diagnosis *Undiagnosed physical disorder:* particularly those with variable, multi-system presentations (e.g. SLE, AIDS, porphyria, tuberculosis, multiple sclerosis). Onset of multiple symptoms for the first time in patients over 40 should be presumed to be due to unexposed physical disease. *Psychiatric disorder:* major affective and psychotic illnesses may initially present with predominately somatic complaints. Diagnosis is by examination of other psychopathology, however over half of somatisation disorder patients exhibit psychiatric comorbidity. *Other somatoform disorders*: distinguish from: hypochondriasis (presence of firm belief in particular disorder), somatoform pain disorder (pain rather than other symptoms is prominent), conversion disorder (functional neurological loss without multi-system complaints). In practice the main distinction is between the full and severe somatisation disorder and somatisation as a symptom of other disorders.

Assessment (see p. 740). Establish reasons for referral, experience of illness, attitudes to symptoms, personal and psychiatric history, family perspective.

Initial management (see general principles, pp. 740–1) Make, document, and communicate the diagnosis. Acknowledge symptom severity and experience of distress as real but emphasise negative investigations and lack of structural abnormality. Reassure patient of continuing care. Attempt to reframe symptoms as emotional. Assess for and treat psychiatric comorbidity as appropriate. Reduce and stop unnecessary drugs. Consider case conference involving GP and treating physicians.

On-going management

- Regular review by single, named doctor.
- Reviews should be at planned and agreed frequency, avoiding emergency consultations.
- Symptoms should be examined and explored with a view to their emotional 'meaning'.
- Avoid tests 'to rule out disease', investigate objective signs only.
- All secondary referrals made through one individual.
- Disseminate management plan.
- These patients can exhaust a doctor's resources—plan to share the burden over time.

Some evidence for the effectiveness of patient education in symptom re-attribution, brief contact psychotherapy, group therapy, or CBT if the patient can be engaged in this.

Prognosis Poor in the full disorder; tendency is for chronic morbidity with periods of relative remission. Treatment of psychiatric comorbidity and reduction of iatrogenic harm will reduce overall morbidity.

Somatoform pain disorder

In somatoform pain disorder (pain disorder in DSM-IV) there is a complaint of persistent severe and distressing pain which is not explained or not adequately explained by organic pathology. The causation of the symptom is attributed to psychological factors. This disorder is diagnosed where the disorder is not better explained by somatisation disorder, another psychiatric diagnosis, or 'functional overlay' of organic disease.

All pain is a subjective sensation and its severity and quality as experienced in an individual is dependant on a complex mix of factors including the situation, the degree of arousal, the affective state, the beliefs about the source, and meaning of the pain. The experience of pain is modified by its chronicity and associations and there is a 'two-way' relationship with affective state, with chronic pain predisposing to depressive illness, while depressive illness tends to worsen the subjective experience of pain.

Comorbidity In common with the other somatoform disorders there is substantial overlap with major depression (~40% in pain clinic patients) and anxiety disorders. Substance abuse (including iatrogenic opiate dependency) and personality disorder patients are over-represented.

Epidemiology No population data are available. The prevalence of patients with medically unexplained pain varies by clinical setting; higher in inpatient settings, particularly surgery, and highest in pain clinic patients.

Differential diagnosis Elaboration of organic pain, malingering, substance abuse, sickle cell crisis, angina.

Assessment History from patient and informants, length of history (may be minimised), relationship to life events, general somatisation, experience of illness, family attitude to illness, periods of employment, treatments, beliefs about cause, comorbid psychiatric symptoms. CSA.

Management (see general principles, pp. 740–1). It is important to recognise and treat occult comorbid depression. It is often helpful to adopt an atheoretical approach: 'let's see what works', and to resist pressure for 'all or nothing' cure or a move to investigation by another speciality. Opiates not generally effective in chronic pain of this type and add the risk of dependence. *Psychological treatments*: these are directed towards enabling the patient to manage and 'live with' the pain, rather than aspiring to eliminate it completely; can include relaxation training, biofeedback, hypnosis, group work, CBT. *Pain clinics*: these are generally anaesthetist-led with variable psychiatric provision. They offer a range of physical treatments such as: antidepressants, TENS, anti-convulsants, and local or regional nerve-blocks.

Conversion (dissociative) disorders

A loss or disturbance of normal function which initially appears to have a physical cause but is attributed to a psychological cause. The disturbance conforms to the patient's conception of pathological processes. These disorders were initially explained by psychodynamic mechanisms—repression of unacceptable conscious impulses and their 'conversion' to physical symptoms, sometimes with symbolic meaning. In ICD and DSM the presumed psychodynamic mechanisms are not part of the diagnosis. Symptoms are not produced intentionally and the presence of 'secondary gain' is not part of the diagnosis.

Classification ICD-10 and DSM-IV classify these disorders differently. In ICD-10 dissociation and conversion are used synonymously, with dissociation preferred as it does not imply a definite psychological explanation. All expressions of such disorders are classified together under the heading 'F44, dissociative (conversion) disorders'. In DSM-IV 'conversion' refers to motor or sensory deficit, while 'dissociation' refers to disturbance in function of consciousness. Conversion disorders are classified with the somatoform disorders, while dissociative disorders are classified separately (see pp. 932–3).

Clinical features These vary depending on the area affected but the following are commonly seen:

- **Paralysis** One or more limbs or one side of the face or body may be affected. Flaccid paralysis is common initially but severe, established cases may develop contractures. Often active movement of the limb is impossible during examination but synergistic movement is observed (e.g. Hoover's test: the patient is unable to raise the affected limb from the couch but is able to raise the unaffected limb against resistance with demonstrable pressing down of the heel on the 'affected' side).
- **Loss of speech (aphonia)** There may be complete loss of speech, or loss of all but whispered speech. There is no defect in comprehension and writing is unimpaired (and becomes the main method of communication). Laryngeal examination is normal and the patient's vocal cords can be fully opposed while coughing.
- **Sensory loss** The area of loss will cover the patient's beliefs about anatomical structure rather than reality (e.g. 'glove' distribution, marked 'midline splitting').
- **Seizures** Non-epileptic seizures are found most commonly in those with genuine epilepsy. The non-epileptic attacks generally occur only in the presence of an audience, no injury is sustained on falling to the ground, tongue biting and incontinence are rare, the 'seizure' consists of generalised shaking, rather than regular clonic contractions, and there is no post-ictal confusion or prolactin rise.

Diagnosis The diagnosis will usually be suspected due to the non-anatomical or clinically inconsistent nature of the signs. It is established by 1) excluding underlying organic disease, or demonstrating minor disorder insufficient to account for the symptoms; 2) finding of 'positive signs' (i.e. demonstration of function thought to be absent); 3) a convincing psychological explanation for the deficit.

Treatment Supportive psychotherapy, explanation that symptoms were initially organic but now problems are due to maladaptive response, perhaps with physiotherapy involvement. Treatment of psychiatric comorbidity.

Prognosis For acute conversion symptoms, especially those with a clear precipitant, the prognosis is good, with expectation of complete resolution of symptoms (70–90% resolution at follow-up). Poorer outcomes for longer-lasting and well-established symptoms.

Hypochondriasis

Hypochondriasis is the preoccupation with the fear of having a serious disease which persists despite negative investigations and causes distress and impaired function.

Clinical features The central and diagnostic clinical feature is the pre-occupation with the idea of having a serious medical condition, usually one which will lead to death or serious disability. The patient may repeatedly ruminate on this possibility and minor insignificant bodily abnormalities, normal variants, normal functions, and minor ailments will be interpreted as signs of serious disease. The patient will consequently seek medical advice and investigation but is unable to be reassured in a sustained fashion by negative investigations.

The form of the belief is that of an over-valued idea; the patient may be able to accept that his worries are groundless but nonetheless be unable to stop dwelling and acting on them. Where the belief in illness is of delu-sional intensity, the patient should be treated as for *delusional disorder* (p. 234).

Aetiology As in somatisation disorder there may be a history of child-hood illness, parental illness, or excess medical attention-seeking in the parents. CSA and other emotional abuse or neglect are associated. In one aetiological model, individuals with combination of anxiety symptoms and predisposition to misattribute psychical symptoms, seek medical advice. The resulting medical reassurance provides temporary relief of anxiety which acts as a 'reward' and makes further medical attention seeking more likely.

Epidemiology Equal sex incidence. Very variable prevalence depending on group studied, (0.8%–10.3%), higher in secondary care.

Differential diagnosis The main differentiation is from the feared physical disease. In most cases this is straightforward, but the possibility of an early, insidious disease with vague physical signs and normal baseline investigations should be considered.

Comorbidity High (>50%) incidence of generalised anxiety disorder. Hypochondriasis may also coexist with major depressive illness, OCD, and panic disorder. Examination of the time course of symptom develop-ment and most prominent clinical features helps to distinguish primary hypochondriasis from a secondary clinical feature of these disorders.

Management *Initial* Allow patient time to ventilate their illness anxiet-ies. Clarify that symptoms with no structural basis are real and severe. Aim to plan continuing relationship and review, not contingent upon new symptoms. Explain negative tests and resist the temptation to be drawn into further exploration. Patients will in the early stages often change or expand symptomatology. Emphasise aim to improve function. Break cycle of reassurance and repeat presentation—family education may help in this. *Pharmacological* Uncontrolled trials demonstrate antidepressant benefit, even in the absence of depressive symptoms. Try fluoxetine 20mg, increasing to 60mg, or imipramine up to 150mg. *Psychotherapy* Behavioural therapy (response prevention and exposure to illness cues); CBT (identify and challenge misinterpretations, substitution of realistic interpretation, graded exposure to illness-related situations, and modification of core illness-beliefs), 75% symptom reduction in one controlled trial[1].

1 Warwick HM, Clark DM, Cobb AM, Salkovskis PM (1996) A controlled trial of cognitive-behavioural treatment of hypochondriasis. *BJP* **169**, 189–95.

Dysmorphic disorder

The core clinical feature of dysmorphic disorder is preoccupation with the belief that some aspect of physical appearance is markedly abnormal, unattractive or pathological. This preoccupation causes distress and has the characteristics of an over-valued idea, it is not amenable to reassurance. The bodily part is found to be normal, or if abnormal is only trivially so compared with the degree of distress.

It is an unusual condition which has only relatively recently come prominently to clinical attention. It rarely presents directly, but such individuals may present requesting plastic surgery or mutilating surgical procedures, and hence come to psychiatric attention. There are many similarities to OCD in terms of clinical features and treatment response.

Clinical features There is preoccupation with the idea that some specified aspect of their appearance is grossly abnormal, markedly unattractive, or diseased. Any part of the body may be affected, most usually the face, head, and secondary sexual characteristics. Patients believe that the supposed deficit is noticeable to others and attempt to hide or minimise it. These beliefs may develop delusional intensity. There is associated functional impairment, agoraphobia, and risk of suicide. Comorbid behaviours such as skin picking, rubbing, topical applications may cause worse secondary problems. Clinically significant disorder causes severe functional impairment, restriction of relationships and employment opportunities, and the risk of iatrogenic morbidity by unwarranted surgical procedures.

Aetiology Begins in late childhood or early adolescence, overlap with normal worries at this age.

Epidemiology Equal sex incidence. Less than 1% prevalence but markedly over-represented in some groups (e.g. plastic surgery (10%) and dermatology). 10% incidence in first-degree family members.

Comorbidity 60% risk of major depression.

Differential diagnosis There is a significant overlap in terms of symptom profile with social phobia, hypochondriasis, OCD, somatic delusions in schizophrenia, and anorexia nervosa. Where the concerns are persistently delusional, ICD-10 reclassifies as delusional disorder, while DSM-IV allows diagnosis of a delusional form.

Treatment
- **Operative** Plastic surgery to the affected part is generally not indicated, even successful surgery risks being followed by a new preoccupation or a focus on surgical scarring.
- **Pharmacological** Evidence for clinical effectiveness of SSRI, try fluoxetine 20mg increasing to 60mg. If ineffective try clomipramine up to 300mg. If delusional features, add antipsychotic.

• **Psychological** Evidence for CBT, treatment focused on response prevention, challenging cognitive errors, and behavioural tasks.

Prognosis Chronic course with fluctuating symptom severity. Partial rather than full remission.

Factitious disorder (Munchausen's Syndrome)

In factitious disorder patients intentionally falsify their symptoms and past history and fabricate signs of physical or mental disorder with the primary aim of obtaining medical attention and treatment. The diagnostic features are the intentional and conscious production of signs, falsification, or exaggeration of the history and the lack of gain beyond medical attention and treatment. Three distinct sub-groups are seen.

- **Wandering:** mostly males who move from hospital to hospital, job to job, place to place, producing dramatic and fantastic stories. There may be aggressive personality or dissocial PD and comorbid alcohol or drug problems.
- **Non-wandering:** mostly females; more stable lifestyles and less dramatic presentations. Often in paramedical professions; overlap with chronic somatisation disorder. Association with borderline PD.
- **By proxy:** mostly female. Mothers, carers, or paramedical and nursing staff who simulate or prolong illness in their dependants—here the clinical focus must be on the prevention of further harm to the dependant.

The behaviours can mimic any psychical and psychiatric illness. Behaviours include: self-induced infections, simulated illnesses, interference with existing lesions, self-medication, altering records, reporting false physical or psychiatric symptomatology. Early diagnosis reduces iatrogenic morbidity and is facilitated by: awareness of the possibility; a neutral interviewing style using open rather than closed questions; alertness to insistencies and abnormalities in presentation; use of other available information sources; and careful medical record keeping.

Differential diagnosis Any genuine medical or psychiatric disorder. Somatisation disorder (no conscious production of symptoms and no fabrication of history), malingering (secondary gain for the patient e.g. compensation, avoiding army service), substance misuse (also gain i.e. the prescription of the drug), hypochondriasis, psychotic and depressive illness (associated features of the primary mental illness).

Aetiology Unknown, there may be a background of childhood sexual abuse or childhood emotional neglect. Probably more common in men and those with a nursing or paramedical background. Association with personality disorder. Production of psychiatric symptoms associated with borderline PD, CSA or emotional abuse.

Management

There are no validated treatments. Patients are often reluctant to consider psychiatric assessment and may leave once their story is questioned. Management in these cases is directed towards reducing iatrogenic harm caused by inappropriate treatments and medications.

- **Direct challenge** Easier if there is direct evidence of feigned illness; the patient is informed that staff are aware of the intent to feign illness and the evidence is produced. This should be in a non-punitive manner with offer of ongoing support.

- **Indirect challenge** Here the aim is to allow the patient a face-saving 'way out', while preventing further inappropriate investigation and intervention. One example is the 'double bind' 'if this doesn't work then the illness is factitious'.
- **Systemic change** Here the understanding is that there is no possibility of change in the individual and the focus is on changing the approach of the health care system to assessing them in order to minimise harm. These strategies can include dissemination of the patient's usual presentation and distinguishing marks to regional hospitals, 'black-listing', 'Munchausen's registers', etc. As these strategies potentially break confidentiality and can decrease the risk of detecting genuine illness, they should be drawn up in a multidisciplinary fashion involving senior staff.

Chronic fatigue syndrome

Chronic fatigue syndrome (CFS) is the current preferred name for a clinical syndrome whose central feature is severe fatigue, unrelated to exertion and unrelieved by rest. Fatigue is a symptom characterised by a subjective feeling of lethargy, lack of energy, exhaustion, and a feeling of 'increased effort to do anything'. Patients also complain of aching muscles, poor unrefreshing sleep, aching joints, and headaches. They may date the symptoms very precisely to an episode of viral infection with sore throat, fever, and tender lymph nodes. CFS is currently preferred to the names myalgic encephalomyelitis (ME) and post-viral fatigue syndrome as it doesn't imply knowledge of underlying pathology or aetiology.

It should be understood that CFS is not a disorder in the conventionally accepted sense, but a characteristic clinical syndrome. The syndrome shows diagnostic overlap with major depression, somatisation disorder, and hypochondrias but cannot be subsumed into these diagnoses because of substantial areas of lack of fit. Any criteria for CFS will be contentious and will include many people with chronic organic illnesses. Patients with this syndrome will often have passionately held beliefs about the cause of their symptoms and the appropriate management. A practical, pragmatic approach is advised from the doctor.

A separate diagnosis of CFS does not appear in DSM-IV; patients not meeting criteria for somatisation disorder would be categorised as 'undifferentiated somatoform disorder'.

Aetiology Unknown; a minority of cases have confirmed onset with viral illness but ongoing viral replication or chronic infection is not the cause. At the moment is understood in terms of an acute reaction to stress or minor illness in vulnerable individual with a persisting clinical syndrome caused by deconditioning and other secondary phenomena. Vulnerable individuals are those with abnormal symptom attribution, increased awareness of normal bodily processes, cognitive errors, and perfectionist personality types.

Comorbidity Many patients with CFS will meet the criteria for another psychiatric diagnosis, most commonly major depression. Arguments exist for calling CFS a form of atypical depression; however this is untenable in a significant minority of cases. Not only do patients resist a 'psychiatric' diagnosis, but many do not have anhedonia or pervasively low mood, and attribute any mood disturbance to the restriction on their activities caused by their illness. Nonetheless, treatment of comorbid depressive or anxiety symptoms can produce clinical improvement.

Investigation findings Non-specific subjective cognitive impairment similar to that found in depression. Normal muscle function with poor performance on tolerance testing related to deconditioning. No characteristic blood abnormalities or immune system abnormalities. Possible cortisol depression? There are no definite and replicable abnormal findings. Do minimum indicated tests.

Assessment Establish the diagnosis and identify comorbid psychiatric disorders. Avoid confrontation with the patient and attempt to agree a common understanding of the disorder. Acknowledge the severity of the symptoms and the consequent disability. Aim to take the focus of the interview towards potentially beneficial interventions and away from unwarranted investigations.

Management

- **Medication** Give antidepressant treatment trial even where no clear-cut evidence of affective symptoms. Try SSRI first (e.g. paroxetine 20mg) as this patient group is intolerant of side-effects.
- **Graded exercise** Establish via diary record the patient's daily activity level, establish with them their maximal tolerable level *even on their worst day*, and encourage them to perform this level of activity every day, no more and no less, with gradual negotiated increase over time. The aim is to break the cycle of inactivity, brief excess activity, and consequent exhaustion.
- **Psychotherapy** Some evidence for the effectiveness of CBT.

Prognosis Poor for established cases with continuing ill-health of fluctuating nature.

Illnesses related to childbirth

▶ **Always ask about thoughts of self-harm or harming the baby.**

Despite the significant life event that pregnancy is, psychiatric admission and completed suicide are less common in pregnancy than at other times. There may be sub-clinical mild anxiety or mood disturbance, worse in the third and first trimesters. 10% risk of clinical depression in the first trimester associated with past history of depression, previous abortion, previous intra-uterine loss, unwanted pregnancy. Third trimester depression may persist as postpartum depression. Avoid drug treatment in the first trimester.

'Baby blues'

Up to 3/4 of new mothers will experience a short-lived period of tearfulness and emotional lability starting two or three days after birth and lasting one to two days. This is common enough to be easily recognisable by midwifery staff and requires only reassurance and observation towards resolution. There is weak evidence that it may be related to post-partum reductions in levels of oestrogen, progesterone, and prolactin (which do occur around 72 hrs after the birth).

Postnatal depression (PND)

A significant depressive episode, temporally related to childbirth, occurring in 10–15% of women within 6 months post-partum (peak 3–4 weeks). The clinical features are similar to other depressive episodes, although thought content may include worries about the baby's health or her ability to cope adequately with the baby. There may be a significant anxiety component. 90% of cases last less than 1 month; 4% greater than one year. **Risk factors** Personal or family history of depression, older age, single mother, poor relationship with own mother, ambivalence towards or unwanted pregnancy, poor social support, significant other psycho-social stressors, severe 'baby blues', previous post-partum psychosis, (no evidence for association with obstetric complications). **Management** Early identification and close monitoring of those 'at risk' (use of Edinburgh Postnatal Depression Scale in primary care setting—see opposite); prevention by education, support, and appropriate pharmacological intervention; depressive episode treated in usual way with antidepressants and/or brief CBT, if severe or associated with thoughts of self-harm or harm to baby, may require hospital admission.

Postpartum psychosis

An acute psychotic episode, occurring following 1.5/1000 live births, peak occurrence at 2 wks postpartum. Aetiology is unknown, but may relate to reduction of oestrogen (leading to DA super-sensitivity), cortisol levels, or postpartum thyroiditis. **Symptoms** 3 common clinical presentations: *prominent affective symptoms* (80%)—mania or depression with psychotic symptoms; *schizophreniform disorder* (15%); *acute organic psychosis* (5%). Common features include: lability of symptoms; insomnia; perplexity; bewilderment, and disorientation; thoughts of suicide or infanticide. **Risk factors** Personal or family history of major psychiatric disorder; lack of social support; single parenthood; previous postpartum psychosis (30% risk of psychosis; 38% risk of PND). **Management** *Prevention* identification, education, support, and treatment of 'at risk' individuals; *Treatment* admission to hospital (specialist mother-baby unit if possible); for major affective disorder there is good evidence for ECT, mood stabilisers (esp. carbamazepine), and early use of antidepressants; psychotic symptoms should be treated with usual protocol (see pp. 198–201).

Edinburgh Postnatal Depression Scale (EPDS)[1]

As you have recently had a baby, we would like to know how you are feeling. Please UNDERLINE the answer which comes closest to how you have felt IN THE PAST 7 DAYS, not just how you feel today.

I have been able to laugh and see the funny side of things.
As much as I always could/Not quite so much now/Definitely not so much now/Not at all
I have looked forward with enjoyment to things.
As much as I ever did/Rather less than I used to/Definitely less than I used to/Hardly at all
* **I have blamed myself unnecessarily when things went wrong**.
Yes, most of the time/Yes, some of the time/Not very often/No, never
I have been anxious or worried for no good reason.
No, not at all/Hardly ever/Yes, sometimes/Yes, very often
* **I have felt scared or panicky for not very good reason**.
Yes, quite a lot/Yes, sometimes/No, not much/No, not at all
* **Things have been getting on top of me**.
Yes, most of the time I haven't been able to cope at all/
Yes, sometimes I haven't been coping as well as usual/
No, most of the time I have coped quite well/
No, I have been coping as well as ever
* **I have been so unhappy that I have had difficulty sleeping**.
Yes, most of the time/Yes, sometimes/Not very often/No, not at all
* **I have felt sad or miserable**.
Yes, most of the time/Yes, quite often/Not very often/No, not at all
* **I have been so unhappy that I have been crying**.
Yes, most of the time/Yes, quite often/Only occasionally/No, never
* **The thought of harming myself has occurred to me**.
Yes, quite often/Sometimes/Hardly ever/Never

Response categories are scored 0, 1, 2, and 3 according to increased severity of the symptoms. Items marked with an asterisk are reverse scored (i.e. 3, 2, 1, and 0). A total score of 12+ is regarded as significant.

1 Cox JL, Holden JM, Sagovsky R (1987) Detection of postnatal depression. Development of the 10-item Edinburgh Postnatal Depression Scale. *BJP* **150**, 782–6.

Transsexualism

Transsexualism is characterised by the feeling of one's gender being different from one's biological sex. The characteristic statement made by male to female transsexuals is 'I feel like a woman trapped in a man's body'. This describes the core clinical feature of these patients which is an enduring belief that they are 'really' of the opposite sex. This is associated with marked unhappiness and discomfort in the birth sex and a persistent desire to live and be treated as a member of the opposite sex.

Transsexuals usually come to psychiatric attention, not because they wish to change these feelings, but in order to gain the psychiatrist's support for undertaking sex reassignment surgery (SRS). SRS is a contentious treatment whose early reported successes have been disputed. In addition it is expensive and irreversible and so if it is to be considered, extreme care in the selection process is required. Assessment should be by a specialist in gender identity disorders, working in close liaison with the surgical team. The aim is to make the diagnosis, to offer alternative treatments, to provide supportive psychotherapy, and to supervise the real-life test.

Aetiology Unknown primary cause. Most transsexuals report that their beliefs about their gender were present from early childhood. Karyotype and phenotypic development is normal.

Epidemiology Prevalence of 1 in 30 000 for male to female (MTF) transsexuals and 1 in 100 000 for female to male (FTM) transsexuals. MTF to FTM ratio is 3–4:1 in most samples.

Differential diagnosis Transvestism (the wearing of clothes of the opposite sex for sexual or other purposes, not associated with the core belief of incorrect gender found in the transsexual); intersexed condition (ruled out by normal karyotyping and normal primary and sexual characteristics for the birth sex); schizophrenia (occasionally associated with a delusion that the patient is the wrong sex or is changing sex).

Comorbidity Deliberate self-harm and suicidal gestures are common and may be directed at underscoring the need for surgery. Genital mutilation is rare. Some MTF transsexuals work in the sex industry and have consequent increased risk of STDs and HIV infection.

Assessment Many such patients will arrive with their diagnosis ('I am a transsexual') and preferred treatment option (hormones and sex reassignment surgery) already fixed in their minds. The aim of assessment is to establish the diagnosis with certainty. Contraindications to treatment are psychotic illness, major depression, substance misuse, and personality disorder.

Treatment

- **Psychological treatments** Aimed at altering the core beliefs. Ineffective in the majority of cases and are generally not welcomed by the patient. If the diagnosis of transsexualism is made then the psychiatrist's role is supervision of the transition, with liaison with the primary care and surgical teams and psychological support during the inevitable difficulties.

- **Real-life test** Most centres require a successful 'real-life test' of at least one year prior to consideration for surgery. During this time the patient undertakes to live full time and attempt to find employment in the new sex. Patients will change their name and 'come out' to friends and family.
- **Hormones** Oestrogen treatment in MTF transsexuals produces diminished libido and erectile function, some breast and hip development, and skin softening; there is no effect on voice pitch and speech therapy may be required to produce an acceptable female vocal pattern. Androgen treatment in FTM transsexuals produces muscle development, some lowering of vocal pitch, male pattern of bodily hair development, and amenorrhoea.
- **Surgery** For MTF patients surgery involves orchidectomy and penectomy with vaginoplasty using penile skin. The cosmetic results can be good, although candidates vary in their ability to be orgasmic post-surgery. For FTM patients surgery involves bilateral mastectomy, hysterectomy, and bilateral salpingo-oopherectomy. Phalloplasty is undertaken in less then half of patients as current techniques are neither cosmetically acceptable or functional for penetration.

Prognosis No RCT are available comparing SRS with other treatment. Cohort follow-up studies report >90% of patients reporting improvement following SRS on measures of psychological adjustment, absence of regret, and vocational adjustment.

Assessment prior to liver transplantation

For patients with end-stage liver disease, a liver transplantation offers the prospect of significant improvement in their mortality and quality of life. There is no equivalent in liver failure to kidney dialysis and the supply of donor livers is less than the number of potential recipients. Because of this, patients requiring liver transplantation will suffer declining health while awaiting transplantation and 10–20% of listed patients will die while awaiting transplant. This places a responsibility on the assessing team to consider carefully each potential candidate for listing for transplantation in order to ensure the best use of the donor livers.

Psychiatric assessment of patients prior to listing for liver transplantation may be requested in the following situations:
• Fulminant liver failure following overdose (usually paracetamol)
• Liver disease secondary to alcoholic liver disease (ALD)
• Patients with history of mental illness
• Patients with previous or current drug misuse.

The involvement of the psychiatrist in the assessment prior to listing for transplantation *should in no sense be a moral judgement* as to the patient's suitability. The issues are whether there are psychiatric factors which would jeopardise the survival of the donor liver. The psychiatric opinion may have the most profound implications for the patient and so assessment should be as thorough as time allows. In addition to taking psychiatric history and MSE, family members, GP, and hospital case records should be consulted.

Fulminant liver failure This will often follow on from a late presenting paracetamol overdose. At the point patients are seen it is often unclear whether they are going to recover or to deteriorate to the point of requiring transplant. They should be seen as soon as possible after presentation as encephalopathy may develop as their condition worsens. The issue is whether there is: ongoing intent to die or refusal of transplant (which would normally preclude transplantation); or whether there is a history of repeated overdoses in the past, significant psychiatric disorder, or ongoing drug or alcohol misuse (which would be relative contraindications).

Liver disease secondary to ALD Suitably selected patients transplanted for ALD have similar outcomes in terms of survival and quality of life to patients transplanted for other indications. Units will have individual policies regarding these patients which should be consulted if available. The issue is whether the patient, who has already damaged one liver, will damage a second. There is a wider issue of maintaining the public confidence in the appropriate use of donated organs. Consider:
• How long have they been abstinent (is there independent verification of this)?
• Do they accept alcohol as the cause of liver failure?
• Do they undertake to remain abstinent post-transplant?
• Do they have a history of dependence or harmful use?

- What is their history of involvement in alcohol treatment services and in the past, how have they responded to relapse?
- When were they told that their drinking was causing liver damage, and what was their response?

Given the above findings and your routine psychiatric assessment, the transplant team will seek your opinion as to:
- The patient's psychiatric diagnosis.
- Their risk of relapse.
- Their risk of re-establishing harmful/dependant drinking.
- The potential for successful intervention should this occur.

History of mental illness/drug misuse Generally speaking a diagnosis of mental disorder (other than progressive dementia) will not preclude transplant. The important issues are whether the mental disorder will affect compliance or longer-term mortality in its own right. Close liaison with the patient's normal psychiatrist is clearly crucial here. Ongoing substance dependence is generally a contraindication to transplantation and should be addressed before listing.

Psychotherapy

Introduction

Psychotherapy is the 'talking cure'—the attempt to alter abnormal thinking and behaviour by a dialogue taking place within a relationship. Psychotherapeutic methods are used both to conceptualise abnormal mental states (to understand why symptoms have developed in this patient at this particular time) and to treat the attendant disorders. There are a variety of different psychotherapeutic methods, each usually initially associated with a single individual or centre. In its broadest sense—of achieving understanding of symptoms and effecting their improvement by means of a therapeutic relationship—psychotherapy is at the heart of all medical and therefore all psychiatric treatment.

Types of psychotherapy

- **Supportive psychotherapy** Aims to offer practical and emotional support, opportunity for ventilation of emotions, and guided, problem-solving discussion. Used where fundamental behavioural change is not aimed for, or where patient factors (e.g. learning difficulty, psychotic illness) preclude exploratory therapies. Examples include counselling, general psychiatric follow-up.
- **Exploratory psychotherapy** Aims to effect change in the individual's abnormal thinking and behaviour by exploration of underlying causes.
  - *Dynamic therapies* Based on psychoanalytic theory. Focus of clinical attention is childhood experience and exploration of the unconscious mind.
  - *Cognitive/behavioural therapies* Based on learning theory and cognitive theory. Focus of clinical attention is the 'here and now': current behaviours and thoughts, and their modification.

Common factors to different psychotherapies

- A theory of illness or symptom development.
- Empirical or case-based evidence to support this theory.
- A rationale for treatment.
- Prescribed roles for the therapist and patient.
- A form of structured therapy—sometimes in the form of a manual.
- Takes place in a setting recognised as a 'place of healing'.

Psychotherapeutic training As a psychiatric trainee you will be expected to gain experience in at least one type of psychotherapy during your training. This will usually be via supervised long and short case experience. You may also undertake a period of basic or higher training in a psychotherapeutic centre during one of your clinical attachments. Following suitable personal and tutorial based training in the method, you will take on a case under the supervision of an individual with the requisite experience. It is only through the process of therapy and supervision that you will really understand psychotherapeutic techniques. These notes on general concepts and specific psychotherapies aim to familiarise you with concepts, guide your referrals, and assist you in explaining the process to patients.

Assessment for psychotherapy

Psychotherapeutic methods can be useful in the treatment of mild to moderate depressive illness, neurotic disorders, behavioural disorders, and personality disorders. Specific therapies may have a place in the management of learning disability, sexual problems, substance misuse, and chronic psychotic symptoms. They are generally contraindicated for acute psychosis, severe depressive illness, dementia/delirium, and conditions where there is acute suicide risk.

Selection criteria for psychotherapy

- **'Psychological-mindedness'** The ability to understand problems in psychological terms.
- **Motivation for insight and change** Includes the ability to form a 'therapeutic alliance', which requires a degree of introspectiveness, average intelligence, and verbal fluency.
- **Adequate 'ego strength'** Includes the ability to sustain feelings and fantasies without impulsively acting upon them, being overwhelmed by anxiety, or losing the capacity to talk rationally. The individual should be capable of maintaining a therapeutic alliance and there should be no impairment of 'ego boundaries' due to psychosis or severe depression.
- **Able to form and sustain relationships** Where there is inability to enter into trusting relationships, (e.g. in paranoid personality disorder) or where there is inability to maintain relationship boundaries (e.g. in borderline personality disorder), this may preclude exploratory methods.
- **Able to tolerate change and a degree of frustration** As with any potentially powerful treatment, psychotherapy has the potential to exacerbate symptoms, particularly as maladaptive coping mechanisms are examined and changed.

Selection of psychotherapeutic method

- **Local availability** In practice, often the main determinant of therapy choice is local availability and the practical availability determined by the length of the waiting list. The waiting times associated with most forms of therapy should encourage all practitioners to exercise care in patient referral.
- **Practitioner experience** In some cases the treating doctor will take on therapy themselves and utilize the method with which they are familiar.
- **Illness factors** The exact suitability of each of the therapy methods has yet to be clearly established. Nonetheless, some therapies are indicated for particular disorders, (e.g. behaviour therapy for simple phobias, CBT for anorexia nervosa).
- **Patient choice** Patients may express a preference for a particular therapeutic model because of previous positive experience or having read or been told about the approach of different methods. A method which 'makes sense' to the patient given their understanding of their symptoms is desirable.

Counselling

Counselling may be thought of as a method of relieving distress undertaken by means of a dialogue between two people. The aim is to help the client or patient find their own solutions to problems, while being supported to do so and being guided by appropriate advice. In Western countries over the last fifty years, counselling has emerged as a profession in its own right and individual forms of specific counselling have been developed. In its more general sense—helping others by the provision of advice, non-judgemental reflection, and emotional support—counselling takes place all over the world in the guise of family members, priests, tutors, teachers, etc.

Counselling skills are integral to the practice of medicine, particularly in primary care and psychiatry, where counselling techniques are useful in history taking, assessing and ensuring compliance, etc. Counselling should not be thought of as 'cut-down' or 'half-price' psychotherapy. There is clearly overlap in the methods and skills of a psychotherapist and a counsellor. However, the decision to use counselling as a specific treatment, (e.g. for postnatal depression) should be made after considering both the disorder and the patient. There are a variety of counselling services in the voluntary and private sectors, some directed towards specific problems and some more general.

Rationale Behaviour and emotional life are shaped by previous experience, current environment, and the relationships the individual has. Many life problems can be viewed as arising from resolvable difficulties in one of these three areas, rather than as an 'illness'. People have a tendency towards positive change and fulfilment which can be retarded by 'life problems'. A collaborative relationship with a counsellor (however defined) is one method of addressing these issues. This relationship will proceed according to agreed rules, towards a goal, and will be based on developing the client's strengths.

Techniques

- **Information giving** Key to all psychiatric treatment and psychotherapeutic work. Information should be provided in a form the patient can understand and information giving should not be a 'one off' but should continue throughout counselling.
- **Client-focused discussion** The client should 'lead' the sessions particularly beyond the early information gathering sessions. Time constraints may hinder this.
- **Problem solving** A variety of techniques, particularly those borrowed from cognitive behavioural therapy are employed here. The basic goal is to use the session time to explore current and potential future problems and to help the client consider the optimum solution.

Different types of counselling

- **Information sharing/discussion** In some contexts is also called psychoeducation. Aim is to properly inform a client prior to them making their own decision. Techniques of guided learning, providing verbal and written information, collaborative enquiry (cf. CBT).

- **Crisis management** Views crisis as stressor providing both risk and opportunity to change/learn/develop. Short term, immediately follows trauma (first few weeks). Facilitates adaptive and normal emotional responses, discourages maladaptive responses. Focus on end-point of intervention. Alternative to hospital admission in some cases. Should have access to alternative treatments if necessary.
- **Problem-based counselling** Directed towards a specific primary problem, (e.g. drug misuse, CSA). Counsellor may or may not have had similar experiences themselves.
- **Risk counselling** Used to guide an informed decision (e.g. pre-natal interventions, genetic counselling). Differentiated from other forms of counselling by the fact that the counsellor is clearly 'the expert' and has access to specialist information. Nonetheless, the basic goal, of enabling the patient to come to their own decision, with appropriate information and support, remains the same.

Indications Absolute advice limited by lack of comparative trials and tendency for local availability of services to be the main factor in the decision to use counselling methods. Clinical usefulness in:
- Adjustment disorder.
- Mild depressive illness.
- Normal and pathological grief.
- Sequelae of childhood sexual abuse.
- After other forms of trauma (e.g. rape, accidents).
- Postnatal depression.
- Pregnancy loss and stillbirth.
- Drug and alcohol problems.
- Reaction to chronic medical conditions.
- Prior to decision such as undergoing genetic testing or HIV testing.

A brief history of Sigmund Freud

Freud remains far and away the world's best-known psychiatrist and his image, of a scholarly, bearded man sitting behind a distressed patient lying on a couch, is many lay-people's archetype for our profession. He made a huge contribution to our understanding of the mind, but many of his ideas are now so much a part of our general view of the world that it is easy to overlook the breakthroughs they originally were.

He was born in 1856 in Moravia (now part of the Czech republic, but then part of the Austro-Hungarian Empire). He moved to Vienna when he was a child and lived there until his last year. On entering medical training he was influenced by scientific empiricism—the belief that through careful observation the un-understandable could be understood. On qualification he began laboratory work on the physiology of the nervous system under Brücke, later entering clinical medical practice after his marriage in 1882. He chose neurology as his specialty and received a grant to study at the Salpêtrière in Paris where he was exposed to the ideas of Charcot who interested Freud in the study of hysteria and the use of hypnosis. In Paris with Charcot, and later in Nancy with Liébault, he studied the behaviour of hysterical patients under hypnosis and developed his ideas of the unconscious mind and its role in normal and disordered behaviour.

Returning to Vienna, Freud began collaboration with Josef Breuer on the study of hysteria. The subsequent development of psychoanalysis was prompted by the case of Anna O., treated by Breuer between 1880 and 1882. This patient, a 21-year-old woman (real name Bertha Pappenheim) presented with a range of hysterical symptoms including paralysis, visual loss, cough, and abrupt personality change. These symptoms had developed while her father was terminally ill. Breuer observed that her symptoms resolved during hypnotic trances. Breuer also noted that not only did the symptoms recur after the sessions ended, but that after he terminated the treatment relationship she suffered a full-blown relapse. Breuer wrote up the case after discussing it with his younger colleague. Later they published *Studies in Hysteria*, detailing their ideas on the aetiology and treatment of hysterical symptoms. This book postulated that trauma is unacceptable to the patient and hence repressed from conscious memory. This repression produces an increase in 'nervous excitation'—which is expressed eventually as hysteria—with a conscious remnant, often in a disguised form, which can be accessed and resolved during hypnosis.

Freud explored these ideas during his clinical practice in the 1890s, using a variety of methods to uncover the repressed memories. Later he developed the technique of *free association*, where the patient is encouraged to say whatever comes to mind. He noted that some patients developed powerful feelings towards him and called this phenomenon *transference*.

Experience in the 1890s led Freud to develop the ideas of *repression* of unacceptable memories and their expression as hysterical symptoms. The initial memory was generally of a sexual nature. At first Freud thought this was a real assault, but later realised that in the majority of cases the patients were describing a sexualised fantasy towards parental figures. Freud described these ideas in his most famous book, *The Interpretation of Dreams*, published in 1900. It described the basis of his psychoanalytic technique including analysis of the content of dreams, descriptions of defence mechanisms, and his *topographical model* of the mind. Freud's early insights tended to come directly from clinical experience, particularly patients with hysteria. His later ideas were more theoretical and related to developing a complete understanding of the normal and abnormal development of mind through psychoanalytical ideas. His drive theory postulated the existence of basic drives, which included the *libido*, the sexual drive, and the *eros* and *thanatos* (the drives towards life and death). He described the *pleasure principle*, the drive to avoid pain and experience pleasure, and its modification through the *reality principle*.

In 1905 he published *Three essays on the Theory of Sexuality*, describing his theories regarding childhood development including the ideas of developmental phases and the Oedipal and Electra complexes and their relationship with the development of adult neuroses. *The Ego and the Id*, published in 1923, saw the replacement of the topographical with the structural model of the mind. He described his theories of ego psychology and the production of anxiety symptoms in *Inhibitions, Symptoms and Anxiety* in 1926. Although he recognised the importance of unconscious defences in response to anxiety, the first systematic account of these mechanisms was written by Freud's daughter Anna in *The Ego and the Mechanisms of Defence* in 1936. Freud's repeated revision of his own theories was mirrored by repeated disagreements and splits in the psychotherapeutic movement and the formation of separate psychotherapeutic 'schools', usually strongly associated with one charismatic individual. Freud died from cancer in England in 1939 after fleeing Vienna following the rise to power of the Nazis. His daughter Anna continued to refine and publicise her father's work.

Later developments

Jung Expanded drive theory to include drives other than sexual. Ideas of 'collective unconscious' and personality archetypes. Ideas of extroversion and introversion.

Klein Theories of childhood development including primitive defence mechanisms such as 'splitting'. Methods of play therapy.

Winnicott Object relations theory—gratification through relationships as well as through satisfaction of desires. Described transitional objects and the idea of the 'Good enough mother'.

Erikson Described alternative model of psychosocial development based on the crises at each developmental stage.

Rogers Client-centred therapy. Importance of therapeutic attributes of genuineness, unconditional positive regard, and accurate empathy.

Berne Transactional analysis. Examination of 'games' and 'scripts' which characterise relationships.

Basic psychoanalytic theory (1)

Freudian theories of symptom development

'Psychic abscess' theory In the treatment of his early patients, described in *Studies on Hysteria*, Freud conceived of hysterical symptoms as arising as an indirect result of a previous traumatic event in the patient's life. The memory of this trauma was painful and the emotions associated with its recall gave rise to unacceptable contradictions in the patient's beliefs about themselves. They were therefore *repressed* from consciousness. Although the memories were not recalled directly, the powerful associated emotions were expressed as hysterical symptoms, sometimes with symbolic connection to the initial traumatic event. The hysterical symptoms could be treated (and the 'psychic abscess lanced') by forcing the memories into consciousness by abreaction.

Topographical model of the mind Described in *The interpretation of dreams*, later superseded by the structural model. In this model the mind consists of the unconscious, the preconscious, and the conscious. Only those ideas and memories in the conscious mind are within awareness. The preconscious performs a 'censorship' function by examining unconscious ideas and memories and repressing those which are unacceptable. The unconscious mind acts according to the 'pleasure principle'—the avoidance of pain and the seeking of gratification. This is modified by the 'reality principle' of the conscious mind.

Structural model of the mind Proposed in 1923. It consisted of the Id, the Ego, and the Superego. The Id pursues its own desires and is heedless of external reality or moral constraints. A new born baby's mind is conceived as all Id. The Ego emerges during infancy and is the personality which moderates the desires of the Id. The Superego (the 'conscience') is the internalisation of the morals and strictures of society, which provides judgements on what behaviours are acceptable and which are 'bad'. When the Ego is unable to successfully moderate between the Id and Superego it may defend the individual's sense of self by repressing the impulse to the unconscious where its presence may produce disturbance.

Ego defence mechanisms

Freud conceived the idea of the repression of unacceptable thoughts from conscious awareness. Subsequently a number of other 'defence mechanisms' were described, viewed as developing to prevent conflict between the conscious mind and the unconscious desires.

Repression Preventing unacceptable aspects of internal reality coming to conscious attention by unconscious 'forgetting' of the painful memory or unacceptable impulse. (e.g. in adult life, no longer being able to recall episodes of childhood sexual abuse) The associated emotional reaction may remain in the conscious mind but divorced from its accompanying idea.

Regression Responding to emotional stresses by reverting to a level of functioning of a previous maturational point.

Denial Preventing unacceptable aspects of external reality coming to conscious attention by refusal to consciously acknowledge events or truths which are obvious to other people.

Distortion Similar to denial. Dealing with a reshaped version of external reality rather than the true version.

Projection Attributing one's own unacceptable ideas and impulses to another person.

Projective identification Similar to projection. Here the individual attributes his negative response to another as a justifiable response to the attitudes he perceives them as having.

Isolation/intellectualisation Dealing with emotion-laden memories or ideas by considering them in an logical manner, divorced from emotion.

Reaction formation The expression externally of attitudes and behaviours which are the opposite of the unacceptable internal impulses.

Displacement Transferring the emotional response to a particular person, event, or situation to another where it doesn't belong but which carries less emotional 'risk'.

Rationalisation Justifying behaviour or feelings with a plausible explanation after the event, rather than examining their underlying, consciously unacceptable explanation.

Undoing Performing an action which has the effect of unconsciously 'cancelling out' an unacceptable internal impulse. The action may have an obvious symbolism related to the internal impulse.

Splitting Separating the good and bad aspects of a person or situation in one's mind in order to avoid the ambivalence felt towards the whole person.

Turning against the self Unacceptable feelings of internal hostility or aggression towards others are expressed in harm to oneself.

Compensation The conscious development of abilities in response to a deficit.

Sublimation Regarded as the most 'healthy' of the defence mechanisms. The external expression of unacceptable internal impulses in socially acceptable ways.

Transference reactions
Transference The development, in the patient, of feelings and patterns of behaviour towards the therapist which unconsciously partly recapitulate earlier relationships in their lives. **Counter-transference** Describes the equivalent reaction in the therapist towards the patient. The examination of the transference and counter-transference is a central part of dynamic psychotherapy and guides diagnostic formulation and the exploration of the patient's neurosis in therapy.

Basic psychoanalytic theory (2)

Freudian theory of psychosexual development

Freud believed that the psychological conflicts which produced morbidity arose during infancy and childhood. He developed a theory which attempted to explain the development of sexuality in children. He visualised four phases, characterised by particular satisfactions and conflicts. Inability to resolve conflicts at a particular stage would lead to subsequent adult problems.

- **Oral stage** Birth to ~18 months. Pleasure comes from suckling and investigation of objects by placing them in the mouth.
- **Anal stage** 18 months to 3 years. Pleasure comes from anal sensations and the ability to withhold and to appropriately produce faeces.
- **Phallic stage** 3 to 6 years. Pleasure comes from manipulation of the phallus. This behaviour is not socially sanctioned and may be associated with shame and concealment. In addition, Freud postulated a range of anxieties related to the child's evolving ideas about itself and about gender and sexuality, including the Oedipus and Electra complexes.
  - **Oedipus complex** The young boy focuses his erotic attraction towards his mother and develops resentment towards his father who blocks his total possession of her. Because of his hostility towards his father and following his observation of the difference between males and females, he imagines his father may take revenge by castrating him (*castration anxiety*). This anxiety leads to repression or resolution of the desire for exclusivity in maternal relations and the child enters the latent phase.
  - **Electra complex** In young girls there is also an erotic desire for the mother and initial hostility towards the father as a rival. Due to her absence of a penis there is *penis envy* which becomes expressed as hostility towards the mother who she feels has handicapped her in her desires. This envy leads to an acceptance that she cannot compete with her father due to her lack of a penis and so the desire is transformed into a desire to have a baby as a penis substitute. The young girl then develops an Oedipal attachment towards her father as a potential father for this baby before again repressing these desires and entering the latent phase. Lack of the spur of castration anxiety leads to the conflict being harder to resolve in females than males.
- **Latency phase** 6 years until puberty. Period of relative quiescence of sexual thoughts between the resolution of the Oedipus/Electra complex and the awaking of adult sexuality.
- **Genital phase** Period of mature adult sexuality. During this period, improper resolution of previous phases may be manifest in symbolic ways.

The story of Oedipus (Sophocles ~430 B.C.)

King Laius of Thebes is told by the oracle at Delphi that his son will kill him and marry his wife. When his wife Jocasta gives birth to a boy, Oedipus, he orders a slave to abandon the child on a mountain. The slave takes pity on the child and, instead of leaving him to die, gives him to a shepherd, who brings him to the King of Corinth who is childless. Oedipus grows up thinking that Polibus, King of Corinth is his father.

As a youth, Oedipus visits the oracle at Delphi and is told that he will grow up to kill his father and marry his mother. At this, Oedipus vows never to return to Corinth and sets out for Thebes instead. On a narrow part of the road he meets an old man in a chariot who angrily orders him aside and strikes him with a spear. Oedipus seizes the spear to defend himself and strikes the old man on the head, killing him. The man is Laius, King of Thebes, his real father.

Approaching Thebes, Oedipus meets the Sphinx which is terrorising the city. The monster is stopping all passers-by and challenging them with its riddle; those who fail to answer the riddle are devoured. Oedipus solves the riddle of the Sphinx and the monster jumps to its death. He enters the city as a hero. He is told that the king has been murdered and is offered the throne, together with the hand of Jocasta in marriage.

Oedipus is a wise and successful king and Jocasta bears him two sons and two daughters. Many years later Thebes is afflicted by a terrible plague. The people appeal to Oedipus to save them and he sends his brother-in-law to the oracle at Delphi for advice. The oracle states that the plague will abate when the murderer of Laius is banished. Oedipus promises to bring the murderer to justice and forbids the people of Thebes from offering him any shelter.

Oedipus asks the prophet Teiresias to help him discover the killer's identity. Teiresias tries to dissuade him from pursuing the matter but the king persists, eventually accusing the prophet of being a fraud. Teiresias them angrily tells him that before nightfall he will find himself 'both a brother and a father to his children'. The king is bewildered and Jocasta tries to comfort him by telling him about the prophecy given to Laius—it was prophesied that he would be killed by his son, when in fact his son had died as an infant and he had been killed by bandits—hence prophecies could not be trusted. This story only increases Oedipus's worry and he suspects that he murdered Laius but does not yet realise that Laius was his father.

A messenger arrives to inform him of the death of the King of Corinth. The messenger also reveals that Oedipus was adopted. He begins to suspect that he is the son of Laius and continues to investigate, ignoring the pleas of Jocasta who has already realised the whole truth. Eventually he finds the shepherd who took him to the household of the King of Corinth and the full truth is revealed. At this point he hears anguished cries coming from the palace and rushes to his apartments. Oedipus breaks down the door of the royal bedchamber to find the queen, his wife and mother, has hung herself. He seizes her dress pin and gouges out his eyes so as not to have to look at the atrocity he has unwittingly committed. He enters into exile, having failed to avoid the fate laid out for him.

Dynamic psychotherapy

A method of therapy derived from the theories and practice of Sigmund Freud. Psychoanalytic theories have been repeatedly refined and reviewed over the last century, however the principles of dynamic psychotherapy remain similar—the gradual exploration with the patient of thoughts and conflicts not previously directly accessible to the conscious mind.

How illness is viewed Overt symptoms are merely the external expression of underlying psychic abnormality. Symptoms continue, despite the suffering they cause to the individual because of what Freud called *primary gain*. This is the benefit to the individual of not having unacceptable ideas in the conscious mind.

Rationale Traumatic experiences, particularly those in early life, give rise to psychological conflict. The greater part of mental activity is unconscious and the conscious mind is protected from the experience of this conflict by in-built defences, designed to decrease 'unpleasure' and to diminish anxiety. These defences are developmentally appropriate but their continuation into adult life results in either psychological symptoms or in a diminished ability for personal growth and fulfilment. Conflict can be examined with regard to the anxiety itself, the defence, or the underlying wish or memory. The individual's previous family and personal relationships will have symbolic meaning and be charged with powerful emotions. Representations of these relationships will emerge during therapy and provide a route towards understanding and change.

Techniques

- **Free association** The process of free association is the main route for the exploration of the unconscious. The 'fundamental rule' of psychoanalysis is that the patient agrees to reveal everything which comes to mind during free association, no matter how embarrassing or socially unacceptable (i.e. 'speaking without self-censorship'). Areas where free association 'breaks down' and areas of resistance to further associative thought suggest important areas to be explored at future sessions.
- **Examination of dreams** Dreams are viewed as being formed by an admixture of daytime memories, nocturnal stimuli, and representations of unconscious desires. This admixture, the 'latent dream', is converted to the 'manifest dream' by 'dream work'—a process of symbolisation and elaboration. This process can be consciously unravelled with a therapist to reveal something of the unconscious desire.
- **Examination of parapraxes** A parapraxis is a slip of the tongue, commonly now known as a 'Freudian slip'. Occasionally it reveals unconscious meaning, particularly in affect-laden situations.
- **Examination of the symbolism of neurotic symptoms** Individual patient symptoms may have symbolic meaning in the context of the patient's history, which can be usefully explored.
- **Exploration of transference/counter-transference** The most important areas of repression find expression in the transference relationship.
- **Interpretation** Expression of the therapist's understanding of the meaning of what is currently happening in therapy. May be about the

current defence mechanisms, explanation for current anxiety, or the presumed underlying desire.

- **Neutrality** The withholding of emotional support and directive advice.

Phases of treatment 1–5, 1-hour sessions per week. Therapy may last years rather than months.

- **Diagnostic and assessment sessions** Psychodynamic formulation of case. Assess patient suitability and motivation. Explore potential risk factors and formulate plan for dealing with these (e.g. potential development of suicidal behaviour in a socially unsupported patient). Explain methods of therapy. Establish ground rules
- **Early sessions** Formulation of problems. Identify unconscious defence mechanisms, key conflicts, style, and defects in personal development.
- **Later sessions** Balance between supportive techniques and interpretive techniques (which may increase anxiety). Clarification and guided exploration. Exploration of regression and resistance. Examination of counter-transference and review with supervisor. Interpretation.

Indications and contraindications See general indication for psychotherapy (p. 766). Used in patients where there are severe emotional symptoms which can be understood in psychological terms (e.g. personality disorder, mild to moderate depressive illness, significant impairment in social or interpersonal function). Relatively contraindicated for drug or alcohol dependency, harmful or suicidal 'acting out' behaviours, psychotic illness, or in those with severe depressive features.

Efficacy There is a lack of standardisation in diagnosis, method, control groups, and improvement measures in psychotherapeutic trials. Suggestive of enduring benefits in expressed symptoms, treatment-seeking, and need for medication. Long-term and enduring improvements noted, associated with length and completeness of treatment.

Training Involves education in psychoanalytic history, theory and practice; supervised case work; and personal psychoanalysis. In the UK practitioners are accredited with either the United Kingdom Council for Psychotherapy (UKCP) or the British Confederation of Psychotherapists (BCP).

Brief psychodynamic psychotherapy

Freud regarded the open-ended, non-time-limited method of therapy relying on non-guided free association as 'pure gold'. Nonetheless he recognised that practical considerations would see this alloyed with the 'bronze' of a briefer method where interpretation and guidance played a role. Brief psychodynamic therapy is an intervention where the concepts of symptom development and methods of therapy are based on those of psychoanalysis, but where the timescale and number of sessions are reduced. Although driven by economic factors, this is more similar to Freud's initial practice, where intervention was generally for less than one year. It involves 'active therapy', where the therapist attempts to guide free association on more focused topics.

Rationale Essentially that the benefits to the patient of the insights and opportunity for change and growth available from long-term psychoanalysis can be achieved in a shorter time scale and that introducing directive elements and focus on particular topics does not necessarily reduce overall treatment effectiveness.

How illness is viewed According to psychoanalytic theory.

Techniques The methods employed are those of dynamic psychotherapy but are more focused on the 'here and now'—the patient's current experience of the world, and techniques are employed to accelerate the process of therapy. These include:

- **Goal setting** Explicit identification of the anxiety and defences which are to be tackled.
- **Focus choosing** Identification of currently active problem. Repetitive behaviour or emotional response usually related to single transference figure. Explore symptom precipitants and associated early trauma and avoidance.
- **Active interpretation** Therapist may guide therapy by use of interpretation at an earlier point than in more prolonged methods.

Phases of treatment Lasts up to one year, usually 20–25 sessions with the termination date decided at outset.

- **Initial assessment** Diagnosis, consideration of appropriateness of this method of therapy in this patient (psychologically minded, ability to introspect and contemplate change, availability of external support, absence of psychotic or suicidal features). Consideration of appropriate use of medication.
- **Early sessions** Identification of 'central issue': an enduring and developmentally relevant anxiety which is stable over time and occurs in different situations. Limited comments from therapist. Usually there is positive transference due to expectation of 'magical' change. Identification of main defences, coping styles, and ability to accept and work with interpretations.
- **Middle sessions** Exploration of transference. Usual development of resistance.
- **Closing sessions** Anticipation of termination. Arrangements for aftercare. Management of the patient who 'reveals' new information near the end of therapy.

Indications and contraindications As for dynamic psychotherapy, appropriate in those individuals with emotional problems which can be understood in psychological terms. This briefer therapy may be more appropriate in those with clear and easily identifiable goals, problems which can be understood as a focal conflict, and where there are recent rather than chronic or life-long problems.

Efficacy Evidence for treatment effectiveness as measured in length of illness and global functional measures. Trials comparing effectiveness with other brief therapies (e.g. CBT and IPT) are required.

Group therapy

Psychotherapy can be defined as treatment based on a dialogue within a relationship. Group therapy methods involve a relationship with a specially created community, with the dialogue occurring between group members as well as with a therapist. Group methods were developed in the early 20th Century following observations of beneficial group effects in TB patients. Groups vary as to whether their patient population has single or multiple diagnoses; whether the therapist is actively involved or supervisory; whether the membership is closed or open after the group starts; and whether they exist for a fixed term or are ongoing.

Types of group

- **Activity groups** Used for patients unsuitable for other group activities. Focuses may be art, gardening, computing, etc. Used in LD, chronic psychosis, and other disorders with chronic functional impairment. Fosters social skills, adaptive behaviours, and allows confrontation of anxiety and phobias.
- **Support groups** Peer support in LD, chronic illness, and also for those caring for others. Therapist may have a psychoeducational role.
- **Problem-focused groups** E.g. alcohol or drug dependence, 'Hearing voices', sexual deviancy. No analytic work. Focus on mutual support with addition of group examination of strategies for change. Peers may be experts at identifying resistance and rationalisation for avoiding change in other group members. Where the problem is a chronic illness the therapist may again take on a psychoeducational role.
- **Psychodynamic groups** All of the above elements plus aim of lasting change through exploratory therapy. (Therapy may be viewed as individual therapy which takes place in the group setting, or as psychotherapy of the group as a whole.)

Techniques

- Free-ranging discussion—the group form of free association.
- Psychoeducation.
- Allowing the opportunity for individual members to confront the effects of their behaviour on others while providing a supportive milieu during change.
- Encouraging group specific process: *mirroring* (duplication of experience), *amplification* (increase in emotional resonance by sharing), *catharsis* (supported ventilation of emotion).
- Analysis of group dynamics (e.g. leadership, group structure, individual roles) to understand reasons for progress (or the lack of it).
- Clarification/interpretation/confrontation with individuals.
- Group curative factors described by Yalom[1] are: installation of hope, universality, imparting information, altruism, corrective of early family group, development of socialisation, imitation of adaptive behaviour, interpersonal learning, group cohesion, catharsis, existential factors.

Phases of therapy

- **Early sessions** Set-up and engagement, formulation of rules and establishment of goals, focus on leader.

- **Middle sessions** Adaptation, potential for conflict, discussion of authority, establishment, intimacy, and group coherence
- **Closing sessions** Negotiation of termination, agreement that goals have been achieved, reflection on experience of group.

1 Yalom I (1975) *The theory and practice of group psychotherapy.* Basic Books. New York.

Basic learning theory

Behavioural psychology is a method for understanding the development of knowledge and behaviours in organisms. In an individual organism these are shaped by environmental influences and can change as a result of experience. Learning theory concerns the testing of methods to produce behavioural change through changing environmental influences. The two basic learning processes are *classical (Pavlovian) conditioning*—learning what goes with what, and *operant (Skinnerian) conditioning*—learning to obtain reward and avoid punishment. Although most abnormal mental processes and mental illnesses are not amenable to understanding purely in terms of conditioning, understanding of learning theory is helpful in conceptualising the development and maintenance of abnormal mental processes and provides a rationale for behavioural and cognitive behavioural treatment approaches.

Classical conditioning In the initial experiment, Pavlov presented a dog with food which produced the response of salivation. Here the food is the unconditioned stimulus (US) and the salivation is the unconditioned response (UR). A neutral stimulus such as a bell ringing is not associated with any unconditioned response. However if a bell is rung immediately before the food is presented, after a number of repetitions the dog will salivate in response to the bell alone. Now the bell is a conditioned stimulus (CS) producing a conditioned response (CR), the salivation.

Acquisition The development of the association between the UR and the US producing a CR. In animal experiments this can take between 3 and 15 pairings. Where there is sufficient emotional involvement acquisition can occur with as few as one pairing.

Extinction The loss of the association between the CR and the CS. Occurs when the CS is repeatedly *not* followed by the US.

Generalisation The phenomenon where similar stimuli to the initial CS produce the response.

N.B. For emotional disorders the response is usually an emotion rather than a behaviour. For example, an initial encounter with a large, barking dog which bites the individual can produce the CR of fear to the generalised CS of seeing a dog. The affected individual may then avoid all contact with dogs and so avoid the unpleasant CR. However, because there is no occasion when the CS of seeing a dog is not paired with the CR of fear, there is no opportunity for extinction to take place.

Techniques based on classical conditioning concepts
- *Systematic desensitisation* (p. 784) Presentation of situations more and more similar to the CS are paired with relaxation techniques, in order to eventually break the association between the CS and the CR.
- *Flooding* (p. 784) Presentation of the full CS without the possibility of withdrawal from the situation. The initial unpleasant experience of the CR gradually diminishes.

Operant conditioning The experimental techniques and rules of operant conditioning were developed by Thorndike and refined by

Skinner. The basic principles of operant conditioning are that if a response to a stimulus produces positive consequences for the individual it will tend to be repeated, while if it is followed by negative consequences it will tend not to be repeated. In the original experiments rats were placed in a box containing a lever which, when pressed delivered a pellet of food. Eventually the rat would press the lever and be rewarded. The rat would then press the lever with increasing frequency. (Note that operant conditioning doesn't rely on insight on the part of the rat.)

Acquisition The linkage of the response (pressing the lever) with the reinforcer (receiving the food).

Reinforcement Can occur after every response (continuous reinforcement) or only after some responses (partial reinforcement). Behaviours conditioned by partial reinforcement extinguish at a much slower rate than those conditioned by continuous reinforcement.

Extinction Occurs when the response is no longer followed by the reinforcer.

Techniques based on operant conditioning concepts
* Behaviour modification (p. 784).
* Aversion therapy (p. 784).

Behaviour therapy

Techniques based on learning theory are utilised in order to extinguish maladaptive behaviours and substitute adaptive ones.

Systematic desensitisation Holds as a central tenant the principle of *reciprocal inhibition* (i.e. anxiety and relaxation cannot coexist). Systematic graded exposure to the source of anxiety is coupled with the use of relaxation techniques (the 'desensitisation' component). Effective for simple phobias, but less so for other phobic/anxiety disorders (e.g. agoraphobia). Process in a typical case is as follows:

• Patient identifies the specific fear (e.g. cats).
• Patient and therapist develop *hierarchy* of situations provoking increasing levels of anxiety, (e.g. stroking a cat on one's knee > touching a cat > having a cat in the room > looking at pictures of cats > thinking about cats).
• Patient is instructed in relaxation technique.
• Patient experiences the lowest item on the hierarchy while practising the relaxation technique *and remains exposed to the item until the anxiety has diminished*.
• The process is repeated until the item no longer produces anxiety.
• The next item in the hierarchy is tackled in similar fashion.

Flooding/implosive therapy High levels of anxiety cannot be maintained for long periods, and a process of 'exhaustion' occurs. By exposing the patient to the phobic object and preventing the usual escape or avoidance, there is extinction of the usual (maladaptive) anxiety response. This may be done *in vivo* (flooding) or in imagination (implosion).

Behaviour modification Based on operant conditioning. Behaviour may be *shaped* towards the desired final modification through the rewarding of small, achievable intermediate steps. This can be utilised in behavioural disturbance in children and patients with learning disability. Other forms of behavioural modification include the more explicit use of secondary reinforcement, such as 'token economy', in which socially desirable/acceptable behaviours are rewarded with tokens that can be exchanged for other material items or privileges, or 'star charts' where children's good behaviour is rewarded when a certain level is achieved.

Aversion therapy and covert sensitisation The use of negative reinforcement (the unpleasant consequence of a particular behaviour) to inhibit the usual maladaptive behavioural response (extinction). True 'aversion' therapy (e.g. previously used to treat sexual deviancy) is not used today, however, covert techniques (e.g. the use of Antabuse in alcohol dependency) can be (at least partially) effective.

Cognitive behaviour therapy

Cognitive behaviour therapy (CBT) was developed by Beck in the 1960s and described in *Cognitive Therapy of Depression*[1]. Its development was prompted by the observation that patients referred for psychotherapy often held ingrained, negatively skewed views of themselves, their future, and their environment. Treatment is based on the idea that disorder is caused not by events, but by the view the patient takes of events. It is a short-term, collaborative therapy, focused on current problems, whose goals are symptom relief and development of new skills.

Rationale Behaviours and emotions are determined by the person's cognitions. Some pathological emotions are as a result of 'cognitive errors'. While underlying emotions are not amenable to examination and behavioural change, the cognitions are. If the person can be helped to understand the connection between cognitive errors and distressing emotion, they can try methods of change. CBT aims to 'change the way you feel by changing the way you think'.

How illness is viewed In some personality types and in mental illness there are errors in the perception of risk, logical errors, and errors in the processing of information (i.e. cognitive distortions). These distortions relate to self, world, and future (Beck's cognitive triad). The model is: events → faulty cognitive appraisal → emotional response → maladaptive behaviour → (behaviours/emotions) = pathology. Cognitive errors thus lead to dysphoria and maladaptive behaviour. These errors originate in childhood learning, internalised family/cultural attitude, and early traumatic experiences. The cognitive model is a guide for therapy, not a comprehensive model of illness causation, and does not preclude neurochemical or other factors as important in symptom development nor preclude the use of pharmacological treatments.

Techniques The therapist is very active in CBT. The patient and the therapist are viewed as working together in spirit of scientific enquiry to explore the problem and solutions—'collaborative empiricism'. The therapist aims to assist the patient to: monitor cognitions; identify cognitive errors; understand maladaptive schema; and explore with them strategies to challenge and change these and examine the resultant symptomatic effects. CBT makes use of behavioural, cognitive, and experimental techniques to treat patients.

- **Behavioural techniques** Activity scheduling; graded assignments; exposure; response prevention; distraction; relaxation training; assertiveness/social skills training.
- **Cognitive techniques** Psychoeducation, including reading assignments (e.g. 'Coping with depression'); identifying automatic thoughts; Socratic questioning ('If that were true, what would it mean... and what would *that* mean... etc.?'); role play; thoughts diary; examining the evidence (e.g. 'let's suppose that's true—what happens then?'); 'working through the options'; thought rehearsal.

Phases of treatment A short-term treatment, with the initial assessment being followed by 6–20, hour-long sessions. Clinical attention is primarily focused on events in the 'here and now'. Each session generally proceeds as follows: deal with emergencies; jointly set agenda; review homework task; feedback; focus on specific items guided by current problems; suggestion of cognitive or behavioural techniques to challenge automatic thoughts/core schema; give homework.

Indications and contraindications CBT is considered as an active treatment requiring patient understanding and collaboration. Patients should therefore be motivated and be able to link thought and emotions. In addition to the general contraindications to psychotherapy (p. 766), CBT is contraindicated in LD and dementia. Indicated in:
- Mild to moderate depressive illness.
- Eating disorders (anorexia nervosa and bulimia nervosa).
- Anxiety disorders.
- In selected patients, may have a role in personality disorder, substance abuse, and in the management of chronic psychotic symptoms.

Efficacy There is good evidence for effectiveness in depressive illness, eating disorders and anxiety disorders. CBT is at least as effective as pharmacotherapy[2] in mild to moderate depression and may be more effective in long-term follow-up (e.g. at preventing relapse).

Cognitive errors
CBT identifies two levels of cognitive errors: *automatic thoughts* and *core schemas*. Automatic thoughts can be perpetuated by never being challenged consciously or by novel experience. Schemas are a person's 'rules' for behaving, based on fundamental beliefs and shaped by previous (and current) experiences.

Automatic thoughts
- Selective abstraction
- Arbitrary inference
- All or nothing thinking
- Magnification/minimisation
- Personalisation
- Catastrophic thinking
- Overgeneralisation

Fundamental beliefs (in schema)
- Basic rules for making sense of environmental information, (e.g. 'a person must do every thing right to be successful', 'a good person always retains emotional control').

---

1 Beck AT, Rush AJ, Shaw BF, *et al.* (1979) *Cognitive therapy of depression.* New York, Guilford.

2 Dobson KS (1989) A meta-analysis of the efficacy of cognitive therapy for depression. *J Consult Clin Psychol* **57**, 414–19.

Rational emotive therapy

Developed by Albert Ellis in 1955. A 'reality-based', short-term therapy aimed at 'cognitive re-structuring', with many similarities to the later developed CBT.

Rationale Harmful emotions and personally dysfunctional behaviours can arise as a result of irrational thinking (see opposite). Individuals retain responsibility for their own emotions and actions and can effect change to their patterns of irrational thinking. As well as reducing harmful emotions and behaviours, this change in thinking can produce greater personal satisfaction, potential for growth, and ability to resolve future negative events successfully.

How illness is viewed Emotional suffering is a secondary problem to the primary practical problems which are inevitable and part of life. It is the person's emotional reaction to an event, rather than the event itself, which determines the degree of distress. Irrational ideas can cause emotional suffering in the absence of external trauma.

Techniques Therapy proceeds by guiding the patient to identify, challenge, and change their irrational thoughts. These can be viewed as a series of 'musts' relating to oneself, others, and the environment. So, for example:

* 'I must always be on top of things or else I'm no good at what I do'
* 'Others must be there for me, otherwise they don't care at all'
* 'Life must be free of worry otherwise I won't be able to cope'

The therapist aims to encourage the patient to examine their basic beliefs; to encourage the replacement of irrational with rational thinking; and to examine the resultant change in their emotional response. Therapy is active, focused on the 'here and now', and is largely a teaching and learning process. The therapist uses guided discussion, logic, real-life challenges, and appropriate humour to challenge irrational thinking.

Phases of treatment

* **Early sessions** Explain rationale for therapy and explore current stresses and negative events. Explore 'musts' and question their basis. Direct patient towards activities which question irrational beliefs.
* **Middle sessions** Go beyond awareness of irrational thinking and explore the maintenance of emotional disturbance and self-defeating patterns of thinking.
* **Later sessions** Guide the development of new patterns of thinking and enable the patient to observe and minimise the development of future maladaptive thinking patterns.

Indications and contraindications Useful in mild to moderate depression, anxiety disorders, eating disorders. Contraindications are those to any psychotherapy (p. 766).

Efficacy There is evidence that RET is better than placebo or 'treatment as usual' for mild to moderate depression and anxiety disorders[1].

1 Engels GI, Garnefski N, Diekstra RF (1993) Efficacy of rational-emotive therapy: a quantitative analysis. *J Consult Clin Psychol.* **61**, 1083–90.

However, its similarity to CBT means that most recent meta-analyses include RET with CBT when looking at outcomes, making comparisons with other cognitive/behavioural or pharmacological therapies difficult.

Ellis identified 12 basic irrational beliefs

- Everyone should love and approve of me for me to be lovable at all.
- I should always be successful and 'on top of things'; if I'm not, I'm a failure.
- People who are bad should be made to 'pay the price'.
- I can't stand it when things do not go the way planned.
- External events cause most of my unhappiness and as I don't have any control over these things I can't do anything about my problems.
- When the situation is going badly I can't help worrying all the time.
- It is easier for me to avoid thinking about tense situations.
- I need someone to be with and lean on.
- Things have been this way so long, I can't do anything about these problems now.
- When my close friends and relatives have serious problems it is only natural that I get very upset too.
- I don't like the way I'm feeling but I can't help it. I just have to accept it.
- I know there is an answer to every problem and I should be able to find it.

Most of these fall into 4 basic categories: **unwarranted conclusions, misattribution of cause, catastrophising**, and **overgeneralising**.

Interpersonal therapy

Interpersonal therapy (IPT) was developed in the 1970s by Klerman and Weissman as a treatment for depressive illness and later developed for use in other disorders. It is a time-limited and disorder-focused therapy which deals with symptoms in the 'here and now'. It is described in a manual for practitioners[1] and a guide for patients[2].

Rationale The development of psychopathology can be understood as a result of life events occurring at any time in life. Emotional problems are best understood by studying the interpersonal context in which they arise. Life events related to illness development include: grief, interpersonal disputes, change of role, and interpersonal deficits. These events are not viewed as directly causing the episode of illness, but helping the patient to understand their role in the evolution of illness and resolving the interpersonal problem is seen as a route to recovery. The therapy's role in various disorders is rooted in RCT evidence for efficacy.

How illness is viewed Illnesses are viewed as medical disorders and are diagnosed according to standard criteria (e.g. DSM-IV) and rated in severity by rating scales (e.g. BDI). The patient is diagnosed as ill and explicitly given the 'sick role' with its benefits (freedom from guilt at condition, time-out from normal social role) and responsibilities (to seek treatment and get better).

Techniques The focuses of treatment are the current interpersonal relationships and their relationship to the development of illness. Interventions are directed at dysfunctions in social relationships rather than underlying beliefs (cf. CBT). Basis for planning treatment is inventory of all close relationships. Focus is on role transitions (e.g. new mother, job loss) or role dispute (e.g. work difficulties, relationship problems).

Phases of treatment Treatment lasts for 12–16, hour-long weekly sessions, roughly divided into three phases:
- **Phase one (sessions 1–2)** Standard psychiatric history; risk assessment; diagnosis and communication of diagnosis to patient; establishment of the 'sick role'; explanation of rationale for treatment and its aims and processes; assessment of need for psychotropic medication and prescription if indicated; completion of interpersonal inventory (description of current relationships); and psychotherapeutic formulation based on identifying the extent of problems in any of four areas mentioned above.
- **Phase two (sessions 3–11)** Each session begins with enquiry as to events since the last session. The therapist is directive and hopeful about the possibility of change which may be minimised by a depressed patient. The patient is encouraged to identify and carry through change in interpersonal relationships and to test the possibility of consequent improvement in their symptoms. Therapeutic techniques are specific to the problem under review; they include role-play, catharsis, facilitation of grief, and relationship problem-solving. 'Role disputes' can be resolved by renegotiation, acceptance of impasse, or dissolution.
- **Phase three (sessions 12-end)** Assessment of improvement; plan for termination of therapy or exploration of other form of treatment; identification and planning for the possibility of re-emerging symptoms.

Indications
- Mild to moderate depressive illness
- Bulimia nervosa
- Dysthymic disorder

Patients without significant social dysfunction do best. Possibly indicated especially in atypical depression. It is not indicated in the treatment of substance abuse or as monotherapy in patients with severe depression or psychotic features.

Efficacy The efficacy of IPT is currently being assessed in panic disorder, bipolar disorder, borderline PD, and somatisation disorder, and indications may broaden in the future. RCT evidence of similar outcome to imipramine treatment in major depression with improved psychosocial functioning at 1-year follow-up.

1 Klerman GL, Weissman MM, Rounsaville BJ, Chevron ES. (1984) *Interpersonal therapy of depression.* Basic books, New York.

2 Weissman MM. (1995) *Mastering depression: a patient guide to interpersonal psychotherapy.* Graywind Publications, Albany, New York.

Cognitive analytic therapy

Cognitive analytic therapy (CAT) is a relatively new therapy method introduced by Anthony Ryle in 1990. It aims to bring together ideas from both dynamic and behavioural therapies by attempting to explain psychoanalytic ideas in cognitive terms.

Rationale Problems such as depression, anxiety disorders, and interpersonal difficulties cause emotional suffering and also hinder the ability of the individual to make positive change. These problems can often be understood in the context of an individual's history and early experiences and can be prolonged by habitual coping mechanisms. Through collaborative therapy these mechanisms can be identified, understood, and changed.

How illness is viewed Traumatic childhood and adolescent experiences can give rise to coping mechanisms to protect the individual from conscious distress. These maladaptive mechanisms can be inappropriately maintained into adult life when they give rise to emotional symptoms such as anxiety and depression and destructive behaviours such as self-harm. Although harmful these behaviours are maintained by 'neurotic repetition'. Neurotic repetition has 3 essential patterns:

- **'Traps'**—negative assumptions generate acts that produce consequences, which in turn reinforce assumptions.
- **'Dilemmas'**—a person acts as if available actions or possible roles are limited and polarised (called 'false dichotomy') and so resists change.
- **'Snags'**—appropriate goals or roles are abandoned either because others would oppose them or they are thought to be 'forbidden' or 'dangerous' in light of personal beliefs.

Techniques The 'three Rs' of CAT are recognition of maladaptive behaviour and beliefs, reformulation of these (the main 'work' of therapy), and revision. The reformulation is agreed between therapist and patient and documented in a 'psychotherapy file'. This reformulation is expressed in narrative and diagrammatic form and considers both past history and current problems. It is used throughout therapy to guide the active focus, to set homework, and to enable recognition of transference/countertransference.

Phases of treatment Therapy involves active participation from both parties.

- **Assessment** Explanation of rationale of method of therapy. Planning of number and timing of sessions (8–24 sessions, normally 12).
- **Early sessions** *(1–3)* Patient asked to begin 'psychotherapy file' exploring common traps, dilemmas, and snags. Diary keeping to monitor moods and behaviours. Recapitulation of early experiences and narrative of current relationships.
- **Middle sessions** *(4–8)* Agreement on reformulation of problems with written and diagrammatic description of 'target problem procedures'. Exploration of methods of change, (called 'exits') via work in sessions and in homework.
- **Ending sessions** *(9–12)* Identification and recapitulation of key themes which emerged during therapy. Both therapist and patient

write 'goodbye' letters summarising progress and formally closing the relationship. There may be a planned 3-month review appointment.

Indications and contraindications As for other cognitive therapies.

EfficacyOngoing RCTs examining effectiveness in personality disorders and comparing CAT with other methods.

Dialectical[1] behavioural therapy

Dialectical behaviour therapy (DBT) is an integrative therapy drawing on ideas from behavioural, cognitive and psychodynamic therapies, as well as from Eastern philosophy and meditation techniques. It was introduced in 1991 by Marsha Linehan[2,3] and colleagues as a treatment for borderline personality disorder.

Rationale Patients with borderline personality disorder suffer from significant psychiatric morbidity and a mortality related to completed suicide. They are a difficult group of patients to treat as their characteristic patterns of behaviour tend to challenge therapeutic progress and exhaust therapist resources ('burnout'). Such individuals can however learn more adaptive responses later in life, with subsequent improvement in functioning and quality of life and reduction in morbidity and mortality.

How illness is viewed A combination of abnormal early experiences ('invalidating environment') and currently poorly understood biological factors leaves some individuals with abnormal emotional reactions to life events and interpersonal crises. They also have less well-developed methods of coping with their own emotional responses (less 'emotional modulation') and a habitual pattern of maladaptive behaviours, (e.g. self-harm). Lack of emotional modulation means that the person will look to others to assist with emotional stress but will also have a limited ability to maintain relationships.

Techniques

Hierarchical view of treatment aspirations

* Reduction in behaviours which cause harm (DSH and suicidal).
* Reduction in behaviours which interfere with therapy.
* Reduction in behaviours which diminish quality of life and personal relationships.

Cognitive and behavioural methods

* Person of, and relationship with, the therapist seen as the main 'reinforcer' of adaptive behaviour and in-therapy analysis of maladaptive behaviour seen as aversive.
* DBT involves a variety of approaches: individual therapy group skills training (emotional understanding, tolerance of distress, Eastern meditation techniques), availability of the therapist for telephone contact between appointments.
* Key techniques include: *validation* (recognising distress and behaviours as legitimate and understandable but ultimately harmful) and *problem solving* (agreeing with patient a more appropriate approach given all the evidence).

Preserving therapist morale Therapist supported by group of other DBT therapists.

Phases of treatment

- **Assessment** Orientation and commitment to therapy. Commitment to therapy for specific period. Aim at reduction of DSH and suicidal behaviours. Specific attention to those behaviours which inhibit successful therapy. Attendance at other therapies as directed.
- **Stage 1** Focuses on suicide and DSH prevention with recording of episodes, exploration of internal and external antecedents. Weekly DBT skills group introduces basic skills (e.g. 'mindfulness training', focusing on the 'here and now', and learning to tolerate aversive states). DSH may be viewed as understandable in the context of the patient's current situation but the therapist always argues on the side of life and ways of making it more tolerable.
- **Stage 2** Focuses on emotional processing of previous traumatic experiences. Underlying historical causes of dysfunction. Memories of abuse. Flashbacks. Exposure and distress tolerance techniques.
- **Stage 3** Aims to develop self-esteem and establish future goals. Self-esteem and adaptive behaviours are individual agreed goals.

Indications and contraindications DBT methods are described specifically for patients with borderline personality disorder.

Efficacy The original DBT group produced RCT evidence of reduced DSH, reduced admission, and improved retention in therapy compared with 'treatment as usual'.

1 'Dialectic' refers to a means of arriving at the truth by examination of the argument (the 'thesis' the contradictory argument—the 'antithesis') and resolving them into a coherent 'synthesis';

2 Linehan MM (1993) *Cognitive-Behavioral Treatment of Borderline Personality Disorder*. New York: The Guilford Press.

3 Linehan MM (1993) *Skills Training Manual for Treating Borderline Personality Disorder*. New York: The Guilford Press.

Legal and ethical issues

Introduction

To practise psychiatry one needs to have some knowledge of several areas of law which relate to people with mental disorders. Broadly this could all be called 'forensic psychiatry' (see definition on p. 624), but in this book areas of criminal law relevant to psychiatry are covered in Chapter 15 on forensic psychiatry, and other legal issues (which could broadly be labelled 'civil matters') are covered here.

This chapter deals broadly with two areas:

- Mental health legislation: the compulsory treatment of people with mental disorder.
- Other civil matters: consent, confidentiality, and driving.

As mentioned in Chapter 15 on forensic psychiatry, law is parochial and dynamic. The practitioner needs to be aware of the current law in their jurisdiction. This chapter will focus on the UK and the Republic of Ireland. The same abbreviations for the four main jurisdictions will be used as in Chapter 15 (i.e. E&W, Scot, NI, and RoI). As this is written, we are in the middle of reform of mental health and/or incapacity legislation in all these jurisdictions (p. 624).

Mental health legislation—general principles and background

Why do we have mental health legislation?

There are three main reasons for the existence of legislation allowing and regulating the compulsory treatment of mental disorder:

- Mental disorder may impair ability to make decisions about treatment.
- Provision of safeguards and protection for vulnerable patients.
- Prevention of harm to self and others.

The development of mental health legislation

Mental health legislation in the UK and RoI has its origins in 18th-century vagrancy laws allowing the confinement of the 'furiously mad and dangerous' and in laws regulating private madhouses. The former primarily arose out of concerns about potential harm and the latter out of concerns regarding the interests of vulnerable patients. Impaired ability to make decisions about treatment has not featured explicitly in consideration of mental health legislation until recent years.

Treatment of patients with mental illness (lunacy and insanity) and learning disability (idiocy, imbecility, feeble-mindedness) was largely institutional in asylums until the second half of the 20th Century. Laws developed to regulate the detention of patients and the scrutiny of their care. Voluntary treatment in hospital was not available until 1930.

Current legislation in the UK has its origins in the Report of Lord Percy's 'Royal Commission on the Law relating to Mental Illness and Mental Deficiency' (1957). This led to very similar legislation in E&W, Scot, and NI, which arose in the context of optimism about the treatment of mental disorder, emphasis on voluntary treatment where possible, and the beginning of treatment in the community. Concerns about patient's rights led to updates of legislation in the 1980s leading to the current Acts in the UK.

In the RoI, developments were similar to the UK until the mid 20th Century when the Mental Treatment Act 1945 was enacted. However, there has been little significant change in Irish mental health legislation until very recently.

What's in a Mental Health Act?

A modern Mental Health Act should cover the following areas:

- *Definition* of mental disorder: who are the individuals covered by the Act?
- *Criteria* for compulsion: under what conditions can involuntary measures be used when treating these individuals?
- *Compulsory interventions*: what can be done when individuals meet these criteria? This includes procedures for emergency detention, longer-term detention/compulsion, and for the giving of specific treatment.
- *Safeguards*: Limits, scrutiny, and review of whether the individual should be subject to compulsion and of the compulsory measures authorised.
- *Bodies to monitor operation of Act*: For example legal forum for appeal and review, and independent commission to monitor and scrutinize.

Using mental health legislation

When using mental health legislation the following points should be borne in mind:

- Be aware of the current legislation in your jurisdiction.
- Codes of practice, guidance, and/or notes are available that give practical guidance on the use of legislation.
- Have a detailed knowledge of the parts of the legislation you need to use day to day, and particularly in emergency situations.
- Know where to go for further information and advice (e.g. guidance material, senior colleagues, legal personnel, commission).
- Be wary of mental health 'lore'. Much misinformation about legislation is promulgated without reference to what is actually correct. For example, many believe that UK legislation does not permit the detention of someone who is drunk, even if they are also depressed or acutely psychotic.
- The law cannot resolve clinical dilemmas. For example, if a detained patient takes an overdose, mental health legislation cannot be used to impose physical treatment. This does not mean that you can do nothing knowing that you are acting (or not acting) legally. In this situation common law may allow, and medical ethics may dictate, that physical treatment be imposed.
- Although it is useful, and essential, to have access to the relevant statute, it is impossible to get an understanding of how the law works in practice through reading legislation alone. This develops through experience, training, consulting guidance material, and discussion with colleagues.

Reform of mental health legislation

Mental health legislation is in the process of being renewed in all the jurisdictions under consideration in this chapter. Scot and the RoI have new Acts which are in the process of implementation. E&W have a draft bill which is controversial and has missed two Queen's speeches; there is uncertainty as to the form and timing of a new Act. In NI, legislation is currently being reviewed.

In this chapter the main provisions of the most recently passed legislation for each jurisdiction will be described.

Mental health legislation—England and Wales (1)

Introduction

The Mental Health Act 1983 sets out relevant procedures for E&W. There has been a process of review of mental health legislation, culminating in a draft Bill in 2002[1]. However, this has not been well received, mainly due to its overemphasis on public protection and underemphasis on the rights of individuals with mental disorder.

Principles

The Act itself does not set out any guiding principles, but some are set out in the Code of Practice: recognition of basic human rights under the European Convention of Human Rights (ECHR); respect for individuality without discrimination; taking needs fully into account, but recognising that, within available resources, it may not always be practicable to meet them in full; giving any necessary treatment or care in the least restrictive environment; promoting, self-determination and personal responsibility, consistent with patients' needs and wishes; discharging patients from detention or other powers as soon as it is clear that their application is no longer justified.

Definition of mental disorder

'Mental disorder' is defined under section 1(2) as meaning 'mental illness, arrested or incomplete development of mind, psychopathic disorder and any other disorder or disability of mind'.

There are four recognised categories of mental disorder:

- Mental illness which is not further defined.
- Severe mental impairment defined as 'a state of arrested or incomplete development of mind which includes severe impairment of intelligence and social functioning and is associated with abnormally aggressive or seriously irresponsible conduct on the part of the person concerned'.
- Mental impairment defined as 'a state of arrested or incomplete development of mind (not amounting to severe mental impairment) which includes significant impairment of intelligence and social functioning and is associated with abnormally aggressive or seriously irresponsible conduct on the part of the person concerned'.
- Psychopathic disorder defined as 'a persistent disorder or disability of mind (whether or not including significant impairment of intelligence) which results in abnormally aggressive or seriously irresponsible conduct on the part of the person concerned'.

The following are *excluded* if they are the *only* 'conditions' present: promiscuity, other immoral conduct, sexual deviancy, dependence on alcohol or drugs.

Other definitions

Approved doctor Under section 12(2) the Secretary of State may approve a registered medical practitioner as having special experience in the diagnosis and treatment of mental disorder. This is done in practice through the regional health authority. Some sections require one of the recommendations from an approved doctor.

Responsible medical officer (RMO) The registered medical practitioner in charge of the patient's treatment, usually the consultant.

Approved social worker (ASW) A social worker who has undergone specific training and assessment and is appointed for the purposes of the Act as having competence in dealing with individuals with mental disorder (section 114).

Nearest relative Usually determined by who is first on the following list (section 26(1)): husband or wife, son or daughter, father or mother, brother or sister, grandparent, grandchild, uncle or aunt, nephew or niece. If two relatives are of equal standing then the elder prevails. If a patient lives with a relative, or has lived with a non-relative as a spouse for 6 months, then that person is the nearest relative.

Mental Health Review Tribunal (MHRT) Legal forum to which a patient or a nearest relative can appeal against detention (p. 809). The MHRT has 3 members: a legally qualified chairperson, a medical practitioner, and a lay member. It must discharge a patient if the criteria for detention no longer apply.

Mental Health Act Commission (MHAC) The body that monitors and regulates the operation of the Act (p. 805).

Second Opinion Appointed Doctor (SOAD) An independent doctor appointed by the Secretary of State (in practice by the Mental Health Act Commission), who gives a second opinion regarding treatment which can be given without the patient's consent under Section 57 or Section 58.

Criteria for compulsory intervention

The criteria for compulsory intervention are less stringent for emergency or shorter-term measures (i.e. sections 2, 4, 5) than for longer-term measures (i.e. section 3). The criteria for detention under section 3 are:

- The person suffers from at least one of the four categories of mental disorder (the category must be specified) of a nature or degree which makes it appropriate for the person to receive medical treatment in hospital.
- If the category is psychopathic disorder or mental impairment then such treatment should be likely to alleviate or prevent a deterioration in the condition.
- It is necessary for the health or safety of the patient or for the protection of other persons that the person should receive such treatment and it cannot be provided unless he is detained.

For sections 2, 4, and 5 the category of mental disorder does not need to be specified and the nature or degree of the disorder should warrant detention for assessment (rather than treatment).

1 See http://www.dh.gov.uk/PublicationsandStatistics/Publications/PublicationsLegislation/PublicationsLegislationArticle/fs/en?CONTENT_ID=4008466&chk=HBBEEq.

Mental health legislation—England and Wales (2)[1-4]

Compulsory measures

The main procedures allowing compulsory detention in hospital are section 2 (admission for assessment), section 3 (admission for treatment), section 4 (emergency admission), and section 5 (2) (emergency detention of informal inpatient). Compulsory admission should usually be under section 2 or 3; section 4 should only be used rarely, in a genuine emergency where an approved doctor is not available soon enough.

Emergency detention Section 4 allows the emergency detention of patients who have not yet been admitted to hospital (this includes those in accident and emergency, outpatients, and day hospitals); section 5(2) is similar but applies to patients who have already been admitted to hospital (whether in a psychiatric or non-psychiatric ward).

For section 4 the application is made by the nearest relative or ASW and requires a recommendation from one registered medical practitioner.

For section 5(2) the medical recommendation must be by the RMO or his nominated deputy; this will usually be the duty SHO, but the nomination should be made before the relevant period of duty. Involvement of the nearest relative or ASW is not required for section 5(2).

The duration of detention is 72 hours, during which an assessment must be undertaken to determine if detention under section 2 or 3 is warranted.

Section 5(4) allows nurses (of the prescribed class) to hold an informal inpatient in hospital for up to 6 hours to allow for a medical assessment.

Admission for assessment An application for detention under section 2 may be made by the nearest relative or ASW and requires two medical recommendations, one of which must be by an approved doctor. Duration of detention is 28 days. Following the section 2 an application may be made for detention under section 3. Alternatively the patient may remain in hospital informally or be discharged.

Admission for treatment An application for detention under section 3 is made in a similar manner to section 2. Duration of detention is initially 6 months, which may be renewed for a further 6 months, and then 12 monthly thereafter.

Guardianship Section 7 allows for a patient to be placed on guardianship if they suffer from a specified mental disorder, are over 16 years old, and it is necessary for their welfare or the protection of others. The application procedure and renewal is similar to section 3. The guardian (the local authority or someone acceptable to them) may specify where the person should reside.

Treatment of patients subject to compulsion

- A patient detained in hospital (except under emergency provisions) may be given *medication* for mental disorder for up to 3 months, whether they consent and/or have capacity or not.
- Under section 58, *medication* for over 3 months or *ECT* requires the patient's consent (the RMO completes form 38) or, if the person

refuses or is incapable of consenting, agreement of a SOAD (who issues a form 39).
- Under section 62, *treatment that is urgently necessary* may be authorized by the RMO without consent or a second opinion; this is usually used for giving ECT to severely ill and at-risk patients while awaiting a second opinion.
- Under section 57, the patient's consent and agreement of a SOAD are required if any patient (whether detained or informal) is to receive *neurosurgery for mental disorder* or surgical implantation of hormones to reduce male sex drive.

Leave, absconding, and transfer

Procedures allow for patients to be granted leave of absence with the authorisation of the RMO (section 17); for patients to be taken into custody and returned to hospital if they abscond (section 18); and for patients to be transferred between hospitals (section 19).

Review

Patients subject to emergency detention have no right of appeal. Patients detained under section 2 or 3, or subject to guardianship under section 7, may appeal to a MHRT. The nearest relative may also appeal against section 3 or 7. One appeal is allowed during each period of compulsion. The RMO may terminate a patient's detention at any point. Hospital managers and nearest relative (if not opposed by RMO) may also discharge a patient.

Mental Health Act Commission

The MHAC monitors the use of the MHA and the care of patients subject to it. It also investigates certain complaints, appoints second opinion doctors, and maintains the Code of Practice. It produces a biennial report.

---

1 Bartlett, P. and Sandland, R. (2000) *Mental Health Law—policy and practice.* London: Blackstone Press Ltd.

2 Cope, R. (1995) Mental Health Legislation. In *Seminars in Practical Forensic Psychiatry* (eds. Chiswick D and Cope R). London: Gaskell.

3 Department of Health and Welsh Office (1999) *Mental Health Act 1983 Code of Practice* (3rd edition). London: The Stationery Office.

4 Hogett, B. (1996) *Mental Health Law.* London: Sweet and Maxwell.

Mental health legislation—England and Wales (3)

Aftercare following detention

Care programme approach and section 117 aftercare

Section 117 places a statutory duty on health and social services to provide aftercare for patients who have been discharged from detention under sections 3, 37, 47, or 48 (the last 3 are sections used for mentally disordered offenders, see Chapter 15). The framework within which this aftercare is planned and implemented is the Care Programme Approach (CPA) which was introduced in 1991, but has been significantly modified recently. The CPA should be used for all patients where appropriate, even if they have not been detained in hospital. For patients in hospital the CPA process should start well before discharge.

The key aspects of CPA are:
- A coordinated assessment of the patient's health and social care needs.
- The development of a care plan addressing the identified needs, which will be agreed by the patient and any carers who are involved.
- An identified care coordinator who will be the main contact and will monitor the care plan.
- Regular reviews of the care plan with changes as necessary.

The CPA should be integrated with care management (the process of care coordination used by social services).

There are two levels of CPA: *standard* and *enhanced*:
- *Standard CPA* may be appropriate for patients who: require the support or intervention of one agency or discipline; require only low-key support from more than one agency or discipline; are more able to self-manage their mental health problems; have an active informal support network; pose little danger to themselves or others; are more likely to maintain appropriate contact with services.
- *Enhanced CPA* may be appropriate for patients who: have multiple care needs requiring inter-agency coordination; are only willing to cooperate with one professional or agency but have multiple care needs; may be in contact with a number of agencies (including the criminal justice system); are likely to require more frequent and intensive interventions; are more likely to have mental health problems coexisting with other problems such as substance misuse; are more likely to be at risk of harming themselves or others; are more likely to disengage with services.

Supervision registers, which identify patients particularly at risk to themselves or others, have been abolished with the introduction of enhanced CPA.

A patient may not be compelled to accept or participate in any aspect of aftercare under section 117. When the aftercare services are no longer required the section 117 duty ends.

Supervised discharge

The Mental Health (Patients in the Community) Act 1995 introduced 'aftercare under supervision' (also called supervised discharge), inserted as sections 25A–25J of the 1983 Act. Essentially, this may be used to add a degree of compulsion to section 117 aftercare.

The grounds for an application are:
• The patient has at least one of the four forms of mental disorder.
• There would be a substantial risk of serious harm to the health or safety of the patient, or the safety of other persons, or of the patient being seriously exploited, if they were not to receive the aftercare services provided.
• Being subject to supervised discharge is likely to help to secure that the patient does actually receive the aftercare services

Requirements which can be imposed on the patient include:
• That the patient lives at a specified place.
• That the patient attends at specified places and times for the purpose of medical treatment (but treatment cannot be given without consent), occupation, education, and/or training.
• That the following people may be given access to the patient at their place of residence: the supervisor who is named in the application, any doctor, any ASW, any other person authorised by the supervisor.

An application is made by the RMO to the Health Authority supported by recommendations from an ASW and the potential community RMO (CRMO). Consultation with a number of people involved with the patient is required before applying for, varying, or renewing the order. The order lasts for 6 months commencing when the patient ceases to be liable to detention. Renewal, appeal to MHRT, and discharge are similar to sections 3 and 7. Procedures allow for detention in hospital where the person meets criteria for detention (p. 804), but not solely on the basis of a breach of the conditions of the order.

Mental health legislation—Scotland (1)

Introduction

The Mental Health (Care and Treatment) (Scotland) Act 2003[1] replaces the Mental Health (Scotland) Act 1984[2]. The main provisions of the 2003 Act will be implemented in 2005, so until then the 1984 Act will operate. As the 2003 Act is in the process of implementation there is no practical guidance or experience available at the time of writing, although a Code of Practice should be available in 2004.

Principles

The new Act emphasises the protection of the rights of mentally disordered patients and shifts the emphasis from detention in hospital to treatment for mental disorder, whether in hospital or the community. A number of principles to guide the use of the Act are set out under sections 1&2: taking into account the patient's past and present wishes; taking into account the views of the named person, carer, guardian, or welfare attorney; allowing the patient to participate as fully as possible; providing maximum benefit to the patient; not discriminating against the patient; providing appropriate services; taking into account the needs and circumstances of carers; using the least restrictive measures possible; and, if the patient is a child, best securing their welfare.

Definition of mental disorder

Section 328 defines 'mental disorder' as 'any mental illness, personality disorder or learning disability' however caused or manifest. None of these terms are further defined.

The following are excluded if they are the only 'conditions' present: sexual orientation; sexual deviancy; transsexualism; transvestism; dependence on, or use of, alcohol or drugs; behaviour that causes or is likely to cause, harassment, alarm, or distress to any other person; acting as no prudent person would act.

Other definitions

Approved medical practitioner (AMP) Under section 22 these are doctors with the necessary qualifications and experience, who have undertaken training, and are approved by a Health Board as having special experience in the diagnosis and treatment of mental disorder.

Responsible medical officer (RMO) The registered medical practitioner in charge of the patient's treatment, usually the consultant.

Mental health officer (MHO) A social worker, with the necessary registration, experience, education, training, and competence in dealing with individuals with mental disorder; appointed under section 32 of the Act.

Designated medical practitioner (DMP) Medical practitioners appointed by the MWC to give second opinions regarding the medical treatment of patients subject to compulsion.

Care plan A document that sets out the care, treatment, and services that it is proposed that a patient subject to compulsion should receive. It will include compulsory and non-compulsory measures.

Named person Someone nominated by a person under section 250 to support them and protect their interests. Entitled to be informed about certain decisions and to act on the patient's behalf in certain circumstances. If one has not been nominated then it is the primary carer or nearest relative. For a child under 16 it is a parent.

Advance statement May be made under sections 275 and 276. When making this the person must have capacity and must make it in writing with a witness. It may be withdrawn at any point if the person has capacity. When carrying out duties under the Act must 'have regard to the wishes specified in the advance statement'. If act against these wishes this must be recorded in writing with reasons, and a copy of this record must be sent to patient, named person, welfare attorney, guardian, MWC.

Advocacy Under section 259 every person with mental disorder has right of access to independent advocacy, and it is the duty of local authority and health board to ensure availability of this.

Mental Health Tribunal (MHT) The legal forum (replacing the Sheriff Court) for making decisions regarding applications for certain compulsory orders, proposals to amend compulsory orders, and appeals against compulsory orders. Three members: legal, medical, and general.

Mental Welfare Commission (MWC) Similar to the MHAC for E&W but has wider remit and powers (p. 811).

Criteria for compulsory intervention

Less stringent for emergency and shorter-term measures (i.e. parts 5 and 6) than they are for longer-term measures (i.e. part 7). The criteria for compulsion under a part 7 compulsory treatment order (CTO) are:
- The person has a mental disorder.
- Medical treatment is available which would be likely to prevent that disorder worsening or be likely to alleviate the symptoms or effects of the disorder.
- There would be a significant risk to the patient's health, safety, or welfare, or to the safety of another person if such treatment were not provided.
- The patient's ability to make decisions about the provision of medical treatment is significantly impaired because of their mental disorder.
- The making of the order is necessary.

For short-term (part 6) or emergency (part 5) detention it only has to be likely that the criteria apply, and the second criterion above regarding treatability does not need to be considered.

---

1 Scottish Executive (2003) *An introduction to the Mental Health (Care and Treatment) (Scotland) Act 2003*. Edinburgh: Scottish Executive. (For information about the implementation of the 2003 Act see *http://www.scotland.gov.uk/health/mentalhealthlaw*)

2 This is not described here—for information on the 1984 Act see the Addendum for Scotland by Chiswick in: Cope R (1995) Mental Health Legislation. In *Seminars in Practical Forensic Psychiatry* (eds. Chiswick D and Cope R). London: Gaskell.

Mental health legislation—Scotland (2)

Compulsory measures

The main compulsory orders are set out under part 5 (emergency detention), part 6 (short-term detention), and part 7 (compulsory treatment order).

Emergency detention Under part 5 any fully registered medical practitioner may grant a certificate authorising the detention of a person in hospital for 72 hours. Consent from a MHO is necessary (unless this is impracticable), the situation must be urgent and such that making arrangements for short-term detention under part 6 would involve 'undesirable delay'. There are not separate procedures for inpatients and outpatients. As soon as is practicable the patient should be assessed by an AMP to determine if detention under part 6 should be applied or if the patient should be dealt with informally.

Nurses' holding powers (section 299) may be used for up to 2 hours and continue for 1 hour after the doctor has arrived.

Short-term detention Under part 6 any AMP may grant a certificate authorising the detention of a person in hospital for 28 days. Consent from a MHO is necessary in all cases. At the end of the order the patient may be discharged, remain as an informal patient, or may be placed on a CTO.

Compulsory treatment order (CTO) Under part 7 an application may be made to a MHT for a patient to be made subject to a CTO authorising compulsory treatment in hospital or in the community for 6 months. The application is made by a MHO and has three components: two medical reports (one by an AMP and the other by the patient's GP or another AMP), a report prepared by the MHO, and a proposed care plan (prepared by the MHO in consultation with the RMO and others who will be involved in the care and treatment of the patient).

The MHT must be satisfied that the criteria for a CTO (see above) are met; if there are issues that require clarification the MHT may grant an interim compulsory treatment order for 28 days instead. A CTO in the community may make requirements as to residence, attendance for treatment and other services, access of staff to the patient's residence, and acceptance of medication for mental disorder (see below). A CTO may be renewed for 6 months, then annually thereafter, without further application to a MHT unless some variation to the order is proposed.

If a patient on a community-based CTO refuses medication then they may be taken to hospital and detained there for up to 6 hours to receive this. If the patient is non-compliant with other aspects of the order, then detention in hospital for up to 72 hours can be authorised by the RMO; this may be extended by a further 28 days with the approval of the RMO and MHO to allow an assessment as to whether an application should be made for the CTO to be varied.

Treatment of patients subject to compulsion (part 16)

• A patient subject to compulsion (except under emergency provisions) may be given *medication* for mental disorder for up to 2 months, whether they consent and/or have capacity or not. Patients under compulsion in the community cannot be given medication using physical force.

- Medication for over 2 months requires the patient's consent or, if the person refuses or is incapable of consenting, authorisation by a DMP.
- ECT may only be given if a patient can and does consent, or if incapable of consenting with the authorisation of a DMP. ECT cannot be given, even in an emergency to a patient with capacity who refuses.
- Treatment that is *urgently necessary* may be authorised by the RMO without consent or a second opinion; this may be used for giving ECT to severely ill and at-risk patients lacking capacity while awaiting a second opinion and for giving medication to acutely disturbed patients on emergency detention.
- To receive *neurosurgery for mental disorder* there must be an independent opinion from a DMP that the treatment will be beneficial, two opinions from lay people appointed by the MWC that the person has capacity and consents, or if they do not have capacity, that they do not object. If the person has incapacity but is not objecting, the treatment must be authorised by the Court of Session.

Leave, absconding, and transfer

Procedures allow for 'suspension of detention' of patients detained in hospital so that they may leave hospital; the taking into custody and return of patients who abscond either from hospital or the residence specified in a community based CTO; and for patients to be transferred to other hospitals.

Review

A patient or their named person may appeal to the MHT against being subject to a CTO or short-term detention (but not emergency detention), against transfer to another hospital, and against being held in conditions of excessive security (from May 2006). This may happen once during each renewed period of compulsion for CTOs. An RMO must refer a case to the MHT if a variation is proposed in an order (e.g. from a community-based to hospital-based order). The MWC may also refer cases to the MHT. If the MHT has not reviewed a case for 2 years then it must do so without a specific referral being made. The MHT must cancel an order if the criteria for compulsion are no longer met. The RMO and MWC also have the power to cancel an order at any point if the criteria for compulsion are no longer met.

Mental Welfare Commission

The MWC has a statutory duty to protect individuals with mental disorder whether they are liable to detention or not. It also has the power to discharge patients subject to compulsion. It has a responsibility to visit and inspect services and the power to conduct enquiries into deficiencies in care. It has new duties to monitor the operation of the Act and promote best practice.

Mental health legislation—Northern Ireland (1)

Introduction

The Mental Health (Northern Ireland) Order 1986 sets out relevant procedures. There is currently a wide ranging review of mental health issues including a review of legislation (see http//www.rmhldni.gov.uk).

Definition of mental disorder

Article 3 defines 'mental disorder' as meaning 'mental illness, mental handicap and any other disorder or disability of mind'. There are further definitions of types of mental disorder:

- 'Mental illness'—'a state of mind which affects a person's thinking, perceiving, emotion or judgement to the extent that he requires care or medical treatment in his own interests or the interests of other persons'.
- 'Mental handicap'—'a state of arrested or incomplete development of mind which includes significant impairment of intelligence and social functioning'.
- 'Severe mental handicap'—'a state of arrested or incomplete development of mind which includes severe impairment of intelligence and social functioning'.
- Severe mental impairment defined as 'a state of arrested or incomplete development of mind which includes severe impairment of intelligence and social functioning and is associated with abnormally aggressive or seriously irresponsible conduct on the part of the person concerned'.

The following are excluded if they are the only 'conditions' present: personality disorder, promiscuity or other immoral conduct, sexual deviancy, or dependence on alcohol or drugs.

Other definitions

Mental Health Review Tribunal for Northern Ireland (MHRTNI) Legal forum to which a patient or a nearest relative can appeal against detention (p. 815). The MHRT has 3 members: a legally qualified chairperson, a medical practitioner, and a lay member. It must discharge a patient if the criteria for detention no longer apply.

Mental Health Commission for Northern Ireland (MHCNI) Like MWC in Scot has broader remit than the MHAC in E&W (p. 815).

Appointed doctor The MHCNI appoints medical practitioners for the purposes of Part II (compulsory admission to hospital and guardianship). These doctors are analogous to approved doctors in E&W. Doctors may also be appointed for the purposes of Part IV (consent to treatment). The term 'appointed doctor' on these pages is used to refer to Part II.

Responsible medical officer (RMO) The registered medical practitioner in charge of the patient's treatment, usually the consultant.

Approved social worker (ASW) A social worker who has undergone specific training and assessment and is appointed for the purposes of the Order as having competence in dealing with individuals with mental disorder.

Nearest relative The person caring for the patient who is first on the following list (article 32): spouse, child, parent, brother or sister, grandparent, grandchild, uncle or aunt, nephew or niece. If there was no carer, then the first person on the list is the nearest relative. If two relatives are of equal standing then the elder prevails.

Criteria for compulsory intervention

The criteria for compulsory intervention are less stringent for emergency and shorter-term measures (i.e. articles 4 and 7(2)) than they are for longer-term measures (i.e. article 12). The criteria for compulsion under article 12 are:

- The patient is suffering from mental illness or severe mental impairment of a nature or degree which warrants his detention in hospital for medical treatment.
- Failure to so detain the patient would create a substantial likelihood of serious physical harm to himself or to other persons.
- Consideration has been given to whether other methods of dealing with the patient are available and to why they are not appropriate.

For article 4 the type of mental disorder does not need to be specified, and for article 7(1) it must appear that the article 4 criteria are met.

Mental health legislation—Northern Ireland (2)

Compulsory measures

Article 4 allows detention in hospital for assessment which may be followed by detention for treatment under article 12. Article 7(2) allows for the detention of a patient already in hospital.

Admission for assessment An application for detention under article 4 may be made by the nearest relative or ASW and requires one medical recommendation. This should be by the patient's GP or a doctor who knows the patient, if this is practicable, and should not, except in urgent cases, be by a doctor on the staff of the admitting hospital. Immediately on admission to hospital the patient must be examined by the RMO, an appointed doctor, or another doctor, who must submit a report to the responsible authority. They may then be detained for 7 days from the point of admission (this is limited to 2 days where the examination is not by the RMO or an appointed doctor, during which the RMO should examine the patient). Detention may be extended by a further 7 days on one occasion following a further report from the RMO. Following detention under article 4 a patient may be detained under article 12, remain informally, or be discharged.

Assessment of patient already in hospital Under article 7(2), where a person is a voluntary inpatient, if it appears to a doctor on the staff of the hospital that an application for assessment ought to be made, then a report may be furnished to the responsible authority, allowing detention for 48 hours. This may be followed by detention under article 4.

Detention for treatment Where a patient has been detained under article 4, they may be further detained for 6 months under article 12. This requires a recommendation from an appointed doctor (not the doctor who made the assessment recommendation). This may be renewed for a further 6 months and annually thereafter.

Guardianship Article 18 allows for guardianship. The application is made by the nearest relative or ASW, and there must be two medical recommendations and an ASW recommendation. The patient must be suffering from mental illness or mental handicap, and guardianship should be necessary in the interest of the patient's welfare. Renewal is as for article 12.

Nurses' holding powers Article 7(3) allows nurses (of the prescribed class) to detain an inpatient in hospital for up to 6 hours to allow for a medical assessment regarding detention. Detention under article 7(3) ends when the doctor arrives.

Treatment of patients subject to compulsion

Articles 62–69 set out very similar provisions regarding consent to treatment as set out for E&W by the 1983 Act (p. 804).

Leave, absconding, and transfer

Procedures allow for patients to be granted leave of absence with the authorisation of the RMO (article 15); for patients to be taken into custody and returned to hospital if they abscond (article 29); and for patients to be transferred between hospitals (article 28).

Review

MHRTNI operates in a very similar way to E&W, but must review a detained patient if they have not been reviewed for 2 years. After reviewing a case the MHCNI may refer a patient to the MHRTNI or may recommend that the patient be discharged. The RMO may discharge a patient at any point. Nearest relative may also discharge a patient if not opposed by RMO.

Mental Health Commission for Northern Ireland

The functions of the MHCNI are very similar to those of the MWC in Scot: the duty to protect individuals with mental disorder whether they are liable to detention or not; the power to recommend discharge of patients subject to compulsion; the responsibility to visit and inspect services; and the power to conduct enquiries into deficiencies in care.

Mental health legislation—Republic of Ireland (1)

Introduction

There is new legislation, the Mental Health Act 2001. This has not been fully implemented yet, but in effect replaces the Mental Treatment Act 1945 and various modifying Acts passed in 1953, 1961, and 1981. As the 2001 Act is in the process of implementation there is no practical guidance or experience available at the point of writing, although a Code of Practice will be available[1].

Principles

Section 4 sets out some principles to be considered in operating the Act. The best interests of the person should be the principle consideration with due regard being given to the interests of others who may be at risk of serious harm; the person should be notified of proposals and should be allowed to make representations regarding these which should be given due consideration; any decision should give due regard to the right of a person to dignity, bodily integrity, privacy, and autonomy.

Definition of mental disorder and criteria for compulsion

Section 3 sets out the definition of mental disorder, which also includes the criteria for compulsory detention.

'Mental disorder' is defined as 'mental illness, severe dementia, or significant intellectual impairment where—

(a) because of the illness, disability or dementia, there is a serious likelihood of the person concerned causing immediate and serious harm to himself or herself or to other persons, or

(b) (i) because of the severity of the illness, disability or dementia, the judgment of the person concerned is so impaired that failure to admit the person to an approved centre would be likely to lead to a serious deterioration in his or her condition or would prevent the administration of appropriate treatment that could be given only by such admission, and

(ii) the reception, detention and treatment of the person concerned in an approved centre would be likely to benefit or alleviate the condition of that person to a material extent.'

- 'Mental illness' means a state of mind of a person which affects the person's thinking, perceiving, emotion, or judgement and which seriously impairs the mental function of the person to the extent that he or she requires care or medical treatment in his or her own interest or in the interest of other persons.
- 'Severe dementia' means a deterioration of the brain of a person which significantly impairs the intellectual function of the person thereby affecting thought, comprehension, and memory and which includes severe psychiatric or behavioural symptoms such as physical aggression.
- 'Significant intellectual disability' means a state of arrested or incomplete development of mind of a person which includes significant impairment of intelligence and social functioning and abnormally aggressive or seriously irresponsible conduct on the part of the person.

Under section 8 the following are *excluded* if they are the *only* conditions present: personality disorder, being 'socially deviant', and being addicted to drugs or intoxicants.

Other definitions

Approved centre Hospitals or other inpatient facilities for the treatment of people suffering from mental disorder. Must be registered with the MHC.

Review tribunal The legal forum which reviews the making of every admission and renewal order. Has three members: a legally qualified chairperson, a consultant psychiatrist, and another member.

Mental Health Commission (MHC) The body responsible for monitoring the standards of mental health services and protecting detained patients. Has a more direct role in the latter than similar bodies in the UK (see below).

Inspector of Mental Health Services Consultant psychiatrist appointed by MHC to visit and inspect approved centres and to review mental health services. Will also review individual cases when visiting centres.

Mental health commission

The MHC was established in April 2002. Its main purpose is to promote, encourage, and foster the establishment and maintenance of high standards and good practices in the delivery of mental health services, and to protect the interests of detained patients. It is notified of every episode of detention and renewal, appoints tribunals, maintains a panel of consultants to undertake independent examinations, appoints an Inspector of Mental Health Services, maintains a register of approved centres, makes regulations as to the use of seclusion and restraint, and prepares codes of practice and other documents.

1 For further information see: *http://www.irishstatutebook.ie/ZZA25Y2001.html* or *http://www.oasis.gov.ie/health/mental_health/mental_health_act_2001.html*

Mental health legislation—Republic of Ireland (2)

Compulsory measures

Application for involuntary admission (section 9)

An application for admission may be made under section 9 by a spouse or relative, an authorised officer (of the health board), a Garda, or any other person (with certain exclusions applying). The applicant must have seen the person within the last 48 hours.

Medical assessment (section 10)

Within 24 hours of the application being made a medical practitioner (who does not work at the approved centre where the person may be admitted) should examine the person. The doctor should inform the person about the purpose of the examination, unless this would be detrimental to the person. If the doctor considers the person to be mentally disordered then a recommendation may be made allowing involuntarily admission to an approved centre. This remains in force for 7 days.

Power of the Garda to detain and apply for involuntary admission (section 12)

The Garda make take a person into custody if they have reasonable grounds to believe that the person is mentally disordered and because of this there is a serious likelihood of the person harming themselves or others. They may forcibly enter premises if necessary. The Garda would then follow the usual application for involuntary admission procedure (section 9). If this application is granted the Garda must take the person to the approved centre.

Removal to an approved centre (section 13)

The applicant is responsible for getting the person to the approved centre. If not possible then the doctor making the recommendation may request that staff from the centre do this. The Garda may be asked for assistance.

Admission to approved centre (sections 14 and 15)

When the person is admitted to the approved centre a consultant psychiatrist must examine them (section 14). They may be held for 24 hours to allow this examination. If this psychiatrist is satisfied that the person is suffering from mental disorder then an 'admission order' is made.

Under section 15 an admission order authorises the detention and treatment of the patient in the centre for 21 days. This may be renewed (as a 'renewal order') for 3 months initially, then 6 months, and then annually thereafter. The consultant responsible for the patient must make the renewal following an examination in the week before making the renewal order. When an order (admission or renewal) is made the consultant must send a copy to the MHC and a written notice to the patient (section 16).

Voluntary patients wishing to leave an approved centre

Previously a voluntary patient had to give 3 days' notice of intention to leave. Under section 23 a voluntary patient may leave hospital at any point unless a consultant psychiatrist or doctor or nurse on the staff considers that they suffer from mental disorder. If this is the case they may be detained for up to 24 hours. During this period the responsible consultant must either discharge the patient or arrange an examination by another consultant. If this consultant is of the opinion that the patient is mentally disordered then they issue a certificate and the patient is detained as they would be under an admission order (section 14).

Treatment of patients subject to compulsion (Part 4)

The consent of a patient to treatment is required except where the consultant psychiatrist considers that the treatment is necessary to safeguard the life of the patient, to restore his or her health, to alleviate his or her condition, or to relieve his or her suffering, and the patient is incapable of giving such consent because of mental disorder.

- Neurosurgery for mental disorder may not be performed unless the patient consents and it is authorised by a tribunal.
- ECT may not be given unless the patient gives consent, or where the patient is unable or unwilling to give consent, the therapy is authorised by the responsible consultant psychiatrist and another consultant psychiatrist.
- Medication for the amelioration of the mental disorder for more than 3 months cannot be given unless the patient consents or, where the patient is unable or unwilling to give consent, the continued medication is authorised by the consultant psychiatrist responsible for the patient and by another consultant psychiatrist. This must be renewed every 3 months.

Review

When the MHC receives a copy of an order it must refer the case to a tribunal, assign a legal representative to the patient if they do not have one, and direct that a member of the panel of consultant psychiatrists appointed by the MHC reviews the case (section 17).

Within 21 days of the making of the order the tribunal must review the detention. The tribunal may affirm or revoke the order depending on whether the criteria for detention are met (section 18). An appeal against a tribunal's decision may be made to the Circuit Court (section 19).

Leave, absconding, and transfers

Procedures allow for patients to be allowed to be absent from the approved centre with the authorisation of the consultant responsible for their care (section 26); for patients to be taken into custody and returned to an approved centre if they abscond (section 27); and for patients to be transferred to other approved centres and hospitals (sections 20, 21, and 22).

Consent to treatment

Forms of consent

Treatment of a patient must be with their consent (or in Scotland with the consent of a proxy). To proceed without consent is an assault. For consent to be valid it must be *informed*, (i.e. the patient has fully understood the details and implications of what is proposed). Consent may be *implied* (i.e. the patient does not object to and cooperates with the procedure) or may be *express* (i.e. oral or written permission is explicitly asked for and recorded, often as a detailed consent form). Generally, express consent is obtained for non-trivial or invasive procedures, and for some interventions is mandatory.

Reviewing consent Even if there is a signed consent form, always review the patient's decision close to the time of treatment, particularly when:

- Significant time has elapsed between obtaining consent and the start of treatment.
- There have been material changes in the patient's condition or in any aspects of the proposed treatment plan which might invalidate the patient's existing consent.
- New, potentially relevant information has become available (e.g. about the risks of the treatment or about other treatment options).

Points to note

- Always respect the patient's autonomy—they have a right to decide whether or not to undergo any medical intervention even where a refusal may result in harm to themselves or in their own death.
- Patients must be given sufficient information, in a way that they can understand, to enable them to exercise their right to make informed decisions about their care.
- This right is protected in law, and you are expected to be aware of the legal principles set by relevant case law in this area (if in doubt, consult your medical defence union or other professional body e.g. BMA, GMC—see 'Useful addresses' p. 919)
- Effective communication is the key to enabling patients to make informed decisions. Take appropriate steps to find out what patients want to know and ought to know about their condition and its treatment. This will strengthen the quality of the doctor/patient relationship and lead to a more satisfactory collaborative working relationship.
- Always document any discussions, the decision(s) taken, and the form of consent given, in the medical records.

Advance statements

Sometimes, in cases where a patient has a progressive disease, although they currently lack **capacity** (p. 822) to consent or refuse treatment, they may have previously indicated their preferences in an advance statement ('advance directives' or 'living wills'). These wishes should be given due regard provided:

- The decision in the advance statement is clearly applicable to the present circumstances.
- There is no reason to believe that the patient has changed his/her mind.

If you act against an advance statement, then you should be able to justify this. Where such a statement is not available, the patient's known wishes should be taken into account using the principles outlined in **'Best interests'** (p. 823).

Emergencies

In emergency situations, it may not be possible to obtain consent (e.g. in an unconscious RTA victim requiring drainage of an extradural haematoma). Under **common law** (p. 822) 'necessity' provides a defence against a potential criminal charge that you have assaulted a patient by giving non-consentual treatment. A doctor may therefore give emergency treatment to preserve life and prevent significant deterioration in health. However, any valid advance refusal which you know about, or is drawn to your attention, should be considered. It is also good practice to inform the patient what has been done, and why, as soon as they are sufficiently recovered to understand.

Treatment without consent

The issue of treating patients without consent (p. 12) arises frequently in a psychiatric context. In general, the principles and scope of compulsory treatment for mental disorder are covered in mental health legislation (pp. 800–19). However, in certain circumstances in all fields of medicine, situations may arise where decisions must be made regarding issues of acting against the patient's wishes, treatment without consent, and capacity. Often a psychiatrist's opinion will be sought—particularly in a liaison setting—because, by the nature of their work, most psychiatrists will have greater knowledge of, and familiarity with, legal issues than their medical counterparts. Often a patient's reasons for withholding consent may be thought to be due to a (possibly undiagnosed) mental disorder. Where this is the case, other professionals may not feel they have the clinical skills to make this diagnosis. When making these difficult decisions, several key principles should be understood:

Common law is the law not derived from statutes (Acts of Parliament). It mainly comprises rulings of judges in cases where the existing law is not sufficiently comprehensive—'test cases'. Common law differs between various jurisdictions.

Emergency treatment As noted on p. 821, in *common law* 'necessity' may provide a doctor with a defence against assault where non-consensual treatment is given. There may be situations (e.g. the use of sedation in a patient with acute behavioural disturbance [p. 896] where there is a suspected physical or psychiatric cause) when the doctor has to act against a patient's wishes, in order to adequately carry out their *duty of care* (see below). Treatment in these situations is given under *common law* even if the patient fulfils the criteria for detention under emergency mental health legislation (p. 821).

Capacity is a legal concept meaning the ability to enter into valid contracts. It is gained on adulthood and is presumed to be present throughout the lifespan unless permanently or temporarily lost. To treat a capable patient without consent would be an assault. Although capacity is a legal concept, doctors may be called on to give an assessment of capacity in order to decide on the ability of the patient to give informed consent or enter into another contract (e.g. to make a will). To be capable the patient must be able to:

• understand the decision
• understand the alternative courses of action
• assess which courses of action would be reasonable
• retain memory of decisions and the reasons for them
• communicate their intent

Scotland (currently) stands alone in the UK in having specific legislation covering incapacity (Adults with Incapacity [Scotland] Act 2000[1]), allowing for the issuing of a 'certificate of incapacity' to replace consent in adults who do not meet the above criteria. It is completed by the 'medical practitioner primarily responsible for the medical treatment of an adult' and gives authority to 'do what is reasonable in the circumstances, in relation to the medical treatment, to safeguard or promote the physical or mental health of the adult'. It does not cover emergency situations, which remain guided by principles of *common law*. Any decisions about treatment should be guided by the principles noted under **'Best interests'** (see below).

Duty of care Medical negligence occurs where there is a duty of care to a patient, where there is a breach of that care, and where harm results as a result of that breach. Any patient is owed a duty of care by the doctors treating them. A breach of that care is a standard of care that falls below what would be expected of a doctor at that level of experience (i.e. the standard is lower for an SHO than a consultant). It is often helpful in making decisions to consider risk of being accused of negligence against risks of being accused of other things. For example, if an elderly man recovering after hip replacement becomes confused and demands to leave the ward, the decision is between (1) agreeing to his demand (and being vulnerable to accusations of negligence for not providing an adequate standard of care for a delirious post-op patient) and (2) confining him to the ward (and accepting the risk of being accused of false imprisonment/ assault/misuse of the Mental Health Act).

'Best interests' When determining what treatment may be in the best interests of a patient who lacks capacity to decide, consider:

- Only those options for treatment or investigation which are *clinically* indicated (i.e. likely to be of benefit to the patient).
- Which option least restricts the patient's future choices—in cases where there is more than one option (including non-treatment) that could be viewed as reasonable and in the patient's best interests.
- Any evidence of the patient's previously expressed preferences, including any advance statements (p. 820), or the views of significant third parties (e.g. the patient's partner, family, carer, guardian [Scotland] or a person with parental responsibility).
- Any knowledge you (or other health professionals) are aware of regarding the patient's background (e.g. cultural, religious, or employment considerations).

Always:
- Be open to the views of others, particularly members of the health care team and next of kin.
- Consider the patient's views in respect of areas of decision making for which they may have 'residual capacity'.

Applications to the court In difficult situations (e.g. where a patient's capacity to consent is in doubt, or where differences of opinion about 'best interests' cannot be resolved satisfactorily), consult more experienced colleagues and, where appropriate, seek legal advice on whether it is necessary to apply to the court for a ruling. The court's approval is always necessary where a patient lacks capacity to consent to a medical intervention which is controversial (e.g. sterilisation, organ donation, withdrawal of life support).

1 For detailed information, the text of the Act is available at: *http://www.scotland-legislation.hmso.gov.uk/legislation/scotland/acts2000/20000004.htm*, with guidance notes on Part 5 (Medical treatment and research) at: *http://www.scotland.gov.uk/health/cmo/mcpasprint.pdf*.

Issues of confidentiality

'Whatever ... I may see or hear in the lives of men which ought not to be spoken abroad I will not divulge, as reckoning that all such should be kept secret.'

Hippocratic Oath

Patients' right to confidentiality

Patients have a right to expect that information about them will be held in confidence by their doctors. Confidentiality is central to trust between doctors and patients. Without assurances about confidentiality, patients may be reluctant to give doctors the information they need in order to provide good care. If you are asked to provide information about patients you should:

- Seek patients' consent to disclosure of information wherever possible, whether or not you judge that patients can be identified from the disclosure.
- Anonymise data where this will serve the intended purpose.
- Keep disclosures to the minimum necessary.
- Always document and be prepared to justify your decisions.

Protecting information

- Doctors have a professional responsibility to ensure patient information is effectively protected against improper disclosure at all times.
- Many improper disclosures are unintentional—do not discuss patients where you can be overheard or leave patients' records, either on paper or on screen, where they can be seen by other patients, unauthorised health care staff, or the public (see table opposite).
- Allowing for issues of personal safety, ensure that as far as possible your consultations with patients are private.

Sharing information with others providing care

- Make sure that patients are aware that personal information about them will be shared within the health care team, and of the reasons for this.
- Respect the wishes of any patient who does not wish specific information to be shared in this way, unless to do so would put others at risk of death or serious harm.
- Where patients have consented to treatment, express consent is not usually needed before relevant personal information is shared to enable the treatment to be provided safely and ensure continuity of care (e.g. medical secretaries typing letters to GPs, referrals for further investigations, referrals to other specialists).

Medical reports

This includes both specific requests for a particular report on *current* medical problems and disclosure of information from existing medical records for a third party (e.g. court report, insurance claim, benefits claim). In these circumstances:

- Satisfy yourself that the patient has been told about the purpose of the examination and/or disclosure, the extent of the information to be disclosed, and the fact that relevant information cannot be concealed

or withheld. (Showing the form or letter of request to the patient may assist in ensuring the patient understands the scope of the information requested.)
- Obtain evidence of written consent to the disclosure from the patient or a person properly authorised to act on the patient's behalf.
- Disclose only information relevant to the request made.
- Include only factual information you can substantiate, presented in an unbiased manner.
- Always check whether the patient wishes to see their report (The Access to Medical Reports Act 1988 entitles patients to see reports written about them before they are disclosed, in most circumstances.)
- Disclosures without consent to employers, insurance companies, or any other third party, can be justified only in exceptional circumstances (e.g. to protect others from risk of death or serious harm—see 'Breaking confidentiality').

Recent developments

In its report in 1997 the Caldicott Committee made a number of recommendations aimed at improving the way the NHS handles and protects patient information. A key recommendation was the establishment of organisational guardians to oversee access to patient-identifiable information. These 'Caldicott Guardians' have been established and are responsible for internal protocols and policies on the use of such information, and on its disclosure. A key principle is that of 'the need to know'.

Confidentiality expectations—the reality

Despite confidentiality being one of the main foundations of the 'privileged' doctor-patient relationship, expectations about where personal information may be reasonably disclosed varies amongst patients and medical professionals at different stages of their training:

Where information revealed	Patients	House staff	Medical students
Large professional meeting	69%	94%	81%
To office nursing staff	50%	69%	83%
Identified by name to other physicians	23%	60%	55%
Told as a story at a party:			
To other physicians	18%	60%	57%
To non-physicians	9%	36%	45%
Told to spouse or 'friend'	17%	51%	70%

Weiss B (1982) Confidentiality expectations of patients, physicians, and medical students. *JAMA* **247**: 2695.

Breaking confidentiality

Personal information should not be disclosed to a third party (e.g. relative, partner, solicitor, police officer, or officer of a court) without the patient's express consent, except in the circumstances described below. If you decide to disclose confidential information against a patient's wishes, you must document this decision in the patient's notes and be prepared to explain/justify your decision (and communicate this decision to the patient).

Disclosures to protect the patient or others

In this case, the risk to third parties is so serious that it outweighs the patient's privacy interest, and the appropriate person or authority should be informed without undue delay. Examples of such circumstances include:

- Where a colleague, who is also a patient, is placing patients at risk as a result of illness or other medical condition. (If you are in doubt about whether disclosure is justified, consult an experienced colleague, or seek advice from a professional organisation. The safety of patients must come first.)
- Where a patient continues to drive, against medical advice, when unfit to do so. In such circumstances you should disclose relevant information to the medical adviser of the Driver and Vehicle Licensing Agency without delay. Fuller guidance is given on pp. 828–32.
- To assist in the prevention or detection of a serious crime (i.e. where someone may be at risk of death or serious harm) (e.g. threats of violence—see 'The Tarasoff Case' opposite) or suspected child abuse (p. 614).

Disclosure in connection with judicial or other statutory proceedings

Under certain circumstances disclosure of information is required by law:

- Notification of a known or suspected communicable disease.
- If ordered to do so by a judge or presiding officer of a court (unless the information appears to be irrelevant e.g. details of relatives or partners of the patient not party to the proceedings).
- To assist a Coroner, Procurator Fiscal, or other similar officer in connection with an inquest or fatal accident inquiry (only *relevant* information should be provided).
- An official request from a statutory regulatory body for any of the health care professions, where disclosure is necessary in the interests of justice and for the safety of other patients.

Difficult situations

- Children and other patients who may lack competence to give consent (see p. 822).
  - Always try to persuade them to allow an appropriate person (e.g. individual with parental responsibility) to be involved in the consultation.
  - Always inform the patient (and their relative or carer) prior to passing on information to other responsible person or statutory agency (e.g. social services).

- Document in the patient's record the steps you have taken to obtain consent and the reasons for deciding to disclose information.
- Where a person lacks capacity, disclosure should be in that person's best interests and follow the other basic principles regarding confidentiality.
- Situations of dual responsibilities (i.e. contractual obligations to third parties, such as companies or organizations) (e.g. occupational health services, insurance companies, benefits agencies, police forensic medical advisors, armed forces, prison services), as well as obligations to patients.
  - Always ensure patients are aware of the purpose of the consultation, and to whom you are contractually obliged to release information (see 'Advice on medical reports', p.00).
- **If in doubt, consult** (in UK):
  - General Medical Council (GMC): guidance may be found at *http://www.gmc-uk.org/standards/secret.htm*
  - Royal College of Psychiatrists (RCP): guidance may be found at *http://www.rcpsych.ac.uk/publications/cr/cr85.htm*
  - *And consult* Your medical defence union (e.g. The Medical Protection Society (MPS): *http://www.mps.org.uk*; The Medical Defence Union (MDU): *http://www.the-mdu.com/*; or The Medical and Dental Defence Union of Scotland (MDDUS): *http://www.mddus.com/*

The Tarasoff Case

On October 27, 1969, Prosenjit Poddar killed his ex-girlfriend, Tatiana Tarasoff. Two months earlier, Poddar had declared his intentions during an outpatient appointment with his psychotherapist, Dr. Lawrence Moore at the University of California at Berkeley's Cowell Memorial Hospital. Dr. Moore tried to have Poddar confined to a mental institution for observation (including asking the university police for assistance). When law enforcement agents decided that Poddar was harmless and released him, Moore's director, Dr. Harvey Powelson, requested that all evidence of contact between Moore and the police department be destroyed. No one, including Dr. Moore, pursued the case further.

After the murder, Tatiana's parents became aware of this prior knowledge and sued the university regents, hospital, and police department, claiming that, at least, a warning should have been issued to her. On July 1 1976 (more than 6½ years after the murder) the Supreme Court of California found that the defendants had breached their duty to exercise reasonable care. In other words, physicians and therapists have a duty to warn third parties of threatened danger arising from a patient's violent intentions. As, a final statement, the Court stated that, 'protective privilege ends where public peril begins'.

Note: *Although often quoted when discussing issues of confidentiality, this case has no legal bearing in the UK. Even in the USA the impact of the Tarasoff case has been less dramatic and intrusive than one might expect.*

Fitness to drive

Principles and legal definitions

- The Driver and Vehicle Licensing Authority (DVLA) in the UK sets out minimum medical standards of fitness to drive and the requirements for mental health in broad terms (pp. 830–2).
- A clear distinction is made between the standards needed for Group 1 (cars and motorcycles) and Group 2 (lorries and buses) licences, the latter being more stringent due to the size of vehicle and the greater time spent at the wheel.
- 'Severe mental disorder' is defined by Section 92 of the Road Traffic Act 1988 as 'mental illness, arrested or incomplete development of the mind, psychopathic disorder or severe impairment of intelligence or social functioning'.
- The standards set reflect not only the need for an improvement in the mental state but also a period of stability, such that the risk of relapse can be assessed should the patient fail to recognise any deterioration.
- The standards for patients with misuse of or dependency on alcohol or drugs are detailed on p. 562.

Notes on medication

- Section 4 of the Road Traffic Act 1988 states that 'any person who is driving or attempting to drive on the public highway, or other public place whilst unfit due to any drug, is liable to prosecution'.
- All drugs acting on the central nervous system can impair alertness, concentration, and driving performance. This is particularly so at initiation of treatment or soon after and when dosage is being increased. **Driving must cease if adversely affected**.
- When planning the treatment of any patient (particularly professional drivers e.g. of taxis, lorries, buses, or construction vehicles), always consider adverse side-effect profiles which may impair driving ability:
  - Antidepressants—anticholinergic/antihistaminic effects (sedation).
  - Antipsychotics—both sedation and EPSEs (assess regularly).
  - Benzodiazepines—the most likely psychotropic medication to impair driving performance; avoid long-acting compounds.
  - For all psychotropics—consider the epileptogenic potential.

Duties and other considerations

- **Duty of care** Doctors have a duty to advise their patients of the potential dangers of adverse effects from medication and interactions with other substances, especially alcohol.
- **Confidentiality** When a patient has a condition which makes driving unsafe and the patient is either unable to appreciate this, or refuses to cease driving, GMC guidelines advise breaking confidentiality and informing DVLA (see opposite)
- **Patients detained under the MHA** Similar rules as for *informal* patients (i.e. drivers must be able to satisfy the standards of fitness for their respective conditions and be free from any effects of medication which will affect driving adversely).

GMC guidelines for informing the DVLA

- The DVLA is legally responsible for deciding if a person is medically unfit to drive. They need to know when driving licence holders have a condition which may, now or in the future, affect their safety as a driver.
- Therefore, where patients have such conditions, you should:
  - Make sure that the patients understand that the condition may impair their ability to drive. If a patient is incapable of understanding this advice (e.g. because of dementia), you should inform the DVLA immediately.
  - Explain to patients that they have a legal duty to inform the DVLA about the condition.
- If the patients refuse to accept the diagnosis or the effect of the condition on their ability to drive, you can suggest that the patients seek a second opinion, and make appropriate arrangements for the patients to do so. You should advise patients not to drive until the second opinion has been obtained.
- If patients continue to drive when they are not fit to do so, you should make every reasonable effort to persuade them to stop. This may include telling their next of kin.
- If you do not manage to persuade patients to stop driving, or you are given or find evidence that a patient is continuing to drive contrary to advice, you should disclose relevant medical information immediately, in confidence, to the medical adviser at DVLA.
- Before giving information to the DVLA you should inform the patient of your decision to do so. Once the DVLA has been informed, you should also write to the patient, to confirm that a disclosure has been made.

Further advice on fitness to drive

- Doctors may write to the DVLA (see 'Useful addresses,' p. 920), or may speak to one of the medical advisers during office hours, to seek advice about a particular driver (identified by an M number) or about fitness to drive in general.
- All of the DVLA advice is available online at: *http://www.dvla.gov.uk* (including an e-mail facility for use by medical professionals only.)

DVLA requirements for specific psychiatric conditions

Anxiety or depression

(without significant memory or concentration problems, agitation, behavioural disturbance, or suicidal thoughts)

Group 1 drivers: DVLA need not be notified and driving may continue.
Group 2 drivers: Very minor short-lived illnesses need not be notified.

Severe anxiety or depression

(with significant memory or concentration problems, agitation, behavioural disturbance or suicidal thoughts)

Group 1 drivers: *Driving should cease* pending the outcome of medical enquiry. A period of stability depending upon the circumstances will be required before driving can be resumed. Particularly dangerous are those who may attempt suicide at the wheel.

Group 2 drivers: *Driving may be permitted* when the person is well and stable for a period of 6 months. Medication must not cause side-effects which would interfere with alertness or concentration. Driving is usually permitted if the anxiety or depression is longstanding, but maintained symptom-free on doses of psychotropic medication which do not impair. DVLA may require psychiatric reports.

Acute psychosis (any cause)

Group 1 drivers: *Driving must cease* during the acute illness. Relicensing can be considered when all of the following conditions can be satisfied:
• Has remained well and stable for at least 3 months.
• Is compliant with treatment.
• Is free from adverse effects of medication which would impair driving.
• Subject to a favourable specialist report.

NB Drivers who have a history of instability and/or poor compliance will require a longer period off driving.

Group 2 drivers: *Driving should cease* pending the outcome of medical enquiry. The person must be well and stable for a minimum of 3 years with insight into their condition before driving can be resumed. At that time, DVLA will usually require a consultant examination. Any psychotropic medication should be of minimum effective dosage and not interfere with alertness, concentration, or in any other way impair driving performance. There should be no significant likelihood of recurrence.

Hypomania/mania

Group 1 drivers: *Driving must cease* during the acute illness. Following an *isolated episode*, re-licensing can be reconsidered when *all* the following conditions can be satisfied:
• Well and stable for at least 3 months.
• Compliant with treatment.
• Insight has been regained.

• Free from adverse effects of medication which would impair driving.
• Subject to a favourable specialist report.

NB Hypomania or mania are particularly dangerous to driving when there are repeated changes of mood. Therefore, when there have been 4 or more episodes of mood swing within the previous 12 months, at least 6 months' stability will be required, with evidence of treatment compliance and a favourable specialist report.

Group 2 drivers: *Driving must cease* pending the outcome of medical enquiry. The person must be well and stable for a minimum of 3 years with insight into their condition before driving can be resumed. At that time, DVLA will usually require a consultant examination. Any psychotropic medication should be of minimum effective dosage and not interfere with alertness, concentration, or in any other way impair driving performance. There should be no significant likelihood of recurrence.

Schizophrenia or other chronic psychoses

Group 1 drivers: The driver must satisfy *all* the following conditions:
• Stable behaviour for at least 3 months.
• Adequately compliant with treatment.
• Free from adverse effects of medication which would impair driving.
• Subject to a favourable specialist report.

NB For patients with *continuing symptoms*, even with limited insight, these do not necessarily preclude licensing. Symptoms should be unlikely to cause significant concentration problems, memory impairment, or distraction whilst driving. Particularly dangerous are those drivers whose psychotic symptoms relate to other road users.

Group 2 drivers: *Driving must cease* pending the outcome of medical enquiry. The person must be well and stable for a minimum of 3 years with insight into their condition before driving can be resumed. At that time, DVLA will usually require a consultant examination. Any psychotropic medication should be of minimum effective dosage and not interfere with alertness, concentration, or in any other way impair driving performance. There should be no significant likelihood of recurrence.

Dementia or any organic brain syndrome

It is extremely difficult to assess driving ability in those with dementia. Those who have poor short-term memory, disorientation, lack of insight and judgement are almost certainly not fit to drive. The variable presentations and rates of progression are acknowledged. Disorders of attention will also cause impairment. A decision regarding fitness to drive is usually based on medical reports.

Group 1 drivers: In early dementia when sufficient skills are retained and progression is slow, a licence may be issued subject to annual review. A formal driving assessment may be necessary.
Group 2 drivers: *Refuse or revoke licence.*

Learning disability

Group 1 drivers: Severe learning disability is not compatible with driving and the licence application must be refused. In milder forms, provided there are no other relevant problems, it may be possible to hold a licence, but it will be necessary to demonstrate adequate functional ability at the wheel.

Group 2 drivers: Recommended permanent refusal or revocation if severe. Minor degrees of learning disability when the condition is stable with no medical or psychiatric complications may be compatible with the holding of a licence.

Persistent behaviour disorder
(including post head injury syndrome, psychopathic disorders, and non-epileptic seizure disorder).

Group 1 drivers: If seriously disturbed (e.g. violent behaviour or alcohol abuse) and likely to be a source of danger at the wheel, licence should be revoked or the application refused. Licence will be issued after medical reports confirm that behavioural disturbances have been satisfactorily controlled.

Group 2 drivers: Recommended refusal or revocation if associated with serious behaviour disturbance likely to make the individual a source of danger at the wheel. If the person matures and psychiatric reports confirm stability a consideration would be given to restoration of the licence but a consultant psychiatrist report would be required.

Transcultural psychiatry

Introduction

Psychiatry is undeniably a branch of Western medicine and our conception of psychiatric illness (and how best to treat it) is undoubtedly heavily influenced by Western social and cultural factors. However, the scientific validity of these concepts can be readily tested if they can be shown to cross cultural boundaries.

Emil Kraepelin recognised this argument when he visited Java in 1896, and found that the clinical symptoms of 'dementia praecox' could be seen in patients he met there, just as they were manifest in his own patients in Germany. It was not until the WHO International Pilot Study of Schizophrenia in 1973 that the incidence of schizophrenia (defined by narrow criteria) was found to be 0.7–1.4 per 10 000 aged 15–54 across all nine countries studied worldwide. Despite variations in the *content* of delusions and hallucinations (which were culturally derived), the *form* was found to be the same. These conclusions have been supported by a large number of epidemiological studies and similar results have been found for bipolar affective disorder.

The manifestations of depressive, stress-related, and anxiety disorders show the greatest cultural variations (see pp. 836–7). The myth that these are predominantly Western diseases held sway for a long time (based on views of Western civilisation articulated most eloquently by Freud in *Civilisation and its Discontents (1930)*).

Certain manifestations of emotional distress, termed 'culture-bound syndromes' by P.M. Yap, a former professor of psychiatry in Hong Kong, are particular to different cultures. These present as mixed disorders of behaviour, emotions, and beliefs and many have local names (see pp. 842–7). Some are clear symptom-correlates of disorders found in ICD-10 and DSM-IV; others have no Western equivalent but appear to be variations of somatoform, conversion, or dissociative disorders. Some Western disorders (e.g. anorexia nervosa, deliberate self-harm) are rarely seen in non-Western countries. However, as we move towards a more global society, 'Western influences' appear to be making these types of disorder increasingly frequent in non-Western societies.

Debate continues as to whether Western diagnostic categories are universally valid. Understanding the biological underpinnings of the common disease entities (e.g. schizophrenia, bipolar affective disorder, depression, anxiety) and the development of treatments based upon our understanding of neurophysiological and neuropharmacological mechanisms will inform this debate. However, awareness of cultural issues as they impact upon an individual, their illness (and illness beliefs), and the relationship between psychiatrist and patient, is critical if we are to successfully provide appropriate interventions.

Cultural context and the presentation of psychiatric disorders

Schizophrenia Some apparently psychotic experiences may be normal when viewed within a cultural context. This applies to delusions (e.g. belief in magic, spirits, or demons) and hallucinations (e.g. seeing 'auras', the appearance of divine entities, hearing God's voice). Other evidence of apparent psychosis, such as disorganised speech, may actually reflect local variations in language syntax, or the fact that the person is not completely fluent in the language used by the interviewer. Differences in non-verbal communication (e.g. eye contact, facial expression, body language) may also be misinterpreted. Historically there has been a tendency in the UK and US to diagnose schizophrenia more readily in certain cultural groups (e.g. Afro-Caribbeans). This probably does not reflect differences in the incidence of schizophrenia, but rather a lack of understanding of cultural differences. Some symptoms of schizophrenia (e.g. catatonia) are more common in non-Western countries, and even between Western countries the diagnosis of brief psychoses (e.g. bouffée deliriante) varies. Interestingly the course of schizophrenia appears to be more acute and have better long-term outcome in some developing countries.

Mania Often used colloquially to mean 'changes in normal behaviour', rather than its strict definition. It may be difficult to distinguish periods of frenzied activity (e.g. in *amok*—see p. 842) from increased activity, energy, and reduced need for sleep in a manic episode. This may be particularly difficult when such episodes are preceded by apparent depressive symptoms.

Depression Cultural expressions of depressive symptoms vary across populations. In some cultures there is greater emphasis on somatic terms e.g. 'nerves' or 'headaches' (Mediterranean cultures); 'problems of the heart' (Middle East); 'imbalance', 'weakness', or 'tiredness' (China and Asia). This often makes the use of Western diagnostic classifications difficult, as symptoms may cross diagnostic boundaries (e.g. mood, anxiety, somatoform disorders). Equally difficult may be the interpretation of culturally normal explanations for symptom causation—which may appear delusional (e.g. spirit possession), or associated somatic symptoms (see p. 345)—that need to be distinguished from actual hallucinations.

Anxiety and stress-related disorders

Agoraphobia Social sanctions against members of certain populations (e.g. women) appearing in public may sometimes be confused with agoraphobic symptoms.

Panic attacks In some cultures these may be interpreted as evidence of magic or witchcraft (particularly when they come 'out of the blue').

OCD Religious and cultural beliefs strongly influence the content of obsessions and nature of compulsions. It may often be difficult to assess the significance of ritualistic behaviours unless the clinician has a knowledge of local customs.

PTSD Immigrants may have emigrated to escape military conflict or particularly harsh regimes. They may have had experience of significant traumatic events, but may be unwilling (or unable) to discuss them because of language problems or fears of being sent back.

Somatisation disorder Common types of somatic symptoms vary across cultures (and genders within cultures). These reflect the principle concerns of the population (or individual) e.g. worms/insects in the scalp/ under the skin—seen in South-East Asia and Africa; concern about semen loss—seen in India (see *Dhat* p. 843) and China (see *Shenkui* p. 846).

Conversion and dissociative disorders More common in rural populations, in 'less educated' societies, and may be culturally normal. Certain religious rituals involve alteration in consciousness (including trance states), beliefs in spirit possession, and varieties of socially sanctioned behaviours that could be viewed as conversion or dissociative disorders (e.g. *falling out* p. 843, *spell* p. 846, *zar* p. 847). 'Running' subtypes of culture-bound syndromes have symptoms that would meet criteria for dissociative fugue (p. 746).

Anorexia nervosa More prevalent in Western societies, with an abundance of food, and where there are strong cultural influences promoting thinness as the ideal of body shape. Immigrants from other cultural backgrounds may assimilate this ideal, or may present with primary symptoms other than disturbed body image and fear of weight gain (e.g. stomach pains, lack of enjoyment of food).

Alcohol and substance misuse Cultural factors heavily influence the availability, patterns of use, attitudes about, and even the physiological or behavioural effects of alcohol and other substances.

Alcohol Social, family, and religious attitudes towards the use of alcohol may all influence patterns of use and the likelihood of developing alcohol-related problems. Although it is difficult to separate cause from effect, low levels of education, unemployment, and low social status are all associated with increased misuse of alcohol. In some populations (e.g. Japanese and Chinese) up to 50% may have a deficiency of aldehyde dehydrogenase (complete absence in 10%), with low rates of alcohol problems in these populations because the physiological effects of consuming alcohol may be extremely unpleasant (e.g. flushing and palpaitations due to accumulation of acetylaldehyde). How individuals behave when intoxicated may also be culturally determined, with aggressive and antisocial behaviour (typified by 'football hooligans') not seen to the same extent in cultures where alcohol is more of a 'social lubricant', despite levels of alcohol consumption being similar.

Other substances Use of hallucinogens and other drugs may be culturally acceptable when part of religious rituals (e.g. peyote in the Native American Church, cannabis in Rastafarianism). Equally, secular movements, typified by the hippie movements of the 60s and 70s, or more recently the 'dance culture', provide a context in which psychedelic experiences (e.g. induced by LSD or MDMA) may be experienced without any adverse social sanctions.

Cultural formulation of psychiatric disorders

When there are clear cultural issues impacting upon the presentation of a psychiatric disorder it is important to have a systematic way of describing the nature and form these take. This may help by engaging the patient more directly in the assessment process; identifying other predisposing, precipitating, or perpetuating factors; and allowing any proposed management plans to be more tailored to the individual patient.

Issues that ought to be considered include:

- Cultural identity—how the person regards themselves; affiliations with ethnic or religious subgroups.
- Preferred language.
- If an immigrant—integration into host society and culture.
- Specific psychosocial factors that may be culturally determined.
- Particular social stressors.
- Support within the community (including the role of religious institutions) and from family and friends.
- Availability and access to appropriate services.
- Culturally-determined illness beliefs and behaviour.
- What the patient believes to be wrong with them (the particular illness model used to explain perceived causation and nature of the condition).
- How the patient expresses their symptoms (language used, local idioms, behavioural manifestations).
- How the local community and family view their problems.
- The doctor-patient relationship—differences in culture, perceived social status, communication difficulties (due to language) and how they impact on:
  - Eliciting symptoms and understanding their significance.
  - Forming a 'therapeutic alliance'.
  - Discussing the possible treatment options (when 'disease models' may be at odds with each other).
- The attitude of their culture towards mental illness and the implications of a psychiatric diagnosis (e.g. will preclude marriage in some cultures).

Culture-bound syndromes

Culture-bound or culture-specific syndromes comprise a wide range of disorders occuring in particular localities or ethnic groups. The behavioural manifestations or subjective experiences particular to these disorders may or may not correspond to diagnostic categories in DSM-IV or ICD-10. They are usually considered to be illnesses and generally have local names. They also include culturally accepted idioms or explanatory mechanisms of illness that differ from Western idioms and outside of their cultural setting may be mistaken for psychosis. Awareness of culture-bound syndromes is important to allow psychiatrists and physicians to make culturally appropriate diagnoses.

According to Littlewood and Lipsedge (1987)[1] these disorders share a number of common general characteristics:

- Occur in young men or women who are 'powerless' and socially neglected.
- Usually dramatic with the individual unaware or not responsible.
- The disorder has symbolic cultural significance ('mystical sanction'.)

and show a typical triphasic pattern:

- Dislocation of an individual as a representative of a particular group.
- Emergence of symptoms as an exaggerated form of this extrusion.
- Restitution into normal relationships.

In fact, these features could also be applied to many of the Western neuroses (where 'mystical sanction' is provided by the medical model). Although controversial, some commentators regard the neuroses (including dissociative states, somatoform and conversion disorders) as examples of Western culture-specific syndromes[2]. This would include a range of specific syndromes such as neurasthenia, fugue, and trance states, as well as the more modern neuroses: multiple personality disorder, anorexia nervosa, chronic fatigue syndrome, alien abduction syndrome, recovered memory syndrome, ritual or satanic abuse, Gulf War syndrome, and even shoplifting and overdosing (!)

If culture-bound syndromes are categorised according to primary phenomenology, a number of common subtypes emerge (see opposite). Descriptions of specific syndromes are outlined in the following glossary (pp. 842–7) illustrating the vast range of manifestations[3].

1 Littlewood R and Lipsedge M (1987) The butterfly and the serpent: culture, psychopathology and biomedicine. *Cult Med Psychiatry* **11**, 289–335.

2 Showalter E (1998) *Hystories*, Picador Press.

3 For further reading see: Simons RC and Hughes CC (eds.) (1985) *The culture-bound syndromes: folk illnesses of psychiatric and anthropological interest.* Dordrecht, The Netherlands: D. Reidel Publishing Company.

Subtypes of culture-bound syndromes

- **Startle reaction** e.g. latah, amurakh, irkunii, ikota, olan miryachit, menkeiti, bah-tschi, bah-tsi, baah-ji, imu, mali-mali, silok
- **Genital retraction** e.g. koro, suo yang, jinjinia bemar, rok-joo
- **Sudden assault** e.g. amok, cafard/cathard, mal de pelea, fighting sickness, juramentado, Puerto Rican syndrome, iich'aa, going postal
- **Running** e.g. pibloktoq/arctic hysteria, grisi siknis
- **Semen loss** e.g. dhat, jiryan, sukra prameha, shenkui
- **Food restriction** e.g. anorexia nervosa, bulimia nervosa, anorexia mirabilis/holy anorexia
- **Spirit possession** e.g. bebainan, spell, zar
- **Obsession with the deceased** e.g. ghost sickness, hsieh-ping, shin-byung
- **Exhaustion** e.g. neuraesthenia, chronic fatigue syndrome/ME, brain fag/brain fog, shenjian shuairuo, nervios
- **Suppressed rage** e.g. hwa-byung/wool-hwa-bung, bilis, colera

Glossary of culture-bound syndromes

Amok, Amuck (Malayan males) Literally 'battling furiously': sudden, unprovoked, random acts of violence, for which the subject is amnesic, and after which they may commit suicide. May be preceded by a period of depression or brooding, anxiety, or feelings of hostility following perceived loss of face or being insulted. Also called *Matal/Mata Elap* ('darkened eye'). Similar syndromes are reported in other countries of Southeast Asia, the Philippines, Polynesia (*cafard* or *cathard*), New Guinea (*ahade idzi be*), Puerto Rico (*mal de pelea; fighting sickness; Puerto Rican syndrome*), the Andes of Bolivia, Columbia, Ecuador, and Peru (*colerina*), and the US (*going postal; iich'aa* in Navajo Native Americans).

Amurakh (Siberian women) 'Copying mania' characterised by echopraxia. (See *lata*.)

Artic hysteria (See *piblokto*.)

Ashanti (West African women e.g. Ghana) Consists of two subtypes: *'frenzied guilt and fear' (FGF)* where, sometimes following physical illness and fever, the person believes they are being punished for some offence, becomes frightened, and then frenzied, followed by a period of withdrawal, hallucinations, hebephrenic behaviour, dancing, singing, tearing off, clothes, and eating faeces; and *'depressive' (DP)* where those affected accuse themselves of being witches and harming someone else without conscious intent. In younger women this often follows a difficult childbirth and subsequent illness, or the death of an infant.

Ataque de nervios (Puerto Ricans and other Hispanics) Dissociative trance disorder, usually following an acute stressful event (e.g. death or conflict) with brief symptoms including: a trance-like state (with narrowing of awareness, perceptual distortions, depersonalisation, loss of consciousness, and partial or global amnesia), anxiety, somatic complaints, impulsive behaviour, and depression.

Bangungut (young male Filipinos) 'Oriental nightmare-death syndrome' where a series of terrifying dreams culminate in death from presumed cardiac arrhythmia. (See also *hmong sudden death syndrome*.)

Bebainan (Indonesia) Possession state, believed to be caused by a spirit power, deity, or other person, in which the subject assumes a new identity, associated with stereotyped involuntary movements and amnesia.

Beserk, Berserk, Beserkergang (Northern Europe) 'Fighting fever', very similar to amok.

Bilis and colera (Latin America) An idiom of distress in which physical or mental illness is explained as due to extreme emotion (anger) that upsets the humours (described in terms of hot and cold.)

Brain fag, brain fog syndrome (West African students) 'Brain fatigue', an idiom of distress with symptoms attributed to over-work, tiredness, and 'too much thinking'. The subject complains of reduced concentration, poor memory, blurred vision, and head/neck pain (often described as tightness, pressure, heat, or burning). Symptoms closely resemble anxiety, depressive, or somatoform disorders.

Cathard, cafard (See *amok.*)

Colerina (See *amok.*)

Curanderismo (Mexican Americans and other Spanish-speaking people) Folk medicine in which the healers (curanderos [male] or cunderas [female]) use a combination of herbal infusions, dramatic healing rituals, and prayers to treat a variety of physical and psychological symptoms including: *embrujo* (witchcraft), *empacho* (intestinal distress), *mal ojo* (evil eye), *mal puesto* (hexing), and *susto* (soul loss.)

Delahara (Philippine women) A syndrome similar to *amok.*

Dhat (India, rural areas of Nepal, Sri Lanka, and Bangladesh) Semen-loss syndrome—a belief in the passage of semen in the urine following the breaking of taboos concerning masturbation or sexual intercourse. Associated with somatic symptoms (weakness, exhaustion), severe anxiety, hypochondriasis, whitish discolouration of the urine, and sexual dysfunction. Traditional remedies consist of herbal tonics to restore semen/humoral balance. Similar to *jiryan* (India), *sukra prameha* (Sri Lanka), and *shenkui* (China).

Echul (Native Americans of South California) Sexual anxiety and convulsions following severe stress (e.g. the death of a child).

Evil eye, mal Ojo (See *curanderismo.*)

Falling out, blacking out (African Americans and Afro-Caribbeans) Collapse, without loss of consciousness, sometimes preceded by dizziness. The subject feels paralysed, but can hear and understand, and may claim to be blind. A type of dissociative/conversion disorder, usually following a traumatic event.

Fighting sickness (See *amok.*)

Frenzied anxiety state (Kenya)

Frigidophobia (See *wind illness.*)

Ghost sickness (Native Americans) Preoccupation with death or the deceased. Subjects may say they have been 'bewitched' and complain of nightmares, weakness, dizziness, episodes of collapse, anxiety, poor appetite, hallucinations, confusion, feelings of futility or apprehension, and sometimes a sense of suffocation.

Grisi siknis (Miskito Indians, Nicaragua) Headache, anxiety, anger, and aimless running. Similar to *pibloko.*

Gururumba episode ('wild man behaviour') (New Guinea) Subject (usually male) breaks into houses to steal small items (they believe to be valuable) and then runs off into the forest for some days, later returning (without the items) to their normal life. There is associated amnesia and during the episode they may appear vague, agitated, behave in a clumsy way, and have disturbance of normal hearing and speech.

Hmong sudden death syndrome (Laos) The death of a person whilst sleeping, attributed to being attacked by spirits in a dream, and often following a traumatic event. (See *bangungut* and *voodoo death.*)

Hi-wa itck (Mohave American Indians) Insomnia, depression, loss of appetite, and sometimes suicide associated with unwanted separation from a loved one.

Hsieh-ping (Taiwan) A brief trance state during which the subject is believed to be possessed by an ancestral ghost, who often attempts to communicate to other family members. Symptoms include tremor, disorientation, delirium, and (visual/auditory) hallucinations.

Hwa-byung, wool-hwa-bung, 'anger syndrome' (Korea) Epigastric pain attributed to a mass in the upper abdomen that the patient fears will lead to death. The belief is related to ideas of bodily imbalances caused by anger (cf. *bilis* and *colera.*) Other symptoms may include tiredness, muscular aches and pains, breathlessness, palpitations, insomnia, dysphoria, panic, loss of appetite, and other GI problems (indigestion, anorexia).

Imu (See *lata.*)

Juramentado (Malays and Moros) Marked agitation, indiscriminate assault or stabbing, followed by stupor, and subsequent amnesia on awakening. (Similar to *amok.*)

Kimilue (Native Americans of Southern California) Apathy, anhedonia, loss of appetite, and vivid sexual dreams.

Koro (Malaysia) Literally 'to shrink' or referring to a 'tortoise' (a popular word for penis). 'Genital retraction syndrome'—the fear or delusion that the genitals are retracting into the abdomen, and that death will occur once this has happened. Prodromal depersonalisation usually occurs and elaborate measures may be taken to prevent the penis from retracting (e.g. grasping of the genitals, splints or other devices, herbal remedies, or fellatio). Occurs more frequently in predominantly young, single males, in Asia and the Middle East (epidemics have been described in the Malay Archipelago, Thailand, China, India, Singapore, and Israel.) Sporadic cases have been reported in Africa, Europe, and North America. The female equivalent (fear or delusion that the labia or nipples are retracting) occurs rarely and most reported cases have been during epidemics. There are no specific associations with other psychiatric disorders, although phobic anxiety disorders, depression, schizophrenia, and depersonalisation syndromes are described. Other names for this syndrome include: *suk-yeong/ suo yang* (Chinese: 'shrunken penis'), *kattao* (Indian: 'cut off'), *jinjinia bemar* (Assam), and *rok-joo* (Thailand.)

Lata, latah, lattah (Malay population) Exaggerated startle reaction seen predominantly in young girls. Following sudden fright/trauma, there is a behavioural response consisting of echopraxia, automatic obedience, coprolalia, and dissociative or trance-like behaviour. May be a symptom of disease (e.g. acute psychosis, conversion/dissociative state) or be an isolated behavioural abnormality. Related syndromes include: *amurakh, irkunii, ikota, miryachit, menkeiti,* and *olan/olonism* (Siberia), *imu* (Ainu of Japan), *bah-tschi, bah-tsi,* and *baah-ji* (Thailand), *mali-mali* and *silok* (Philippines), *Lapp panic* (Lapps), the *Jumpers* of New England (a 19th-century Shaker sect), and *jumping Frenchman* (Canada).

Locura (Latin America) Severe form of chronic psychosis, attributed to an inherited vulnerability and/or adverse life events, characterised by incoherent speech, agitation, auditory/visual hallucinations, impaired social interactions, and unpredictable (possibly violent) behaviour.

'Lost hunter' sequence (New Guinea) After period of social withdrawal (following perceived criticism of actions) the person (typically male) goes hunting alone in the bush and describes five episodes of tracking a large game animal, which suddenly disappears, before he is rescued by a search party. He feels he has been led astray by supernatural beings.

Mal de pelea (See *amok*.)

Miryachit, mirachat (Russian: 'to fool' or 'play the fool') (See *lata*.)

Nerfiza, nerves, nervios (Latino populations in United States, Latin America, Egypt, Northern Europe) Chronic somatic, emotional, and behavioural symptoms (e.g. headache, sleep problems, reduced appetite, nausea, fatigue, dizziness, paraesthesia, anxiety, concentration difficulties, and emotional lability/distress). More common in women; associated with anger, emotional distress, and low self-esteem. Usually treated with traditional herbal teas, 'nerve pills', rest, isolation, and increased family support. (Similar to *nevra* in Greece.)

Olonism (See *lata*.)

Pibloko, pibloktoq (Polar Eskimo women) 'Arctic hysteria',—an acute dissociative state (lasting about 30 mins) following the actual (or symbolic) loss of someone or something important to the individual. Usually mild irritability or withdrawal precedes impulsive or dangerous acts (e.g. screaming, tearing off clothes, breaking furniture, shouting obscenities, eating faeces, or rushing out into the snow). May be followed by convulsions and coma (lasting up to 12 hours) with associated amnesia. Although some researchers have suggested it may be due to hypocalcaemic tetany, it is most probably an anxiety state.

Puerto Rican syndrome (See *amok*.)

Qi-gong psychotic reaction (China) 'Excess of vital energy'—an acute episode characterised by dissociative, paranoid, or other symptoms after participation in the health-enhancing practice of qi-gong.

Rootwork (Haiti and Sub-Saharan Africa) A variety of complaints attributed to hexing, witchcraft, sorcery, voodoo, or the evil influence of another person. Symptoms include anxiety, GI complaints, and fear of being poisoned or killed. Can result in death. Associated syndromes: *voodoo death* (Haiti), *mal puesto* or *brujeira* (Latin America), and *hex*.

Sangue dormido, 'Sleeping blood' (Cape Verde Islanders) Somatic symptoms including pain, numbness, tremor, paralysis, convulsions, blindness, and increased risk of heart attack, infection, and miscarriage.

Sar (Somalian women) A possession state attributed to Sar spirits that are said to hate men. The syndrome may legitimise behavioural disturbance in women who feel neglected by their husbands. (See also *zar*.)

Shenjian shuairuo (China) Similar to *neurasthenia*—symptoms include: fatigue, irritability, poor concentration/memory, sleep disturbance, and other somatic symptoms (dizziness, headaches, pain, GI upset, sexual dysfunction, and other signs of autonomic dysfunction). Most cases would meet criteria for depressive or anxiety disorders.

Shenk-k'uei (Taiwan), **shenkui** (China) Anxiety and panic with somatic complaints, especially sexual dysfunction (premature ejaculation and impotence). Symptoms are attributed to excessive semen loss from sexual activity or 'white turbid urine,' which reduces 'vital energy'. It is viewed as a life-threatening condition and described in areas with a Chinese ethnic population. Similar to *dhat* and *jiryan* (India), and *sukra prameha* (Sri Lanka.)

Shin-byung (Korea) Possession (dissociative) state attributed to ancestral spirits with associated anxiety/fear and somatic complaints (generalised weakness, dizziness, insomnia, loss of appetite, and GI problems).

Shinkeishitsu (Japan) Syndrome marked by obsessions, perfectionism, ambivalence, social withdrawal, fatigue, and hypochondriasis.

Spell (Southern United States) A trance state in which individuals 'communicate' with deceased relatives or with spirits, often accompanied by brief periods of personality change. In context, 'spells' are culturally normal and do not indicate psychiatric illness.

Susto, espanto, 'magic fright', 'fallen fontanel syndrome' (Peru) An acute anxiety state, seen in children and adolescents, usually following an acute stressor or violent (often supernatural) fright. Characterised by anxiety, agitation, dejection/apathy, sleep disturbance, significant weight loss, other somatic symptoms, and a belief that the soul has been, or will be, stolen from the body. (See *curanderismo*.) It is also seen in Latinos of the United States, Mexico, and other Central/South American countries. Related syndromes: *lanti* (Philippines), *malgri* (Aborigines of Australia), *mogo laya* (New Guinea), *narahati* (Iran), and *saladera* (in regions around the Amazon).

Tabanka (Trinidad) Depression associated with a high rate of suicide that is seen in men abandoned by their wives.

Taijin kyofusho (Japan) Fear and guilt about embarrassing others with one's appearance or behaviour, prominent in younger people and similar to the Western concept of social phobia.

Ufufuyane, saka (Kenya, Southern Africa; Bantu, Zulu; and affiliated groups) Anxiety state attributed to the effects of magical potions (given to them by rejected lovers) or spirit possession, with characteristic sobbing, repeated neologisms, paralysis, trance-like states, or loss of consciousness. Usually seen in young, unmarried women, who may also experience nightmares with sexual themes, and rarely episodes of temporary blindness. May be related to *aluro* (Nigeria), *phii pob* (Thailand), and *zar* (Egypt, Ethiopia, Sudan).

Uquamairineq (Inuits of the Arctic Circle) Syndrome akin to a sleep-state transition disorder or dissociative disorder in which sudden paralysis is associated with a sleep state, marked anxiety/agitation, and hallucinations. Usually lasts minutes and may be preceded by a transient sound or smell. Traditionally viewed as the result of soul loss, soul wandering, or spirit possession.

Vimbuza (Northern Malawi and Zambia) A culturally specific response to sickness involving herbal medicines and 'vimbuza dancing' that is performed late at night. Often others will dance on behalf of the patient, keeping the rhythm with metal belts, and inducing a trace state from which the 'healed' patient emerges. If the illness is considered severe, the family of the patient may sponsor a 'chilopa'—an entire night of dancing followed by an animal sacrifice at dawn. The patient drinks some of the animal's blood and then begins to dance again. The larger the animal (usually either a chicken, a goat, or a cow), the more effective the expected cure.

Voodoo death (See *hmong sudden death syndrome* and *rootwork*.)

Wacinko (Native American groups—Oglala Sioux—of North America) Anger, withdrawal, mutism, and immobility frequently leading to suicide. Often related to disappointment or interpersonal problems.

Wihtigo, whitigo, witiko, windigo, wendigo (Native American groups e.g. Cree, Algonkian Indians of central and northeastern Canada) The fear or delusion of being transformed into a *wihtigo*, or giant monster that eats human flesh. There is a prodrome of anxiety about physical symptoms (e.g. reduced appetite, nausea and vomiting) and the person may commit suicide or be the target of violence. The existence of this syndrome is questioned as no single case has been described in the psychiatric or anthropological literature.

Wind illness, p'a leng, frigidophobia (China, Southeast Asia) Anxiety/fear of being cold or of the wind; associated with a loss of yang and upset of natural balance in the body (believed to produce fatigue, impotence, and death), leading a person to do everything they can to stay warm. Described in areas with Chinese ethnic populations. May be related to *agua frio, aire frio, frio* of Mexico, Central and South America.

Wild man behaviour (See *gururumba*.)

Zar (East and North Africa, the Middle East e.g. Ethiopia, Somalia, Sudan, Egypt, and Iran) Dissociative symptoms including shouting, laughing, head banging, singing, weeping, and other demonstrative behaviours. The person believes they are possessed by a spirit, and may develop a long-term relationship with the spirit. Other symptoms may include apathy, withdrawal, refusal to eat, and refusal to carry out tasks of daily living. Such behaviour may be regarded as culturally normal (See *sar*.)

Therapeutic issues

Medication adherence

Is adherence important?

- It has been estimated that only one third of patients prescribed medication actually adhere to the treatment plan (this applies to *all* medical problems, not just psychiatric problems) and that ~80% of psychiatric admissions relate to medication non-adherence. Adherence is a particular problem when the illness runs a chronic course and requires the patient to be on medication *for life* (e.g. diabetes, IHD, pulmonary disease, schizophrenia).
- Patients with schizophrenia who comply with a sufficient dosage of antipsychotic medication have only about one fifth the risk of relapse compared to patients who do not take their medication.
- There is good evidence that prophylactic lithium treatment of bipolar disorder reduces the likelihood of (particularly manic) relapse, as well as the risk of suicide.
- Continuation of antidepressant treatment for *at least* six months after symptom resolution significantly reduces the risk of further depressive episodes.

Reasons for non-adherence

It is important to realise that the patient may have understandable reasons for being reluctant to take prescribed medication. Uncovering these reasons may help in negotiation and developing strategies to improve the situation.

- Continued symptoms of the underlying disorder (e.g. delusions, lack of motivation, impaired insight, disorganisation) or comorbid disorders (e.g. substance misuse, personality disorder).
- Negative attitude towards medication in general (versus other forms of treatment) or stigma associated with being 'on medication', particularly where there are external stigmata of treatment such as parkinsonism ('looking like a zombie').
- Unacceptable (or unexpected) side-effects (e.g. weight gain—p. 852, sedation, EPSEs—p. 860, sexual dysfunction—p. 856, perceived loss of 'good' symptoms e.g. hypomania).
- Forgetting (genuine oversight, disorganisation, cognitive impairment).
- Lack of communication (reasons for medication not fully explained or understood).
- Failure to obtain (or renew) prescription (through non-attendance, poor communication or poor relationship with responsible prescriber e.g. GP).
- Belief that the medication is 'not working'.
- Feeling well and no longer seeing the need for medication. The 'reward' of freedom from side-effects may be immediate, while the 'punishment' of relapse may be more distant, not taken seriously, or not directly associated with stopping treatment.

Strategies to improve adherence

Education

- Promote insight and understanding about the illness and the benefits of treatment.
- Provide information about the medication, how to take it, possible side-effects, the length of time needed to see benefits, and the potential problems of suddenly stopping.
- Discuss the reasons for prophylactic or continued treatment, especially when patient feels well (e.g. to reduce risk of relapse and improve long term outcome).
- Encourage discussion of pros and cons of suggested treatment plan.
- Encourage openness about potentially embarrassing issues that may lead to non-adherence (e.g. sexual side-effects).
- Regularly ask about and document side-effects at each review.

Sensible prescribing

- Simplify drug regime—use single-dose where possible (most psychotropic medications have long half-lives and can be given once daily or are available in slow-release preparations).
- Minimise side-effects through choice of a medication with lowest potential for side-effects, and using lowest therapeutic dose,
- If side-effects are problematic, consider a change to an alternative preparation or (where an alternative would be less effective) co-prescribing agents to counter significant problems.
- Rational medication choice based on individual acceptability of side-effects (e.g. any weight gain may be unacceptable to a young female patient).
- Clear communication of any changes in regime both to patient and primary care team (including written instructions for patient and direct communication with GP) especially if the primary care physician is main prescriber.
- Use depot antipsychotic preparations—this may sometimes be requested by the patient, but is more often necessary when the patient lacks insight, or has had significant serious relapses related to non-adherence.
- Regularly review the need for continued medication.

Practical/behavioural measures

- Written information to patient, particularly where regime is complex or where change of dose/medication is planned.
- Establish a regular daily routine for taking medication.
- Use of Dosette® box.
- Supervised administration (e.g. by relative/carer, at pharmacy, in day hospital, by CPN).
- Active monitoring (e.g. tablet count, blood levels—p. 888).

Weight gain with psychiatric medication

General points

Weight gain is a significant cause of non-compliance with psychiatric medication, and patients often complain about increases in weight, even when clinicians may regard it as 'clinically insignificant'. Effects on general health, self-esteem, and social embarrassment should not be overlooked.

Antipsychotics

Proposed mechanisms Sedation (reduced activity), thirst (anticholinergic S/Es), reduced metabolism, fluid retention, endocrine effects (increased prolactin, altered cortisol, altered insulin secretion), increases in leptin levels (changes in 'set-point' weight), and altered neurotransmitters (5-HT$_{2C}$ blockade, histamine affinity, D2 blockade, CCK changes) have all been proposed.

Increased risk Female, previous pattern of overeating, narcissistic traits, family or personal history of obesity.

Effects of specific agents (see opposite).

Management[1]

- Routine measurement of baseline weight.
- Warn patient of possibility.
- Encourage 'healthy diet' (involve dietician if necessary), moderate physical exercise, avoid high-calorie fluids.
- Use lowest therapeutic dose, introduce medication increases slowly, consider intermittent dosing.
- Consider adjunctive prescribing (e.g. clozapine *plus* quetiapine, to allow lowering of clozapine dose).

Antidepressants

Proposed mechanisms Reduced metabolism, carbohydrate craving (NB may be a symptom of depression itself), central serotonin mechanisms in regulating food intake (appetite/satiety).

Effects of specific agents (see opposite).

Management

- General advice about diet and exercise
- Use lowest therapeutic dose
- Consider switching to alternative antidepressant
- Adjunctive prescribing (e.g. naltrexone, ranitidine at night (may reduce 'midnight snacks')).

Lithium[2]

Proposed mechanisms Increased intake of high calorie drinks, hypothyroidism, increased insulin secretion.

Management Counselling and advice about diet and exercise, use of low-calorie drinks, avoidance of salty foods (or adding salt to foods).

Other mood stabilisers

Carbamazepine Weight gain due to increased appetite.

Valproate Weight gain which may be due to increased serum leptin and insulin.

Gabapentin Marked weight gain in some cases (up to 10% above baseline weight).

Weight gain with antipsychotics

Antipsychotic	Average weight gain (kg)
Pimozide	-2.7
Placebo	-1.0
Trifluoperazine	0.3
Ziprasodone	0.3
Haloperidol	0.5
Polypharmacy	0.5
Loxapine	0.7
Non-drug controls	0.8
Fluphenazine	1.1
Risperidone	1.7
Quetiapine	2.5
Thioridazine	2.8
Sertindole	2.9
Olanzapine	4.2
Chlorpromazine	4.2
Clozapine	5.7
Perphenazine	5.8

Fenton (2000) *Evidence Based Mental Health* **3**, 58.

Weight changes with antidepressants

SSRIs Fluoxetine: weight loss; paroxetine, fluvoxamine: slight weight loss; sertraline: limited weight gain; citalopram: no change

TCAs Weight gain (amitriptyline>imipramine>clomipramine)

MAOIs/RIMAs Weight loss (tranylcypromine)—rarely weight gain; weight gain (phenelzine>moclobemide)

Others Mianserin: mirtazepine; weight gain; reboxetine, trazodone: no change; venlafaxine: weight loss

1 Baptista T (1999) Body weight gain induced by antipsychotic drugs: mechanisms and management. *Acta Psych Scand* **101**, 3–16.

2 Baptista T (1995) Lithium and body weight gain. *Pharmacopsychiatry* **28**, 35–44.

Hyperprolactinaemia with antipsychotics

Essence Secretion of prolactin (PRL) by the pituitary is under inhibitory control via dopamine from the hypothalamus. Blockade of dopamine D2 receptors by conventional antipsychotics (plus risperidone) can raise prolactin levels, leading to symptoms of hyperprolactinaemia in both men (erectile dysfunction, loss of libido, and hypogonadism) and women (amenorrhoea, galactorrhoea, infertility, loss of libido, and possibly osteoporosis).

Differential diagnosis Diseases of the pituitary (e.g. prolactin secreting pituitary adenomas) or hypothalamus, severe primary hypothyroidism, liver cirrhosis, end-stage renal disease, stress, high-dose oestrogens, chronic cocaine use, opiates, dopamine depletion (e.g. due to reserpine, tetrabenazine).

Investigations
- Check for signs of chest wall irritation (which can promote galactorrhoea and raise prolactin) and signs of a sellar mass (including checking visual fields).
- Serum levels of TSH (exclude hypothyroidism), creatinine (exclude renal failure), and PRL (may be raised due to stress, after eating, or post-ictally).
  NB Patients may be symptomatic even when PRL in the normal range (i.e. it is the *relative* increase in PRL that matters, not just the *absolute* increase).
- Consider CT/MRI and/or a referral to endocrinology.

Management
- Exclude other possible aetiologies.
- Consider a change of medication to a prolactin-sparing antipsychotic (e.g. clozapine, olanzapine, quetiapine) or reduction in dose if the patient's mental state is stable (monitor closely).
- If problems persist or medication changes are precluded (or not tolerated), consider referral to endocrinology for consideration of other treatments: hormone replacement, amantadine, bromocriptine, etc.
- Pre-menopausal women should be advised about resumption of normal menstrual cycle (and return of fertility) when changing antipsychotics, and the use of contraception should be discussed.

NB Asymptomatic hyperprolactinaemia does not warrant (in itself) changes to medication.

Sexual dysfunction and psychiatric medication

Sexual dysfunction and psychiatric medication

The degree of sexual dysfunction experienced by patients taking psychiatric medication may be a major source of distress and a significant reason for non-compliance. Clinicians are notoriously poor at enquiring about these problems, despite reports that patients regard sexual side-effects as the most troublesome of all medication-related problems.

Antidepressants

Rates of sexual dysfunction seen in clinical practice (commonly **delayed ejaculation** and **orgasmic dysfunction**) may be higher than those reported in product information. Clomipramine, SSRIs (paroxetine, sertraline, citalopram, fluoxetine), and venlafaxine appear to be most likely to cause sexual dysfunction of some form (30–60%). Other TCAs show intermediate risk of dysfunction (10–30%). Bupropion and moclobemide appear much less likely to cause problems (≤10%). Mirtazepine appears possibly to have the lowest rates of sexual side-effects[1]. Problems of reduced libido appear to be associated with SSRIs, whereas TCAs tend to cause (more troublesome) difficulties with sexual performance.

Management[2]

- 'Watchful waiting'—to see if symptoms subside.
- Dose alteration (either up or down) to find effective dose without side-effects.
- 'Drug holidays' or scheduled interruptions in therapy (e.g. weekends).
- Addition of another agent to counteract the sexual side-effects (*combination* e.g. mirtazepine, buspirone, bupropion; or '*as required*' e.g. sildenafil, cyproheptadine, amantadine, yohimbine).
- Switch to another agent known to have fewer adverse sexual effects (e.g. mirtazepine, bupropion).

Antipsychotics

The prevalence of sexual dysfunction associated with antipsychotics ranges from 40–71%, with reports of problems in all groups of antipsychotic medication (usually reduced libido/sexual arousal problems)[3].

- Dysfunction may be related to dopamine blockade, autonomic side-effects, and hyperprolactinaemia.
- The dose of medication, use of anticholinergics, and comorbid depression are significant associations.
- Thioridazine can cause 'dry' or 'retrograde' ejaculation (semen may be present in the urine).
- Clozapine and quetiapine seem to have the lowest risk of sexual side-effects.

Management

- Dose reduction where possible.
- Reduction or discontinuation of drugs with anticholinergic effects.
- Consider switching to alternative agent (e.g. quetiapine, low-dose olanzapine, clozapine).

Mood stabilisers

Lithium therapy may impair desire and arousal, but does not appear to have a major impact on patient self-satisfaction or subjective sense of pleasure during sexual activity[4]. Although the occurrence of sexual dysfunction is estimated as 10–30%, it is usually mild, not a source of distress, and does not lead to non-compliance.

Carbamazepine and **phenytoin** both increase prolactin and decrease dehydroepiandrosterone and other adrenal androgen levels, making sexual dysfunction likely.

Valproate does not cause these changes, and is associated with a low likelihood of sexual dysfunction.

1 Gregorian RS, Golden KA, Bahce A, et al. (2002) Antidepressant-induced sexual dysfunction. Annals of Pharmacotherapy **36**, 1577–89.

2 Gutierrez MA and Stimmel GL (1999) Management of and counseling for psychotropic drug-induced sexual dysfunction. Pharmacotherapy **19**, 823–31.

3 Wirshing DA, Pierre JM, Marder SR, et al. (2002) Sexual side effects of novel antipsychotic medications. Schizophrenia Research **56**, 25–30.

4 Aizenberg D, Sigler M, Zemishlany Z, Weizman A (1996) Lithium and male sexual function in affective patients. Clinical Neuropharmacology **19**, 515–19.

Priapism

Priapism[1] is defined as a sustained, painful erection that cannot be relieved by sexual intercourse or masturbation, and that is frequently unrelated to sexual desire. Without intervention, it usually subsides within a few days, but 50–80% of affected men become permanently impotent. Stasis of blood for more than several hours leads to increased blood viscosity, deoxygenation, and, ultimately, irreversible fibrosis of tissue. Thus, **priapism is a urologic emergency requiring immediate intervention**[2]. (Clitoral priapism has also been reported and may be associated with either pain and discomfort or increased libido and orgasmic response[3].)

Trazodone About 30% of reported cases of priapism are drug-induced, with 80% of those cases involving trazodone. Trazodone-induced priapism is rare, occurring in less than 0.1% of patients taking the drug. It typically is seen within the first month of therapy, occurs in all age groups, and may occur even with low daily doses of 50–100mg.

Other drugs Antipsychotics (haloperidol, clozapine, zuclopenthixol), SSRIs, bupropion, phenelzine, prazosin, buspirone, phenytoin, and intra-cavernosal injection of vasoactive drugs.

Management

In the past, surgical intervention was routine practice, but it resulted in up to 50% of men being permanently impotent. Because trazodone-induced priapism is understood to be due to alpha$_1$-adrenergic blockade, pharmaco-logic treatment is preferred since it carries no risk of permanent sequelae.

- Patients must be aware of the possibility of priapism when taking trazodone, and treatment must be given quickly to minimise the risk of permanent impotence.
- **If less than 24hrs' duration**: Intracavernosal irrigation with an alpha$_1$-adrenergic agonist (successfully causes detumescence in most patients).
- **If more than 24hrs' duration**: Corporeal fibrosis is more likely and drug treatment is less effective. Remove blood from the penis and infuse a solution of an alpha$_1$-adrenergic agonist into the corpus cavernosum. *Preferred agent*: phenylephrine (the most selective and potent alpha$_1$-adrenergic vasoconstrictor); onset of action less than 1 minute and duration of 7–20 minutes; several intermittent injections of 0.1mg/ml solution may be necessary (continuously monitor BP and HR).

Patient counselling Although rare, priapism is a serious medical emer-gency that requires immediate intervention. Since most patients would not attribute the prolonged erection to trazodone, patient counselling about its possibility is necessary for all men beginning therapy with the drug. They should be advised to report prolonged or painful erections to their doctor immediately.

1 "Priapus", the son of Zeus and Aphrodite, was a god with an enormous penis who symbolized the earth's fertility.

2 Banos JE, Bosch F, Farre M (1989) Drug-induced priapism. Its aetiology, incidence and treatment. *Med Toxicol Adverse Drug Exp.* **4**, 46–58.

3 Patel AG, Mukherji K, Lee A (1996) Priapism associated with psychotropic drugs. *British Journal of Hospital Medicine* **55**, 315–319.

Antipsychotic-induced parkinsonism

Essence A frequent adverse effect found in full form in at least 20% of patients treated with antipsychotic medication. Generally occurs within 4 wks of treatment and is a major cause of non-compliance. Examination (p. 214) is generally sufficient to detect the onset of symptoms and should be carried out frequently in the first 3 mths of treatment. Monitoring may help establish the minimally effective dose of antipsychotic needed by individual patients, reducing discomfort and improving compliance.

Symptoms/signs Characterised by tremor, rigidity, and bradykinesia; the presentation is similar to that of idiopathic Parkinson's disease (p. 170), although bradykinesia may be less prominent and symptoms are always bilateral.

Pathophysiology D_2 receptor blockade in the nigrostriatal pathway.

Differential diagnosis Many drugs have been associated with parkinsonism (see opposite) and some may increase the likelihood of problems (e.g. prednisolone). Other differentials include: idiopathic Parkinson's disease, dementia (e.g. DLB), negative symptoms of schizophrenia, psychomotor retardation (e.g. in depression).

Treatment Several strategies may be used, including:
• Dose reduction.
• Switching to another antipsychotic agente e.g. olanzapine, quetiapine, risperidone (<8mg/day), clozapine.
• Use of anticholinergic agents (e.g. biperiden, procyclidine, orphenadrine, trihexphenidyl) or amantadine.

NB Anticholinergic agents are often used in younger patients. However, older patients may not be able to tolerate the side-effects of blurred vision, dry mouth, constipation, urinary retention, and particularly cognitive impairment. This has led to the use of amantadine, which is better tolerated, or more frequent use of the newer antipsychotics, especially when patients already have early signs of Parkinson's disease.
• When treatment is by depot, there is some evidence that pipothiazine palmitate, flupenthixol, or zuclopenthixol decanoate may be better tolerated. Risperidone depot is also now available, and may be considered as another option.

Follow-up
• If anticholinergics have been used, the need for continued treatment ought to be kept under review.
• Their slow withdrawal should be attempted after the acute phase of treatment, or following any lowering of antipsychotic dose, as drug-induced parkinsonism tends to resolve over time and additional medication may no longer be needed.

Drugs reported to cause parkinsonism
- antidepressants (e.g. SSRIs, MAOIs, TCAs)
- lithium
- anticonvulsants (e.g. carbamazepine, valproate)
- analgesics (e.g. NSAIDs, opiates)
- drugs of abuse (e.g. cocaine, PCP)
- cardiovascular drugs (e.g. amiodarone, diazoxide, diltiazem, methyldopa, metirosine, mexilitine, nifedipine, tocainide)
- GI drugs (e.g. cimetidine, domperidone, metoclopramide, prochlorperazine)
- anti-infection drugs (e.g. acyclovir, cephaloridine, chloroquine)
- respiratory drugs (e.g. antihistamines, salbutamol, terbutaline)
- hormones (e.g. medroxyprogesterone)
- cytotoxics (e.g. cyclosporin, interferons)
- others (e.g. cyclizine, ondansetron, levodopa, tetrabenazine)

Akathisia

Essence Akathisia usually occurs in the context of antipsychotic treatment. It may manifest in acute, chronic, withdrawal-related, or tardive (late-onset) forms. It is an unpleasant, distressing side-effect of medication and may be confused with agitation or worsening of psychiatric symptoms. When it is severe, patients may act aggressively, leading to inappropriate increases in antipsychotic medication. Careful assessment, including detailed history and review of medication, is essential.

Symptoms/signs Although there is no universally accepted definition of akathisia, the disorder characteristically manifests with:

- a **subjective component**—a feeling of inner restlessness (with the drive to engage in motor activity, esp. lower limbs and trunk).
- an **objective component**—movements: such as pacing constantly; inability to stand, sit, or lie still; rocking; crossing/uncrossing legs.

Pathophysiology Not yet fully understood. Theories include: dopaminergic/noradrenergic interactions (e.g. inhibition of presynaptic D_2 heteroreceptors on NA nerve terminals, with net increase in NA release), imbalance of dopaminergic/cholinergic transmission (causing compensatory increased NA or 5HT release), low serum iron/ferritin.

Epidemiology Prevalence ranges reported in schizophrenic patients on antipsychotic medication are quoted as 41% (mild symptoms), 21% (moderate-severe symptoms), up to 24% (for chronic symptoms (inpatient population)). For atypical agents, the reported incidence is up to 6%.

Risk factors Use of high-dose and/or high-potency antipsychotics, chronic use of antipsychotics, rapid increase/sudden withdrawal of antipsychotics, use of depot intra-muscular preparations, history of organic brain disease (e.g. dementia, alcoholism, HIV), history of previous akathisia, concomitant use of predisposing drugs (e.g. lithium, SSRIs).

Differential diagnosis Anxiety/agitation (primary or secondary to other psychiatric disorders), other withdrawal/discontinuation syndromes, acute confusional states, encephalitis/meningitis, parkinsonism/dystonia/dyskinesia, serotonergic syndrome (early symptoms), toxicity due to other drugs (e.g. recreational drugs—amphetamine, MDMA, cocaine; antidepressants; antihistamines; sympathomimetics; salicylate), restless legs syndrome, iron deficiency anaemia, endocrine disorders (e.g. thyrotoxicosis, hypo/hyperglycaemia, phaeochromocytoma).

Investigations General blood screen (FBC, LFTs, U&Es, glucose, TFTs)

Management
- Review history/medication to identify possible causative agent(s).
- Reduce dose or slow increase of potential causative agent.
- If antipsychotic-related, consider use of lower-potency drug.
- If symptoms persist consider specific treatment: first line—propranolol, initially 30mg/d (usual range 30–120mg/d); or pindolol, betaxolol, metoprolol.

- If patient has history of hypotension, diabetes, or associated parkinsonism (or propranolol ineffective) consider use of anticholinergic agents (e.g. benztropine, benzhexol, biperiden, orphenadrine, procyclidine, trihexyphenidyl).
- If ineffective, consider adding or changing to a benzodiazepine (e.g. clonazepam, diazepam, lorazepam).
- For unresponsive, predominantly anxious/agitated patient (without hypotension) consider clonidine 0.2–0.8 mg/d (may be sedative).
- Other possible agents include amantadine, buspirone (may also worsen symptoms), cyproheptadine, mianserin (may also worsen symptoms), tryptophan, piracetam, or even iron supplements.

Course/prognosis Most cases will respond to treatment and usually the response will be seen after a few days. Chronic or tardive cases may be more difficult to treat, and it should be borne in mind that therapeutic benefit (e.g. of propranolol) can take up to 3 months.

Follow-up
- Once the akathisia has settled, any specific treatment ought to be kept under review.
- Slow withdrawal of any additional agent should be attempted after a few weeks (in the case of benzodiazepines) or after several months (for other agents).
- If akathisia recurs, long-term therapy may be necessary. However, little data exists for agents other than propranolol (although original optimism for long-term benefit has not been borne out) or anticholinergics.
- The need for continued use of high-dose, high-potency antipsychotics should also be reviewed in the light of any change in the clinical presentation of the primary psychiatric disorder.

Drugs reported to cause akathisia

Antipsychotics (usually high-potency) Chlorpromazine (less likely), clozapine (rare), haloperidol, olanzapine, pipothiazine, prochlorperazine, promazine, risperidone (withdrawal), thioridazine (less likely), trifluoperazine, trimeprazine, trifluoperazine, zuclopenthixol.

Antidepressants Amoxapine, citalopram, fluoxetine, fluvoxamine, imipramine (and other TCAs), mianserin, paroxetine, sertraline, venlafaxine (withdrawal).

Anxiolytics Alprazolam, buspirone, lorazepam.

Others Diltiazem, alpha-interferon, levodopa, lithium, melatonin (withdrawal), metoclopramide, ondansetron, verapamil.

Tardive dyskinesia

Essence   Late onset (months→years, mean 7yrs) involuntary, repetitive, purposeless movements, occurring with long-term antipsychotic treatment (although also has been reported in *untreated* schizophrenic patients). Also associated with amoxapine, bupropion, buspirone, clomipramine, doxepin, diphenhydramine, fluoxetine, fluvoxamine, lithium, metoclopramide, and phenytoin.

Symptoms/signs   Perioral movements are the most common (e.g. tongue, lips, jaw), hence the alternative terms: **oral-lingual, orofacial, oro-bucco-facial, or buccal-lingual-masticatory dyskinesia**. Other movements may include: **axial**—trunk twisting, torticollis, retrocollis, shoulder shrugging, pelvic thrusting; **limbs**—rapid movements of the fingers or legs, hand clenching (and sometimes slower, choreoform movements). Symptoms can be consciously suppressed, worsen with distraction, are exacerbated by stress and antiparkinsonian agents, and disappear during sleep.

Pathophysiology   Not yet fully understood. Theories include: dopaminergic/cholinergic imbalance, upregulation/supersensitivity of postsynaptic DA receptors in the basal ganglia following chronic blockade, GABA hypofunction leading to enhanced DA transmission.

Epidemiology   Prevalence is ~10% of chronically treated patients but may be as high as 70% in the 'high risk' population.

Risk factors   Chronic use of antipsychotics (particularly in high dose), change/cessation of chronic treatment (especially intermittent treatment), concomitant anticholinergic treatment elderly (over 50), female ($\female : \male$ = 1.7:1), history of organic brain disease (e.g. dementia, learning disability, epilepsy), previous head injury, alcoholism, comorbid mood disorder, negative symptoms of schizophrenia, diabetes mellitus, history of previous drug-induced akathisia/parkinsonism/dystonias, concomitant use of predisposing drugs (e.g. lithium, antidepressants, stimulants).

Differential diagnosis   Stereotypies, tic disorders, other causes of dyskinesia (e.g. Parkinson's disease or use of antiparkinsonian agents), other causes of chorea/athetoid movements (e.g. Sydenham's/Huntington's chorea, Wilson's disease).

Management

- Review history/medication to identify possible causative agent(s).
- Reduce dose of potential causative agent, to achieve minimum effective dose that adequately controls psychotic symptoms.
- Anticholinergic agents will exacerbate the problem and should also be slowly reduced and stopped if possible.
- If residual symptoms can be tolerated, it is best to 'wait and see', as TD tends to improve with time, before considering addition of any specific treatment.
- If residual symptoms are severe, interfere significantly with functional abilities, or may be life-threatening, then temporarily raising the dose of antipsychotic may give immediate relief, whilst addition of a specific treatment may be commenced (dose of antipsychotic should then be reduced again).

- **Specific treatments** First line—biogenic amine (DA) depleting agent: Tetrabenazine 12.5mg to start, titrated to 25–75mg/d, max. 200mg/d.
- **Other possible strategies**
  - dopamine agonists (e.g. low-dose bromocriptine 0.75–7.5mg/d, L-dopa, amantadine)
  - benzodiazepines (e.g. clonazepam (if dystonia also present))
  - adrenergic agents (e.g. propranolol, clonidine)
  - calcium-channel blockers (e.g. nifedipine (high doses), verapamil, diltiazem)
  - anticonvulsants (e.g. valproate, gabapentin)
  - antioxidants (e.g. vitamin E (efficacy disputed))
  - other (e.g. baclofen, buspirone (high dose), cyproheptadine, insulin, ondansetron, piracetam, progabide, pyridoxine).
- If the symptoms are severe and non-responsive to other strategies, then consider an alternative antipsychotic—clozapine (reportedly effective in up to 43% of refractory cases), sulpiride, or an 'atypical' antipsychotic (e.g. olanzapine, risperidone, quetiapine) ECT has also been (anecdotally) shown to be effective.

Course/prognosis
- Symptoms may not progress and remission rates are ~30%/yr with 50% of sufferers clinically improved after 5yrs, even without treatment.
- Most cases will respond to treatment although a balance may need to be struck between reduction in dyskinesia vs. control of psychotic symptoms.

Follow-up
- Residual symptoms should be closely monitored.
- The need for continued antipsychotic treatment should also be regularly reviewed.
- Ensure that occurrence of TD and treatment strategy clearly recorded in case-notes.

Acute dystonic reaction

Essence Acute reaction following exposure to antipsychotic medication with sustained, often painful muscular spasms, producing twisted abnormal postures.

Aetiology Unknown. Usually occur at a time when blood levels of antipsychotics would be falling.

Incidence 3–10% of patients exposed to all antipsychotics (up to 30% with high-potency drugs).

Risk factors Previous/family history of dystonia, younger age group[1], ♂ > ♀ (most likely due to use of higher doses of antipsychotics in men), liver failure, clinically severe schizophrenia (esp. with marked negative symptoms), use of high-potency antipsychotics (up to 10%; for other agents see opposite).

Onset 50% of cases occur within 48hrs, rising to 90% within 5 days.

Symptoms/signs Frequency of occurrence of dystonias: neck (30%), tongue (17%), jaw (15%), oculogyric crisis (neck arched and eye rolled back: 6%), opisthotonus (body arching: 3.5%). Usually more generalised in younger patients (may be confused with fits, esp. in children) and more localised (head and neck) in older patients.

Course May fluctuate over hours, but most last minutes to hours without treatment.

Differential diagnosis May be mistaken for bizarre behaviour motivated by psychotic symptoms or even histrionic personality traits.

Management
- Discontinue suspected agent.
- Emergency treatment with IM/IV anticholinergic agents (e.g. procyclidine 5mg, benztropine 2mg).
- Continue use of anticholinergic for 1–2 days, unless antipsychotic clinically needed—then concomitant anticholinergic should be continued, but tapered off over 2–3 weeks (long term treatment may predispose to TD).
- Alternative treatment includes use of amatadine (fewer SEs than other agents).
- Routine prophylaxis should be considered for patients with a history of previous drug-induced dystonic reaction.

Agents reported to cause dystonias

Antipsychotics

Amoxapine, clozapine (rare/abrupt withdrawal), flupentixol decanoate, haloperidol, loxapine, olanzapine (rare), prochlorperazine, risperidone (rare), trimeprazine, zuclopethixol.

Other psychotropics

Benztropine (rare), bupropion, buspirone, carbamazepine, cocaine (+ withdrawal), disulfiram (rare), fluoxetine, midazolam, paroxetine, phenelzine, sertraline, TCAs.

Other (mostly rare/isolated cases)

Amiodarone, azapropazone, diphenhydramine, domperidone, ergotamine, indomethacin, metoclopramide, nifedipine, penicillamine, prochlorperazine, promethazine, propranolol, sumatriptan.

---

1 Note—in contrast with most medication side-effects, acute dystonias are more common in the young than the elderly. This may be related to asymptomatic loss of dopaminergic neurons in later life.

Neuroleptic malignant syndrome

Essence A rare, life-threatening, idiosyncratic reaction to antipsychotic (and other) medication (see opposite), characterised by: fever, muscular rigidity, altered mental status, and autonomic dysfunction.

N.B. If diagnosed in a psychiatric setting, transfer patient to acute medical services where intensive monitoring and treatment are available.

Pathophysiology Theories: $2°$ to DA activity in the CNS— i.e. striatum (rigidity), hypothalamus (thermoregulation)—by blockade of D_2-receptors or ↓DA availability; impaired Ca^{2+} mobilisation in muscle cells leads to rigidity (like malignant hyperthermia[1]); sympathetic nervous system activation or dysfunction.

Epidemiology Incidence 0.07–0.2% (pooled data); ♀:♂ = 2:1.

Mortality 5–20%—death usually due to respiratory failure, cardiovascular collapse, myoglobinuric renal failure, arrhythmias, or DIC.

Morbidity Rhabdomyolysis, aspiration pneumonia, renal failure, seizures, arrhythmias, DIC, respiratory failure, worsening of primary psychiatric disorder (due to withdrawal of antipsychotics).

Symptoms/signs Hyperthermia (>38°C), muscular rigidity, confusion/agitation/altered level of consciousness, tachycardia, tachypnoea, hyper/hypotension, diaphoresis/sialorrhea, tremor, incontinence/retention/obstruction, ↑CK/urinary myoglobin, leukocytosis, metabolic acidosis.

Risk factors ↑ambient temperature; dehydration; patient agitation or catatonia; rapid antipsychotic initiation/dose escalation; withdrawal of antiparkinsonian medication; use of high-potency agents/depot IM preparations; history of organic brain disease (e.g. dementia, alcoholism), affective disorder, previous NMS; predisposing drugs (e.g. lithium, anticholinergic agents).

Differential diagnosis (Lethal) catatonia (see opposite); malignant hyperthermia; encephalitis/meningitis; heat exhaustion; parkinsonism/acute dystonia; serotonergic syndrome; toxicity due to other drugs (e.g. amphetamine, MDMA, cocaine, antidepressants, antihistamines, sympathomimetics, salicylates); DTs; rhabdomyolysis; septic shock; haemorrhagic stroke; tetanus; phaeochromocytoma; strychnine poisoning.

Investigations FBC, blood cultures, LFTs, U&Es, calcium and phosphate levels, serum CK, urine myoglobin, ABGs, coagulation studies, serum/urine toxicology, CXR (if aspiration suspected), ECG; consider head CT (intracranial cause), LP (to exclude meningitis).

Management

- Benzodiazepines for acute behavioural disturbance (p. 896) (NB: Use of restraint and I/M injection may complicate the interpretation of serum CK.)
- Stop any agents thought to be causative (esp. antipsychotics), or restart antiparkinsonian agents.
- Supportive measures: oxygen, correct volume depletion/hypotension with IV fluids, reduce the temperature (e.g. cooling blankets, antipyretics, cooled IV fluids, ice packs, evaporative cooling, ice-water enema).

- Rhabdomyolysis—vigorous hydration and alkalinisation of the urine using IV sodium bicarbonate to prevent renal failure.
- Pharmacotherapy to reduce rigidity—dantrolene (IV 0.8–2.5mg/kg qds; PO 50–100mg bd), lorazepam (up to 5mg); *2nd line:* bromocriptine (PO 2.5–10mg tds, increase to max. 60mg/day), amantidine (PO 100–200mg bd); *3rd line:* nifedipine; consider ECT (NB ↑risk of fatal arrhythmias).

Course May last 7–10 days after stopping oral antipsychotics and up to 21 days after depot antipsychotics (e.g. fluphenazine).

Prognosis In the absence of rhabdomyolysis, renal failure, or aspiration pneumonia, and with good supportive care, prognosis is good.

Follow-up Monitor closely for residual symptoms. Once symptoms have settled allow 2+wks (if possible) before restarting medication (use low-dose, low-potency, or atypical agents). Consider prophylaxis (bromocriptine). Inform patient about risk of recurrence if given antipsychotic medication. Ensure this is recorded prominently in their medical notes.

Drugs reported to cause symptoms characteristic of NMS

Antipsychotics Chlorpromazine, clozapine (rarely), flupenthixol, fluphenazine, haloperidol, loxapine, olanzapine, promazine, quetiapine (rarely), risperidone, thioridazine.

Antiparkinsonian agents Amantadine (+withdrawal), anticholinergics (withdrawal), levodopa (+withdrawal).

Antidepressants Amoxapine, clomipramine, desipramine, phenelzine, trimipramine, venlafaxine.

Other Carbamazepine (+withdrawal), ganciclovir, ferrous sulphate, lithium, methylphenidate, metoclopramide, oral contraceptives.

Differentiating NMS from catatonia

Feature	NMS	Catatonia
Patient taking antipsychotics	Usually	Not usually
Catatonic symptoms:		
Echo phenomena	Rare	Yes
Ambitendency	Rare	Yes
Posturing	Rare	Yes
Hyperthermia	Usually before stupor	Usually before/during severe agitation
Muscle rigidity	Yes	Yes
Raised WCC	Yes	No
Raised CK	Yes	Yes

1 A rare disorder associated with exposure to inhaled aesthetics and succinylcholine. Genetic linkage found to chromosome 19. Possibly due to a muscle membrane defect, leading to ↓intracellular Ca^{2+} and intense muscle contractions. Temperature rises rapidly (up to 1°C/5mins).

Serotonin syndrome

Essence A rare but potentially fatal syndrome occuring in the context of initiation or dose increase of a serotonergic agent, characterised by altered mental state, agitation, tremor, shivering, diarrhoea, hyperreflexia, myoclonus, ataxia, and hyperthermia. Although SSRIs are commonly linked to SS, many other drugs (e.g. amphetamines, MAOIs, TCAs, lithium) have the potential of causing hyperserotonergic symptoms. SS can occur as a result of overdose, drug combinations (including over the counter medications), and rarely with therapeutic doses.

Pathophysiology A variety of mechanisms can potentially increase the quantity or activity of serotonin: ↑production of serotonin due to ↑availability of precursors (L-tryptophan–containing substances); ↓metabolism of serotonin (MAOIs, selegiline); ↑release of stored serotonin (amphetamine, cocaine, fenfluramine, MDMA, meperidine); reuptake inhibition (SSRIs, TCAs, SNRIs, NaSSAs, MDMA, dextromethorphan, meperidine, St. John's Wort); direct stimulation of serotonin receptors (buspirone, LSD); unknown mechanisms (lithium).

Epidemiology Incidence ~1% for SSRIs (moderate/major symptoms; mild symptoms may be common, but tend to go unreported); mortality <1 in 1000 cases.

Symptoms/signs (see opposite) Psychiatric/neurological Confusion, agitation, coma. **Neuromuscular** Myoclonus, rigidity, tremors (including shivering), hyperreflexia (usually lower rather than upper limbs), ataxia. **Autonomic** Hyperthermia (may be 2° to prolonged seizure activity, rigidity, or muscular hyperactivity), GI upset (nausea, diarrhoea), mydriasis, tachycardia, hyper/hypotension.

Differential diagnosis NMS (see opposite), malignant hyperthermia, infections (encephalitis/meningitis, sepsis), metabolic disturbances, substance abuse (cocaine)/withdrawal/overdose (LSD, PCP).

Investigations FBC, U&Es, LFTs, glucose, pH, biochemistry (including calcium, magnesium, phosphate, anion gap), CK, drug toxicology screen, CXR (if evidence of respiratory distress/possible aspiration), ECG monitoring (arrhythmia/conduction problems—prolonged QRS or QTc interval).

Treatment

- If severe, requires immediate transfer to emergency department for supportive treatment and active management.
- If overdose, consider gastric lavage and/or activated charcoal.
- IV access—to allow volume correction (dehydration: insensible fluid loss due to hyperthermia) and reduce risk of rhabdomyolysis.
- **Rhabdomyolysis** should be dealt with quickly, with emphasis on maintaining a high urine output combined with alkalinisation using sodium bicarbonate (target urine pH of 6). If necessary, reduce the temperature (e.g. cooling blankets, antipyretics, cooled IV fluids, ice packs, evaporative cooling, ice-water enema).

- **Pharmacotherapy** Agitation, seizures, and muscular rigidity/myoclonus best managed using a *benzodiazepine* (e.g. lorazepam IV (slow) 1–2mg every 30 mins; clonazepam). *Serotonin receptor antagonists* may be considered in selected cases (e.g. cyproheptadine PO 4–8mg every 2–4 hrs (max 0.5mg/kg/d), chlorpromazine (risk of reduced seizure threshold), mirtazepine, methysergide, propranolol (mild 5HT antagonist)). *Antihypertensives* are usually unnecessary unless the hypertension is persistent and clinically significant (e.g. nitroglycerin IV 2mg/kg/min).

Course and prognosis Onset is usually acute, However, recurrent mild symptoms may occur for weeks before the appearance of severe symptoms. Most cases resolve without sequelae within 24–36 hours with adequate supportive measures. Following an SSRI overdose, a patient who remains asymptomatic for several hours is unlikely to need further medical management.

Sternbach's diagnostic criteria[1]

- Other potential causes excluded (e.g. infection, metabolic, substance abuse, withdrawal).
- No concurrent antipsychotic dose changes prior to symptom onset.
- At least three of the following:
  - Agitation/restlessness
  - Sweating
  - Diarrhoea
  - Fever
  - Hyperreflexia
  - Ataxia
  - Mental state changes (confusion, hypomania)
  - Myoclonus
  - Shivering
  - Tremor

Distinguishing SS from NMS

Although the clinical presentation of these 2 syndromes is very similar (i.e. autonomic dysfunction, alteration of mental status, rigidity, and hyperthermia), differentiation is very important as specific management may differ (e.g. use of chlorpromazine in SS, which may worsen NMS).

	NMS	SS
Associated Rx	Antipsychotics (Idiosyncratic/normal dose)	Serotonergic agents (OD/drug combination)
Onset	Slow (days to weeks)	Rapid
Progression	Slow (24–72 hrs)	Rapid
Muscle rigidity	Severe ('lead pipe')	Less severe
Activity	Bradykinesia	Hyperkinesia

1 Sternbach H (1991) The serotonin syndrome. *AJP* **148**, 705–13.

SSRI[1] withdrawal (discontinuation) syndrome[2]

The incidence and prevalence of this syndrome are currently unknown. Rates of occurrence vary from 12–85%, depending both on the SSRI used and the underlying condition being treated. The few available discontinuation studies indicate minor forms of the syndrome may be common and severe forms unusual. There may be less risk with certain drugs (e.g. fluoxetine—perhaps due to longer half-life) and possibly greater risk with paroxetine (perhaps due to cholinergic rebound), although symptoms of discontinuation have been reported with *all* the SSRIs.

Clinical features

Neurologic symptoms—most common: dizziness, vertigo, lightheadedness, and gait instability.

Somatic complaints—nausea/emesis, fatigue and headache; insomnia. Less frequently reported: shock-like sensations, paraesthesia, visual disturbances, diarrhoea, flu-like symptoms (myalgias and chills).

Non-specific symptoms—agitation, impaired concentration, vivid dreams, depersonalisation, irritability, and suicidal thoughts have also been reported.

Course and duration Usually develop after 1 month of SSRI treatment, within 2–5 days after SSRI discontinuation or dose reduction. If untreated, duration is variable (one to several weeks) and ranges from mild-moderate intensity in most patients, to extremely distressing in a small number.

Aetiology The biological mechanisms underlying this syndrome are not well understood, although an acute decrease in synaptic serotonin in the face of down-regulated or desensitised serotonin receptors has been postulated.

Risk factors Appears to be idiosyncratic with no specific associations with age, sex, diagnosis, or dose of SSRI (both low and high doses have been reported).

Differential diagnosis The syndrome may be easily confused with *recurrence* of symptoms after inadequate duration of SSRI treatment, particularly in the anxiety disorders. Other possibilities (e.g. infection, metabolic, withdrawal from drugs of abuse/alcohol) should be excluded. If the syndrome occurs when cross-tapering from one SSRI to another antidepressant, be aware of the possibility of serotonin syndrome (see p. 870).

Management

- Tapering SSRIs may help reduce the risk of developing the syndrome (use of liquid preparations may be helpful in allowing greater flexibility). However, guidelines on the optimum rates of dose reduction are at best *empirical* (see p. 275) and a cautious approach is advised (slowly over a number of weeks).
- If severe, re-introduction of the SSRI rapidly resolves the symptoms. However, the syndrome may recur in up to 75% of patients when the same SSRI is later discontinued.

- Awareness of some of the more unusual symptoms, such as dizziness and shock-like sensations, and education of patients prior to stopping or tapering an SSRI, should prevent unnecessary and expensive medical investigations.
- When symptoms are mild-moderate and short-lived they can generally be tolerated by the patient, allowing for successful discontinuation of the SSRI.

1 The 'special case' for differentiating an 'SSRI discontinuation syndrome' is debatable, since withdrawal syndromes have been described with most antidepressants including TCAs and SNRIs (venlafaxine)—all with similar symptoms to those described for SSRIs. In general, gradual tapering of antidepressants is recommended and abrupt stopping should be avoided (see p. 274).

2 Zajecka J, Tracy KA, Mitchell S (1997) Discontinuation symptoms after treatment with serotonin reuptake inhibitors: a literature review. *Journal of Clinical Psychiatry* **58**, 291–7 (& suppl. 7).

Hyponatraemia and antidepressants

Essence Low serum sodium is a rare, idiosyncratic side-effect of antide-pressants which may have serious consequences if undiagnosed.

Aetiology Incompletely understood, but probably due to the syndrome of inappropriate secretion of anti-diuretic hormone (SIADH).

Risk factors Previous SIADH/history of hyponatraemia; age >80yrs; comorbidity: diabetes mellitus, hypertension, impaired renal function, COAD; other medication (e.g. diuretics).

Clinical features Depend upon the severity, duration, and rate of change in serum sodium. May be asymptomatic, or display symptoms and signs (e.g. lethargy, confusion, nausea, weight loss, muscle cramps/weakness, hypertension, cardiac failure, oedema, seizures).

Investigations U&Es (serum Na^+<125mmol/l), 24hr urine collection (urinary Na^+>20mmol/l and osmolality>100mosml/kg). Alternatively there may be low plasma osmolality (<260mmol/kg) without hypovolaemia, oedema, or diuretics.

Differential diagnosis *Malignancy* e.g. lung small-cell; pancreas; prostate; lymphoma. *CNS disorders* e.g. meningoencephalitis; abscess; stroke; subarachnoid/subdural haemorrhage; head injury; Guillain-Barré; vasculitis. *Respiratory disorders* e.g. TB; pneumonia; abscess; aspergillosis. *Metabolic disease* e.g. porphyria; trauma. *Drugs* e.g. opiates; chlorpropramide; cytotoxic agents.

Management

- *Prevention* Baseline U&Es prior to commencing antidepressant, with monitoring for those at high risk (initially monthly, or after any dose change, once treatment dose established—every 3–6mths).
- *Treatment*
  - Withdraw suspected agent immediately.
  - If serum Na^+ remains <125mmol/l, refer to specialist medical care (to eliminate other possible causes, and to treat more intensively—e.g. with fluid restriction and occasionally with demeclocycline).
  - If serum Na^+>125mmol/l, continue to monitor U&Es daily until >135mmol/l.
  - Consider alternative antidepressant (usually from a different class—low dose, gradual increase, close monitoring) or, if treatment urgent, ECT may be an option.

Paradoxical reactions to benzodiazepines[1]

Essence Paradoxical or 'disinhibitory' reactions to BDZs occur in a minority of patients (less than 1% of general population) and are characterised by acute excitement and altered mental state:

- increased anxiety
- vivid dreams
- hyperactivity
- sexual disinhibition
- hostility and rage ('aggressive dyscontrol')

Recognition is important as behavioural disturbance may be exacerbated by inappropriate use of higher doses of BDZs. NB Similar types of reaction are described for most CNS depressants (e.g. alcohol, barbiturates).

Aetiology Incompletely understood; theories include: 'release behaviour' due to loss of frontal lobe inhibition through GABA$_A$ mechanism; BDZ related reduction in 5HT neurotransmission; BDZ related reduction in ACh neurotransmission.

Risk factors Children, learning disability, history of brain injury, dementia, borderline PD, antisocial PD, history of aggression/poor impulse control, family/personal history of paradoxical reaction, use of high-dose/high-potency BDZs (e.g. alprazolam, clonazepam, flunitrazepam, triazolam), IV/intranasal administration.

Management

- Nurse in safe environment, with constant supervision.
- Use sedative antipsychotic to treat acute behavioural disturbance if necessary.
- In extreme cases consider use of IV flumazenil (may require repeated doses).
- Clearly record occurrence of paradoxical reaction so that future episodes of acute behavioural disturbance are managed appropriately.

1 Paton C (2002) Benzodiazepines and disinhibition: a review *Psychiatric Bulletin* **26**, 460–2.

Prescribing in pregnancy

Data is limited (and often conflicting) regarding the safety of psychotropic drugs in pregnancy. Many clinicians prefer to use older agents as they have more experience with these compounds.

Antipsychotics

- All drugs carry a moderate risk and should be used with caution, although there is little clear evidence for teratogenicity of most compounds. (Some evidence for increased risk of organ dysgenesis with the phenothiazines.)
- Depot formulations should be avoided as gradual withdrawal prior to delivery is complicated (and neonatal withdrawal may be more severe).
- Specific advice from the manufacturer (Novartis) should be sought regarding the use of clozapine (although it does not appear to be a major teratogen).

Antidepressants

- There is relatively more data establishing the safety of older compounds (e.g. imipramine, amitriptyline). However, serum monitoring and dose adjustment may be necessary.
- Of the SSRIs, fluoxetine is the most studied with no good evidence of teratogenicity (and only a slight increased possibility of miscarriage—similar to TCAs).

Benzodiazepines

- Neonatal respiratory depression, hypothermia, hypotonia ('floppy baby syndrome') and withdrawal syndromes may occur when BDZs are used close to delivery.
- High doses and use in the first trimester increase the teratogenic risk.
- There may be an association between BDZs (esp. diazepam) and increased risk of facial clefts (detailed ultrasonography at 16–18wks indicated).
- Short-term use and minimum effective dose are advised if BDZs are necessary. Promethazine is often preferred.

Mood stabilisers

- All commonly used mood stabilisers are teratogenic and, where possible, should be avoided in the first trimester.
- **Lithium** has been associated with an increased risk (1:1000) of Epstein's anomaly (downward displacement of the tricuspid valve into the right ventricle) and detailed ultrasound/foetal echocardiography is indicated at 16–18wks.
  - Relapse rates on discontinuation (50% within 2–10wks) are generally regarded to preclude stopping lithium therapy in pregnancy.
  - Serum monitoring, dosage adjustment, and ensuring adequate hydration are essential (particularly after delivery).
  - Neonatal problems include 'floppy baby syndrome', non-toxic goitre, hypothyroidism, nephrogenic diabetes insipidus, and cardiac arrhythmias.

- **Valproate**, and to a lesser extent **carbamazepine**, are associated with neural tube defects (hence folic acid supplementation is recommended for women of child-bearing age—although evidence for benefit is inconclusive). Valproate has recently been associated with increased risk of hypospadias.
  - Detailed ultrasonography should be carried out at 16–18wks, and maternal serum alpha-fetoprotein (AFT) levels measured.
  - There is also an increased risk of neonatal haemorrhage, and vitamin K should be given to mothers in the last month of gestation (and to neonates at birth).
- Little data is available for gabapentin, lamotrigine, or other newer anticonvulsants and the risk/benefit needs to be carefully considered.

Guiding principles[1]

For all women of child-bearing age
- Always consider (and ask about) the possibility of pregnancy.
- Before starting any medication, a pregnancy test is recommended.
- Counsel the patient about the necessity of adequate contraception.
- Advise further consultation if pregnancy is planned.

For a planned conception
- Discuss the risks/benefits of discontinuation/continuation of medication (e.g. relapse vs. teratogenicity, the possible time it may take to conceive, no decision is risk-free).
- Avoidance of all drugs during the first trimester is ideal (but often not achievable).

In pregnancy
- Consider switching to a lower risk drug if possible, use the lowest dose possible, avoid polypharmacy, and monitor closely.
- Pregnancy may alter the pharmacokinetics of drugs, hence dosages may need to be adjusted (e.g. lithium).
- Gradual withdrawal of some compounds (e.g. BDZs, TCAs, SSRIs) in the weeks prior to delivery may help avoid 'withdrawal' effects in the newborn baby.

---

1 Adapted from Bazire S (2001) *Psychotropic Drug Directory 2001/02*, p 206. Bath Press, UK.

Prescribing in lactation

⚠ Absolute contraindications

Breastfeeding should be avoided when the mother is concurrently taking MAOIs, lithium, and clozapine, or there is evidence in the infant of renal, hepatic, cardiac, or neurological disorders.

General points

- All psychotropic medication should be regarded as passing into breast milk (to a greater or lesser degree).
- Of the limited studies examining this problem, the general findings are that levels of most psychotropic drugs in breast milk are relatively low, and infant blood levels may be *undetectable*.
- Although infant exposure may be relatively low from breast milk (much lower than *in utero* exposure if mother was taking medication during pregnancy), there is a risk of both withdrawal symptoms and adverse effects on development.
- Evidence may be lacking for *specific* risks, nonetheless caution should be exercised.
- Monitoring of the infant should include biochemical (renal and liver function tests) and behavioural measures, with the involvement of a paediatrician to ensure development is within normal parameters.

Choice of medication in nursing mothers

- Where possible, consider non-pharmacological treatments.
- If medication is necessary, the lowest effective therapeutic dose should be used and polypharmacy should be avoided.
- A recent review of the topic[1] concludes that 'the findings to date suggest that provided that infants are healthy at the outset it is likely that the benefits of breast-feeding will outweigh potential hazards if their mothers are taking established tricyclic drugs at recommended dose levels. Much less is known about risks associated with SSRI antidepressants or about antipsychotic drugs such as phenothiazines and butyrophenones or mood stabilizers such as carbamazepine'.

Antipsychotics Low doses of chlorpromazine (max. 200mg/day), haloperidol (max. 10mg/day), and trifluoperazine (max. 20mg/day) may be used cautiously, with close monitoring of the infant.

Antidepressants Most evidence exists for the TCAs (esp. imipramine and nortriptyline). SSRIs have not been shown to have major adverse effects on the infant. Newer antidepressants should not be used, unless the mother has taken them during the pregnancy.

Mood stabilisers Lithium should be avoided. Carbamazepine and valproate may be used cautiously, preferably given as a single dose in slow-release form.

Strategies to minimise infant exposure

- Breastfeeding should be avoided at the time when serum levels in the mother are likely to be at their peak (check drug information for these values).

- If possible, medication should be given as a single dose before the infant's longest sleep period.
- Breastfeeding should occur immediately *before* taking the next due dose.
- Alternatively, breast milk may be expressed when serum levels are at their lowest.

1 Yoshida K, Smith B, Kumar R (1999) Psychotropic drugs in mothers' milk: a comprehensive review of assay methods, pharmacokinetics and of safety of breast-feeding. *J Psychopharmacol.* **13**, 64–80.

Prescribing for patients with cardiovascular disease

General points

In considering a suitable psychotropic drug the main issues revolve around the propensity of that drug to interact with other medications the patient may be taking, to affect blood pressure, or lead to cardiac conduction problems (see opposite). Due to the unpredictability of drug interactions, polypharmacy is best avoided.

Specific contraindications

BDZs and chlormethiazole in pulmonary insufficiency, disulfiram (Antabuse) and lithium in heart failure or sick sinus syndrome, lofexidine in post-MI patients. Pimozide is best avoided in most conditions.

Myocardial infarction

Antidepressants Best avoided in the first 2 months; if clinically indicated—SSRIs rather than TCAs, with exception of fluvoxamine and citalopram. If sedation required consider use of a small dose of trazodone at night.

Antipsychotics High doses should be avoided; phenothiazines are generally more hypotensive than butyrophenones; clozapine should be used with caution in the 1st yr post MI; of the newer antipsychotics, olanzapine may offer best risk-benefit balance.

Heart failure

Where possible, hypotensive agents (β-blockers, clozapine, risperidone, TCAs) and drugs causing fluid retention (carbamazepine, lithium) should be avoided.

Angina/IHD

Avoid hypotensive agents (see above) and those known to cause tachycardia (phenothiazines, clozapine, risperidone).

Hypertension

Avoid agents that may raise blood pressure (low-dose TCAs, phenothiazines, clozapine, high-dose venlafaxine).

Arrhythmias (see opposite)

Antidepressants SSRIs should be first choice (but not fluvoxamine or citalopram).

Antipsychotics High doses should be avoided; risperidone may be least likely to cause conduction problems.

The QT^c question

Awareness of QT prolongation, as measured by the *corrected QT interval* (QT^c), has been heightened because of the potential (but relatively rare) risk of fatal arrhythmias (e.g. torsade de pointes), highlighted recently by the withdrawal of thioridazine as a first-line antipsychotic (and now contraindicated in patients with a history of, or at risk of, arrhythmias) and the restricted use of droperidol.

QT^c is derived by dividing the QT interval by the square root of the cycle length i.e.:

$$QT^c = \frac{QT}{\sqrt{(R-R)}}$$

Normal QT^c is 380–420ms; if prolonged to 450ms—some concern; if >500–520ms—'at risk'.

Causes of prolonged QT interval: acute myocardial ischaemia, myocarditis, bradycardia (e.g. AV block), head injury, hypothermia, electrolyte imbalance (K$^+$↑ , Ca^{2+}↓ , Mg^{2+}↓), congenital, sotalol, quinidine, antihistamines, macrolides (e.g. erythromycin), amiodarone, antipsychotics (esp. phenothiazines), antidepressants (esp. TCAs).

General advice: good practice dictates use of routine ECG prior to commencement of antipsychotic medication (esp. pimozide, zotepine, thioridazine, and other phenothiazines), and regular monitoring, particularly with use of high doses (p. 216).

Prescribing for patients with liver disease

General points

- Almost all psychotropic drugs are metabolised by the liver.
- Exceptions to this rule include lithium, gabapentin, sulpiride, and amisulpiride, which have minimal (or no) liver metabolism.
- Most drugs are highly protein-bound (with the exception of citalopram, sulpiride, and amisulpiride) and plasma levels may be *increased* in liver disease.
- In liver disease, when using drugs with high 1st pass clearance (e.g. imipramine, amitriptyline, desipramine, doxepin, haloperidol) initial doses should be low.
- Where possible, phenothiazines (e.g. chlorpromazine) and hydrazine MAOIs (may be hepatotoxic) should be avoided.
- If in doubt, closely monitor LFTs, particularly during dose changes.

Antidepressants (always start with lowest possible dose)

- **TCAs** Best evidence for use of imipramine.
- **SSRIs** Some evidence for paroxetine; avoid sertraline.
- **MAOIs** When clinically necessary, use 30–50% usual dose.
- **Others** Venlafaxine (use 50% usual dose), mirtazepine (cautious use), reboxetine (extensively metabolised, very low starting dose).

Antipsychotics

- Best evidence for haloperidol (considered 'drug of choice'), with sulpiride a close second (only 5% liver metabolism).
- Few problems reported with flupenthixol/zuclopenthixol.
- Clozapine dose should be kept low (some evidence of hepatotoxicity).
- Amisulpiride is predominantly excreted by the kidneys, but there is little literature on its use in liver disease.
- For the newer agents recommendations suggest:
  - Olanzapine (up to 7.5mg) may be safe (but does induce transaminases).
  - Risperidone doses should be kept low (start 0.5mg bd, max 4mg/d).
  - Quetiapine is extensively metabolised (hence start low—25mg).
  - Zotepine should only be used with caution (start 2.5mg bd, max 75mg/d, monitor LFTs weekly for at least 3mths).

Mood stabilisers

- Lithium is the 'drug of choice', with gabapentin as second choice.
- Valproate is *contraindicated* in severe liver disease, but may be used with caution in mild-moderate impairment.
- Similarly caution should be exercised with carbamazepine, and lamotrigine is *contraindicated* in severe disease.

Anxiolytics

- Where necessary, use low doses of short-acting BDZs (e.g lorazepam, oxazepam).
- If chlormethiazole is to be used, the dose should be reduced to ~30%.

Prescribing for patients with renal impairment

General points

- Renal impairment generally leads to accumulation of drugs (or active metabolites) that are predominantly cleared by the kidneys. This will lead to higher serum levels and increased risk of dose-related side-effects (e.g. pick up hypotension, sedation, EPSE).
- Hence, all psychotropic agents should be started at a low (or divided) dose pressed slowly, and carefully monitored for efficacy and side-effects.
- When patients are receiving dialysis, seek specific advice from manufacturer—doses should usually be reduced by at least 50% and dosing separated in time from dialysis itself.

Classification of chronic renal failure (CRF)

- Renal... classified as mild (GFR 30–50mL/min), moderate (GFR 10–30mL/min), severe (GFR <10mL/min) or end-stage (GFR < ...mL/min). See opposite for estimation of GFR.

Antidepressants

- In severe renal failure avoid fluoxetine, venlafaxine and reboxetine (unless the patient is on dialysis).
- Otherwise, cautious use, beginning low and gradually increasing the dose is advised.
- No specific therapeutic dose adjustments are necessary for MAOIs (except for isocarboxazid), RIMAs, mianserin, tryptophan, trazodone, or TCAs.

Antipsychotics

- Lower doses are recommended to avoid dose-related side-effects (particularly with the phenothiazines), which may be best avoided.
- Clozapine is contraindicated in severe renal impairment.
- Greater care is necessary with amisulpride, sulpiride, risperidone and zotepine.
- Loxapine appears to have few specific problems.
- Some authorities recommend haloperidol, but accumulation is possible, so careful monitoring is still necessary.

Mood stabilizers

- Lithium is relatively contraindicated in renal failure. However, if its use may often be necessary, and dose reduction (e.g. to 50–75% for mild-moderate and 25–50% for severe renal failure) with close monitoring of plasma levels is recommended. In dialysis 600mg 3× week (after dialysis) has been shown to maintain therapeutic plasma levels.
- No specific problems are reported for valproate or carbamazepine, although in severe renal failure, serum levels should be monitored.
- Gabapentin requires specific dose adjustments and manufacturer's recommendations should be sought.
- Lamotrigine should be used cautiously, particularly in severe renal impairment.

Prescribing for patients with renal impairment

General points

- Renal impairment generally leads to accumulation of drugs (or active metabolites) that are predominantly cleared by the kidney. This will lead to higher serum levels, and increased risk of dose-related side-effects (e.g. postural hypotension, sedation, EPSEs).
- Hence, all psychotropics should be started at a low (or divided) dose, increased slowly, and carefully monitored (for efficacy and tolerability).
- When patients are receiving dialysis seek specific advice from manufacturer—dosages should usually be reduced by at least 50% and dosing separated in time from dialysis itself.

Classification of chronic renal failure (CRF)

CRF may be classified as **mild** (GFR 30–50ml/min), **moderate** (GFR 10–29ml/min), **severe** (GFR <10ml/min), or **end-stage** (GFR <5ml/min). **See opposite for estimation of GFR.**

Antidepressants

- In severe renal failure avoid fluoxetine, venlafaxine, and lofepramine (unless the patient is on dialysis).
- Otherwise cautious use, beginning low and gradually increasing the dose is advised.
- No specific therapeutic dose adjustments are necessary for MAOIs (except for isocarboxazid), RIMAs, mianserin, tryptophan, trazodone, or TCAs.

Antipsychotics

- Lower doses are recommended to avoid dose-related side-effects (particularly with the phenothiazines, which may be best avoided).
- Clozapine is contraindicated in severe renal impairment.
- Greater care is necessary with amisulpiride/sulpiride, risperidone, and zotepine.
- Loxapine appears to have few specific problems.
- Some authorities recommend haloperidol, but accumulation is possible, so careful monitoring is still necessary.

Mood stabilisers

- Lithium is relatively contraindiciated in renal failure. However, its use may often be necessary, and dose reduction (e.g. to 50–75% for mild-moderate and 25–50% for severe renal failure) with close monitoring of plasma levels is recommended. In dialysis, 600mg ×3/wk (after dialysis) has been shown to maintain therapeutic plasma levels.
- No specific problems are reported for valproate or carbamazepine, although in severe renal failure, serum levels should be monitored.
- Gabapentin requires specific dose adjustments and manufacturer's recommendations should be sought.
- Lamotrigine should be used cautiously, particularly in severe renal impairment.

Anxiolytics/hypnotics

- BDZs (with the exception of chlordiazepoxide) tend to accumulate, with increasing CNS side-effects (particularly sedation)—hence use low doses.
- Buspirone is contraindicated in moderate-severe renal failure.
- β-blockers should be started at low dose as they may complicate renal failure by reducing renal blood flow.
- Zopiclone and zaleplon require no dosage adjustment. However, the half-life of zolpidem may be doubled in renal failure.

Others

- Anticholinergics, disulfiram—cautious use.
- Acamprosate—contraindicated if serum creatinine >120µmol/l.
- Anticholinesterases—no reported problems.

Estimating glomerular filtration rate (GFR)

Creatinine clearance is a measure of GFR, the volume of fluid filtered by the glomeruli per minute (ml/min). Normal value is approx. 125ml/min. Urine is collected over a 24-hr period for urinary creatinine (mmol/l), along with a blood sample for serum creatinine (µmol/l).

Urine creatinine concentration = **u** mmol/l
Plasma creatinine concentration = **p** µmol/l
24-hr urine volume = **v** mls

Creatinine clearance $(ml/min) = (u \times 0.7) \times \left(\dfrac{v}{p}\right)$

NB Always check the **units** are correct for each variable in the equation.

For an estimate of creatinine clearance[*] based only on the serum creatinine, the following formula can be used:

Creatinine clearance $(ml/min) = \dfrac{(140 - \text{age in year}) \times (\text{wt in kg})}{72 \text{ serum creatinine in mg/dl}}$

NB To convert µmol/l to mg/dl, divide µmol/l by 88.4.

[*] For women, the above estimate should be multiplied by 0.85. This estimate assumes stable renal function, absence of obesity and/or oedema.

Prescribing for patients with epilepsy

General points

In considering a suitable psychotropic there are 2 related considerations:
- The propensity of that drug to interact with other medications the patient may be taking (justifying serum monitoring where possible).
- The risk of lowering seizure threshold and exacerbating the condition.

As these effects appear dose-related, the daily dose of any drug should be kept as low as possible. Greater caution is necessary when:
- Other psychotropics are also being given (e.g. regular *plus* 'as required' antipsychotics).
- Patients may be withdrawing from CNS depressants (e.g. BDZs, barbiturates, or alcohol).

Antidepressants

- All TCAs appear to lower seizure threshold, although there appears to be greater risk with amitriptyline and clomipramine.
- Tetracyclics (maprotiline and amoxapine) also appear pro-convulsant, as does bupropion.
- The other antidepressants appear less likely to cause problems, and a usual first choice is often an SSRI.

Antipsychotics

- Greatest risk of seizures is associated with the use of phenothiazines (esp. chlorpromazine), loxapine, zotepine, olanzapine, and particularly clozapine.
- The risk of seizures with clozapine rises from 1% (at doses <300mg/d), to 2.7% (300–600mg/d), to 4.4% (>600mg/d). EEG changes are seen in up to 75% of people taking clozapine, with ~40% showing paroxysmal discharges[1]. Because of this risk it is quite common to cover high doses of clozapine with concomitant use of valproate. Hence, greater caution is needed when clozapine is used in individuals with epilepsy.
- Lowest risk is associated with haloperidol, sulpiride, zuclopenthixol, amisulpiride, pimozide, quetiapine, and risperidone.

Mood stabilisers

- Lithium does cause seizures in overdose. However, therapeutic doses appear safe.
- If in doubt, anticonvulsants provide useful alternatives. However, clinical efficacy must be weighed against any *potential* risks of using lithium.

Anxiolytics/hypnotics

- Generally these drugs are *anticonvulsant*.
- Exceptions include buspirone, zolpidem, and β-blockers—although there is no evidence that they are epileptogenic.

Others

- Anticholinergics, acamprosate—no reported problems.
- Disulfiram—caution recommended.
- Anticholinesterases—care is needed with donepezil and rivastigmine. However, galantamine appears safe.

1 Pacia SV and Devinsky O (1994) Clozapine-related seizures: experience with 5,629 patients. *Neurology* **44**, 2247–9.

Plasma level monitoring

There are a limited number of drugs with well-established plasma levels that equate with efficacy. Plasma monitoring is a regular procedure only for lithium therapy. However, there may be a number of other reasons for requesting plasma levels (bear in mind that assays for *specific* drugs may not be locally available and may need special arrangements.) Many psychiatric drugs have marked variations in metabolism, or large numbers of active metabolites, making plasma levels difficult to interpret.

Reasons for monitoring

- Established therapeutic plasma levels (see below).
- Monitoring of any changes in plasma level that might affect efficacy (e.g. due to drug interactions, inter-current illness, pregnancy, or altered pharmacokinetics over time).
- Clinical evidence of toxicity (e.g. lithium, anticonvulsants).
- Where there is doubt about patient compliance (e.g. lack of effect despite adequate or even high-dose treatment).
- In cases where the patient may be unable to report adverse effects (e.g. children, severe LD, dementia).
- After overdose, to confirm it is safe to restart medication.

Reference ranges for selected drugs	
Lithium *(see p. 328)*	0.8–1.2mmol/L
	(0.6–0.8mmol/L—as an augmentative agent)
Valproate *(see p. 332)*	50–125mg/L
Carbamazepine *(see p. 334)*	4–12mg/L
	(>7mg/L may be more efficacious in BAD)
Clozapine *(see p. 218)*	350–500mcg/L (0.35–0.5mg/L)
Nortriptyline	50–150mcg/L

Chapter 22

Difficult and urgent situations

Dealing with psychiatric emergencies

It is a common misconception that there are no *real* emergencies in psychiatry. The billowing white coat may be gone, but then so is the backup of the arrest team. Dealing with acute situations can feel like a lonely business, and doubts about the best management of given situations may prevent you getting that much needed rest period.

As a psychiatrist, you are primarily a doctor, and you should ensure that you are up to date with basic resuscitation procedures. Familiarise yourself with the procedures in place for the management of medical emergencies in your hospital, as the level of on-site facilities will vary.

There is no substitute for experience, but hopefully some of the guidance in the following section (and the other pages they refer to) will allow a rational approach to a number of common (and not so common) difficult and urgent situations in a psychiatric setting.

Keep the following principles in mind:

Primum non nocere

('*Above all, do no harm*')
- Always ensure your own and other staff's safety.
- Remember—patient confidentiality does not override issues of threatened harm to themselves or other individuals.
- Always suspect (and as far as possible eliminate) potential organic causation for psychiatric presentations.
- If necessary facilities or expertise are not available, make appropriate arrangements to get the patient to them as soon as possible.

Assess

- Always make the fullest assessment possible—do not fail to ask about important issues just because you feel a person may not wish to talk about them.
- Ensure that you have the best quality information available. If other sources of information are available (e.g. previous notes, 3rd party information), use them!
- Don't dawdle—if a situation requires immediate action, act.

Consult

- Do not *assume* anything. If in doubt, consult a senior colleague. Remember you are part of a team, and if there is a difficult decision to make, do not make it alone.

Keep contemporaneous records

- Clearly record your assessment, decisions made (*and* reasons), and the names of any other colleagues involved or consulted. Legally, if it's not been recorded, it's not been done.

What to do if summoned to a crisis situation/negotiation principles

First principles

- Speak to the staff who originated the call.
- Obtain as much information as possible about the situation prior to seeing the patient.
- Establish what your expected role is.
- Keep your own safety uppermost in your mind (no heroics).

General aims

- Attempt to put the patient at their ease; explain who you are and why you have been asked to speak to them.
- Be clear in any questions you need to ask.
- Elicit useful information.
- Achieve a safe, dignified resolution of the situation.

Important communication principles

- Be conscious of both verbal and non-verbal language.
  - Listen actively—assimilate and understand what is actually being said and interpret the various underlying meanings and messages.
  - Feedback—go back over what the patient has said with them to assure them that you understand what they are saying.
  - Empathy—show you appreciate them sharing their thoughts, feelings, and motives.
  - Content and feeling—note any difference between what is said verbally and what message is really being given.
- Use checkpoint summaries—brief reviews of the main points discussed, about issues, and any demands.

Important suggestions

- Use open questions to give the patient an opportunity to ventilate what is on their mind (this may help relieve tension, keep the patient talking, and allow you to assess the mental state).
- Listen carefully to what the patient is saying.
  - This may provide further clues as to their actions.
  - It also demonstrates concern for the patient's problem.
- Be honest, upfront, and sincere—try to develop a trusting relationship.
- Be neutral—avoid approval or disapproval unless absolutely necessary.
- Orient the patient to looking for alternative solutions together, without telling them how to act (unless asked).
- Try to divert any negative train of thought.
- Check with other team members before making any commitments.
- If the police have been called, present the reason for their presence realistically, but neutrally.
- Do not involve family members in negotiations.

Some suggestions for dealing with particular patients
(See opposite)

The patient responding to paranoid ideas/delusion

- Avoid prolonged eye contact and do not get too close.
- The patient's need to explain may allow you to establish a degree of rapport. Allow them to talk, but try to stay with concrete topics.
- Do not try to argue them out of their delusions—ally yourself with their perspective without sounding insincere (e.g. 'What you are saying is that you believe…x…y…z')
- Avoid using family members who may be part of the delusional system.
- Try to distance yourself from what may have happened in the past (e.g. 'I'm sorry that was your experience before…maybe this time we could manage things better…').
- Be aware that your offer of help may well be rejected.

The patient with antisocial traits

- A degree of flattery may facilitate discussion of alternative solutions (e.g. you understand their need to communicate, how important their opinions are to you, your desire to work together to resolve things).
- Encourage them to talk about what has led up to this situation.
- Try to convince them that other ways of achieving their aims will be to their advantage—keep any negotiation reality-oriented.
- Focus their attention on you as the means to achieve their aims.

The patient with borderline traits

- Provide 'understanding' and 'uncritical acceptance'.
- Help them find a way to sort things out without having 'failed again'.
- Try to build self-esteem (e.g. 'You have done well coping with everything up to now…'.)
- Once trust has been gained, it may be possible to be more directive.
- Use the patient's desire to be accepted (e.g. 'I really think it would be best if we…').
- Bear in mind that often the behaviour will be attention-seeking, and it may be worth asking: 'What is it you feel you need just now?'
- Do not be surprised if the patient acts impulsively.

The depressed patient

- Psychomotor retardation may make response time slow—be patient.
- The presence of friends or relatives may worsen their feelings of worthlessness and guilt.
- Focus on the 'here and now'—avoid talking abstractly.
- Acknowledge that they probably cannot imagine a positive future.
- Be honest and straightforward—once rapport has been established, it may be appropriate to be explicitly directive.
- Try to postpone the patient's plans, rather than dismiss them (e.g. 'Let's try this…and see how you feel in the morning…').
- Be prepared to repeat reassurances.

The patient experiencing acute stress

- Allow ventilation of feelings.
- Try to get them to describe events as objectively as possible.
- Have them go back over the options they have ruled out.
- Review the description of events, and present a more objective, rational perspective.

Managing suicide attempts in hospital

Attempted overdose

In psychiatric wards, the most likely means of attempted self-poisoning involves building up a stock of prescribed medication or bringing into the ward tablets to be taken at a later date (e.g. while out on pass). Often patients will volunteer to trusted nursing staff that they have taken an overdose, or staff will notice the patient appears overtly drowsy and when challenged the patient admits to overdose.

- Try to ascertain the type and quantity of tablets taken (look for empty bottles, medication strips, etc.)
- Establish the likely time-frame.
- If patient is unconscious or significantly drowsy, arrange immediate transfer to emergency medical services.
  - Inform medical team of patient's diagnosis, current mental state, current status (informal/formal), any other regular medications.
- If patient asymptomatic, but significant overdose suspected, arrange immediate transfer to emergency services.
  - Do not try to induce vomiting.
  - If available, consider giving activated charcoal (single dose of 50g with water) to reduce absorption (esp. if NSAIDs/paracetamol).
- If patient asymptomatic, and significant overdose unlikely:
  - Monitor closely (general observations, level of consciousness, evidence of nausea/vomiting, other possible signs of poisoning).
  - If paracetamol or salicylate (aspirin) suspected: perform routine bloods (FBC, U&Es, LFTs, HCO_3, INR) and request specific blood levels (4h post-ingestion for paracetamol).
  - If other psychiatric medications may have been taken, consider urgent blood levels (e.g. lithium, anticonvulsants—see p. 888).
  - Be aware that LFTs may be abnormal in patient on antipsychotic or antidepressant medication.
- If in doubt, get advice, or arrange for medical assessment.

Deliberate self-harm

Most episodes of deliberate self-harm involve superficial self-inflicted injury (e.g. scratching, cutting, burning, scalding) to the body or limbs. These may be easily treated on the ward with little fuss (to avoid secondary reinforcement of behaviour).

- Any more significant injuries (e.g. stabbing, deep lacerations) should be referred to emergency medical services, with the patient returning to the psychiatric ward as soon as medically fit.
- Medical advice should also be sought if:
  - You do not feel sufficiently competent to suture minor lacerations.
  - Lacerations are to the face/other vulnerable areas (e.g. genitals) or where you cannot confirm absence of damage to deeper structures (e.g nerves, blood vessels, tendons).
  - The patient has swallowed/inserted sharp objects into their body (e.g. vagina, anus).
  - The patient has ingested potentially harmful chemicals.

Attempted hanging

Most victims of attempted hangings in hospitals do not use a strong enough noose or sufficient drop height to cause death through spinal cord injury ('judicial hanging'). Cerebral hypoxia through asphyxiation is the probable cause of death and should be the primary concern in treatment of this patient population.

On being summoned to the scene

- Support the patient's weight (if possible enlist help).
- Loosen/cut off ligature.
- Lower patient to flat surface, ensuring external stabilisation of the neck and begin usual basic resuscitation (ABCs, IV access, etc.)
- Emergency airway management is a priority:
  - Where available, administer 100% O_2
  - If competent and indicated: use nasal or oral endotracheal intubation.
- Assess conscious level, full neurological examination, and degree of injury to soft tissues of the neck.
- Arrange transfer to emergency medical services as soon as possible.

Points to note

- Aggressive resuscitation and treatment of post-anoxic brain injury is indicated even in patients without evident neurological signs.
- Cervical spine fractures should be considered if there is a possibility of a several foot drop or evidence of focal neurological deficit.
- Injury to the anterior soft tissues of the neck may cause respiratory obstruction. Close attention to the development of pulmonary complications is required.

Attempted asphyxiation

- Remove source (ligature, polythene bag, etc.)
- Give 100% O_2
- If prolonged period of anoxia, or impaired conscious level, arrange immediate transfer to emergency medical services.

After the event

Patient

- Once the patient is fit for interview, formally assess mental state and conduct assessment of further suicide risk (pp. 730–3).
- Establish level of observation necessary to ensure patient's safety, clearly communicate your decision to staff and make a record in the patient's notes. (NB Hospitals policy may vary, but levels of observation will range from timed checks (e.g. every 15mins) to having a member of staff within arm's length of the patient 24hrs/day).

Staff

- For particularly traumatic events, it may be necessary to arrange a "critical incident review" (at a later date) where all staff involved participate in a confidential debriefing session. This is not to establish blame, but rather to review policy and to consider what measures (if any) might be taken to prevent similar events occurring in the future.

Severe behavioural disturbance

This covers a vast range of presentations, but will usually represent a qualitative acute change in a person's normal behaviour, that manifests primarily as antisocial behaviour—e.g. shouting, screaming, increased (often disruptive/intrusive) activity, aggressive outbursts, threatening violence (to others or self).

In extreme circumstances (e.g. person threatening to commit suicide by jumping from a height (out of a window, off a roof), where the person has an offensive weapon, or a hostage situation), this is a *police* matter and your responsibility does not extend to risking your own or other people's lives in trying to deal with the situation.

Common causes

- Acute confusional states (see delirium p. 734).
- Drug/alcohol intoxication.
- Acute symptoms of psychiatric disorder (anxiety/panic—p. 344, mania—p. 318, schizophrenia/other psychotic disorders—p. 198).
- 'Challenging behaviour' in brain-injured or LD patients (pp. 716–18).
- Behaviour unrelated to primary psychiatric disorder—this may reflect personality disorder, abnormal personality traits, or situational stressors (e.g. frustration).

General approach

- Sources of information will vary depending on the setting (e.g. on the ward, in outpatients, emergency assessment of new patient). Try to establish the context in which the behaviour has arisen.
- Follow the general principles outlined on pp. 890–3.
- Look for evidence of possible psychiatric disorder.
- Look for evidence of possible physical disorder.
- Try to establish any possible triggers for the behaviour— environmental/inter-personal stressors, use of drugs/alcohol, etc.

Management

This will depend upon assessment made:
- If physical cause suspected:
  - Follow management of delirium (p. 734)
  - Consider use of sedative medication (see opposite) to allow proper examination, facilitate transfer to medical care (if indicated), or to allow active (urgent) medical management.
- If psychiatric cause suspected:
  - Consider pharmacological management of acute behavioural disturbance (see opposite).
  - Consider need for compulsory detention.
  - Review current management plan, including observation level.
- If no physical or psychiatric cause suspected, and behaviour is dangerous or seriously irresponsible, inform security or the police to have person removed from the premises (and possibly charged if a criminal offence has been committed e.g. assault, damage to property).

Pharmacological approach to severe behavioural disturbance

Numerous local guidelines are available. Be aware of these and ensure that, if involved in control and restraint, you are adequately trained to carry out these duties responsibly.

The following is a suggested aid to pharmacological management. The doses quoted are appropriate for young, physically fit patients who have previously received antipsychotic medication. In patients who are elderly, have physical health problems, or are 'antipsychotic naïve', dosage should at least be halved (refer to BNF for further guidance).

First-line treatments:

Option 1: Intramuscular haloperidol 10–20mg and 1–2mg lorazepam
Intramuscular olanzapine may also be an alternative[1]
Repeat if necessary

Option 2: Diazepam 10mg by slow intravenous bolus
Repeat if necessary. N.B. Ensure flumazenil available.

Second-line treatments:

Option 3: Intramuscular chlorpromazine 25–100mg
N.B. Danger of postural hypotension and fatality if given inadvertently by **intravenous** injection.

Option 4: Zuclopenthixol acetate 50–150mg. (This is rapidly acting, sedating, depot antipsychotic which is best avoided in antipsychotic naïve or inexperienced patients because of long half-life.)

Third-line treatments

Other treatments (e.g. paraldehyde) or combinations of the above may be suggested in some centres. Always consult senior medical advice before administering these interventions.

The evidence base is relatively weak for the superiority of any compound over another, although benzodiazepines may have a shorter time to onset and are generally safe[2].

Aftercare

Respiration, pulse, and blood pressure should be monitored within an hour of drug administration and regularly thereafter. Look for extrapyramidal side-effects, particularly acute dystonia. Remember: fatalities have occurred in the context of emergency restraint.

Note on consent: Giving emergency medication for acute behavioural disturbance is essentially treatment under common law (p. 822). The justification rests on the judgement that no other management options are likely to be effective, and that tranquillisation will prevent the patient harming themselves or others. Harm may include behaviour that is likely to endanger the physical health of the patient (e.g. not consenting to urgent treatment or investigations that are likely to be life-saving) when capacity to give consent is judged to be impaired (p. 822).

1 www.nice.org.uk

2 TREC Collaborative Group (2003) Rapid tranquillisation for agitated patients in emergency psychiatric rooms: a randomised trial of midazolam versus haloperidol plus promethazine. *BMJ* **327**, 708–13.

The catatonic patient

Catatonia is certainly less common in current clinical practice, thanks to the advent of effective treatments for many psychiatric disorders and earlier interventions. Nonetheless the clinical presentation may be a cause for concern, particularly when a previously alert and oriented patient becomes mute and immobile. The bizarre motor presentations (e.g. posturing) may also raise concerns about a serious acute neurological problem (hence these patients may be encountered in a medical/liaison setting), and it is important that signs of catatonia are recognised. Equally, the 'excited' forms may be associated with sudden death ('lethal' or 'malignant' catatonia), which may be preventable with timely interventions.

Clinical presentation
Characteristic signs
- Mutism
- Posturing
- Negativism
- Staring
- Rigidity
- Echopraxia/echolalia

Typical forms
- Stuporous/retarded
- Excited/delirious

Common causes
- **Mood disorder** More commonly associated with mania (accounts for up to 50% of cases) than depression. Often referred to as manic (or depressive) stupor (or excitement).
- **General medical disorder** Often associated with delirium:
  - Metabolic disturbances
  - Endocrine disorders
  - Viral infections (including HIV)
  - Typhoid fever
  - Heat stroke
  - Autoimmune disorders
  - Drug-related (antipsychotics, dopaminergic drugs, recreational drugs, BDZ withdrawal, opiate intoxication)
- **Neurological disorders**
  - Postencephalitic states
  - Parkinsonism
  - Seizure disorder (e.g. non-convulsive status epilepticus)
  - Bilateral globus pallidus disease
  - Lesions of the thalamus or parietal lobes
  - Frontal lobe disease
  - General paresis
- **Schizophrenia** (10–15% of cases) Classically catalepsy, mannerisms, posturing, and mutism ('Catatonic schizophrenia', p. 185).

Differential diagnosis

- **Elective mutism** (p. 596) Usually associated with pre-existing personality disorder, clear stressor, no other catatonic features, unresponsive to lorazepam.
- **Stroke** Mutism associated with focal neurological signs and other stroke risk factors. 'Locked-in' syndrome (lesions of ventral pons and cerebellum) is characterised by mutism and total immobility (apart from vertical eye movements and blinking). The patient will often try to communicate.
- **Stiff-person syndrome** Painful spasms brought on by touch, noise, or emotional stimuli (may respond to baclofen, which can induce catatonia).
- **Malignant hyperthermia** Occurs following exposure to anaesthetics and muscle relaxants in predisposed individuals (p. 868).
- **Akinetic parkinsonism** Usually, in patients with a history of parkinsonian symptoms and dementia—may display mutism, immobility, and posturing. May respond to anticholinergics, not BDZs.

Other recognised catatonia (and catatonia-like) subtypes

- **Malignant catatonia** Acute onset of excitement, delirium, fever, autonomic instability, and catalepsy—may be fatal.
- **Neuroleptic malignant syndrome (NMS)**—p. 868.
- **Serotonin syndrome (SS)**—p. 870.

Management

Assessment

- Full history (often from 3rd party sources), including recent drug exposure, recent stressors, known medical/psychiatric conditions.
- Physical examination (including full neurological).
- Investigations—T°, BP, pulse, FBC, U&Es, LFTs, glucose, TFTs, cortisol, prolactin, consider CT/MRI and EEG.

Treatment

- Symptomatic treatment of catatonia will allow you to assess any underlying disorder more fully (i.e. you will actually be able to talk to the patient).
- Best evidence for use of BDZs (e.g. lorazepam 500mcg-1mg oral/IM—if effective, given regularly thereafter), barbiturates (e.g. amobarbital [amytal] 50–100mg), and ECT.
- Alone or in combination these effectively relieve catatonic symptoms regardless of severity or aetiology in 70–80% of cases[1,2].
- Address any underlying medical or psychiatric disorder.

---

1 Bush G, Fink M, Petrides G, *et al.* (1996) Catatonia II: treatment with lorazepam and electroconvulsive therapy. *Acta Psychiatr Scand* **93**, 137–43.

2 Ungvari GS, Kau LS, Wai-Kwong T, Shing NF (2001) The pharmacological treatment of catatonia: an overview. *Eur Arch Psychiatry Clin Neurosci* **251 (suppl 1)**, 31–4.

Medication or drug-related problems requiring immediate action

There are a number of presentations related to both prescribed and recreational drugs that may present acutely and require urgent attention. These include:

Prescribed medication

- Acute dystonic reaction (p. 866)
- Neuroleptic malignant syndrome (p. 868)
- Serotonin syndrome (p. 870)
- Lithium toxicity (p. 330)
- Clozapine 'red' result (p. 220)
- Paradoxical reactions to benzodiazepines (p. 875)

Recreation drugs

- Acute opiate withdrawal (p. 538)
- Acute benzodiazepine withdrawal (p. 540)
- Acute alcohol withdrawal (p. 518)

The manipulative patient (1)

Manipulation is a term that is generally used pejoratively, although some ethologists regard manipulative behaviour as 'selfish but adaptive' (i.e. the means by which we use others to further our own aims—which may be entirely laudable). In the context of psychiatric (and other medical) settings, manipulative behaviours are usually maladaptive and include:

- **Inappropriate or unreasonable demands**
  - More of your time than any other patient receives.
  - Wanting to deal with a *specific* doctor.
  - Only willing to accept one particular course of action (e.g. admission to hospital, a *specific* medication or other form of treatment).
- **Behavioural sequelae of failing to have these demands met**
  - Claims of additional symptoms they failed to mention previously.
  - Veiled or explicit threats of self-harm, lodging formal complaints, litigation, or violence.
  - Passive resistance (refusing to leave until satisfied with outcome of consultation).
  - Verbal or physical abuse of staff/damage to property.
  - Actual formal complaints relating to treatment (received or refused), or false accusations of misconduct against medical staff.

Key points

- Patients DO have the right to expect appropriate assessment, care, and relief of distress.
- Doctors DO have the right to refuse a course of action they judge to be inappropriate.
- Action should always be a response to clinical need (based on a thorough assessment, diagnosis, and best evidence for management), NOT threats or other manipulative behaviours.
- It is entirely possible that a patient who demonstrates manipulative behaviour DOES have a genuine problem (it is only their way of seeking help that is inappropriate).
- Some of the most difficult patients tend to present at 'awkward' times (e.g. the end of the working day, early hours of the morning, weekends, public holidays, intake of new staff)—this is no accident!
- Admitting a patient to hospital overnight (when you are left with no other option) is not a failure—some patients are very good at engineering this outcome. At worst it reinforces inappropriate coping behaviours in the patient. (Critical colleagues would probably have done the same themselves in similar circumstances.)
- If you have any doubts about what course of action to take, consult a senior colleague and discuss the case with them.

Management principles:

1. New case

- Make a full assessment to establish:
  - Psychiatric diagnosis and level of risk (to self and others).
  - Whether other agencies are required (e.g. specific services: drug/alcohol problems; social work: housing/benefits/social supports;

counseling: for specific issue—debt/employment/bereavement/alleged abuse).
- Ask the patient what they think is the main problem.
- Ask the patient what they were hoping you could do for them, e.g.:
  - Advice about what course of action to take.
  - Wanting their problem to be 'taken seriously'.
  - Wanting to be admitted to hospital (below).
  - Wanting a specific treatment.
- Discuss with them your opinion of the best course of action, and establish whether they are willing to accept any alternatives offered (e.g. other agencies, outpatient treatment).

2. The 'frequent attender'/chronic case
- Do not take short cuts—always fully assess current mental state and make a risk assessment.
- When available—always check previous notes, any written care plan, or 'crisis card'.
- Establish the reason for presenting *now* (i.e. what has changed in their current situation).
- Ask yourself 'Is the clinical presentation significantly different so as to warrant a change to the previously agreed treatment plan?'
- If not, go with what has been laid out in the treatment plan.

Pitfalls (and how to avoid them)
- Try not to take your own frustrations (e.g. being busy, feeling 'dumped on' by other colleagues, lack of sleep, lack of information, vague histories) into an interview with a patient—your job is to make an objective assessment of the person's mental state and to treat each case you see on its own merits.
- Try not to allow any preconceptions or the opinions of other colleagues colour your assessment of the *current* problems the patient presents with (people and situations have a tendency to change with time, and what may have been true in the past may no longer be the case).
- Watch out for the patient who appeals to your vanity by saying things like: 'You're much better than that other psychiatrist I saw…I can really talk to you …I feel you really understand…' They probably initially said the same things to 'that other psychiatrist' too!
- Do not be drawn into being openly critical of other colleagues; remember you are only hearing one side of the story. Maintain a healthy regard for the professionalism of those you work beside—respect their opinions (even if you really don't agree with them).
- If you encounter a particularly difficult patient, enlist the support of a colleague and conduct the assessment jointly.
- NEVER acquiesce to a 'private' consultation with a patient of the opposite sex; do not make 'special' arrangements; and NEVER give out personal information or allow patients to contact you directly.

The manipulative patient (2)

Specific situations

Patient demanding medication

- There are really only two scenarios where there is an urgent need for medication:
  - The patient who is acutely unwell and requires admission to hospital anyway (e.g. with acute confusion, acute psychotic symptoms, severe depression, high risk of suicide).
  - The patient who is known and has *genuinely* run out of their usual medication (for whom a small supply may be dispensed to tide them over until they can obtain a repeat prescription).

Patient demanding immediate admission

- Clarify what the patient hopes to achieve by admission, and decide whether this could be reasonably achieved, or if other agencies are better placed to meet these requests (see p. 6).
- If the patient is demanding admission due to drug/alcohol dependence, emphasise the need for clear motivation to stop, and offer to arrange outpatient follow-up (the next day) (see p. 514).
- Always ask about any recent trouble with the police; it is not uncommon for hospital to be sought as a 'sanctuary' from impending court appearance (but remember this can be a significant stressor for patients with current psychiatric problems).

Additional complications

Demanding relatives/other advocates

- Assess the patient on their own initially, but allow those attending with the patient to have their say (this may clarify the 'why now' question, particularly if it involves the breakdown of usual social supports).
- Ask the patient for their consent to discuss the outcome of your consultation with those accompanying them (to avoid misunderstandings and improve compliance with the proposed treatment plan).

Patient 'raising the stakes'

- If a patient is dissatisfied with the outcome of your consultation, they may try a number of ways to change your mind (see p. 902); They may even explicitly say: What do I have to do to convince you… before resorting to other manipulative behaviours.
- This type of response only serves to confirm any suspicions of attempted manipulation and should be recorded as such in the notes (verbatim if possible).
- Stick to your original management plan, and if the behaviour becomes passively, verbally or physically aggressive, clearly inform them that unless they desist, you will have no other option than to have them removed (by the police, if necessary).
- Equally, any threats of violence towards individuals present during the interview or elsewhere should be dealt with seriously and the police (and the individual concerned) should be informed—patient confidentiality does not take precedence over ensuring the safety of others.

Suspected factitious illness

- Try to obtain corroboration of the patient's story (or confirmation of your suspicions) from 3rd party sources (e.g. GP, relative, previous notes, including other hospitals they claim to have been seen at).
- If your suspicions are confirmed, directly feed this information back to the patient, and clearly inform them of what course of action you plan to take (e.g. recording this in their notes, informing other agencies, etc.)
- Do not feel 'defeated' if you decide to admit them to hospital. Record your suspicions in the notes and inform the psychiatric team that the reason for admission is to assess how clinically significant the reported symptoms are (it will soon become clear in a ward environment and it may take time to obtain 3rd party sources).

Patient threatening suicide by telephone

- Keep the person talking (see advice, pp. 890–3).
- Try to elicit useful information (name, where they are calling from, what they plan to do, risk to anyone else).
- If you judge the patient to be at high risk of suicide, encourage them to come to hospital—if they refuse or are unable to do so, organise for emergency services to go to their location and bring them to hospital.
- If the patient refuses to give you any information, inform the police who may have other means to determine the source of the call and respond.
- Always document 'phone calls in the same way as you would any other patient contact (see below).

Closure

- Clearly document your assessment, any discussion with senior colleagues, the outcome, and any treatment plan.
- Record the agreement/disagreement of the patient and any other persons attending with them.
- If appropriate, provide the patient with written information (e.g. appointment details, other contact numbers) to ensure clear communication.
- Ensure that you have informed any other necessary parties (e.g. keyworkers/psychiatric team already involved with the patient, source of referral—which may be the GP, other carers, social workers, etc.)
- If the assessment occurs out of hours, make arrangements for information to be passed on to the relevant parties in the morning (ideally try to do this yourself).
- If you have suggested outpatient follow-up for a new patient, make sure you have a means of contacting the patient, to allow the relevant service to make arrangements to see them as planned.
- If you think it is likely the patient will re-present to other services, inform them of your contact with the patient and the outcome of your assessment.

Issues of child protection

The treating doctor has a responsibility to consider the welfare not only of their patient, but of the patient's dependants (in most cases, their children). Where there are concerns relating to the welfare of children, this responsibility may be discharged both through actions you take yourself (e.g. admitting the patient to hospital), and through involvement of appropriate statutory agencies (e.g. child and family social services). Each case should be individually assessed, however a number of scenarios can be recognised:

- **Necessary absence** When a patient is brought into hospital (e.g. for emergency assessment) the admitting doctor should clarify whether they have dependent children, and if so, what arrangements have been made for their care. If these are unsatisfactory, or are disconcertingly vague (e.g. 'with a friend'), child and family social services should be consulted.
- **Neglect of childcare responsibilities** In some circumstances, as a result of mental disorder, patients' ability to provide the appropriate level of physical or emotional care may be impaired. This may relate to functional impairments (e.g. poor memory), continuing symptomatology (and medication side-effects), or dependence on drugs or alcohol. Having a mental disorder does not preclude being a parent—what is important is that individual patients receive appropriate assessment to ascertain the type of additional support they may need and the level of monitoring required.
- **Risk of positive harm to child** Certain disorders carry the risk of harm to the child by acts of *commission*, rather than *omission*. These include:
  - Psychotic disorders in which the patient holds abnormal beliefs about their child.
  - Severe depressive disorder with suicidal ideas, which involve killing the child (usually for altruistic reasons).
  - Drug misuse where there are drugs or drug paraphernalia left carelessly in the child's environment.

In these cases, a joint approach should be adopted involving mental health (optimising the patient's management) and social services (addressing issues of child protection and welfare).

Patients acting against medical advice

In certain situations, doctors are faced with deciding whether or not to act against a patient's stated wishes. This most commonly occurs when:
- A patient does not consent to a particular treatment plan.
- A patient wishes to leave hospital, despite medical advice that this is not in their best interests.

Fundamental principles
- An adult has the right to refuse treatment or to leave hospital should they wish.
- Doctors have a responsibility to discuss what they are proposing with the patient fully, to ensure that the patient is informed of the options, risks, and the preferred management (but not to enforce or coerce).

Special circumstances

In some circumstances, doctors have the power to act without the patient's consent or override a patient's expressed wishes when:
- Consent cannot be obtained in an *emergency* situation (pp. 821, 822) and treatment may be given under *common law* (p. 822).
- A patient's *capacity* is either temporarily or permanently impaired (p. 822) and they are unable to give *informed* consent. The responsible doctor should act in the patient's *best interest* (p. 823)—use of the Adults with Incapacity Act (2002) in Scotland (p. 822).
- They are suffering from a mental disorder and their capacity to take decisions is impaired. Use of the MHA may be necessary to ensure their own (or other persons') safety.

Points to note
- When a *capable* patient disagrees with a proposed course of action, this should be recorded clearly in the notes (with the reasons given by the patient). If this involves discharge from hospital, a 'discharge against medical advice' form may be useful (as a written record of the patient's decision), even though such forms have no special legal status.
- In emergency situations, the definition of 'mental disorder' is that of a layperson, not whether ICD-10 or DSM-IV criteria are satisfied.
- Judging a person *incapable* does not allow for detention in hospital; equally detaining someone under the MHA does not allow for treatment (either physical or psychiatric) such *emergency* interventions are covered by common law.
- Always consider the balance of risks: ask yourself 'what am I more likely to be criticised (or sued) for?'
- Although the final decision in non-mentally ill, capable adults rests with them, in 'close-call' situations it is better to err on the side of safety, and review again later. (Such situations should always be discussed with a senior colleague.)

Patient wanting to leave a psychiatric ward

The duty psychiatrist is often called to psychiatric wards when patients wish to take their own discharge. Although *not* wanting to be in a psychiatric ward may often seem the most rational response—particularly when there are other more behaviourally disturbed patients in the same ward— a pragmatic approach should be adopted (i.e. balancing the need for assessment/inpatient treatment against the additional stress caused by admission). Follow the general principles detailed above, focusing on managing risk and acting in the patient's 'best interests'. Note especially:

* Deciding whether a patient is permitted to leave the ward will be informed by both an assessment of their current mental state and knowledge of any established management plans.
* Often decisions regarding the course of action to take will have already been discussed by the responsible consultant with nursing staff. When there are concerns, the default position is often reassessment at the time the patient is asking to leave.
* When a patient does elect to leave against medical advice, record this clearly in the notes with, at the very minimum, an agreement for a planned review (e.g. as an outpatient, by the GP) and the recommendation that, should the patient (or their relatives) feel the situation has become unsustainable at home, they should return to the hospital.

Some examples of clinical scenarios

52-yr-old ♂ admitted with chest pain, who ought to remain in the hospital for overnight telemetry, cardiac enzymes, and repeat ECG (in the morning), but does not wish to do so. He is not incapable and not suffering from a mental disorder.
The decision rests with him (he has a right to refuse—even if you think he is acting foolishly).

22-yr-old ♀ who admits to ingesting 56 aspirin, brought to GP by a concerned friend, now refusing to get in an ambulance to go to hospital.
Most people would agree that she is possibly suffering from a mental disorder (suggested by her recent OD), hence there are grounds for use of MHA, with emergency treatment under common law.

18-yr-old ♀ admitted after a paracetamol overdose who needs further treatment but wishes to leave. She has some depressive features and may possibly be under the influence of alcohol.
There is sufficient suspicion of mental disorder to detain under the MHA (perhaps more than in the previous scenario); treatment would be under common law.

34-yr-old ♀ with long history of anorexia nervosa, current weight under 6st, with clear physical complications of starvation (and biochemical abnormalities), refusing admission for medical management.
Clear mental disorder, as well as 'risk to themselves'—detain under the MHA; emergency treatment under common law.

53-yr-old ♂ Previously seen in A&E following a fall whilst intoxicated, brought back up to A&E 6 days later by spouse with fluctuating level of consciousness (also has been drinking heavily)—suspected extradural, but angrily refusing CT head.
Capacity impaired both by alcohol and potentially serious underlying treatable physical disorder. Necessary urgent investigation warranted as in patient's best interests—with use of sedation (if necessary) under common law.

67-yr-old ♂ with post-operative URTI who presents as confused, wishing to leave the ward because he is 'late for his brother's wedding'.
There is a clear mental disorder and he ought to be detained under the MHA; treat under common law (sedate if necessary).

23-yr-old ♂ admitted with psychotic illness, who wants to go home to confront the neighbours whom he believes have conspired with the police to get him 'banged up in a nut hut'.
Clear mental disorder—detain under MHA; emergency treatment if required under common law.

The mental health of doctors

'Quis custodiet ipsos custodes?'
('Who will watch the watchmen?')

In general, doctors are in a pretty good state of health, with a lower prevalence of smoking, cardiovascular disease, cancer, and a longer life expectancy than the general population. With respect to mental health, however, the situation is reversed—with the incidence of most psychiatric disorders *higher* in doctors:

- Surveys have found ~25% of doctors to have significant depressive symptoms, with : = 1:2 and increased risk in: junior house officers/interns; junior doctors in O&G and psychiatry; radiologists, anaesthetists, surgeons, and paediatricians.
- Suicide rates are high, with depression, alcohol, and drug misuse significant contributory factors. Specialties over-represented include anaesthetics, GP, psychiatry, and emergency medicine.
- Problems of drug and alcohol dependence may affect as many as 1 in 15 doctors in the UK.

Why are doctors more likely to have mental health problems?
Individual factors

- Personality—many of the qualities that make a 'good doctor' may also increase the risk of psychiatric problems: (e.g. obsessionality, perfectionism, being ambitious, self-sacrifice, high expectations of self, low tolerance of uncertainty, difficulty expressing emotions).
- Ways of thinking/coping styles e.g. being overly self-critical, denial, minimisation, rationalisation, drinking culture, need to appear competent ('no problems').

Occupational factors

- Long and disruptive work hours.
- Exposure to traumatic events—dealing with death, ethical dilemmas.
- Lack of support (particularly from senior colleagues).
- Competing needs of patients and family.
- Increasing expectations with diminishing resources.
- Professional and geographic isolation.

Barriers to seeking help

Doctors are notoriously bad at seeking help for their own medical problems—particularly psychiatric problems—often only presenting when a crisis arises. Reasons for this include:

- Symptom concealment due to fears of hospitalisation, loss of medical registration, exposure to stigmatisation.
- Negative attitudes to psychiatry, psychiatrists, and people with psychiatric problems.
- Lack of insight being a feature of many psychiatric disorders.

This may lead to delayed referral, misdiagnosis, and not receiving the benefits of early interventions.

What to do if you suspect a colleague has a problem

You have a duty to take action (see below), both in the interests of patient care and of your colleague's health (such actions are both ethically responsible and caring). Not to do so could both put patients at risk and potentially deny your colleague treatment which might prevent further deterioration in health and performance. Usually a staged approach works best:

- Confirm your suspicions through informal discussion with other colleagues.
- If a clear pattern of behaviour is present, first consider discussing this observation with the colleague in question.
- It is better if face-to-face discussion is conducted by someone of the same grade.
- If face-to-face discussion yields no results, speak to an impartial senior colleague and/or seek further advice about local procedures (see below).
- If the colleague is YOU, remember: *responsible* physicians put their patients first and take pride in looking after their own health (see p. 912).

'If you have grounds to believe that a doctor or other healthcare professional may be putting patients at risk, you must give an honest explanation of your concerns to an appropriate person from the employing authority, such as the medical director, nursing director or chief executive, or the director of public health, or an officer of your local medical committee, following any procedures set by the employer. If there are no appropriate local systems or local systems cannot resolve the problem, and you remain concerned about the safety of patients, you should inform the relevant regulatory body [*] . If you are not sure what to do, discuss your concerns with an impartial colleague or contact your defence body, a professional organisation or the GMC for advice.'

General Medical Council (2001) Good medical practice. London. para 27.

* It is worth noting that doctors referred to the GMC because of mental health problems can continue to practice, provided their problems are not judged to affect their professional abilities, and they are suitably supervised in an agreed treatment regime.

Looking after your own mental health

You have a duty to yourself and your patients to act promptly if you feel there are early warning signs that your health may be affecting your performance.

Signs to watch out for

- Difficulties sleeping.
- Becoming more impatient or irritable.
- Difficulties concentrating.
- Being unable to make decisions.
- Drinking or smoking more.
- Not enjoying food as much.
- Being unable to relax or 'switch off'.
- Feeling tense (may manifest as somatic symptoms e.g. recurrent headache, aches and pains, GI upset, feeling sweaty, dry mouth, tachycardia).

Developing good habits

- **Learn to relax** This can involve learning methods of progressive relaxation, or simply setting aside time when you are not working to relax with a long bath, a quiet stroll, listening to music. It also means living life less frantically—going to bed at a regular time and getting up 15–20 minutes earlier to prevent the feeling of 'always being in a rush'.
- **Take regular breaks at work** This includes regular meal breaks (away from work). Even when work is busy, try to give yourself a 5–10 minute break every few hours.
- **Escape the pager** In the day and age of being always obtainable, it is a good idea to be 'unobtainable' once or twice a week, to give yourself time to be alone and reflect.
- **Exercise** There is no doubt that regular exercise helps reduce levels of stress. It will also keep you fit, helps prevent heart disease, and improve quality of sleep.
- **Drugs** Tobacco and other recreational drugs are best avoided. Caffeine and alcohol should be used only in moderation.
- **Distraction** Finding a pursuit that has no deadlines, no pressures, and which can be picked up or left easily can allow you to forget about your usual stresses. This might be a sport, a hobby, music, the movies, the theatre, or books. The important point is that it is not work-related.

Organising your own medical care

- Register with a GP ! (two-thirds of junior doctors have not done this)!
- Allow yourself to benefit from the same standards of care (including expert assessment, if this is felt to be necessary) you would expect for your patients.
- If you are having difficulties related to stress, anxiety, depression, or use of substances, consult your GP sooner rather than later.
- Be willing to take advice. In particular, do not rely on your own judgement of your ability to continue working.
- If your GP suggests speaking to a psychiatrist, and you feel uncomfortable with being seen locally, ask for an out-of-area consultation.

- Utilise other sources of help and advice—both informal (friends, family, self-help books) and formal (see below). Remember you are certainly not the first doctor to have encountered these sorts of difficulties.

Sources of support and advice

- The **National Counselling Service for Sick Doctors** is a confidential independent service supported by the Royal Colleges, the Joint Consultants Committee, the BMA, and other medical professional bodies. Tel: 0870 21 0535
- The **Doctors' Support Network.** Tel: 07071 223 372.
- The **BMA** offers free expert advice for members who may be affected by illness through **'Doctors for doctors'** (Tel: 020 7383 6739) and a free telephone counselling service (Tel: 0645 200 169).
- The **Sick Doctors' Trust** runs a 24 hr helpline for doctors with addiction problems. Callers are put in touch with the nearest member of the **Addicted Physicians Programme (APP)** an independent and free service. The **British Doctors and Dentists Group** is an affiliated organisation, running support groups in local areas throughout the UK and Eire. For further information contact: Isis, 126 Weybourne Road, Farnham, Surrey, GU9 9HD (Tel: 020 7487 4445; Fax: 01252 350242; Helpline: 01252 345163).

Chapter 23

Useful addresses

Useful patient-related addresses (UK)

Age Concern
Astral House
1268 London Road
London
SW16 4ER
Information line tel: 0800 009966
Web: *http://www.ace.org.uk/*

Alcohlics Anonymous (AA)
PO Box 1
Stonebow House
Stonebow
York
YO1 7NJ
Helpline tel: 0845 769 7555
Admin tel.: 01904 644026
Web: *http://www.alcoholics-anonymous.org.uk*

Al-Anon Family Groups UK and Eire
61 Great Dover Street
London
SE1 4YF
Tel: 020 7403 0888
Fax: 020 7378 9910
Web: *http://www.al-anonuk.org.uk*

Other Information Services in the UK and Eire:

Al-Anon Information Centre
Mansfield Park Building
Unit 6
22 Mansfield Street
Partick
G11 5QP
Tel: 0141 339 8884
(Helpline 24 hours)

Al-Anon Information Centre
Peace House
224 Lisburn Road
Belfast
BT9 6GE
Northern Ireland
Tel: 028 9068 2368

Al-Anon Information Centre
Room 5
5 Capel Street
Dublin 1
EIRE
Tel: 00353 1 873 2699

Alzheimer's Society (UK, not Scotland)
Gordon House
10 Greencoat Place
London
SW1P 1PH
Tel: 020 7306 0606
Fax: 020 7306 0808
Email: enquiries@alzheimers.org.uk
Web: http://www.alzheimers.org.uk

Alzheimer Scotland—Action on Dementia
22 Drumsheugh Gardens
Edinburgh
EH3 7RN
Tel: 0131 243 1453
Fax: 0131 243 1450
Email: alzheimer@alzscot.org
Web: http://www.alzscot.org

CRUSE Bereavement Care (CBC)
Cruse House
126 Sheen Road
Richmond
Surrey
TW9 1UR
Helpline tel: 0870 167 1677
Admin tel: 020 8939 9530 (UK); 01738 444 178 (Scotland)
Web: http://www.cruselochaber.freeuk.com/canhelp.html

Manic Depression Fellowship (MDF)
21 St George's Road
London
SE1 6ES
Admin tel: 020 7793 2600
Admin fax: 020 7793 2639
Email: mdf@mdf.org.uk
Web: http://www.mdf.org.uk

MIND
15–19 Broadway
London
E15 4BQ
Helpline tel: 08457 660 163
Admin tel: 020 8519 2122
Admin fax: 020 8522 1725
Email: contact@mind.org.uk
Web: http://www.mind.org.uk

...cotics Anonymous (NA)

Service Office
2 City Road
London
EC1V 2PH
Tel: 020 7251 4007
Fax: 020 7251 4006
Email: ukso@ukna.org
UK helpline: 020 7730 0009
Email: helpline@ukna.org
Web: *http://www.ukna.org*

Rethink (previously National Schizophrenia Fellowship)

Head Office
30 Tabernacle Street
London
EC2A 4DD
General enquiries: Tel: 0845 456 0455 or Email: info@rethink.org
National advice line: Tel: 020 8974 6814 or Email: advice@rethink.org
Web: *http://www.rethink.org/contact.html*

Samaritans

Tel: 08457 90 90 90
Email: jo@samaritans.org
Web: *http://www.samaritans.org.uk/*

SANE

1st Floor
Cityside House
40 Adler Street
London
E1 1EE
Helpline tel: 0845 767 8000
Admin tel: 020 7375 1002
Admin fax: 020 7375 2162
Email: london@sane.org.uk
Website: *http://www.sane.org.uk*

Young Minds

102–108 Clerkenwell Road
London
EC1M 5SA
Helpline tel: 0800 018 2138
Admin tel: 020 7336 8445
Admin fax: 020 7336 8446
Email: enquiries@youngminds.org.uk
Web: *http://www.youngminds.org.uk*

Useful websites (professional)

British National Formulary
http://www.bnf.org.uk

British Association for Behavioural and Cognitive Psychotherapists

Directory of accredited cognitive behavioural psychotherapists.
http://www.babcp.org.uk

British Association for Counselling

Directories and other information.
http://www.bac.co.uk

British Association for Psychopharmacology

Journal, membership, and training events.
http://www.bap.org.uk

British Confederation of Psychotherapists
http://www.bcp.org.uk

British Medical Association

http://www.bma.org.uk

British Psychological Society

The professional body for psychologists in the UK.
Directory of chartered psychologists (with areas of expertise and geographical area).
http://www.bps.org.uk

National Institute for Clinical Excellence (NICE)

Special health authority for England and Wales which develops 'best practice' guidelines.
http://www.nice.org.uk

NHS Quality Improvement Scotland (NHS QIS)

Similar to NICE; develops guidelines for Scottish practice.
http://www.nhshealthquality.org

Royal College of Psychiatrists

The professional and educational body for psychiatrists in the UK and Republic of Ireland.
http://www.rcpsych.ac.uk

Useful professional contacts

Clozaril Patient Monitoring Service (CPMS)
General enquiries: 0845 769 8269
Out of hours: 01276 692504
Fax: 0845 769 8379
Supplies: 0845 769 8357
Toxicology: 0207 771 5365/5361

Driver and Vehicle Licensing Agency (DVLA)
The Senior Medical Advisor
DVLA
Driver Medical Unit
Longview Road
Morriston
Swansea
SA99 1TU
Tel: 01792 761 119
http://www.dvla.gov.uk/dvla.htm

NHS 24
Tel: 0845 24 24 24
http://www.nhs24.com

Poisons Information Services (UK)
Will direct callers to relevant local centre.
Tel: 0870 600 6266

Exam-related sites of interest

All the relevant information for the MRCPsych exam (dates, cost, syllabus, format, etc.) can be found at the Royal College site:
http://www.rcpsych.ac.uk/traindev/exams/

Other useful sites for exam preparation include:
http://www.irishpsychiatry.com/osce_doc.html
http://mrcpsych-help.com/
http://www.mrcpsych.com/
http://www.psychejam.com/
http://www.psychexam.co.uk/
http://www.superego-cafe.com/
http://www.trickcyclists.co.uk/

Bibliotherapy resources

It is useful to have a list of good self-help or educational books addressir. general principles of good mental health or dealing with specific disorders. Whilst in no way exhaustive, patients and/or their carers may find the following books helpful:

General

Butler, G. & Hope, T. (1995) *Manage your mind: mental fitness guide.* Oxford Paperbacks.

Schizophrenia

Torrey, F. (2001) *Surviving schizophrenia: a family manual.* HarperCollins.

Depression

Padesky, C. & Greenberger, D. (1995) *Mind over mood.* Guilford Press.
Tanner, S. & Ball, J. (1989) *Beating the blues: a self-help approach to overcoming depression.* Sydney: Doubleday.

Bipolar disorder

Goodwin, F.K. & Jamison, K.R. (1990) *Manic-depressive illness.* New York: Oxford University Press.

Anxiety disorders

Barlow, D.H. & Craske, M.G. (1989) *Mastery of your anxiety and panic.* Albany: University of Albany, State University of New York.

Eating disorders

Schmidt, U. & Treasure, J. (1993) *Getting better bit(e) by bit(e): a survival guide for sufferers of bulimia nervosa and binge eating disorders.* Psychology Press.

Sleep problems

Bearpark, H. (1994) *Overcoming insomnia.* Rushcutters Bay, Sydney: Gore & Osment Publications.

Alcohol problems

Robertson, I. & Heather, N. (1998) *So you want to cut down your drinking? A self help guide to sensible drinking.* Health Education Board for Scotland (HEBS).

Chapter 24

ICD-10/DSM-IV index

ICD-10 Classification of Mental and Behavioural Disorders (1992)

The following index provides ICD-10 coding information with the 'equivalent' DSM-IV coding, and a page reference (where available).

As 'mental and behavioural disorders due to psychoactive substance abuse' is so dissimilar in organisaton to DSM-IV (i.e. separate coding for substance use and substance-induced disorders), equivalent codings have not been included (see p. 926).

0–F09 Organic, including symptomatic, mental disorders

ICD-10	DSM-IV	Disorder	Page
F00	**290**	**Dementia in Alzheimer's disease**	*134*
F00.0	290.10	Early onset	
F00.1	290.0	Late onset	
F00.2	294.1	Atypical or mixed type	
F00.9	294.1	Unspecified	
F01	**290.40**	**Vascular dementia**	*144*
F01.0	290.40	Acute onset	
F01.1	290.40	Multi-infarct	
F01.2	290.40	Subcortical	
F01.3	290.40	Mixed cortical and subcortical	
F02.0	**290.10**	**Dementia in Pick's disease**	*142*
F02.1	**290.0**	**Dementia in Creutzfeldt-Jakob disease**	*146*
F02.2	**294.1**	**Dementia in Huntington's disease**	*172*
F02.3	**294.1**	**Dementia in Parkinson's disease**	*170*
F02.4	**294.9**	**Dementia in HIV disease**	*165*
F02.8	294.1	Dementia in other specified diseases	
F03	294.8	Unspecified dementia	
F04	**294.0**	**Organic amnesic syndrome, not induced by alcohol and other psychoactive substances**	*148*
F05	**293.0**	**Delirium**	*734*
F05.0	293.0	Delirium not superimposed on dementia	
F05.1	293.0	Delirium superimposed on dementia	
F06	**293.8**	**Mental disorders due to brain damage, dysfunction, and physical disease**	
F06.0	293.82	Hallucinosis	
F06.1	293.89	Catatonic disorder	*898*
F06.2	293.81	Delusional (schizophrenia-like) disorder	*130*
F06.3	293.83	Mood (affective) disorders	*130–1*
F06.4	293.84	Anxiety disorder	*131*
F06.5	293.9	Dissociative disorder	*746*
F06.6	293.9	Emotionally labile (asthenic) disorder	
F06.7	294.9	Mild cognitive disorder	

0–F19 Mental and behavioural disorders due to psychoactive substance abuse

Notes:

A 4th character denotes the clinical condition and a 5th modifies it:

F1x.0—Acute Intoxication
F1x.0—.00 uncomplicated
F1x.0—.01 with trauma or other bodily injury
F1x.0—.02 with other medical complications
F1x.0—.03 with delirium
F1x.0—.04 with perceptual distortions
F1x.0—.05 with coma
F1x.0—.06 with convulsions
F1x.0—.07 pathological intoxication

F1x.1—Harmful use

F1x.2—Dependence syndrome
F1x.2—.20 currently abstinent
F1x.2—.21 currently abstinent but in a protected environment
F1x.2—.22 on a clinically supervised maintenance or replacement regime
F1x.2—.23 currently abstinent, but receiving treatment with aversive or blocking drugs
F1x.2—.24 currently using
F1x.2—.25 continuous use
F1x.2—.26 episodic use

F1x.3—Withdrawal state
F1x.3—.30 uncomplicated
F1x.3—.31 convulsions

F1x.4—Withdrawal state with delirium
F1x.4—.40 with convulsions
F1x.4—.41 without convulsions

F1x.5—Psychotic disorder
F1x.5—.50 schizophrenia-like
F1x.5—.51 predominantly delusional
F1x.5—.52 predominantly hallucinatory
F1x.5—.53 predominantly polymorphic

F1x.5—.54 predominantly depressive
F1x.5—.55 predominantly manic
F1x.5—.56 mixed
F1x.6—Amnestic disorder
F1x.7—Residual and late-onset psychotic disorder
F1x.7—.70 flashbacks
F1x.7—.71 personality or behavioural disorder
F1x.7—.72 residual affective disorder
F1x.7—.73 dementia
F1x.7—.74 other persisting cognitive impairment
F1x.7—.75 late-onset psychotic disorder

F20–F29 Schizophrenia, schizotypal and delusional disorders

ICD-10	DSM-IV	Disorder	
F20	295	Schizophrenia	
F20.0	295.30	Paranoid	
F20.1	295.10	Hebephrenic	
F20.2	295.2	Catatonic	
F20.3	295.90	Undifferentiated	
F20.4	311	Post-schizophrenic depression	
F20.5	295.60	Residual	
F20.6	295.90	Simple	
F21	301.22	Schizotypal disorder	226
F22	297	Persistent delusional disorder	230
F22.0	297.1	Delusional disorder	
F22.8	297.1	Other persistent delusional disorders	
F23		Acute and transient psychotic disorders	236
F23.0	298.9	Acute polymorphic psychotic disorder without symptoms of schizophrenia	
F23.1	295.40	Acute polymorphic psychotic disorder with symptoms of schizophrenia	
F23.2	295.40	Acute schizophrenia-like psychotic disorder	
F23.3	297.1	Other acute predominantly delusional psychotic disorders	
F24	297.3	Induced delusional disorder	238
F25	295.7	Schizoaffective disorder	228
F25.0	295.70	Manic type	
F25.1	295.70	Depressive type	
F25.2	295.70	Mixed type	
F28	298.9	Other non-organic psychotic disorders	239
F29	298.9	Unspecified non-organic psychosis	

Notes:

Schizophrenia—a 5th character denotes course : continuous (1), episodic with progressive deficit (2), episodic but stable deficit (3), episodic remittent (4), incomplete remission (5), complete remission (6), other (8) and period of observation less than one year (9)

Acute and transient psychotic disorders—a 5th character may be used to identify the presence (1) or absence (0) of acute stress.

–F29 Schizophrenia, schizotypal, and lusional disorders

CD-10	DSM-IV	Disorder	Page
F20	**295**	**Schizophrenia**	186
F20.0	295.30	Paranoid	
F20.1	295.10	Hebephrenic	
F20.2	295.2	Catatonic	
F20.3	295.90	Undifferentiated	
F20.4	311	Post-schizophrenic depression	
F20.5	295.60	Residual	
F20.6	295.90	Simple	
F21	**301.22**	**Schizotypal disorder**	226
F22	**297**	**Persistent delusional disorder**	230
F22.0	297.1	Delusional disorder	
F22.8	297.1	Other persistent delusional disorders	
F23		**Acute and transient psychotic disorders**	236
F23.0	298.9	Acute polymorphic psychotic disorder without symptoms of schizophrenia	
F23.1	295.40	Acute polymorphic psychotic disorder with symptoms of schizophrenia	
F23.2	295.40	Acute schizophrenia-like psychotic disorder	
F23.3	297.1	Other acute predominantly delusional psychotic disorders	
F24	**297.3**	**Induced delusional disorder**	238
F25	**295.7**	**Schizoaffective disorder**	228
F25.0	295.70	Manic type	
F25.1	295.70	Depressive type	
F25.2	295.70	Mixed type	
F28	**298.9**	**Other non-organic psychotic disorders**	239
F29	**298.9**	**Unspecified non-organic psychosis**	

Notes:

Schizophrenia—a 5th character denotes course : continuous (1), episodic with progressive deficit (2), episodic but stable deficit (3), episodic remittent (4), incomplete remission (5), complete remission (6), other (8) and period of observation less than one year (9).

Acute and transient psychotic disorders—a 5th character may be used to identify the presence (1) or absence (0) of acute stress.

Mood (Affective) Disorders

Mood (Affective) Disorders

ICD-10	DSM-IV	Disorder
F34		**Persistent mood (affective) disorders**
F34.0	301.13	Cyclothymia
F34.1	300.4	Dysthymia
F38		**Other mood (affective) disorders**
F38.0	296.90	Other single mood (affective) disorders
F38.1	296.90	Other recurrent mood (affective) disorders
F38.8	296.90	Other specified mood (affective) disorders
F39	**296.90**	**Unspecified mood (affective) disorders**

F49 Neurotic, stress-related and somatoform disorders

ICD-10	DSM-IV	Disorder	
F40		**Phobic anxiety disorders**	
F40.00	300.22	Agoraphobia without panic disorder	
F40.01	300.21	Agoraphobia with panic disorder	
F40.1	300.23	Social phobias	
F40.2	300.29	Specific (isolated) phobias	
F41		**Other anxiety disorders**	
F41.0	300.01	Panic disorder (episodic paroxysmal anxiety)	344
F41.1	300.02	Generalised anxiety disorder	356
F41.2	300.00	Mixed anxiety and depressive disorder	
F41.3	300.00	Other mixed anxiety disorders	
F42		**Obsessive-compulsive disorder**	358
F42.0	300.3	Predominantly obsessional thoughts or ruminations	
F42.1	300.3	Predominantly compulsive acts (obsessional rituals)	
F42.2	300.3	Mixed obsessional thoughts and acts	
F43		**Reaction to severe stress and adjustment disorders**	
F43.0	308.3	Acute stress reaction	362
F43.1	309.81	Post-traumatic stress disorder	368
F43.2	309.9	Adjustment disorders	364
F44		**Dissociative (conversion) disorders**	746
F44.0	300.12	Dissociative amnesia	
F44.1	300.13	Dissociative fugue	
F44.2	300.15	Dissociative stupor	
F44.3	300.15	Trance and possession disorders	
F44.4	300.15	Dissociative motor disorders	
F44.5	300.15	Dissociative convulsions	
F44.6	300.15	Dissociative anaesthesia and sensory loss	
F44.7	300.15	Mixed dissociative (conversion) disorders	
F44.8)	300.11	Ganser syndrome	93
F44.81	300.14	Multiple personality disorder	96
F44.82	300.11	Transient dissociate (conversion) disorders occurring in childhood and adolescence	

F49 Neurotic, stress-related, and somatoform disorders

-10	DSM-IV	Disorder	Page
•0		**Phobic anxiety disorders**	
F40.00	300.22	Agoraphobia without panic disorder	350
F40.01	300.21	Agoraphobia with panic disorder	350
F40.1	300.23	Social phobias	354
F40.2	300.29	Specific (isolated) phobias	352
F41		**Other anxiety disorders**	
F41.0	300.01	Panic disorder (episodic paroxysmal anxiety)	344
F41.1	300.02	Generalised anxiety disorder	356
F41.2	300.00	Mixed anxiety and depressive disorder	
F41.3	300.00	Other mixed anxiety disorders	
F42		**Obsessive-compulsive disorder**	358
F42.0	300.3	Predominantly obsessional thoughts or ruminations	
F42.1	300.3	Predominantly compulsive acts(obsessional rituals)	
F42.2	300.3	Mixed obsessional thoughts and acts	
F43		**Reaction to severe stress and adjustment disorders**	
F43.0	308.3	Acute stress reaction	362
F43.1	309.81	Post-traumatic stress disorder	368
F43.2	309.9	Adjustment disorders	364
F44		**Dissociative (conversion) disorders**	746
F44.0	300.12	Dissociative amnesia	
F44.1	300.13	Dissociative fugue	
F44.2	300.15	Dissociative stupor	
F44.3	300.15	Trance and possession disorders	
F44.4	300.15	Dissociative motor disorders	
F44.5	300.15	Dissociative convulsions	
F44.6	300.15	Dissociative anaesthesia and sensory loss	
F44.7	300.15	Mixed dissociative (conversion) disorders	
F44.80	300.11	Ganser syndrome	93
F44.81	300.14	Multiple personality disorder	96
F44.82	300.11	Transient dissociate (conversion) disorders occurring in childhood and adolescence	

ICD-10	DSM-IV	Disorder	
F45		**Somatoform disorders**	
F45.0	300.81	Somatisation disorder	
F45.1	300.82	Undifferentiated somatoform disorder	
F45.2	300.7	Hypochondriacal disorder	748
F45.3	300.82	Somatoform autonomic dysfunction	
F45.4	307.80	Persistent somatoform pain disorder	744
F48		**Other neurotic disorders**	
F48.0	300.82	Neurasthenia	754
F48.1	300.6	Depersonalisation-derealisation syndrome	372

Notes:

Somatoform autonomic dysfunction—5th character denotes organ or system: unspecified (0), heart and cardiovascular system (1), upper gastrointestinal tract (2), lower gastrointestinal tract (3), respiratory system (4), genitourinary system (5), other (8), multiple (9).

59 Behavioural syndromes
ciated with physiological
turbance and physical factors

F55	305	**Abuse of non-dependence-producing substances**
F55.0	305.90	Harmful use of antidepressants
F55.1	305.90	Harmful use of laxatives
F55.2	305.90	Harmful use of analgesics
F55.3	305.90	Harmful use of antacids
F55.4	305.90	Harmful use of vitamins
F55.5	305.90	Harmful use of steroids or hormones
F55.6	305.90	Harmful use of specific herbal or folk remedies
F55.8	305.90	Harmful use of other substances that do not produce dependence
F59	**300.9**	**Unspecified behavioural syndromes associated with physiological disturbances and physical factors**

69 Disorders of adult
onality and behaviour

ICD-10	DSM-IV	Disorder
F66		Psychological and behavioural disorders associated with sexual development and orientation
F66.0	302.6	Sexual maturation disorder
F66.1	302.6	Egodystonic sexual orientation
F66.2	302.6	Sexual relationship disorder
F68		Other
F68.0	300.9	Elaboration of physical symptoms for psychological reasons
F68.1	300.19	Intentional production or feigning of symptoms or disabilities, either physical or psychological

Notes:

For F66—Psychological and behavioural disorders associated with sexual development and orientation—a 5th character denotes orientation (.x0 heterosexuality, .x1 homosexuality, .x2 bisexuality, .x8 other, including prepubertal).

F70–F79 Mental retardation

ICD-10	DSM-IV	Disorder	Page
F70	317	Mild mental retardation	686
F71	318.0	Moderate mental retardation	686
F72	318.1	Severe mental retardation	686
F73	318.2	Profound mental retardation	686
F78	319	Other mental retardation	
F79	319	Unspecified mental retardation	

Notes:

A 4th character may be employed to specify the extent of associated behavioural impairment:

F7x .0 none or minimal

F7x .1 significant, requiring attention or treatment

F7x .8 other impairments of behaviour

F7x .9 unspecified (without mention of impairment of behaviour)

F98 Behavioural and emotional disorders with onset usually occurring in childhood and adolescence

8 Behavioural and emotional ...ders with onset usually occuring ...ildhood and adolescence

...-10	DSM-IV	Disorder	Page
...90		**Hyperkinetic disorders**	576
F90.0	314.9	Disturbance of activity and attention	
F90.1	312.81	Hyperkinetic conduct disorder	
F90.8	314.9	Other hyperkinetic disorders	
F91	**312.8**	**Conduct disorders**	580
F91.0	312.89	Confined to the family context	
F91.1	312.89	Undersocialised conduct disorder	
F91.2	312.89	Socialised conduct disorder	
F91.3	313.81	Oppositional defiant disorder	581
F91.8	312.89	Other conduct disorders	
F92		**Mixed disorders of conduct and emotions**	
F92.0	312.89	Depressive conduct disorder	
F92.8	312.89	Other mixed disorders of conduct and emotions	
F93		**Emotional disorders with onset specific to childhood**	
F93.0	309.21	Separation anxiety disorder of childhood	590
F93.1	300.29	Phobic anxiety disorder of childhood	597
F93.2	300.23	Social anxiety disorder of childhood	596
F93.3	V61.8	Sibling rivalry disorder	
F93.8	313.9	Other childhood emotional disorders	
F94		**Disorders of social functioning with onset specific to childhood and adolescence**	
F94.0	313.23	Elective mutism	596
F94.1	313.89	Reactive attachment disorder of childhood	590
F94.2	313.89	Disinhibited attachment disorder of childhood	590
F94.8	313.9	Other childhood disorders of social functioning	
F95		**Tic disorders**	602
F95.0	307.21	Transient tic disorder	
F95.1	307.22	Chronic motor or vocal tic disorder	
F95.2	307.23	Combined vocal and multiple motor tic disorder (de la Tourette)	
F95.8	307.20	Other tic disorders	

ICD-10	DSM-IV	Disorder	
F98		**Other**	
F98.0	307.6	Non-organic enuresis	5
F98.1	307.7	Non-organic encopresis	588
F98.2	307.59	Feeding disorder of infancy and childhood	589
F98.3	307.52	Pica of infancy and childhood	589
F98.4	307.3	Stereotyped movement disorders	
F98.5	307.0	Stuttering (stammering)	586
F98.6	307.9	Cluttering	586
F98.8	313.9	Other specified behavioural and emotional disorders with onset usually occurring in infancy or childhood	

ICD-10 multiaxial system

...tiaxial diagnosis, a patient's problems are viewed within a broader ...ext, which includes: clinical diagnosis, assessment of disability, and ...chosocial factors. In ICD-10, multiaxial diagnoses are made along ...ree axes, as follows:

Axis I—clinical diagnoses

This includes all disorders, both psychiatric and physical, including learning disability and personality disorders.

Axis II—disabilities

Conceptualised in line with WHO definitions of impairments, disabilities, and handicaps (p. 688), this covers a number of specific areas of functioning which are rated on a scale of 0 ('no disability') to 5 ('gross disability'):

- **Personal care** Personal hygiene, dressing, feeding, etc.
- **Occupation** Expected functioning in paid activities, studying, home-making, etc.
- **Family and household** Participation in family life.
- **Functioning in a broader social context** Participation in the wider community, including contact with friends, leisure, and other social activities.

Axis III—contextual factors

The factors considered to contribute to the occurrence, presentation, course, outcome, or treatment of the present Axis I disorder(s). They include problems related to:

- negative events in childhood
- education and literacy
- primary support group, including family circumstances
- social environment
- housing or economic circumstances
- (un)employment
- physical environment
- certain psychosocial circumstances
- legal circumstances
- family history of disease or disabilities
- lifestyle or life-management difficulties

Index

Urgent detention under mental health legislation

Which section?

Jurisdiction	Legislation	Outpatient[1]	Inpatient[2]
England and Wales (p. 804)	Mental Health Act 1983	s. 2 or 3 should be used rather than s. 4* unless the situation is such an emergency that to do so would be unsafe.	s. 5(2)* can be used immediately. In some cases s. 2 or 3 would be used directly instead.
Scotland (p. 810)	Mental Health (Scotland) Act 1984	s. 24*	s. 25(1)*
	Mental Health (Care and Treatment) (Scotland) Act 2003	Part 5* if arranging Part 6 would involve undesirable delay.	Part 5* if arranging Part 6 would involve undesirable delay.
Northern Ireland (p. 814)	Mental Health (Northern Ireland) Order 1986	a. 4**	a. 7(2)* In some cases patient may be detained directly under a. 4**
Republic of Ireland (p. 818)	Mental Treatment Act 1945	s. 184	s. 184
	Mental Health Act 2001	s. 9 and 10**	s. 23*

[1] Patient not admitted to hospital yet—includes day hospital, outpatient department, accident and emergency, and patients attending wards who have not been admitted to a bed yet.

[2] Patient in psychiatric or non-psychiatric unit, except for RoI where patient must be in an approved centre (i.e. a psychiatric unit).

* Indicates procedures where medical recommendation does not need to be by an approved doctor (E&W, Scot) /appointed doctor (NI) or consultant psychiatrist (RoI).

** Indicates procedures which may be initiated by recommendations from doctors who are not appointed (NI) or consultant psychiatrists (RoI), although soon after admission an assessment from such a doctor is required for the order to stand.

n.b. for the procedures marked * and ** the doctor should be a registered medical practitioner (i.e. not a pre-registration house officer) but need not be a psychiatrist or psychiatric trainee.

Other issues to consider when detaining patients

- Before seeing a patient (especially an outpatient) if it seems likely from the available information that detention will be necessary make appropriate arrangements (e.g. booking a bed, arranging for the necessary medical and social work personnel to arrive at the same time, having staff available to convey the patient, liaising with the police if indicated)
- Patients should only be detained if it is necessary and there is no alternative less restrictive option
- Make sure that the proper procedure is followed (e.g. the making of the application (or gaining consent in Scotland), the medical recommendations, the appropriate timings)
- In some cases getting the person to hospital will be straightforward. However in more difficult cases nursing staff and an ambulance, and where there is potential for violence, the police will be required.

nacological approach to severe
avioural disturbance

erous local guidelines are available. Be aware of these and ensure
, if involved in control and restraint, you are adequately trained to
ry out these duties responsibly.

he following is a suggested aid to pharmacological management. The
doses quoted are appropriate for young, physically fit patients who have
previously received antipsychotic medication. In patients who are elderly,
have physical health problems, or are 'antipsychotic naïve', dosage should
at least be halved (refer to BNF for further guidance).

First line treatments:

Option 1:   Intramuscular haloperidol 10-20mg and 1-2mg lorazepam
Intramuscular olanzapine may also be an alternative
Repeat if necessary

Option 2:   Diazepam 10mg by slow intravenous bolus
Repeat if necessary. **Ensure flumazenil available**

Second line treatments:

Option 3:   Intramuscular chlorpromazine 25–100mg
**Danger of postural hypotension and fatality if given inadvertently by intra-
venous injection**

Option 4:   Zuclopenthixol acetate 50-150mg. (This is rapidly acting,
sedating, depot antipsychotic which is best avoided in antipsychotic naïve
or inexperienced patients because of long half life).

Third line treatments

Other treatments (e.g. paraldehyde) or combinations of the above may be
suggested in some centres. Always consult senior medical advice before
administering these interventions.

The evidence base is relatively weak for the superiority of any compound
over another, although benzodiazepines may have a shorter time to onset
and are generally safe.

Aftercare

Respirations, pulse and blood pressure should be monitored within an
hour of drug administration and regularly thereafter. Look for extrapyramidal side effects, particularly acute dystonia. Remember: fatalities have
occurred in the context of emergency restraint.

Note on consent: Giving emergency medication for acute behavioural disturbance is essentially
treatment under common law (p. 822). The justification rests on the judgement that no other
management options are likely to be effective, and that tranquillisation will prevent the patient
harming themselves or others. Harm may include behaviour that is likely to endanger the physical
health of the patient (e.g. not consenting to urgent treatment or investigations that are likely to be
life-saving) when capacity to give consent is judged to be impaired (p. 822).